"A broader and more international collection of writing on embodiment and psychotherapy is currently unimaginable. This new collection should serve as an authoritative source for embodied psychotherapy practitioners for many years to come. The coverage provided by the thirty-seven chapters that cover dance movement psychotherapy and body psychotherapy practice is unprecedented and offers a truly wide range of opinion and approach. This work may serve to bring these related but different approaches closer and establish greater understanding. Kudos to the editors, this volume is a true achievement!"

—**Robyn Flaum Cruz, PhD**, BC-DMT; Professor,
Lesley University PhD Program in Expressive Therapies, USA

"The editors of this volume bring together an illustrious group of international leaders in both dance movement psychotherapy and body psychotherapy to share their wisdom on embodied therapeutic practice. Vast in its scope, original in its perspective, and comprehensive in its inclusion of diverse points of view, this book is a treasure trove of practical and theoretical riches. For all who honor the role of the body's natural intelligence in healing from trauma and attachment inadequacies, this book is an essential resource."

—**Pat Ogden, PhD;** founder of Sensorimotor Psychotherapy Institute
and author of *Trauma and the Body: A Sensorimotor Approach
to Psychotherapy* and *Sensorimotor Psychotherapy:
Interventions for Trauma and Attachment*

"This book is an important contribution to the growing science of mind-body interaction in psychotherapy. It is unique in its wide range of views of the importance of the body and will be invaluable for those working in psychotherapy and counselling."

—**Prof. Dr. phil. Claire Schaub-Moore, CPsychol,**
AFBPsS, WiAP, Wiesbaden, Germany

W0113254

THE ROUTLEDGE INTERNATIONAL HANDBOOK OF EMBODIED PERSPECTIVES IN PSYCHOTHERAPY

There is a growing interest in embodied approaches to psychotherapy internationally. This volume focuses on the respective focal professions of dance movement psychotherapy (DMP) and body psychotherapy (BP), addressing the psychotherapeutic need for healing throughout the lifespan. Within embodied clinical approaches, the therapist and client collaborate to discover how the body and movement can be used to strengthen positive relational skills, attending to the client's immediate and long-term needs through assessment, formulation, treatment and evaluation. Both DMP and BP are based upon the capacity and authority of the body and non-verbal communication to support and heal patients with diverse conditions, including trauma, unexplained bodily symptoms and other psychological distress, and to develop the clients' emotional and relational capacities by listening to their bodies for integration and wellbeing.

In *The Routledge International Handbook of Embodied Perspectives in Psychotherapy*, world leaders in the field contribute their expertise to showcase contemporary psychotherapeutic practice. They share perspectives from multiple models that have been developed throughout the world, providing information on theoretical advances and clinical practice, as well as discourse on the processes and therapeutic techniques employed individually and in groups. Presented in three parts, the book covers underpinning embodiment concepts, potentials of dance movement psychotherapy and of body psychotherapy, each of which is introduced with a scene-setting piece to allow the reader to easily engage with the content. With a strong focus on cross- and interdisciplinary perspectives, readers will find a wide compilation of embodied approaches to psychotherapy, allowing them to deepen and further their conceptualization and support best practice.

This unique handbook will be of particular interest to clinical practitioners in the fields of body psychotherapy and dance movement psychotherapy as well as professionals from psychology, medicine, social work, counselling/psychotherapy and occupational therapy, and to those from related fields who are in search of information on the basic therapeutic principles and practice of body and movement psychotherapies and seeking to further their knowledge and understanding of the discipline. It is also an essential reference for academics and students of embodied psychotherapy, embodied cognitive science and clinical professions.

Helen Payne, PhD, MPhil; UKCP Reg., ADMP-UK Reg., is Professor of Psychotherapy, specializing in dance movement psychotherapy, adverse childhood experiences and medically unexplained symptoms, at the University of Hertfordshire, UK.

Sabine Koch, PhD, MA, BC-DMT, is a psychologist and dance movement therapist. She is director of the Research Institute for Creative Arts Therapies at Alanus University, Germany, and Professor of Dance Movement Therapy of the Master Program at SRH University Heidelberg, Germany.

Jennifer Tantia, PhD, MS, BC-DMT, LCAT, is a somatic psychologist and dance movement psychotherapist, specializing in trauma and medically unexplained symptoms in the US. Dr. Tantia is former chair of the United States Association for Body Psychotherapy research committee and currently serves on the board of the American Dance Therapy Association as chair of Research and Practice.

Thomas Fuchs, PhD, MD, is Karl Jaspers Professor for Philosophical Foundations of Psychiatry and Psychotherapy at the University of Heidelberg and the Psychiatric University Hospital, Germany.

ROUTLEDGE INTERNATIONAL HANDBOOKS

For more information about this series, please visit: www.routledge.com/Routledge-International-Handbooks/book-series/RIHAND

THE ROUTLEDGE INTERNATIONAL HANDBOOK OF EMBODIED PERSPECTIVES IN PSYCHOTHERAPY

Approaches from Dance Movement and Body Psychotherapies

Edited by Helen Payne, Sabine Koch and Jennifer Tantia, with Thomas Fuchs

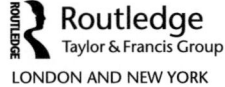

Routledge
Taylor & Francis Group

LONDON AND NEW YORK

First published 2019
by Routledge
2 Park Square, Milton Park, Abingdon, Oxon OX14 4RN

and by Routledge
52 Vanderbilt Avenue, New York, NY 10017

Routledge is an imprint of the Taylor & Francis Group, an informa business

British Library Cataloguing-in-Publication Data
A catalogue record for this book is available from the British Library

Library of Congress Cataloging-in-Publication Data
Names: Payne, Helen, 1951– editor. | Koch, Sabine C., editor. | Tantia, Jennifer, editor. | Fuchs, Thomas, 1958– editor.
Title: The Routledge international handbook of embodied perspectives in psychotherapy : approaches from dance movement and body psychotherapies / Helen Payne, Sabine Koch, Jennifer Tantia and Thomas Fuchs.
Other titles: International handbook of embodied perspectives in psychotherapy
Description: New York : Routledge, 2019. | Series: Routledge international handbooks | Includes bibliographical references and index.
Identifi ers: LCCN 2018033556 (print) | LCCN 2018046606 (ebook) | ISBN 9781315159416 (Masterebook) | ISBN 9781351659482 (Adobe Reader) | ISBN 9781351659475 (ePub) | ISBN 9781351659468 (Mobipocket) | ISBN 9781138065758 (hardback)
Subjects: LCSH: Mind and body therapies. | Dance therapy. | Movement therapy.
Classifi cation: LCC RC489.M53 (ebook) | LCC RC489.M53 R683 2019 (print) | DDC 616.89/1655—dc23
LC record available at https://lccn.loc.gov/2018033556

ISBN: 978-1-138-06575-8 (hbk)
ISBN: 978-1-032-37616-5 (pbk)
ISBN: 978-1-315-15941-6 (ebk)

Typeset in Bembo
by Apex CoVantage, LLC

CONTENTS

Contents

FIGURES

TABLES

CONTRIBUTORS

Jessica Acolin received her MA in Dance/Movement Therapy and Counselling from Drexel University. She is a counsellor and advocate at Victim Services Centre of Montgomery County in Norristown, PA. Her interests include embodiment research, dance/movement therapy theory, and trauma.

Ursula Bartholomew, consultant psychiatrist and psychotherapist, Berlin, Germany. EMDR (Eye Movement Desensitisation Recovery) therapist (EMDRIA). Functional relaxation therapist and instructor for functional relaxation. Author of various publications in psychosomatic medicine, psychotherapy and functional relaxation.

Teresa Bas, Clinical Psychologist, Psychotherapist and DMT. MA in Constructivist Psychotherapy, MA in Dance Movement Therapy by Universitat Autònoma de Barcelona. For eight years, she was member of the training team of the MA Danza Movimiento Terapia at Universitat Autònoma de Barcelona, coordinated by Dr. Heidrun Panhofer (as a group co-therapist, tutor and co-supervisor). Has 18 years of experience as a psychotherapist and over 12 years as DMT, working with children, families, adolescents and adults in private practice in Barcelona. She is a facilitator of groups of body awareness and DMT for self-growth. She also lectures in DMT in different organizations and is a DMT supervisor. She is practitioner and facilitator of groups of Authentic Movement and currently training in Body-Mind Centering. She is a Registered Supervising Member of the Asociación Española Danza Movimiento Terapia and former Treasurer (ADMTE); Registered Member of Federación Española de Asociaciones de Psicoterapia; Registered Psychologist in the Col·legi Oficial de Psicòlegs de Catalunya. Full member of the Barcelona Network of English Speaking Therapists (Barcelona NEST).

Asaf Rolef Ben-Shahar, PhD, is an Israeli psychotherapist, supervisor, trainer and writer. He founded two relational body psychotherapy programmes, in Israel (Psychosoma) and the UK, and is regularly teaching worldwide. Asaf published many papers and book chapters on psychotherapy, hypnosis, relationality and body. His latest books include *Touching the Relational Edge* (Karnac, 2014), *When Hurt Remains—Relational Perspectives on Therapeutic Failure* (co-edited with Rachel Shalit, Karnac, 2016) and *Speaking of Bodies* (co-edited with Liron Lipkies and Noa Oster, Karnac, 2016). He is on the international board of advisors for *Body, Movement and Dance* *in Psychotherapy, Self and Society*, and *Psychotherapy and Politics International*. Asaf is a father to two girls, a novice DJ, bird watcher, and loves dancing and hiking.

David Boadella, DSc hon., MEd, BA, (born 1931) became interested in Reich's work in the 1950s. He subsequently trained in Vegetotherapy with Paul Ritter, in England, and with Ola Raknes, who was educated by Reich. His major contributions to embodied psychotherapy were: (a) his founding of the journal *Energy and Character* which was one of the early (only) journals available in Europe in the 1970s; (b) three published books: *Wilhelm Reich: the evolution of his work*; *In the Wake of Reich*; and *Lifestreams: an introduction to Biosynthesis*; and (c) the founder of Biosynthesis therapy. In the early 1980s, he started to travel worldwide, teaching and training in Body Psychotherapy-Biosynthesis, before settling down in Switzerland in 1985 and founding the International Institute for Biosynthesis, together with his wife, Dr. Silvia Boadella. He was elected as first President of the European Association for Body Psychotherapy in 1989. Since then, he has continued to contribute massively to the field of Body Psychotherapy; teaching Biosynthesis internationally, presenting at conferences, writing articles. In 1995, he was awarded an honorary Doctor of Science degree from the Open International University of Complementary Medicine. www.biosynthesis.org.

Iris Bräuninger, PhD, DMT practitioner, supervisor (BTD, European Association of Dance Movement Therapy), is a researcher and lecturer at the University of Applied Sciences of Special Needs Education in Zurich. She received her PhD from the University of Tuebingen and studied DMT at the Laban Centre/City University. She teaches internationally and at the DMT Master Program at the Autonomous University Barcelona. Iris was a former researcher and deputy head of the DMT department at the University Hospital of Psychiatry Zurich and a post-doctoral researcher at the Stress and Resilience Research Team at the University of Deusto Bilbao. Iris is a DMT supervisor with the German (BTD) and Spanish Association (ADMTE), a Kestenberg Movement Profile (KMP) notator and holds the European Certificate for Psychotherapy. Her research focuses on DMT efficacy and interventions and psychomotor therapy. Iris has published extensively, for example in: *The Arts in Psychotherapy* "DMT group intervention in stress treatment: A randomized controlled trial," 2012, 39, 443–450 and "The efficacy of DMT group on improvement of quality of life: A randomized controlled trial," 2012, 39, 296–303. In: *Current Opinion in Psychiatry*, "*Zeitschrift für Sportpsychologie*" [DMT in treatment of cancer], 2017, 24, 54–64, and "Provision of arts therapies for people with severe mental illness," 2017, 30, 306–311.

Gillat Burckhardt-Bartov, MSc, is a clinical psychologist, with a specialization in Psychogerontology, who trained in psychoanalysis in the C.G. Jung Institute of Zurich. She practices psychotherapy in the Oberberg-clinic, in the Black Forest (Germany). Becoming a psychologist had a lot to do with her ascetic, emotionally distant childhood, growing up in a Kibbutz in The Valley of Jesrael. Bourgeois concepts such as parenting were adamantly discouraged and in retrospect she believes that we, the children of the dream, carried into our adulthood a painful longing for private rather than collective attachments. Her longings were later personalized in painting and in the discovery of similar longings in others. Her philosophy studies and later psychology and psychotherapy taught her to cherish the privilege to accompany people in their journey out of the labyrinth.

Christine Caldwell, PhD, LPC, BC-DMT, NCC, ACS Professor, Graduate School of Counseling and Psychology Somatic Counseling Naropa University, is the founder and former director of the Somatic Counseling Program at Naropa University, USA. She currently teaches coursework in somatic counseling theory and skills, clinical neuroscience, research, and diversity issues at Naropa. Her work began 35 years ago with studies in anthropology, dance therapy, bodywork and Gestalt therapy, and has developed into innovations in the field of body-centered psychotherapy. She calls her work the Moving Cycle. This system goes beyond the limitations of therapy and emphasizes lifelong personal and social evolution through trusting and following body states. The Moving Cycle spotlights natural play, early physical imprinting, and the transformational effect of fully sequenced movement processes. She has taught at the University of Maryland, George Washington University, Concordia, Seoul Women's University, Southwestern College, and Santa Barbara Graduate Institute, and trains, teaches and lectures internationally. She has published over 30 articles and chapters, and her books include *Getting Our Bodies Back*, and *Getting in Touch*. She had two books published in 2018, *The Body and Oppression*, and *Bodyfulness*.

Michael Changaris, PsyD, is a clinical psychologist with a specialty in the biological bases of behaviour, stress physiology, and the neuroanatomy of PTSD, and is currently the training coordinator for an integrated health psychology program. Dr. Changaris completed his dissertation research on the efficacy of Somatic Experiencing in treating adults who were homeless. He also has worked extensively with elders with and without neurodegenerative disorders and developed treatments and trainings to address the unique needs of this population. Dr. Changaris has training in multiple body-based modalities and has a specialty in neuroscience of touch. He has presented several papers with the USABP on Somatic Experiencing with elders, family, and the neurobiology of touch. He serves on the board of the Somatic Experiencing Trauma Institute.

Diana Cheney is a practicing Movement Psychotherapist for over 15 years who has worked with children in school settings, in psychiatry with adults and with children, adolescents and adults with learning disabilities who suffered from trauma and abuse. She currently works with adolescents in a tier 4 inpatient adolescent unit (CAMHS/NHS) and in a school setting, her interest lying in the area of developmental trauma. Diana also has some experience working in forensic psychotherapy. After training as a Movement Psychotherapist Diana did a Masters in Psychoanalytic Observational studies at the Tavistock Clinic where she did a two-year infant observation as well as a one year toddler observation. She is especially interested in how the pre-verbal and non-verbal relates to and supports (or not) the verbal language both in human development and in the clinical setting.

Maci Daye, EdM, EdS, is a Licensed Professional Counselor, Certified Hakomi Trainer, and Certified Sex Therapist. She has a master's degree from Harvard University and an Educational Specialist Degree from Georgia State University. Ms. Daye was the Editor of the Hakomi Therapy Association newsletter for a decade and moderated a discussion on Embodiment for Somatic Perspectives in Psychotherapy. She is the creator of Passion and Presence® couple's retreats. Her article, "Have We Forgotten About Sex" was published in *Somatic Therapy Today* and her work is featured on Somatic Perspectives in Psychotherapy. Ms. Daye wrote the Introduction and the chapter, "The Experimental Attitude in Hakomi Therapy: Curiosity in Action," in *Hakomi Mindfulness-Centered Somatic Psychotherapy*.

Marianne Eberhard-Kaechele is a registered dance movement therapist, trainer, supervisor, teaching therapist German Dance Therapy Association. European Certificate of Psychotherapy,

KMP notator. Published 50 articles and book chapters. Lecturer, researcher and administrator at the German Sport University, Cologne, department of neurology, psychosomatics and psychiatry. Academic head of the Langen Institute for Dance Therapy in Düsseldorf, private practice in Leverkusen. 35 years of clinical experience. Co-editor "körper-tanz-bewegung," journal for body psychotherapy, and vice-president of the German National Association for Arts Therapies.

Haguit Ehrenfreund, PhD in psychopathology, MA in dance-movement therapy, Switzerland, supervisor and private practitioner. Haguit was an accomplished dancer before she turned to DMP and academic research. Her work focuses on the meta-psychology of movement, using psychoanalytical concepts to theorize body action. She has taught in various programs in Europe and Israel and is the coordinator of "Creavie" art-therapy school in Lausanne. She is now starting to teach her therapeutic approach, concentrating on the integration of conscious movement and psychosomatic balance.

Radwa Said Abdelazim Elfeqi, Psychiatrist/Creative Arts Therapist with focus on DMT/ Researcher at Cairo University Hospital-Faculty of Medicine, Egypt. Graduate of Contemporary Dance School at Cairo Opera House (2002–2005). Graduate of Creativity Centre Workshop at Cairo Opera House (2005–2010). Supervised by Dr. Jill Bunce Head of Dance Movement Therapy at Derby University UK (2004), studied at Brecha (Buenos Aires) 240 hours of intensive workshops on Dance Movement Therapy (2004–2007). Studied at Lesley University CAGS and PhD programs on Expressive Therapies (2013–2015). Published over 40 abstracts in WCP (2000–present). Participated in and led over a hundred workshops and symposia in national and international contexts, on Creative Arts Therapies and DMT (2001 till present) in Egypt, Europe, US, and Latin America. Represented Egypt several times on the international Panel of ADTA. Most recent publication in *Current Opinion* July 2017, Vol. 30, N4 with Dr. Iris Bräuninger (Fenner et al., 2017).

Diana Fischman, PhD, BC-DMT, Licensed psychotherapist and educator, is founder director of Brecha (Buenos Aires Dance Movement Therapy Training Institute), the first Spanish speaking DMT training in the world. She is an academic advisor and professor at the DMT Master at Universidad Nacional del Arte—UNA, Argentina. She also teaches at Universidad Autónoma de Barcelona—DMT Master Program. Dr Fischman is the founder president of Argentina Association of Dance Therapy. Her dissertation for Universidad de Palermo was on Kinesthetic Empathy. It was published by Editorial Académica Española as Embodied Empathy. She directs Cali, Colombia Dance Movement Therapy Training and Mar del Plata—CICDAI. ORG Dance Therapy Training. Dr Fischman lectures and teaches internationally. She also directs a research line on movement patterns and social interaction at Universidad Nacional del Arte. Dr Fischman has a private practice with adults, couples, families and DMT trainees. dfischman@ brecha.com.ar.

Thomas Fuchs, MD, PhD, Karl Jaspers Professor for Philosophical Foundations of Psychiatry and Psychotherapy, Head of the Section "Phenomenological Psychopathology and Psychiatry," University Clinics Heidelberg, Co-Director of the Interdisciplinary Forum for Biomedicine and Cultural Studies (IFBK), MD in History of Medicine (Munich), PhD in Philosophy (Munich), Habilitation in Psychiatry (Heidelberg), Habilitation in Philosophy (Heidelberg). thomas.fuchs@ med.uni-heidelberg.de.

Shaun Gallagher, PhD, is the Lillian and Morrie Moss Professor of Excellence in Philosophy at the University of Memphis, and Professorial Fellow at the Faculty of Law, Humanities and the Arts, University of Wollongong; Honorary Professor at Tromsø University. He is currently a Humboldt Foundation Anneliese Maier Research Fellow (2012–2018). Publications: *Enactivist Interventions* (2017); *The Neurophenomenology of Awe and Wonder* (2015); *Phenomenology* (2012); *The Phenomenological Mind* (with Dan Zahavi, 2012); *How the Body Shapes the Mind* (2005).

Sylvie Garnero, Doctor in medicine, psychiatrist for children and adolescents, and modern dance performer and teacher, combined her interests developing dance workshops for psychiatric patients. Attended University College Los Angeles to study Dance Movement Therapy. After studying social anthropology and ethnology at postgraduate level (D.E.A, E.H.E.S.S., Paris), she evolved research interests in the field of body and dance anthropology. She has several years of clinical experience as a dance therapist in psychiatry with children, adolescents and adults (group sessions, individual therapy) and conducts workshops and creation projects to suburban teenagers. Since 1998 she delivers the DMT programme at the Scholar Cantorum (Paris) and teaches DMT (creative process, authentic movement, theory). She has been the SFDT President for many years until last June.

Ulfried Geuter, PhD, and Honorary Professor of Body Psychotherapy, works as a psycho-therapist in Berlin. He teaches body psychotherapy as an honorary professor at the University of Marburg and as a training psychotherapist at various psychotherapeutic training institutes. Numerous publications on the history of psychology and on body psychotherapy, in English: *The Professionalization of Psychology in Nazi Germany*, 1992; "Experiencing the Body: Experiencing the Self," 2016; contributions to the *Handbook of Body Psychotherapy and Somatic Psychology*, 2015; in German: *Body Psychotherapy. Outline of a Theory for Clinical Practice*, 2015.

Alexander Girshon, PhD, is a dancer, improviser, psychologist, dance and body therapist, and teacher. His first teachers in movement, improvization and contact were Oleg Ignatiev (Yaro-slavl, Russia), Oleg Sulimenko (Russia-Austria), Danny Lepkoff (USA) from 1988; contemporary dance and butoh with Paula Josa-Jones (USA). Studied transpersonal psychology (with Sergey Vsechsvyatsky and Vladimir Kozlov, Russia, 1989–1994), as well as different approaches in personal development (in the Institute of Personal Development, Moscow). Co-founder of Great Net Theater (Yaroslavl, 1988–1992) and Studio for Dance Improvisation (Yaroslavl, 1994–1997). Artistic director of Performance-Trio (1997–2002), and Alexander Girshon Performance Project (Moscow, since 2002). He has participated in numerous local, national and international dance events, festivals and collaborations. One of the first teachers of contact improvization in Russia. Head of the Dance and Movement Therapy Department of the Moscow Institute of Personal Development (Moscow, 1996–2004), International Institute of Integrative Psychology (Moscow, 2004–2007), Institute of Integrative Psychology and Professional Development (since 2007), he developed integrative approaches in dance-movement therapy and still teaches his workshops and long-term programs in Russia, Ukraine, Belorussia, Israel, France, Kazakhstan, Latvia and Lithuania http://girshon.com.

Amber Gray has worked with survivors of relational trauma (war, torture, ritual abuse, domes-tic violence, genocide, terrorism) for 18 years, and has developed a components-based and developmentally-informed DMT framework for working with trauma. Restorative Movement Psychotherapy is the clinical counterpart to this framework and is a trauma informed approach to DMT.

Thomas Heidenreich, PhD, studied psychology at Konstanz University, did his PhD in Clinical Psychology at Frankfurt University in 2000 and was an Assistant Professor at the Clinic of Psychiatry and Psychotherapy of Frankfurt University from 2000 to 2004, from 2000 he was the director of the cognitive behavioural therapy outpatient clinic at the psychological institute of Frankfurt University. Since 2006, he is a full professor of Psychology for social work and nursing at Esslingen University of Applied Sciences.

Michel Coster Heller, PhD, studied developmental psychology in Geneva with Piaget's team, while training in body psychotherapy with Geda Boyesen's team. He became doctor in psychology and sports in Duisburg (Germany), by presenting an experimental study on postural dynamics and social status. During that time, he also practiced body psychotherapy and participated in the development of that field. For more than 10 years he directed a research laboratory on suicidal behaviour in the Geneva Psychiatric institutions. In Lausanne, he has developed his own brand of clinical work, as psychotherapist, supervisor, international trainer, lecturer and author. He is also working in the psychosomatic department of Le Noirmont Clinic in the Swiss Jura. His main publication is *Body Psychotherapy: History, Concepts and Methods*, in French in 2008, translated into English and German. Suggested reading on the general frame used for the case analysis: Heller, MC. (2016). "The Embodied Psyche of Organismic Psychology: A Possible Frame for a Dialogue between Psychotherapy Schools and Modalities." *International Body Psychotherapy Journal*: 15, 1: 20–50. www.ibpj.org Heller, MC. and Westland, G. (2011). "The System of the Dimensions of the Organism (SDO): A Common Vocabulary for Body Psychotherapy." *Body, Movement and Dance in Psychotherapy*, 6, 1: 43–57.

Ingrid Herholz, consultant for psychosomatic medicine and psychotherapy, Cologne, Germany. Psychoanalyst (DPV/IPA) and instructor for Functional Relaxation (AFE). Lectureship at the University of Cologne for Psychosomatic Medicine and Psychotherapy. Editor of books and articles on practice of Functional Relaxation in psychosomatics and prevention.

Rainbow Tin Hung Ho, PhD, is the Director of the Centre on Behavioral Health (CBH), Professor of the Department of Social Work and Social Administration (SWSA), and the Director of the Master of Expressive Arts Therapy and MSocSc (Behavioral Health) programs in the University of Hong Kong. She is a board-certified dance movement therapist, registered somatic movement therapist and expressive arts therapist, certified group psychotherapist and movement analyst, and registered teacher in many dance disciplines. Prof. Ho has been working as a researcher, therapist, teacher, and performing artist for many years. She has published extensively in refereed journals, scholarly books and encyclopaedias and has been the principal investigator of many research projects related to creative and expressive arts therapy, physical exercises, psychophysiology, mind-body medicine, complementary and alternative therapy, as well as spirituality for healthy and clinical populations with different ages. She also works on different community projects related to dance arts and mental wellness. In 2015, Prof. Ho received the Outstanding Achievement Award and Research Award from the American Dance Therapy Association and the Outstanding Teaching Award from the University of Hong Kong. In 2016, she received the Research and Development Award from the Australia and New Zealand Arts Therapy Association.

Daniel D. Hutto, PhD, is Professor of Philosophical Psychology at the University of Wollongong and member of the Australian Research Council College of Experts. He is co-author of the award-winning *Radicalizing Enactivism* (MIT, 2013) and its sequel, *Evolving Enactivism* (MIT,

2017). His other recent books include: *Folk Psychological Narratives* (MIT, 2008) and *Wittgenstein and the End of Philosophy* (Palgrave, 2006). He is editor of *Narrative and Understanding Persons* (CUP, 2007) and *Narrative and Folk Psychology* (Imprint Academic, 2009). A special yearbook, *Radical Enactivism*, focusing on his philosophy of intentionality, phenomenology and narrative, was published in 2006. He is regularly invited to speak not only at philosophy conferences but at expert meetings of anthropologists, clinical psychiatrists/therapists, educationalists, narratologists, neuroscientists and psychologists.

Susan D. Imus, MA, LCPC, BC–DMT, GL–CMA, is an Associate Professor and Chair of the Department of Creative Arts Therapies in the School of Fine and Performing Arts at Columbia College, Chicago. Susan is a licensed clinical professional counsellor, LCPC, a board–certified dance/movement therapist, BC–DMT, and a certified movement analyst at the graduate level, GL–CMA. Susan has practiced, educated, and consulted in dance/movement therapy and the creative arts throughout the US and abroad for 33 years. She is currently the chair of the Education, Research, and Practice Committee for the American Dance Therapy Association (ADTA). She received the first Excellence in Education award by the ADTA in 2006. Susan teaches a course called *Embodiment: A Way to Know Your Patient* in the Bioethics and Humanities Department in the Feinberg School of Medicine at Northwestern University and Rush University Medical College.

Rae Johnson, PhD, RSMT, is a scholar/practitioner working at the intersection of Somatics and social justice. Over the past decade, Rae's research has focused on the embodied experience of oppression and the role of the body in reproducing and transforming oppressive social norms. As a psychotherapist, social worker and somatic movement therapist, clinical practice included working with members of marginalized groups in exploring and reclaiming the lived authority of the body and developing a model to support somatic resilience using movement improvization and the expressive arts. Rae is the author of several books, including *Elemental Movement, Knowing in our Bones*, and the recently released *Embodied Social Justice*, and publishes regularly in scholarly and professional journals in the field. They have held leadership positions in a number of somatic psychology organizations and graduate programs over the years, and currently chairs the somatic studies in depth psychology doctoral program at Pacifica Graduate Institute in Santa Barbara, California. raejohnsonsomatic@gmail.com.

Miyuki Kaji, PsyD, Certified Clinical Psychologist, BC–DMT, is a dance therapist, trained by Amy Wapner, MA, BC–DMT at Hasegawa Hospital in Tokyo. She is a board member of the Japan Dance Therapy Association, and a board–certified dance therapist. She is a coordinator of the Tokyo Dance Therapy Project and organizes workshops and training seminars to establish dance therapy in Japan. Miyuki received a doctoral degree in clinical psychology at Rikkyo University. She also studied the training methods of Clinical Psychologists under Professor Akira Kaito and Associate Professor Yasue Takahashi, with completion of course work at the Graduate School of Education of Kyoto University. She practices psychodynamic psychotherapy for adult and adolescent clients. Her recent research interests include the effect of bodily expression in psychotherapy in terms of Merleau-Ponty's "intercorporéité," which describes an embodied intersubjective relationship between a therapist and a client. She mainly researches this phenomenon though case studies and interviews.

Ekaterina Karatygina is a dance-movement therapist, business coach, dance-psychological training coach Institute of Integrative Psychology for Professional Development, "Integrative dance psychological training and integrative dance movement psychotherapy" course (January 2015).

Sabine Koch, PhD, MA, BC-DMT, Psychologist and Dance Movement Therapist, Director of the Research Institute for Creative Arts Therapies at Alanus University, Alfter, Professor and Head of the DMT Master Program at SRH University, Heidelberg, Germany. Specialized in embodiment research, evidence-based research, Kestenberg Movement Profiling (KMP), and active factors across the creative arts therapies. Meta analyses and randomised controlled trials studies on DMT for schizophrenia, autism, and depression. Research in dance movement therapy (DMT), body-mind approaches, embodiment, nonverbal communication, body memory, movement and meaning, DMT for trauma, dance for Parkinson's disease, Phenomenological Body Psychotherapy, Creative Arts Therapies. sabine.koch@alanus.edu.

Margit Koemeda-Lutz is a licensed psychotherapist in private practice; faculty member of the International Institute for Bioenergetic Analysis (IIBA); coordinating trainer of the Swiss Society's psychotherapy training program (SGBAT). Has been presenting and training in Switzerland, Austria, Germany and the US. Study group member in different research projects; founding member and co-organizer of annual psychotherapy conferences "Breitensteiner Psychotherapiewochen" (1981–2000); author and editor of several books and articles on psychosomatic psychotherapy and its effectiveness. www.sgbat.ch; www.bioenergetic-therapy.com; www.koemeda.ch.

Naomi Lyons studied psychology and Dance-Movement Therapy at the University of Osnabrueck and SRH Heidelberg finishing her psychology degree in 2014. Since 2015 she is a research assistant at the department for clinical psychology and psychotherapy, Witten/Herdecke University.

Helma Mair, PhD, is a somatic psychotherapist who specializes in developmental and attachment trauma. She earned her Master of Arts in Clinical Psychology with a Specialization in Somatic Psychology from Santa Barbara Graduate Institute and her Doctor of Philosophy in Clinical Psychology with a Specialization in Somatic Psychology from The Chicago School of Professional Psychology. A qualified Somatic Experiencing® and NARMTM practitioner as well as a certified Hakomi® therapist, she has served as an assistant for Peter Levine's Somatic Experiencing® training and Steve Hoskinson's Organic Intelligence® training as well as a trainee assistant for Dr. Heller's NARMTM training. Dr. Mair's research focuses on the issue of safety in psychotherapy. She currently works in private practice in Dublin, Ireland.

Johannes Michalak, PhD, studied psychology at Ruhr-University, Bochum. In 1999 he finished his PhD in Clinical Psychology at the Ruhr-University, Bochum. He was an Acting Professor at the University of Heidelberg (Germany, 2005–2006) and at the Ruhr-University, Bochum (Germany, 2009–2010) and Visiting Professor at Queen´s University, Kingston (Canada, 2009). In 2011 he moved as a Full Professor to the University of Hildesheim. Since 2014 he is a Professor for Clinical Psychology and Psychotherapy at Witten/Herdecke University.

Helen Payne, PhD, is a Professor of Psychotherapy, specializing in Dance Movement Psychotherapy, at The University of Hertfordshire where she supervises doctoral students, conducts and teaches research. She holds a PhD and an MPhil, is United Kingdom Council for Psychotherapy (UKCP) registered and is a registered member and Fellow of ADMP UK. She pioneered DMP in the UK leading the professional association, first postgraduate accredited training, research and publications. She is trained in Laban Movement Analysis, Person-Centered Counselling, Group Analysis and the Discipline of Authentic Movement, works with children, adolescents and adults, and examines doctorates nationally/internationally. She is the founding editor-in-chief for the international peer reviewed journal *Body, Movement and Dance in Psychotherapy* published by Taylor and Francis. She has recently been honoured to have been invited to join the National Task Force for Therapies for Medically Unexplained Symptoms. Her recent publication entitled *Essentials of Dance Movement Psychotherapy: International Perspectives on Theory, Research and Practice* was published by Routledge. www.amazon.co.uk/Essentials-Dance-Movement-Psychotherapy-International/dp/113820045X and her website for circles and training in The Discipline of Authentic Movement is: https://authenticmovementcirclesblog.wordpress.com.

Rosa Mª Rodríguez, BSc Physics (UCM, 1991), PhD Physics (UCM, 1997), Degree in Education for Special Needs (UPS, 2005), MA in Dance Movement Therapy (UAB, 2007). Currently she is finishing the Degree in Psychology (UEM). She has kept parallel dance studies (classical and contemporary) for more than 20 years, working as a professional dancer and instructor of dance for several years. Her profile is very interdisciplinary. She is full professor at the Universidad Europea de Madrid (UEM) since 1998, sharing this job with the head of the Volunteer and Cooperation Office at the same university for nine years. Much of her work has been focused on cooperation social projects (as in Morocco, Bolivia and Paraguay) through creative dance and movement. She has been involved in training programs for teachers in higher education. She also collaborates with other institutions in higher education (UAB, UC, ISEP). She has over 30 research publications and chapters of books. She is co-director of Movimiento Atlas (www.movimientoatlas.com)—an association dedicated to the development and dissemination of Somatic Movement Education and Dance Movement Therapy in Spain. She is vice-president of the Spanish Association of Dance Movement Therapy and Delegate for European Association of Dance Movement Therapy.

Rosemarie Samaritter, PhD, is a licensed senior DMT, psychomotor therapist and supervisor. Her work is rooted in her studies in Dalcroze Rhythmics, Modern Dance, Dance Movement Therapy, Integrative Movement Psychotherapy and Experiential Dynamic Therapy. She completed her PhD with Professor Helen Payne at the University of Hertfordshire. Since 1987 she has been working as a DMT and supervisor in outpatient settings in Dutch and German National Health Services and in private practice. She is specialized in DMT intervention in personality disorders, post-trauma treatment (war survivors and sexual trauma) and psychopathology of disturbed sense of self (e.g. attachment trauma, autism). She has been teaching DMT theory in methods since the beginning of various DMT programs in the Netherlands, Finland and Germany. She was founding chair of the dance therapy section in the Association of Creative Arts Therapies in the Netherlands (NVCT) and a member of the board of Dutch Register of Creative Arts Therapists. She is coordinating DMT oriented research in collaboration with Codarts Arts for Health, the Netherlands and is participating in the development of guidelines for the national health service there.

Annette Schwalbe, MA, MSC, RDMP, registered dance movement psychotherapist, UKCP registered, is a UK based Dance Movement Psychotherapist and Somatic Body Mapper. Originally from Germany, she trained at the London School of Economics and the Laban Centre

London during the 1990s. She has since lived and worked as therapist, supervisor, lecturer and trainer in Mali, Pakistan, Uganda and Kenya. She established and taught graduate courses in Dance Movement Therapy at Makerere Univeristy, Kampala. She also co-founded the international consultancy Art2Be based in Nairobi, Kenya. During that time Annette worked with adults and children living with HIV/AIDS, homeless pregnant girls and young mothers, leaders in the LGBTI community, underground artists, and mental health staff in the field of gender-based violence. Since her return to the UK in 2009 she has been pioneering Somatic Body Mapping as an approach to feminine embodiment and empowerment. Her work is informed by a lifelong quest to explore and meet what is different and 'other', a deep respect for the world of the body, and an unflinching trust in the creative process as a way to make inner and outer connections. Annette currently practices in Bath, Southwest England (UK). www.annetteschwalbe. co.uk; mail@annetteschwalbe.co.uk.

Maxine Sheets-Johnstone, PhD, was a dancer/choreographer, professor of dance/dance scholar. In her second and ongoing life, she is a philosopher whose research and writing remain grounded in the moving body. She is an independent interdisciplinary scholar affiliated with the Department of Philosophy at the University of Oregon where she taught periodically in the 1990s and where she now holds an ongoing Courtesy Professor appointment. She has published 80 articles in humanities, science, and art journals. Her ten books include *The Phenomenology of Dance*; *Illuminating Dance: Philosophical Explorations*; the "roots" trilogy—*The Roots of Thinking*, *The Roots of Power: Animate Form and Gendered Bodies*, and *The Roots of Morality*; *Giving the Body Its Due*; *The Primacy of Movement*; *The Corporeal Turn: An Interdisciplinary Reader*; *Putting Movement into Your Life*; *Insides and Outsides: Interdisciplinary Perspectives on Animate Life*. She was awarded a Distinguished Fellowship at the Institute of Advanced Study at Durham University in the UK in the Spring of 2007 for her research on xenophobia, an Alumni Achievement Award by the School of Education, University of Wisconsin in 2011, and was honoured with a Scholar's Session by the Society of Phenomenology and Existential Philosophy in 2012.

Michael Soth is an integral-relational Body Psychotherapist, trainer and supervisor (UKCP), with more than 30 years' experience of practising and teaching from an integrative perspective. Drawing on concepts, values and ways of working from a broad-spectrum range of psychotherapeutic approaches across both psychoanalytic and humanistic traditions, he is interested in the therapeutic relationship as a bodymind process between two people who are both wounded and whole. Having been a training director at the Chiron Centre for Body Psychotherapy in London for 18 years until its closure in 2010, he has been developing a relational-systemic bodymind conception of enactment since the mid-90s. This now forms a cornerstone of his teaching and training through INTEGRA CPD, an organization he founded in 2011. He has written numerous articles and several book chapters and is a frequent presenter at conferences. Extracts from his published writing as well as summaries of presentations and hand-outs are available at www. integra-cpd.co.uk or find him on Facebook and Twitter (INTEGRA_CPD). He is co-editor of the *Handbook of Body Psychotherapy and Somatic Psychology*, published in 2015.

Tina Stromsted, PhD, MFT, LPCC, BC-DMT, RSME/T, is a Jungian Psychoanalyst, board-certified dance therapist, and Somatics educator. Past co-founder and faculty member of the Authentic Movement Institute in Berkeley (1993–2004) and a founding faculty member of the Women's Spirituality Program at the California Institute of Integral Studies, she teaches at the C.G. Jung Institute of San Francisco, the Depth Psychology/Somatics Doctoral program at Pacifica Graduate Institute, and as a core faculty member for the Marion Woodman Foundation.

With over 40 years of clinical experience and a background in dance and theater, she offers programs at universities and healing centers internationally, and has a private practice in San Francisco. Founder and director of Soul's Body Center®, her work in further developing Authentic Movement, Dreamdancing®, Embodied Alchemy®, and other conscious embodiment practices can be found in her numerous articles, book chapters, and webinars which explore the integration of body, brain, psyche and soul in healing and transformation. Dr. Stromsted's work supports individuals in listening for the soul's call and working with obstacles to its fulfilment—a process that can assist women and men in re-inhabiting their bodies, reclaiming their instinctual wisdom, and nourishing their authentic sense of self. www.AuthenticMovement-BodySoul.com.

Maurizio Stupiggia, MD, is a body-psychotherapist, Professor of General Psychology at the University of Genoa, Italy. Dr. Stupiggia works as a trainer in Europe, Japan and Latin America. Beside many articles, he wrote two books, *La terapia biosistemica* and *Il corpo violato*, which were translated into other languages. In collaboration with other authors he published *Il benessere nelle emozioni* (2009), and *Biosistemica, la scienza che unisce* (2015).

Jennifer Tantia, PhD, MS, BC-DMT, LCAT, Licensed Creative Arts Therapist, is a somatic psychologist and dance/movement psychotherapist, specializing in trauma and medically unexplained symptoms. Dr. Tantia is former chair of the United States Association for Body Psychotherapy research committee and currently serves on the board of the American Dance Therapy Association as chair of Research and Practice. She specializes in embodied research, consulting for several master's and doctoral programs, and is a peer-reviewer for several academic journals, including serving as associate editor of the international journal, *Body, Movement and Dance in Psychotherapy*. Dr. Tantia presents and teaches internationally and has authored several publications in both dance/movement therapy and somatic psychology. She has a full-time private practice in Manhattan. www.soma-psyche.com.

Suzi Tortora, EdD, BC-DMT, LCAT, LMHC, CMA, serves as a consultant to the "Mothers, Infants and Young Children of September 11, 2001: A Primary Prevention Project" in the Department of Psychiatry, Columbia University under Dr. Beatrice Beebe and has a dance/movement psychotherapy practice in New York. She designed and is the senior dance/movement therapist of the Integrative Medicine Services Dréas Dream dance/movement therapy program for paediatric patients at Memorial Sloan-Kettering Cancer Center, NYC since its inception in 2003. She has published numerous papers and her book called *The Dancing Dialogue: Using the Communicative Power of Movement with Young Children* is used extensively in national and international DMP training programs. She has been featured in Malcolm Gladwell's book, *What the Dog Saw*. Dr. Tortora received the 2010 Marian Chace Distinguished Dance Therapist award from the American Dance Therapy Association and teaches her "Ways of Seeing" international training programs in Europe, South America and Asia and holds faculty positions in the USA, the Netherlands, the Czech Republic, Argentina and China. She also offers international webinar-based "Ways of Seeing" training programs for dance/movement therapists and allied professionals.

Nick Totton is a body psychotherapist, trainer and supervisor, qualified since 1983. Founder and lead trainer of Embodied-Relational Therapy. Original training in Post Reichian Therapy (William West). Member of EABP. Author or editor of fifteen books, including three directly relevant: *Body Psychotherapy: An Introduction* and *Embodied Relating: The Ground of Psychotherapy*

(2003 and 2015, both authored) and *New Dimensions in Body Psychotherapy* (2005, edited and contributed). Also, author of many papers and chapters, several of them about body psychotherapy.

Tom Warnecke, PgDip, ECP, is a relational body psychotherapist, psycho-social campaigner, artist and tutor at "Re-Vision" in London. He teaches internationally, facilitates small and large group events, and developed a relational-somatic approach to borderline trauma. He is co-editor for the *International Journal for Body, Dance and Movement in Psychotherapy* and his publications include *The Psyche in the Modern World—Psychotherapy and Society* (Karnac, 2015) and most recently, the article "Chronic fatigue phenomena: somatic and relational perspectives". He is a webcast editor for www.psychotherapyexcellence.com and a past Vice-Chair of the UK Council for Psychotherapy.

Halko Weiss, PhD, is a Clinical Psychologist and lecturer (including Tübingen- and Marburg Universities) on mindfulness, couples' therapy and body-centered psychotherapy. He authored 20 professional publications and eight books, as well as more than 50 congress contributions, including keynotes, and was awarded the Alice K. Ladas Research Award by the USABP in 2005. Halko co-founded the Hakomi Institute in Boulder, Colorado, and the Hakomi Institutes of Europe, Australia and New Zealand, and was instrumental in developing the Hakomi Method and its curricula used worldwide. He established a successful coaching training program and an Emotional Intelligence training for executives in Germany. He also developed two comprehensive programs on couples' therapy and interpersonal skills taught internationally.

Gill Westland is Director of Cambridge Body Psychotherapy Centre and a UKCP registered body psychotherapist. She is a full member of the European Association for Body Psychotherapy and an External Examiner for the Karuna Institute in Devon, UK and the London School of Biodynamic Psychotherapy, London, UK. She is a co-editor of the journal *Body, Movement and Dance in Psychotherapy* and an Associate Lecturer on the MA Body Psychotherapy programme at Anglia Ruskin University, Cambridge, UK.

Jennifer Whitley, MS, BC-DMT, LCAT, CMA, is a board-certified Dance/Movement Therapist and Licensed Creative Arts Therapist who received her master's degree, with honours, in Dance Therapy at Pratt Institute in Brooklyn, NY. Additionally, she is a "Ways of Seeing" practitioner, Level II Reiki trained, and Certified as a Laban Movement Analyst. Ms. Whitley has been a DMT at Dancing Dialogue since 2014 working with children and families using "Ways of Seeing" psychotherapeutic multi-arts approach with children with attention deficit hyperactivity disorder, anxiety, family separation, eating disorders, learning difficulties and disruptive behaviour and provides parenting support. Ms. Whitley's experience includes medical DMT at Memorial Sloan Kettering Cancer Center, joining the Integrative Medicine Services team in 2012, with a focus in paediatric oncology alongside Dr. Tortora. Ms. Whitley has continued working with children diagnosed with autism spectrum disorder, downs syndrome, cerebral palsy, among others through group DMT sessions in the therapeutic school setting since 2013. She has taught as interim instructor in The New School's Creative Arts Therapy Certification Program, worked as DMT/Choreographer for Angelight Films, and presented workshops locally, nationally, and internationally.

FOREWORD BY DON HANLON JOHNSON

Ambulant scholarship

The uniqueness of this volume, among all those focusing on embodiment which have been published in recent years, is the confluence of different fields of inquiry each of which has the potential to clarify and enrich the others who are working in this fertile intersection. Somatics, dance and movement therapy represent the world of highly advanced immersion in the silent worlds of moving, sensing, touching, breathing, and feeling. psychoanalytic thought, cognitive science and phenomenology join with these practitioner-scholars in the common task of articulating a 1st- and 2nd person science that honors the irreducibility of direct experience to what is known by instruments and measurements, preserving the authority of subjectivity. At the same time, these scholars work to account for the radical individuality of direct experience and the tenacious vice of self-deception. Without this hard-communal work represented in these chapters, the claims of those working in somatic psychotherapy and dance/movement therapy will continue to be vulnerable to the repetitive charges of remaining in the realm of personal anecdote, not evidence-based generalities.

Developing and refining these works demands that practitioner/thinkers emerge out of silent experiences into the seemingly distant world of language. However, the very nature of our intricate explorations of experience makes it difficult to find words that do justice to that intricacy. Under constant pressure to explain ourselves to others, and to make available to others the riches which we have found, we often reach for words too soon, snaring ones that are already close at hand. Such words can trivialize our findings, and, even worse, they can anchor our discoveries in conventional discourses that diminish the uniqueness of what we have found.

And yet that pressure to verbalize is unavoidable. Most of us practice within the world of healing, making claims that our works have efficacy in one or another realm of dysfunction. To make such claims instantly puts us into the sights of those who are given the task of monitoring the kinds of fraud, deceit, and exaggerated claims that have always plagued the healing professions. To make our living by mounting training programs, academic degree programs certified by governments, and insurance claims, we have to say something about what we do and why anyone else should do it also. Unlike poets, novelists, and people in long-term psychotherapy, we don't have the luxury to wait for exactly the right words. Nor can we be silent about matters of such importance when there are so many suffering people who stand to be helped by what we know.

For these reasons, this is a both a courageous and important volume, joining the many efforts made in the past 50 years to give voice to the scattered subcommunities whose practices and emergent ideas have been shoring up our bodies of knowledge against the seemingly inevitable tide of dissociated thinking and institution-building, a tide whose intensities wash aside the human and earthly in favor of the abstract and profitable.

Susan Leigh Foster, in the collection which she edited on the role of body movement in a scholarly work, crafted a term that is helpful in addressing the dangers of moving from silent experience into theory—"ambulant scholarship." She illustrates that phrase by contrasting Japanese and EuroAmerican puppetry.

> Where the conventions of Western puppet performances hide the puppeteer backstage either above or below the puppet, the Bunraku puppeteers hover just behind the puppet, onstage and in full view. The Western puppet remains an instrumentality, a simulcrum of the body, whereas the Bunraku puppet performs its concrete abstraction . . . fragility, discretion, sumptuousness, extraordinary nuance, abandonment of all triviality, and melodic phrasing of gestures.[1]

This "disappearance" of the author behind the text has created an academic form that has made it particularly difficult for those of us who have devoted our lives to the explorations of fleshy experiential practices to enter into the ethereal realms of academic discourse. It is only slowly that the upsurge of the body's intelligence has found avenues of inserting itself into the conversations that shape the larger world that we now are struggling to cope with. We are not without companions: women throughout the world struggling to emerge from centuries of silence, and the many marginalized groups throughout the world who are reaching for words to express their unique experiences in such ways that people will listen. Without those languages, the brilliance of these experiential wisdoms is left lurking in the shadows, with our decaying social structures languishing in need of new visions.

In older cultures, there were vocabularies for direct experiences embedded in their rituals, songs, dances, and spiritual teachings: Zen Buddhism, Daoism, Advaita Vedanta, Sufism, Kabbala, the various shamanisms, and many others. In the West, these languages are excised from the 3rd-person syntax of science and academic scholarship, left to the poets, songwriters, and hip-hop artists.

Our challenge, however, is not only to communicate information that lies on the outskirts of conventional understandings, but for the speakers and writers ourselves to engage in what Eugene Gendlin has called "carrying forward." This entails the hard work of recovering a sense that words are not only for telling what we have found, but for actually completing the movements that begin silently within. Finding words is not just a task for relating to some "public," but part of the full process of expanding our souls. Giving words to the complex realizations that emerge in our silent practices actually deepens and anchors those practices so that they expand our possibilities in an ever-growing cycle of experience-verbalization-fresh experiences. We find ourselves more related to each other as well as to ourselves, more kind, compassionate, and ready for engaging the turmoil of the world.

Don Hanlon Johnson, PhD, is the founder of the Somatics Graduate Degree Program at The California Institute of Integral Studies, and author of several books and articles, and editor of several collections in the field, most recently Diverse Bodies, Diverse Practices: Toward an Inclusive Somatics.

Note

1 *Choreographing History* (Bloomington, IN: Indiana University Press, 1995), p. 11.

FOREWORD BY
VASSILIKI KARKOU

Several years back, I think it was 2005, when Helen (Payne) asked me to work with her on editing a new journal on dance movement psychotherapy and body psychotherapy, I was baffled by the fact that, up to that time, these two affiliate disciplines had not had more and closer connections, academic or otherwise. The embodied emphasis in these two types of psychotherapy seemed an obvious common component, still unacknowledged. Since that first discussion, the journal (*Body, Movement and Dance in Psychotherapy*) took off, an international publication by Taylor and Francis with wide circulation around the world. Several years later, publishing a book that talked to these two disciplines seemed to be an obvious way forward. And long overdue.

Similar to the journal, this new publication has a strong international flavour covering almost 40 contributions from practitioners and researchers in Europe, USA, South Africa, Japan and Hong Kong, making it aptly titled as a Routledge International Handbook (one of the series). As expected for a textbook on this topic, the attention to embodiment in the form of 'being a body' or 'moving a body', as discussed by Jennifer Tantia in one of the sections of the introductory chapter of the book, becomes a crucial distinction between the two disciplines. Aspects of these two concepts get unpacked in different ways by the different contributors, adding to existing literature that discuss similarities and differences between the two disciplines (see for example a recent publication by Payne, Westland, Karkou and Warnecke, 2016).

As I am sitting in my garden in Liverpool and writing this brief foreword I am reflecting on my own body sensations. I feel the breeze on my face in this sunny and welcoming day. I feel the sun warming my skin, while my muscles are loosening up as I stretch, turn and twist. As I follow the impulse to attend to my body, I become increasingly aware of my breath, a breath that appears for a moment as if it is carrying the core of my existence, or what Maxine Sheets-Johnson, in the first chapter of the book, refers to as a 'moving embodied self'. I become intensively aware of my rib cage widening and narrowing, while my spine gently moves from side to side; it is me, in Maxine's terms, in 'kinaesthesia'. I look at the plants in the garden. The tomatoes, the herbs and I become one, made out of the same material. I am filled with gratitude for the oxygen they share generously with me and with guilt for what I can only describe as neglect from my part. An internal voice calls: 'Remember to water the plants!'. While I am filled with feelings of gratitude and guilt, I am reminded of Maxine's term 'affective being'; my 'moving embodied self' is clearly an 'affective self'.

I am raising my arms up and down the sides of my body, coordinating this movement with my breath. I am amusing myself with the thought that the ants on the vine leaves are attentively watching me. I need someone to 'witness' my experience, as Tina Stromsted in her chapter argues in the context of the practice of authentic movement; the ants appear to be my 'witnesses' on this occasion. The gentle up and down movement of my arms begin to diversify; the rest of the body follows. I become curious about how each shape I make with my body leads to another. I am becoming both a storyteller and a listener/viewer. I try to squeeze meaning attached to this improvised movement into the words – words that I write, I delete, I replace, none completely doing justice to what I am experiencing and what I am beginning to discover. Altogether however, words and movement, create a movement narrative (maybe a body story?), unique to me and my relationship with the garden. Body stories described in different ways in the chapters by Silvie Garnero, Shaun Gallagher and Dan Hutto, Helma Mair and Christine Caldwell.

I turn to the paper in front on me, free associating: the text, poetic, imaginative; words and images intermingling, while keeping attention and awareness of my body sensations. I am keen, as some of the authors of this book also argue for, to move away from an either/or position and to embrace both mind and body, both object and subject and both my internal and external reality. Jessica Acolin in Chapter 3 reminds us exactly of this: the need to bring these domains together. Creative writing and image-making create this bridge for me today.

I bring a large piece of paper out. As I had asked clients and students to do before (see Athanasiadou and Karkou, 2017) and as discussed in this book by authors such as Annette Schwalbe, I mark my own internal sensations on a human-shaped outline on the paper: a tickling sensation of the arm, the right arm, the one that is doing most of the writing, celebrating a moment of pen/mouse-free experience. A vibrant sense on the sides of the torso, maybe activated after my earlier attention to my breath. And a darker sensation in between, in the centre of my body; all marked with different line qualities on the outlined figure on the paper in front of me. I am reflecting on the dull, dark sensation on my chest: a reference to the news of my cousin's death? It seems raw and vulnerable, maybe sitting on top of other forgotten losses. I add one more mark on the paper, a thin line on my lower back, a reference to sharp but now faint pain. It reminds me of things still unprocessed in my own personal history, completing a temporary fluid map of what Annette Schwalbe refers to as one's body map of the past, present and future.

I search for gravity, regressing to an earlier stage where I feel supported. I, like my dear plants in the garden, search for nutrients and for water, trying to find, as Diane Cheney suggests, what is happening on the floor on a horizontal plane, before I push up to the vertical and get ready for action on the sagittal plane. Resilience, a topic discussed in this book by authors such as Rosemarie Samaritter, together with Alexander Girshon and Ekaterina Karatygina, will allow me to process the pain of my cousin passing away.

I need to move away from the garden first; the midday heat is more than I can take by now. The sun has started burning. I come inside the house. I feel cooler both from the inside and outside. This seems to be an easy solution to dealing with an environment that is no longer friendly to me. I am thinking about clients who do not have the luxury to simply shift from one place to another, physically or emotionally; in some cases, the 'heat' of their emotions remaining permanently high. References of distress in the body are often evident, as contributors to this book suggest. Clients with depression or suicide risk (Johannes Michalak, Naomi Lyons and Thomas Heidenreich; Susan Imus), trauma (Amber Gray; Silvie Garnero; Rae Johnson; Maurizio Stuppigia), eating disorders (Haguit Ehrenfreund; Suzi Tortora and Jennifer Whitley), medically unexplained symptoms or psychosomatic issues (Helen Payne; Ursula Bartholomew and Ingrid Herholz) are all clinical populations with whom embodied approaches to psychotherapy have a lot to offer.

From the approaches discussed, mindful in-depth approaches (Halko Weiss and Maci Daye; Gill Westland), sit side by side with relational models (Amber Gray; Teresa Bas, Diana Fischman and Rosa Mᵃ Rodríguez; Nick Totton; Michael Soth; Rolef Ben-Shahar; and Rae Johnson). Synthesising intrapersonal and interpersonal perspectives also features in the book as seems to be the case with Helen Payne's The BodyMind Approach and David Boadella's biosynthesis. A mosaic of practice that involves, for the first time, so much diversity in shape and colour, reflecting maybe the numerous ways in which one can approach the concept of embodiment.

Vassiliki Karkou, Chair of Dance, Arts and Wellbeing,

Edge Hill University, UK

References

Athanasiadou, F., and Karkou, V. (2017). Establishing Relationships with Children with Autism Spectrum Disorders through Dance Movement Psychotherapy: A Case Study using Artistic Enquiry. In S. Daniel and C. Trevarthen (Eds.), *Rhythms of Relating in Children's Therapies* (pp. 272–293). London: Jessica Kingsley.

Payne, H., Westland, G., Karkou, V., and Warnecke, T. (2016). A comparative analysis of body psychotherapy and dance movement psychotherapy from a European perspective. *Body, Movement and Dance in Psychotherapy, 11*(2–3), 144–166.

FOREWORD BY
BABETTE ROTHSCHILD

Body psychotherapy has been around for more than 100 years. Best known for its historic emphasis on emotional release, in the 1960s and 1970s body psychotherapy was relegated to the fringes of the personal growth movement. Nonetheless, it gained momentum. Thirty years ago, most therapists and clients had never heard of it. Nowadays, most professionals and many consumers have become aware of the importance of paying attention to body as well as mind as a part of successful psychotherapy. In addition, body psychotherapy has grown and matured. While at one time body psychotherapy was mostly concerned with angry pillow pounding and dramatic sobbing catharses, it has now evolved into a legitimate area of study, comprising theories and practices gleaned from the sciences of physiology, anatomy, psychology, neurology, and neurophysiology.

Though many have contributed to the development of the various types of body psychotherapy and somatic psychology that are practiced today, three individuals stand out for providing the foundation upon which this field of study and practice has grown:

- Pierre Janet, the 1880s physician who is commonly claimed as the "father of body psychotherapy," was instrumental in pioneering the observation that mind and body were not, as had been believed to date, separate, independent structures, but intricately linked in the manifestation of physical, mental, and emotional processes.
- Wilhelm Reich, a student of Sigmund Freud's followed closely behind with his interest in dissolving physiological *armor* through expression of held emotions to free the *orgasm reflex*.
- Fritz Perls, co-founder of Gestalt Therapy, was a student of Reich's. He integrated attention to body and mind with core elements of Buddhist meditation and mindfulness putting the greater focus on *awareness* rather than expression.

It is only recently—in the last few decades—that body psychotherapy has gained broad recognition as well as growing respect. The biggest advance in legitimizing the study and practice of body psychotherapy came from the 1994 publication of Bessel van der Kolk's scholarly, bridge-building article, "The Body Keeps the Score: Memory and the Evolving Psychobiology of Post Traumatic Stress," in the *Harvard Review of Psychiatry*. The fact that a mainstream Harvard psychiatrist recognized that the mind and body were intimately bound, one influencing the other, was revolutionary to both the alternative, somatic world of body psychotherapy and the mainstream, cognitive world of psychology and psychiatry. In addition, van der Kolk's article illuminated the work of other researchers and inspired body psychotherapists to integrate scientific theories and findings to further the understanding of the mind/body relationship. Since the 1990s a tidal wave of study initiated a library of publications on the mind/body relationship that continues to grow today. Some (but by no means all) of the seminal works include:

Antonio Damasio, *Descarte's Error*, 1994
Robert Sapolsky, *Why Zebras Don't Have Ulcers*, 1995
Joseph LeDoux, *The Emotional Brain*, 1996
Peter Levine, *Waking the Tiger*, 1997
Daniel Siegel, *The Developing Mind*, 1999
Babette Rothschild, *The Body Remembers*, Volume 1, 2000
Pat Ogden, *Trauma and the Body*, 2006
Stephen Porges, *Polyvagal Theory*, 2011

In this volume, *The Routledge International Handbook of Embodied Perspectives in Psychotherapy: Approaches from Dance Movement and Body Psychotherapies*, editors Helen Payne, Sabine Koch, Jennifer Tantia, and Thomas Fuchs have done a momentous job of gathering a wide variety of views from—literally—all corners of the world. It is, truly, an international handbook! Contributors include many of the most prominent practitioners in their respective fields, including David Boadella who published the first journal *Energy and Character* dedicated to body psychotherapy and founded the European Association of Body Psychotherapy. No compendium on 20th- and 21st-century somatic psychology would be complete without his contribution.

Therapists of all types of somatic approaches as well as those who heretofore have steered clear of the body will find a wealth of innovation, wisdom, and tools ready for integration into existing and beginning practices.

Babette Rothschild, MSW, author of *The Body Remembers*,
Volumes 1 and 2

PREFACE

This book scopes embodied perspectives in psychotherapy framed from phenomenological, psychological and interdisciplinary views, and presents the state-of-the art in the two embodied disciplines of body psychotherapy and dance movement psychotherapy. It is a reference book which scholars, researchers, practitioners and others with an interest in embodied approaches to psychotherapy can access for its wealth of resources and knowledge. In terms of integrative body-mind psychotherapy, it offers answers to many questions, and opportunities for thinking about embodied approaches to psychotherapy.

Authors come from all over the globe to share their in-depth experience in practice, theory and research. The editors have brought to fruition a vast network of practitioners, thinkers and researchers to offer their unique perspectives on embodied approaches to psychotherapy.

This book examines in great detail how these disciplines work, their application to various populations, cutting edge research and scholarly thought based in theoretical and philosophical foundations. The holistic nature of human health is acknowledged, whereby the body is the primary psychotherapeutic resource and entry point of embodied approaches to work on physical issues, emotions, cognitions, relationships, etc. The body offers a prime access to emotions and an autonomous level for therapeutic work through which transformation can occur. The creative and expressive aspects of dance movement therapy are complemented by the physiological and biological elements pertaining to body psychotherapy. The similarities and differences of two related disciplines in embodied psychotherapy are explored in detail in this volume. Following an in-depth description of embodiment by the editors in the first chapter, the overarching chapters at the beginning set the scene for the two disciplines with an introduction to each section providing a summary of the material in that section.

Embodiment is a concept which is growing internationally in a whole range of subjects, for example: neuroscience, psychotherapy, leadership, coaching, education, psychology, philosophy, performance, research methodology and health. It is the editors' vision to encompass significant works from body psychotherapy and dance movement psychotherapy into one volume with a sense of inclusivity. In the current awareness of body/mind integrative therapies, trauma healing and increased interest in personal development, we anticipate the time is right for the body to be honoured and acknowledged for its innate wisdom, and the therapeutic possibilities this can offer for personal growth and transformation.

The book is unique in that it combines various lenses employed by each author which span philosophy and theory, empirical research and clinical practice, not to be found in any other compilation. It shows the wellspring of knowledge which can be derived from the body is fruitful for psychological healing; that embodied experience is the very source of present moment experience and cannot be replaced by thinking about a problem or situation.

It will support and assist students with their assignments and practice placements; therapists with their practice; educators with their teaching; researchers with their conceptual framework. Furthermore, it will help to illuminate the importance of embodiment for professionals from psychiatry, psychology, talking therapies, mental health, community services, social work, arts in health, and other healing arts.

It is with great enthusiasm that the editors bring this volume to completion, as the elements of embodied experience are not only a source of personal knowledge, but are shared across cultures, communities, and nations in that we all have a common bond of embodiment that makes us human.

Hertfordshire, New York and Heidelberg, January 2018
Helen Payne
Jennifer Tantia
Sabine Koch
Thomas Fuchs

ACKNOWLEDGEMENTS

The editors would like to thank all the authors who have worked so diligently to refine their chapters for this volume. Appreciations to clients and patients without whom none of the discourses could take place. Gratitude to those mentors and teachers who have heavily influenced the editors in their professional development, without them this book could not have come to fruition. The publishers at Routledge also played their part brilliantly.

We would particularly like to thank our families who have put up with our focus on this volume over some many months, especially during the last few.

Finally, we would like to acknowledge the contributions to our continuing professional development of the following people relevant to our respective fields in embodied psychotherapy who have, sadly, since passed during the gestation of this book: Jaak Panksepp, Claire Schmais, Linnie Diehl and Eugene Gendlin.

ABBREVIATIONS

ACT	Acceptance and Commitment Therapy
ADHD	Attention deficit hyperactivity disorder
ADMTE	Asociación Española Danza Movimiento Terapia
ADTA	American Dance Therapy Association
AM	Authentic movement
ANS	Autonomic nervous system
B-M-E	Continuum Body-mind-emotion continuum
BMQ	Body Mindfulness Questionnaire
BOPT	Body-Oriented Psychological Therapy
BP	Body Psychotherapy
BPD	Borderline Personality Disorder
BTK	Swiss Association for Movement, Dance and Body Therapies
CAMHS	Children and adolescent mental health service
CAS	Certificates of Advanced Study Degrees
CBH	Centre on Behavioral Health
CBT	Cognitive behavioural therapy
CCC	Columbia College Chicago
CDC	Centers for Disease Control
CICDAI	Cali-Colombia Dance Movement Therapy Training and Mar del Plata
CM	Continuum Movement
CMA	Certified movement analyst
cPTSD	Complex post-traumatic stress disorder
DMP	Dance Movement Psychotherapy
DMT or D/MT	Dance Movement Therapy
DMTC	Dance/Movement Therapy and Counseling
DNA	DeoxyriboNucleic Acid
DSM	American Diagnostic and Statistical Manual of Mental Disorders
EABP	European Association for Body Psychotherapy
EADMT	European Association of Dance Movement Therapy
ECP	European Certificate for Psychotherapy
EMDR	Eye Movement Desensitisation Recovery

ERT	Embodied-Relational Therapy
FE	Functional Relaxation
GAD7	Generalised Anxiety Disorder Scale
GAF	The Global Assessment of Functioning Scale
GP	General Physician
IBS	Irritable bowel syndrome
IFBK	Interdisciplinary Forum for Biomedicine and Cultural Studies
IIBA	International Institute for Bioenergetic Analysis
IPA	Interpretative Phenomenological Analysis
KE	Kinesthetic empathy refers to emotional reactions
KMP	Kestenberg Movement Profile
KS	Kinesthetic seeing refers to body reactions and experiences
LCAT	Licensed Creative Arts Therapist
LMA	Laban movement analysis
MBCT	Mindfulness-based cognitive therapy
MC	Making Connections Suicide Prevention Program
MG	Mobility Gradient
MTS	Movement Thinking Strategies
MUS	Medically unexplained symptoms
MYMOP	Measure Yourself Medical Outcome Profile
NHS	National Health Service, UK
PhQ9	Primary Healthcare Depression Scale
PNS	Parasympathetic nervous system
PTSD	Post Traumatic Stress Disorder
RCT	Randomised controlled trial
RDMP	Registered dance movement psychotherapist
RMP	Restorative Movement Psychotherapy
SAMHSA	Substance Abuse and Mental Health Services Administration
SGBAT	Swiss Society's psychotherapy training program
SHHH	Seen, heard, held, and hugged
SMIFT	Sense, move, imagine, feel, and think
SNS	Sympathetic nervous system
SP	Somatic psychotherapy
SPRC	Suicide Prevention Resource Center
SSD	Somatic Symptom Disorder
SWSA	Department of Social Work and Social Administration
TBMA	The BodyMind Approach
UCLA	University College Los Angeles
UEM	Universidad Europea de Madrid
UK	United Kingdom
UKCP	United Kingdom Council for Psychotherapy
UNA	Universidad Nacional del Arte
UNHCR	United Nations High Commissioner for Refugees
USA	United States of America
WOS	Ways of Seeing
WWII	World War 2
W	Witnessing refers to immediate thoughts and images
ZRM	Zurich Resource Model

INTRODUCTION TO EMBODIED PERSPECTIVES IN PSYCHOTHERAPY

Helen Payne, Sabine Koch, Jennifer Tantia, and Thomas Fuchs

This volume presents a collection of multi-faceted chapters illustrating the recent theoretical shift in psychotherapy that begins to conceptualise the importance of including bodily felt sensations, movement and creative expression as an integrated aspect of being human and therefore an integral part of the psychotherapeutic process. It illustrates that organismic aliveness and health cannot rightfully be sub-divided into psyche and soma.

There are three sections to this book. Section I offers chapters elucidating philosophical and theoretical underpinnings of embodied psychotherapies in psychotherapy. Section II presents chapters from the field of dance movement psychotherapy (DMP), and Section III from the field of body psychotherapy (BP), with their concomitant theory, practice and discourses. Each section has an introduction for ease of access to the reader. All contributions are from leading edge authors from around the globe, providing a truly international flavour to the handbook. It is framed as a reference book and resource for theoreticians, health practitioners, academics, clinicians, students and all others with an interest in psychotherapy and the embodied mind. The community of practice assumes human beings to be subject to unconscious processes, which can be accessed through awareness of the body and via creative, symbolic, and expressive movement. Thoughts, sensations and emotions felt, identified and/or communicated through the body in relational encounters between client and therapist can be utilised to support emotional growth and development, diagnostics, intervention planning and treatment.

Background

Psychotherapists reporting on working with and through the body in the psychotherapy literature come from a variety of different schools in various countries and employ terms such as 'Body Psychotherapy', 'Body-Oriented Psychological Therapy (BOPT)', Body-Oriented (Psycho-) Therapy', 'Somatic Psychology' etc. According to Heller (2012), Body Psychotherapy (BP) is an overall term for the many models of psychotherapy 'that explicitly use body techniques to strengthen the developing dialogue between patient and psychotherapist about what is being experienced and perceived . . . the body is considered a means of communication and exploration' (Heller, 2012, p. 1). Heller, in his book, does not explicitly include dance movement psychotherapy in his analysis of body psychotherapy, as is the conventional conceptualisation in the US and the UK. In the US Johnson and Grand (1998) took on the term 'somatic psychotherapy', based on Hanna's phenomenological theory of Somatics, and Geuter (2015), in Germany, adopted the terminology of body psychotherapy in which dance movement therapy is part of BP (Body Psychotherapy, at its more dynamic pole), as is conventionally conceptualised in Germany.

Dance movement psychotherapy (UK terminology) is known as 'dance therapy' and 'dance movement therapy' (e.g. Germany), 'dance/movement therapy' (US) and 'creative movement therapy' (India); 'expressive movement therapy' and 'movement therapy' in different parts of the world. All terms refer to practices articulated in Section II of the book and all differentiate the practice from the separate discipline of somatic psychotherapy (USA)/body psychotherapy (Europe). For the purposes of this introduction, the two fields will be referred to as body psychotherapy (BP) and dance movement psychotherapy (DMP). However, the book as a whole honours the international variations, acknowledging US authors' terminologies concurrent with dance/movement therapy (DMT) and somatic psychotherapy (SP), and the European tradition (including Israel) with the term dance movement therapy, as well as educating the reader on these differences in nomenclature expanding awareness of how those professions are acknowledged in different parts of the globe.

Although there were some connections between early dance therapists and Wilhelm Reich, and conversely some body psychotherapists who studied with Rudolf von Laban, the two fields of practice, dance movement psychotherapy and body psychotherapy have differing history, training and professional associations (Tantia, 2016), and are therefore considered separate fields of psychotherapeutic practice in the US. In Germany, dance movement therapy is considered one of the body psychotherapies as well as one of the arts therapies, while in the US it is related solely to the arts therapies. It is important to acknowledge that dance movement psychotherapy and body psychotherapy are two different practices, yet with important underpinnings shared between them, such as promoting 'bodymind' integration on the level of clinical practice and theory to evolve beyond the Cartesian body-mind split. Consequently, this volume differentiates between BP and DMP within two sections (both forms of psychotherapy are clearly embodied therapies). However, there are also integrated overarching chapters, which attest to the complex richness and unavoidable integration of many parts of the self when it comes to embodied therapies aiming to resolve health issues in an integrated, holistic way. In this volume the term embodied psychotherapy is employed to include both BP and DMP.

What is embodiment?

The following definition of embodiment provides a basis from which to start:

> Embodiment denominates a field of research, in which the reciprocal influence of the body as a living, animate, moving organism on the one side and cognition, emotion, perception and action on the other side is investigated with respect to the expressive and impressive functions, on three levels: the individual, the interactional, and the extended level.
>
> *(Koch and Fuchs, 2011, p. 276)*

The latter two levels include person-person and person-environment interactions and imply a certain affinity of embodiment approaches to enactive and dynamic systems approaches (Varela, Thompson, and Rosch, 1991).

The concept of 'embodiment' stems from Merleau-Ponty's (1962, 1964) phenomenology, from enactive cognition (Varela et al., 1991), as well as from Bourdieu's (1977) theory of practice. In contrast to Cartesian duality, it links matter and mind in the ongoing enactment of life.

Merleau-Ponty (1964) proposes that perception begins in the body, and, with reflective consciousness, ends in the constitution of independent objects. Perception as a bodily process connects with the notion of somatic modes of attention (Csordas, 1993), which have been identified in a range of cultural practices. Moreover, according to Merleau-Ponty, the lived body is inherently linked to others, thus forming a shared intercorporeality which is also the basis of empathy (Fuchs, 2017). 'Because body and consciousness are one, intersubjectivity is also a co-presence; another's emotion is immediate, because it is grasped pre-objectively, and familiar insofar as we share the same habitus' (Csordas, 1993, p. 151).

Knoblauch (2005) suggests that an expansion of clinical attention should include the embodied experience. She refers to the process of symbolisation as limited in communication within the clinical talking therapies. Moreover, she criticises the displacement effect of language and the futility that language offers as a description of Husserl's 'lived experience' (cited in Wilson and Knoblich, 2005). As Stern states, 'language is a double-edged sword. It makes some parts of our experience less shareable with ourselves and with others' (1985, pp. 162–163), since it is distinct and fixed, and not fuzzy, many-faceted and process-oriented, as sensory and affective experience is. Common verbal expressions at moments of intense experience such as 'words fail me', or 'it goes beyond words', or 'I cannot find the words' indicate this phenomenon as well.

Embodiment as defined in this volume is a genuinely interdisciplinary theoretical and empirical approach that provides a new perspective on the person as a bodily, living, feeling, thinking organism outdating the view of a cognitivist image of the person as an information processor (Smith and Semin, 2004). It integrates a more physical and body-based view of the person as emerging in neuroscience research (Damasio, 1994, LeDoux, 1996; Panksepp, 1998) with a phenomenological concept of the subjective or lived body and its sensations, perceptions (Merleau-Ponty, 1962), movement (Sheets-Johnstone, 1999), and kinaesthesia (Husserl, 1952; Gallagher, 2005). The body is a special category: it is the only 'object' that we can perceive from the inside (interoception) as well as from the outside (exteroception) (Koch and Fuchs, 2011, p. 276). The body has a prototype function for our self- and world understanding, and thus any cognition is primarily situated in the lived body. Embodied cognition, perception, and action often go beyond situated cognition in that many investigated effects generalise across situations, bearing witness to a certain universality (joint principles) of our bodily presence in the world.

Yet, as Wilson (2002) rightfully pointed out, the notion of embodiment is ill-defined, that is, it is often defined differently depending on the context and therefore its meaning is unclear, if not explicitly defined (Wilson, 2002; Ziemke, 2003). Wilson (2002) classified the then emerging embodied cognition research into six claims: (1) cognition is situated, (2) cognition is time-pressured, (3) we off-load cognitive work onto the environment, (4) the environment is part of the cognitive system, (5) cognition is for action, (6) offline cognition is body-based, which, according to Wilson, is the best supported of the claims. However, it is important to note that it is precisely offline cognition (thinking, imagining, etc.) which poses the greatest difficulty to an embodied/enactive approach (see Fuchs, 2018; Glenberg, 1997). Shortly after Wilson, Ziemke (2003) identified six different notions of embodiment, which better relate to clinical reasoning. According to him, embodiment comes in the following forms: as (1) structural coupling between agent and environment, (2) historical embodiment as the result of a history of structural coupling, (3) physical embodiment, (4) organismoid embodiment, i.e. organism-like bodily form (e.g. humanoid robots), (5) organismic embodiment of autopoietic, living systems, and (6) social embodiment. Maxine Sheets-Johnstone (2015) criticised the use of the term embodiment, expressing concern that embodied accounts of mind and cognition neglect 'animate experience', referring to the lived body as defined in phenomenology. She points out that the use of the word 'embodied' and its variations fails to capture the dynamic 'synergies of meaningful movement created by animate organisms' (2015, p. 23); that referring to the 'embodied mind' sounds as if it is all about the mind, which now is burdened with one more aspect, namely the body. Nevertheless, the term is without alternative in present cognitive science (Gibbs, 2005; Koch, 2006).

Four levels of embodiment in clinical practice

Next to the individual level, embodiment influences the person–person and the person–environment interaction. In cognitive science, the so-called '4e's' (embodied, enactive, embedded, extended) are indicative of these interactions using biological and dynamic systems perspectives as well as phenomenological and cultural perspectives.

The *embodied self* is defined by our corporeality (*leiblichkeit*) (Merleau-Ponty, 1962), and mind-body unity. It is empirically investigated by the analysis of the relations between what is conceptualised as body and mind. The embodied self unifies phenomena of embodied cognition, perception, emotion, and action (Niedenthal, 2007; Niedenthal, Barsalou, Winkielman, Krauth-Gruber, and Ric, 2005; Raab, Johnson, and Heekeren, 2009; for clinical applications see Fuchs and Schlimme, 2009; Michalak, Mischnat, and Teismann, 2014; Ramseyer and Tschacher, 2011).

The *enactive self* is conceptualised as a living system following the principles of autonomy, plasticity, self-organisation, sense-making and coupling with the environment (De Jaegher and Di Paolo, 2007; Varela, Thompson, and Rosch, 1991). If applied to person interactions, it also encompasses the self when extended to a dyad or a group constituting a new entity beyond that of the individual embodied self (Fuchs and De Jaegher, 2009; for clinical applications see Koch and Fischman, 2011).

The *embedded self* is the self as connected to an ongoing situation, exploiting its specific circumstances in order to functionally adapt its capacities and to increase its possibilities such as conceptualised in systemic thinking (Schlippe and Schweitzer, 1996; Thelen and Smith, 1994), or in ecological approaches (Gibson, 1966).

The *extended self* (Clark, 1997) is defined by the embodied self's intertwining with and reaching into the environment including cultural externalisation such as in clothing, housing, and artistic expressions through sculptures, pictures, songs, poems, dance, etc. These aspects of embodiment include externalisations and symbolisations of the self, for example in the form of artworks.

Important assumptions of embodiment research

One of the main assumptions of embodiment is the two-way direction between subjective experience (for example, of an emotion or of a situation) and the body's sensations and movements participating in this experience. Hence, the way in which we are moving does not only affect how others understand our nonverbal expressions, it also provides us with our own kinesthetic body feedback (for the physiological basis see Holst and Mittelstaedt, 1950) that helps us perceive and specify, for example, certain emotions (for the psychological basis see Hatfield, Cacioppo and Rapson, 1994). In any case the reciprocal influence of the body and the cognitive-affective system is a simplified construct that has been introduced mainly in order to permit the experimental investigation of body feedback effects on cognition, emotion, perception, and action. We, however, generally conceptualise body and mind, action and perception as a unity, as outlined in Fuchs and Koch (2014), and that it demands original methods for collecting and analyzing embodied data (Ellingson, 2012; Hartelius, 2015; Mehling, et al., 2011; Rennie, 2006; Tantia, 2013a, 2014; Todres, 2007).

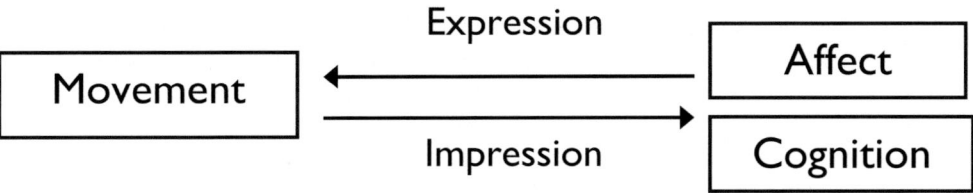

Figure 0.1 Bi-directionality assumption between the cognitive-affective and the motor system
(Koch, 2011, 2014; Wallbott, 1990)

Even though simplified, the bi-directionality assumption is useful to demonstrate various facts and relations (see Figure 0.1 above). It shows how affect and cognition effect changes in movement's expressive function (Darwin, 1872), but also how movement induces change in cognition and affect via feedback effects (impression function; body feedback hypothesis; Laird, 1984; Neumann and Strack, 2000; Wallbott, 1990; Riskind, 1984). In social psychology, such body feedback effects have been investigated from the 1970s on. However, movement as a basic facility of the body has only now become a focus (Koch, 2011, 2014). Such movement feedback can be defined as the afferent feedback from the body periphery to the central nervous system and has been shown to play a causal role in the emotional experience, the formation of attitudes, and, behaviour regulation (Adelman and Zajonc, 1987; Zajonc and Markus, 1984). In a phenomenological understanding, the lived body is the mediator between and the background of the cognitive-affective system and movement. This understanding is reflected in recent clinical embodiment approaches from phenomenology and psychology (Fuchs, 2012, 2018; Fuchs and Schlimme, 2009; Michalak, Troje, Fischer, Vollmar, Heidenreich, and Schulte, 2009). The aforementioned bi-directionality has also been conceptualised as a cycle of embodied affectivity (Fuchs and Koch 2014), linking affection or impression as a centripetal (sensory) component with 'e-motion' or expression as a centrifugal (motor) component. The focus on movement is also the distinctive feature between dance movement therapy and body psychotherapies.

According to embodiment approaches in psychotherapy, movement or movement tendencies can thus directly influence affect and cognition. For example, the mere taking on of a dominant versus a submissive body posture has been shown to cause changes not only in experiencing the self, but also in testosterone levels in the saliva and risk-taking behaviour after the intervention: both indicators were higher in those participants who had assumed a dominant posture (Carney, Cuddy, and Yap, 2010). Arm flexion as an approach movement and arm extension as an avoidance movement have been shown to influence attitudes toward arbitrary Chinese ideographs, causing more positive attitudes in participants of the approach condition (Cacioppo, Priester, and Berntson, 1993). Similarly, different qualities and rhythms of movement have been shown to effect affective and cognitive reactions, such as smooth movement rhythms in handshakes leading to more positive affect and a more open, extrovert and agreeable personality perception than sharp rhythms (Koch, 2011; Koch and Rautner, 2017), or smooth rhythms in embraces signaling indulgence and the wish to continue the embrace versus sharp movement rhythms signaling the wish to separate and end the embrace (Koch and Rautner, 2017). A bidirectional link has also been demonstrated between facial expression of emotions and the comprehension of emotional language: cosmetic injections of botulinum toxin-A, suppressing frowning movements, also hindered processing and understanding of angry sentences and critical texts (Havas, Glenberg, Gutowski, Lucarelli, and Davidson, 2010).

Havas' experiment was based on Conceptual Metaphor Theory (Lakoff and Johnson, 1980, 1999), another influential embodiment approach assuming that all of our abstract (linguistic) concepts are based on our embodiment and our embodied experiences in the world. This is a strong assumption that both philosophers back up with a high amount of convergent empirical evidence. Particularly their image schema concept (container scheme, balance scheme, source-path-goal scheme) is relevant for clinical practice in embodied therapies, since it immediately translates into movement and bodily action. Koch, Fuchs, Summa and Müller (2012) show how image schemas can be helpful in clinical practice in order to identify important embodied metaphors for the client.

Clinical implications

Embodiment provides a holistic approach to lived experience at the interface of psychotherapy and cognitive sciences. It treats the influences of sensations, postures and gestures on perception, action, emotion, and cognition (Barsalou, Niedenthal, Barbey and Ruppert, 2003). Since it emphasises qualitative experience and animation of one's kinesthetic sense, the embodiment concept also suggests approaches considering movement such as dynamic body feedback (Koch, 2011, 2014), or spatial bias (Koch, Glawe, and Holt, 2011), and movement qualities (Kestenberg, 1975; Kestenberg-Amighi, Loman, Lewis, and Sossin, 1999; Laban, 1960; Sheets-Johnstone, 1999). Its enactive and intersubjective aspects are related to concepts such as empathy (Fuchs, 2017; Gallese, 2003), rapport, and outcome in therapeutic interactions (Ramseyer and Tschacher, 2011).

The body is the unifying base of the constant first-person perspective that we 'carry with us'. We cannot escape from this direct experience and thus need to integrate it – with all its biases – into our theorising, empirical research and clinical practice. The study and practice of embodiment provides many opportunities for psychotherapies to build interdisciplinary bridges to the cognitive sciences (not only to cognitive psychology, but also to cognitive linguistics, cognitive anthropology, phenomenology, and even robotics), and to actively contribute to establish the unity of body-mind and the role of movement in cognitive science and beyond. The knowledge of dance movement therapy, for example, may enable embodiment researchers in cognitive sciences to better operationalise their body-based conceptualisations. Dance movement therapists have the potential to contribute to research by sharing their knowledge and practice to refine the operationalisation of movement used by embodiment researchers, because, for example, DMP's degree of differentiation of movement observation and analysis knowledge exceeds that of the average interdisciplinary embodiment researcher. Moreover, dance movement therapists are positioned to pose questions resulting from their applied field to studies from cognitive science and neuroscience.

Likewise, concepts within body psychotherapy such as grounding, centering, and interoceptive awareness described in imaginal shape, colour, texture and other somatic experiences which can offer new knowledge of embodied awareness relating to emotional content unavailable to traditional research methods and language. In addition, there is much that body psychotherapists and somatic clinicians can offer current research paradigms to supplement new knowledge in cognitive science. Conversely, the areas of research that measure physiological mechanisms of the body may also provide opportunities for body psychotherapists to contribute their expertise regarding the phenomenology of the body's psychophysiological process in clinical practice to augment scientific areas of study that are less body-informed.

The basic knowledge embodiment research generates needs to be put to an applied empirical test by, for example, answering questions such as 'can it help the therapeutic progress to explain why a patient feels nauseous every time he carries out an approach in movement toward the therapist?' Or is embodiment just another promise that cannot live up to therapeutic practice? Such questions provide interesting challenges for embodiment researchers. In order to differentiate the suitability of the embodiment approach to body psychotherapy and dance movement therapy as applied empirical disciplines in the service of the client, an important goal is to specify its potential and limitations. It is the hope of the current volume's editors that the fertile interchange between embodied therapies and cognitive science is sustained in the next decade, facilitated by phenomenology and enactive perspectives under the umbrella of embodiment.

Dance movement psychotherapy

'Dance movement psychotherapy is an animate, active form of embodied communication, or inter-corporeality, which can be understood as the vehicle for the co-creation of the therapeutic alliance whereby there is an interplay' [between therapist and client] (Payne, 2017, p. 4).

There are numerous dance movement psychotherapy masters' training programmes across the USA and Europe of which the UK boasts four currently. There is a well established European Association and many countries have professional associations (please see appendix for training and associations details and other resources). In dance movement psychotherapy there are important traditions such as the participatory and interactive approach of Marian Chace (East Coast of the US), Mary Whitehouse (West Coast of the US), Foulkesian approach (Maria Foulkes, Argentina), ethno-dance therapy approaches such as the Philippine stick fighting martial-art of Escrima (Germany), or the Maori dances of Haka (New Zealand), and other approaches from around the world.

The DMT approach, created by Marian Chace, (Chaiklin, 1975; Sandel, Chaiklin, and Lohn, 1993) is a participatory one and derived from humanistic theories of Carl Rogers' Client-Centered Therapy (Rogers, 1951) and Harry Stack Sullivan's Interpersonal Psychiatry Approach (Sullivan, 2013/1955). It was developed with very low functioning psychiatric patients in the 1950s. Chace invited all patients into the circle and, together with music (often Strauss) as an accompaniment, mirrored their movements and movement qualities, picking up their movement and mood, naming who they are and what they do to involve them with each other: 'Can we all move our arms like Mrs. Jackson?', 'Can we all bounce like Mrs. Miller?', or 'Can we all stand with Mr. Turotti?'. She did purposeful variations thereof (maximisation, minimisation, changes in tempo, intensity, and spatial parameters) in order to broaden patients' movement repertoire and thus their flexibility not only on a bodily level, asking 'Can we make this movement bigger/ smaller/stronger/lighter/faster/slower?' After identifying individual movement from each patient, the sessions progressed into the verbal group process which is based on the movement experience. An important principle is to stay on the level of describing movements and sensations as long as possible and only very gradually invite metaphors from the patients such as asking 'What are we doing here? What does it look like? What does it remind you of?' Verbal processing emphasising the embodied experience is an important last part of the session, where again each participant should be heard while the therapist facilitates the holding environment.

Authentic movement (AM) (which does not use music), created by Mary Whitehouse nearly at the same time as Chace was developing her method, is also a practice under the umbrella of dance movement psychotherapy, and facilitates bodily consciousness at our most primordial, underlying awareness of existence (Adler, 2007; Chodorow, 1999; Pallaro, 1999, 2007; Whitehouse, 1999). Mover and witness are in a co-created, intersubjective relationship whereby the mover, with eyes closed, waits for an impulse at a deep cellular level. It is practiced as self-directed movement, with non-judgmental and empathic attitudes from the witness/therapist who sees the mover/client moving. This in turn creates empathy towards self and others. Founded on Jung's concept of active imagination and the collective unconscious, it is influenced by group work and spiritual practice where symbolic meaning is seen in spontaneous, physical expression. Participants learn to engage with the direct experience of the self beyond words and concepts. AM can help a person to develop body awareness, body-mind-spirit connections, therapeutic presence, and kinaesthetic empathy, in which mindfulness is crucial to practice, and which provides a gateway to embodiment (Tantia, 2012, 2013b).

In Europe, there is phenomenologically based integrative dance movement therapy (Willke, Hölter and Petzold, 1991; Willke, 2010), similar to Serlin's phenomenological approach in the US (Serlin, 1985, 1996). There is primitive dance therapy in France (Schott-Billmann, 2015), systemic dance movement therapy by Bender (2015), and medical dance/movement therapy in the US (Goodill, 2006). In Goodill's model of medical dance/movement therapy, she addresses the psychosocial implications of disease phenomenology. She explores the ways in which creativity in movement can facilitate change in negative thoughts and feelings while normalising how anger, depression, and loss of self-esteem are a normal part of a medical condition. Goodill's approach literally mobilises the patient's creativity as a means toward confronting the disease, as well as accepting parts of its effect that cannot be changed. Serlin (1985, 1996) also has an approach to disease phenomenology. She addresses the problem of embodiment in terms of the objectified body, the mute body, and meaningless action and seeks to restore a language of embodiment and an embodied language in terms of the conscious body, action language, and action hermeneutics. The therapeutic task is to restore congruence between thinking, feeling, and action; between psyche, soma, and language; between logos and eros. This is done by grounding therapeutic tradition not in the language of scientific psychology but in an older tradition of rhythm and sound, in image and story, in the arts, and in culture. As a therapeutic method, kinaesthetic imagining is a dynamic embodied form of imagination in which patients as artists compose themselves and transform their lives (Serlin, 1996).

But how can we systematise movement observations in order to investigate effects? Clinical movement analysis differentiates two major categories of *movements*: movement quality and movement shaping (Kestenberg, 1975; Laban, 1960). Quality denominates the changes in the dynamics of the movement, which can be fighting or indulgent, and either occur in tension-flow (the alternations between tension and relaxation, which can be sharp or smooth), in pre-efforts (Kestenberg, 1975), or efforts (Laban and Lawrence, 1974). Shaping denominates shape changes of the body, such as open and closed postures, or growing and shrinking as prototypically observed in inhaling and exhaling. In shaping, the body either expands or shrinks in different directions, in response to an internal or to an external stimulus. These changes can all be described in specific movement terms and notated in writing. Movement rhythms, the earliest most unconscious movement qualities patterns we employ, are graphed by use of kinesthetic empathy (Kestenberg, 1975) which is a bodily attitude that makes use of the resonance of another's movements in one's own body (see also Fuchs and De Jaegher, 2009), bringing movement curves onto paper just like a human seismograph. The fine-grained differentiations and basic dimensions of the Laban and Kestenberg systems need to be considered when investigating the influence of movement on the self empirically.

Body psychotherapy

When Freud's body-based developmental stages began to cause him resistance from critics of his work, Wilhelm Reich, a student of Freud's in the 1920s continued where Freud's observations ceased and began to develop his own theories of the body as an integral part of the psychological healing process. Similar to Freud, Reich held an MD and created a style of therapy based in psychoanalysis known as 'Orgone Therapy'. He also constructed the concepts that Body Armour, or postures and gestures that the body holds as a manifestation of emotional patterning in a patient, can be changed through manual manipulation (Reich, 1945). Fritz Perls (1969), a humanistic psychologist, entered into treatment with Reich while he was creating Gestalt Therapy with his wife, Laura Perls (a dancer who contributed to the movement-based aspects of Gestalt therapy). One can see the influence in some of the body-oriented applications within Gestalt therapy today. Like Freud, Reich also had students and was succeeded by several emerging body psychotherapists who developed methods over the next 40 years: Alexander Lowen's (1975) Bioenergetic Therapy, Ron Kurtz's (2013) Hakomi Method and John Pierrakos' (1990) Core Energetics were among them and are still practiced widely today.

Curious therapists and philosophers in both the US and Europe were roused by this new way of healing, and just as Reich's influence thrived in Europe, Perls travelled from Europe to the US and began to teach and develop Gestalt Therapy at a healing center in California called the Esalen Institute, where he met others who were also integrating embodied experience as a means toward healing during the humanistic era (Kripal, 2007). One philosopher, Thomas Hanna, was developing a system of healing called Somatics. Still today, Body Psychotherapy is known as 'Somatic Psychotherapy' in the US. To clarify the difference between 'body' and 'soma', Hanna stated, 'Somatics is the field which studies the *soma;* namely the body as perceived from within by first-person perception. When a human being is observed from the outside – i.e. from a third-person viewpoint – the phenomenon of a human *body is* perceived' (Hanna, 1986, p. 4).

Body Psychotherapy (somatic psychotherapy) is a psychotherapeutic practice derived from theories of psychoanalysis, developmental psychology, biological neuroscience and attachment theory. In practice, a body psychotherapist identifies a client's sensorial experience as a source of knowledge in the psychotherapeutic process and helps the client to integrate their present embodied experience as a measure of healing. As of today, education in BP is mostly attained through postgraduate certificate programs, although there exists one master's and one doctoral program in the US and one master's in the UK. In the UK there appears to be resistance from the field of psychiatry/mental health to include body psychotherapy as a legitimate form of psychotherapy, and most body psychotherapists must attain a post graduate degree in traditional psychotherapy prior to continuing education toward body psychotherapy practice.

In contrast to the difficulty that body psychotherapists/somatic psychotherapists have in gaining lawful recognition as a profession, recent theories from neuroscience and neurobiology have contributed studies that practically explain the processes at work of both body psychotherapy and dance movement psychotherapy. Five neurobiological distinctions in dance/movement therapy have been made to assess one's organismic state: a) arousal and rest, b) emotion regulation, c) implicit and explicit memory, d) mirror neurons, and e) right/left brain interaction (Homann, 2010). In arousal and rest, Porges (2009) illustrates how the body's natural patterns of activation and relaxation are seen through the change in neurotransmitters, which also change attention (Hart, 2008). Emotional regulation is physiologically realised through the vagus nerve (Porges, 2005), among others; it can be altered by traumatic incidences (Rothschild, 2000) and felt through interoception (Hindi, 2012).

Differences between implicit and explicit memory have been described by Schacter (1987) and Fuchs (2012). Fuchs termed implicit memory 'body memory', thus denoting that procedural and other kinds of implicit memory cannot be attributed to the brain only but are capacities of the body as a whole. The mirror neurons, discovered by Rizzolatti, Fadiga, Gallese and Fogassi (1996), have provided us with a neural basis for intersubjectivity, interpersonal resonance, and ability to feel empathy toward another (Gallese, 2003). The phrenology of right- and left-brain hemispheric processes have since evolved, and neurobiologists now understand brain functioning to be a much more complex process. Today brain processes are not segregated into sections or modules but are conceived of as more interrelated than previously thought, especially when it comes to psychophysiological processes (Fuchs, 2018; Labouvie-Vief, 2015). This current, more integrated way of viewing brain functioning aligns with the very concept of the holistic, integrative embodied healing, giving further support for the clinical study of body psychotherapy.

The chapters

We have invited contributors to discuss some of the underlying principles in the clinical practice, clarify assumptions and add definitions of, for example, embodiment, in order to increase existing theory, knowledge and understanding in the two fields of body and dance movement psychotherapy. The book looks at diverse types of practices and theories to add to our knowledge of how these embodied psychotherapies work and their impact on clients/patients. It offers a new understanding of existing practices and supports state-of-the art and pioneering ways of working. The book explores recent ideas, models and methodologies of body and dance movement psychotherapies and provides an exchange of professional discourses to contribute to improved concepts and practices in the future.

In order to assist the reader each section has an introduction aiming to synthesise the diverse views and practice, clarifying common themes and differences. We highlight questions arising and hope these generate debate and further publications.

This is an academic publication which makes the case for embodied approaches to psychotherapy. The arguments, based on, for example, new theories of embodied social cognition (Barsalou et al., 2003; Niedenthal et al., 2005), and embodied emotion (Niedenthal, 2007), we anticipate will engage the reader in responding to the text from within, from his/her own genuine embodied reactions. The volume is intended as a fundamental source book for all dance movement and body psychotherapy practitioners whether novice or experienced professionals. For training establishments in both disciplines, it will be essential reading on reference lists at every stage of training, from introductory to advanced master's levels. For researchers, it will form the basis for further studies whether in embodiment, cognitive science, philosophy, psychology, counselling/psychotherapy, the arts, health or education. For psychotherapists from all schools, it can enhance an understanding of the role of the body and movement in psychotherapy, complementing any studies during training and beyond on the importance of the body and on non-verbal communication.

There are three sections to this book. The first section introduces some overarching dialogues in current embodied psychotherapy approaches. The two subsequent sections on DMP and BP each span a rich range of embodied clinical approaches, frameworks and applications. We hope you find these chapters of interest and can take knowledge and further understanding from the state-of-the-art scholarship presented in this volume.

References

Adelman, P. K., and Zajonc, R. B. (1987). Facial efference and the experience of emotion. *Annual Review of Psychology, 40,* 249–280.

Adler, J. (2007). From seeing to knowing. In P. Pallaro (Ed.), *Authentic Movement: Moving the Body, Moving the Self, Being Moved* (pp. 260–269). London: Jessica Kingsley.

Barsalou, L. W., Niedenthal, P. M., Barbey, A., and Ruppert, J. (2003). Social embodiment. In B. Ross (Ed.), *The Psychology of Learning and Motivation* (Vol. 43, pp. 43–92). San Diego, CA: Academic Press.

Bender, S. (2015). *Systemische Tanztherapie* [Systemic Dance Therapy]. Munich: Reinhard.

Bourdieu, P. (1977). *Outline of a Theory of Practice* (R. Nice, Trans.). Cambridge: Cambridge University Press.

Cacioppo, J. T., Priester, J. R., and Berntson, G. (1993). Rudimentary determinants of attitudes II: Arm flexion and extension have differential effects on attitudes. *Journal of Personality and Social Psychology, 65,* 5–17.

Carney, D. R., Cuddy, A. J. C., and Yap, A. Y. (2010). Power posing: Brief nonverbal displays affect neuroendocrine levels and risk tolerance. *Psychological Science, 21*(10), 1363–1368.

Chaiklin, S. H. (1975). *Marian Chace: Her Papers.* Columbia, MD: American Dance Therapy Association.

Chodorow, J. (1999). To move and be moved. In P. Pallaro (Ed.), *Authentic Movement: Essays by Mary Starks Whitehouse, Janet Adler and Joan Chodorow* (pp. 267–278). London: Jessica Kingsley.

Clark, A. (1997). *Being There: Putting Brain, Body, and World Together Again.* Cambridge, MA: MIT Press.

Csordas, T. (1990). Embodiment as a paradigm for anthropology. *Ethos, 18*(1), 5–47.

Csordas, T. (1993). Somatic modes of attention. *Cultural Anthropology, 8*(2), 135–156.

Damasio, A. R. (1994). *Descartes' Error: Emotion, Reason, and the Human Brain.* New York: Putnam.

Darwin, C. (1872/1965). *The Expression of Emotions in Men and Animals.* Chicago: University of Chicago Press. (Original work published 1872)

De Jaegher, H., and Di Paolo, E. (2007). Participatory sense-making: An enactive approach to social cognition. *Phenomenology and Cognitive Sciences, 6*, 485–507.

Ellingson, L. (2012). Interview as embodied communication. In J. F. Gubrium, J. A. Holstein, A. B. Marvasti, and K. D. McKinney (Eds.), *The Sage Handbook of Interview Research: The Complexity of the Craft* (2nd ed., pp. 525–540). Thousand Oaks, CA: Sage.

Fuchs, T. (2012). The phenomenology of body memory. In S. C. Koch, T. Fuchs, M. Summa, and C. Müller (Eds.), *Body Memory, Metaphor and Movement.* Amsterdam: John Benjamins.

Fuchs, T. (2017). Intercorporeality and interaffectivity. In C. Meyer, J. Streeck, and S. Jordan (Eds.), *Intercorporeality: Emerging Socialities in Interaction* (pp. 3–24). Oxford: Oxford University Press.

Fuchs, T. (2018). *Ecology of the Brain. The Phenomenology and Biology of the Embodied Mind.* New York: Oxford University Press.

Fuchs, T., and De Jaegher, H. (2009). Enactive intersubjectivity: Participatory sense-making and mutual incorporation. *Phenomenology and the Cognitive Sciences, 8*, 465–486.

Fuchs, T., and Koch, S. (2014). Embodied affectivity: on moving and being moved. *Frontiers in Psychology: Psychology for Clinical Settings, 508*, 1–12.

Fuchs, T., and Schlimme, J. E. (2009). Embodiment and psychopathology. A phenomenological perspective. *Current Opinion in Psychiatry, 22*, 570–575.

Gallagher, S. (2005). *How the Body Shapes the Mind.* Oxford: Oxford University Press.

Gallese, V. (2003). The roots of empathy: The shared manifold hypothesis and neural basis of intersubjectivity. *Psychopathology, 36*, 171–180.

Geuter, U. (2015). *Körperpsychotherapie* [Body Psychotherapy: A Theoretical Outline for Clinical Practice]. Berlin: Springer.

Gibbs, R. W. (2005). *Embodiment and Cognitive Science.* Cambridge, MA: Cambridge University Press.

Gibson, J. J. (1966). *The Senses Considered as Perceptual Systems.* Boston, MA: Houghton Mifflin.

Glenberg, A. M. (1997). What memory is for? *Behavioral and Brain Sciences, 20*, 1–55.

Goodill, S. W. (2006). *An Introduction to Medical Dance Movement Therapy.* London: Jessica Kingsley.

Hanna, T. (1986, Spring/Summer). What is Somatics? *Somatics, 5*, 4.

Hart, S. (2008). *Brain, Attachment, Personality: An Introduction to Neuro-Affective Development.* London: Karnac.

Hartelius, G. (2015). Body maps of attention: Phenomenal markers for two varieties of mindfulness. *Mindfulness Online.* doi:10.1007/s12671-015-0391-x

Hatfield, E., Cacioppo, J. T., and Rapson, R. L. (1994). *Emotional contagion.* Paris: Cambridge University Press.

Havas, D. A., Glenberg, A. M., Gutowski, K. A., Lucarelli, M. J., and Davidson, R. J. (2010). Cosmetic use of botulinum toxin-A affects processing of emotional language. *Psychological Science, 21*, 895–900.

Heller, M. (2012). *Body Psychotherapy: History, Concepts, Methods.* New York: W. W. Norton.

Hindi, F. S. (2012). How attention to interoception can inform dance/movement therapy. *American Journal of Dance Therapy, 34*(2), 129–140.

Holst, E. V., and Mittelstaedt, H. (1950). Das Reafferenzprinzip (Wechselwirkungen zwischen zentralnervensystem und peripherie) [The Re-afference principle: Interaction of CNS and periphery]. *Naturwissenschaften, 37*, 464–476.

Homann, K. B. (2010). Embodied concepts of neurobiology in dance/movement therapy practice. *American Journal of Dance Therapy, 32*(2), 80–99.

Husserl, E. (1952). *Ideen zu einer reinen Phänomenologie und Phänomenologischen Philosophie, Zweites Buch: Phänomenologische Untersuchungen zur Konstitution* [Ideas II]. Den Haag: Nijhoff.

Johnson, D. H., and Grand, I. J. (Eds.). (1998). *The Body in Psychotherapy: Inquiries in Somatic Psychology.* Berkeley, CA: North Atlantic Books.

Kestenberg, J. S. (1975). *Parents and Children.* Northvale: Jason Aronson.

Kestenberg-Amighi, J., Loman, S., Lewis, P., and Sossin, K. M. (1999). *The Meaning of Movement. Clinical and Developmental Assessment with the Kestenberg Movement Profile.* New York: Brunner-Routledge Publishers.

Knoblauch, S. H. (2005). Body rhythms and the unconscious. Toward an expanding of clinical attention. *Psychoanalytic Dialogues, 15*(6), 807–827.

Koch, S. C. (2006). Interdisciplinary embodiment approaches. Implications for creative arts therapies. In S. C. Koch and I. Bräuninger (Eds.), *Advances in Dance/Movement Therapy. Theoretical Perspectives and Empirical Findings* (pp. 17–28). Berlin: Logos.

Koch, S. C. (2011). Basic body rhythms and embodied intercorporeality: From individual to interpersonal movement feedback. In W. Tschacher and C. Bergomi (Eds.), *The Implications of Embodiment: Cognition and Communication* (pp. 151–171). Exeter: Imprint Academic.

Koch, S. C. (2014). Rhythm is it: Effects of dynamic body feedback on affect and attitudes. *Frontiers in Psychology, 10*(5), 537.

Koch, S. C., and Fischman, D. (2011). Embodied enactive dance/movement therapy. *American Journal of Dance Therapy*, 33(1), 57–72.

Koch, S. C., and Fuchs, T. (2011). Embodied arts therapies. *The Arts in Psychotherapy, 38*, 276–280.

Koch, S. C., and Rautner, H. (2017). Psychology of the embrace. How body rhythms communicate the need to indulge or to separate. *Behavioral Science, 7*(4), Basel, 11/29; pii: E80.

Koch, S. C., Fuchs, T., Summa, M., and Müller, C. (2012). *Body Memory, Metaphor and Movement*. Philadelphia: John Benjamins.

Koch, S. C., Glawe, S., and Holt, D. (2011). Up and down, front and back: Movement and meaning in the vertical and sagittal axis. *Social Psychology, 42*(3), 214–224.

Kripal, J. J. (2007). *Esalen: America and the Religion of No Religion*. Chicago: University of Chicago Press.

Kurtz, R. (2013). *Body-Centered Psychotherapy: The Hakomi Method*. Mendocino, CA: LifeRhythms.

Laban, R. V. (1960). *The Mastery of Movement*. London: MacDonald and Evans.

Laban, R. V., and Lawrence, F. C. (1974). *Effort: Economy in Body Movement*. Boston: Plays. (Original was published 1947).

Labouvie-Vief, G. (2015). Emotions and cognition: From myth and philosophy to modern psychology and neuroscience. In G. Labouvie-Vief (Ed.), *Integrating Emotions and Cognition Throughout the Lifespan*. New York: Springer Nature.

Laird, J. D. (1984). The real role of facial response in the experience of emotion: A response to Tourangeau and Ellsworth, and others. *Journal of Personality and Social Psychology, 47*, 909–917.

Lakoff, G., and Johnson, M. (1980). *Metaphors We Live By*. Chicago: University of Chicago Press.

Lakoff, G., and Johnson, M. (1999). *Philosophy in the Flesh. The Embodied Mind and Its Challenge to Western Thought*. New York: Basic Books.

LeDoux, J. (1996). *The Emotional Brain*. New York: Shuster and Schuster.

Lowen, A. (1975). *Bioenergetics: The Revolutionary Therapy That Uses the Language of the Body to Heal the Problems of the Mind*. New York: Penguin.

Mehling, W. E., Wrubel, J., Daubenmier, J. J., Price, C. J., Kerr, C. E., Silow, T., . . . Stewart, A. L. (2011). Body awareness: A phenomenological inquiry into the common ground of mind-body therapies. *Philosophy, Ethics, and Humanities in Medicine, 6*(6). doi:10.1186/1747–5341–6-6

Merleau-Ponty, M. (1962). *Phenomenology of Perception*. London: Routledge.

Merleau-Ponty, M. (1964). *The Primacy of Perception* (C. Smith, Trans.). London: Routledge.

Michalak, J., Mischnat, J., and Teismann, T. (2014). Sitting posture makes a difference – embodiment effects on depressive memory bias. *Journal of Clinical Psychology and Psychotherapy, 21*(6), 519–524.

Michalak, J., Troje, N. F., Fischer, J., Vollmar, P., Heidenreich, T., and Schulte, D. (2009). Embodiment of sadness and depression – gait patterns associated with dysphoric mood. *Psychosomatic Medicine, 71*, 580–587.

Neumann, R., and Strack, F. (2000). Approach and avoidance: The influence of proprioceptive and exteroceptive cues on encoding of affective information. *Journal of Personality and Social Psychology, 79*(1), 39.

Niedenthal, P. M. (2007). Embodying emotion. *Science, 316*, 1002–1005.

Niedenthal, P. M., Barsalou, L. W., Winkielman, P., Krauth-Gruber, S., and Ric, F. (2005). Embodiment in attitudes, social perception, and emotion. *Personality and Social Psychology Review, 9*(3), 194–211.

Pallaro, P. (1999). *Authentic Movement: Essays by Mary Starks Whitehouse, Janet Adler and Joan Chodorow*. London: Jessica Kingsley.

Panksepp, J. (1998). *Affective Neuroscience: The Foundations of Human and Animal Emotions*. New York: Oxford University Press.

Payne, H. (2017). Introduction. In H. Payne (Ed.), *Essentials in Dance Movement Psychotherapy: International Perspectives on Theory, Research and Practice* (pp. 1–17). London: Routledge.

Perls, F. (1969). *Gestalt Therapy Verbatim*. New York: Bantam Books.

Pierrakos, J. (1990). *Core Energetics: Developing the Capacity to Love and Heal*. Mendocino, CA: LifeRhythms.

Porges, S. W. (2005). The vagus: A mediator of behavioral and visceral features associated with autism. In M. L. Bauman and T. L. Kemper (Eds.), *The Neurobiology of Autism* (pp. 65–78). Baltimore: Johns Hopkins University Press.

Porges, S. W. (2009). Reciprocal influences between body and brain in the perception and expression of affect: A polyvagal perspective. In D. Fosha, D. Siegel, and M. Solomon (Eds.), *The Healing Power of Emotion: Affective Neuroscience, Development, and Clinical Practice* (pp. 27–54). New York: W. W. Norton.

Raab, M., Johnson, J. G., and Heekeren, H. (Eds.). (2009). *Mind and Motion: The Bidirectional Link Between Thought and Action. Progress in Brain Research, 174.* New York: Elsevier.

Ramseyer, F., and Tschacher, W. (2011). Nonverbal synchrony in psychotherapy: Relationship quality and outcome are reflected by coordinated body-movement. *Journal of Consulting and Clinical Psychology, 79*(3), 284–290.

Reich, W. (1945). *Character Analysis.* New York: Farrar, Straus and Giroux.

Rennie, D. L. (2006). Embodied categorizing in the grounded theory method: Methodological hermeneutics in action. *Theory and Psychology, 16*(4), 483–503.

Riskind, J. H. (1984). They stoop to conquer: Guiding and self-regulatory functions of physical posture after success and failure. *Journal of Personality and Social Psychology, 47*, 479–493.

Rizzolatti, G., Fadiga, L., Gallese, V., and Fogassi, L. (1996). Premotor cortex and the recognition of motor actions. *Cognitive Brain Research, 3,* 131–141.

Rogers, C. (1951). *Client-Centered Therapy.* Boston: Houghton Mifflin Co.

Rothschild, B. (2000). *The Body Remembers: The Psychophysiology of Trauma Treatment.* New York: W. W. Norton.

Sandel, S. L., Chaiklin, S., and Lohn, A. (1993). *Foundations of Dance Movement Therapy: The Life and Work of Marian Chace.* Marian Chace Memorial Fund of the American Dance Therapy Association.

Schacter, D. L. (1987). Implicit memory: History and current status. *Journal of Experimental Psychology: Learning, Memory, and Cognition, 13,* 501–518.

Schlippe, A. V., and Schweitzer, J. (1996). *Lehrbuch der Systemischen Therapie und Beratung* [Textbook of Systemic Therapy and Counseling]. Göttingen, Germany: Vandenhoeck and Ruprecht.

Schott-Billmann, F. (2015). *Primitive Expression and Dance Therapy: When Dancing Heals* (Explorations in Mental Health). London: Routledge.

Serlin, I. A. (1985). *Kinaesthetic Imagining. A Phenomenological Study.* Unpublished doctoral dissertation.

Serlin, I. A. (1996). Kinesthetic imagining. *Journal of Humanistic Psychology, 36*(2), 25–33.

Sheets-Johnstone, M. (1999). *The Primacy of Movement.* Philadelphia: John Benjamins.

Sheets-Johnstone, M. (2015). *The Phenomenology of Dance.* Philadelphia: Temple University Press.

Smith, E. R., and Semin, G. R. (2004). Socially situated cognition. Cognition in its social context. In M. P. Zanna (Ed.), *Advances in Experimental Social Psychology* (Vol. 36, pp. 53–117). Amsterdam: Elsevier.

Stern, D. N. (1985). *The Interpersonal World of the Infant.* New York: Basic Books

Sullivan, H. S. (2013). *The Interpersonal Theory of Psychiatry.* London: Routledge. (Original work published 1955)

Tantia, J. F. (2012). Authentic movement and the autonomic nervous system: A preliminary investigation. *American Journal of Dance Therapy, 34*(1), 53–73.

Tantia, J. F. (2013a). Body-focused interviewing: Corporeal experience in phenomenological inquiry. In SAGE *Research Methods Cases.* London: Sage. Retrieved from http://srmo.sagepub.com/view/methods-case-studies-2013/n228.xml

Tantia, J. F. (2013b). Mindfulness and dance/movement therapy for treating trauma. In L. Rappaport (Ed.), *Mindfulness in the Creative Arts Therapies* (pp. 96–107). London: Jessica Kingsley.

Tantia, J. F. (2014). Is intuition embodied? A phenomenological study of clinical intuition in somatic psychotherapy practice. *Body, Movement and Dance in Psychotherapy, 9*(4), 211–223.

Tantia, J. F. (2016). The interface between somatic psychotherapy and dance/movement therapy: A critical analysis. *Body, Movement and Dance in Psychotherapy, 11*(2–3), 181–196.

Thelen, E., and Smith, L. B. (1994). *A Dynamic Systems Approach to the Development of Perception and Action.* Cambridge, MA: MIT Press.

Todres, L. (2007). *Embodied Enquiry: Phenomenological Touchstones for Research, Psychotherapy and Spirituality.* New York, NY: Palgrave Macmillan.

Varela, F. J., Thompson, E., and Rosch, E. (1991). *The Embodied Mind. Cognitive Science and Human Experience.* Cambridge, MA: MIT Press.

Wallbott, H. G. (1990). *Mimik im Kontext. Die Bedeutung verschiedener Informationskomponenten für das Erkennen von Emotionen* [Mimics in Context: The Meaning of Different Information Components for Emotion Recognition]. Göttingen: Hogrefe.

Whitehouse, M. (1999). C G Jung and dance therapy: Two major principles. In P. Pallaro (Ed.), *Authentic Movement: Essays by Mary Starks Whitehouse, Janet Adler and Joan Chodorow* (pp. 73–106). London: Jessica Kingsley.

Willke, E. (2010). *Tanztherapie – Theoretische Kontexte und Grundlage der Intervention* [Dance Therapy – Theoretical Contexts and Principles of Intervention]. Bern: Hogrefe/Huber.

Willke, E., Hölter, G., and Petzold, H. (1991). *Tanztherapie. Theorie und Praxis – Ein Handbuch* [Dance Therapy. Theory and Practice – A handbook]. Paderborn: Junfermann.

Wilson, M. (2002). Six views of embodied cognition. *Psychonomic Bulletin and Review, 9,* 625–636.

Wilson, M., and Knoblich, G. (2005). The case for motor involvement in perceiving conspecifics. *Psychological Bulletin, 131,* 460–473.

Zajonc, R. B., and Markus, H. (1984). Affect and cognition: The hard interface. In C. Izard, J. Kagan, and R. B. Zajonc (Eds.), *Emotions, Cognition and Behavior* (pp. 73–102). Cambridge: Cambridge University Press.

Ziemke, T. (2003). What is that thing called embodiment? In *Proceedings of the 25th Annual Meeting of the Cognitive Science Society.* Mahwah, NJ: Erlbaum.

SECTION I

Overview of concepts

Introduction

This first section provides an overview on embodied therapies placing them in present phenom-enological and clinical discourses. Each chapter is summarised and offers a distinct element of embodiment in terms of philosophy, narrative, cognitive psychology, and clinical practice.

Chapter 1 is entitled 'Essential dimensions of being a body' by the philosopher **Maxine Sheets-Johnstone** from the USA, who describes living realities of being a body that are integral to dance, to creative arts therapies, and to body psychotherapy. It specifies and investigates these living realities to begin with in terms of 'the self', specifically, in terms of two notable concep-tions and formulations of the self: both the emergent self and core self as described by infant psychiatrist and clinical psychologist Daniel Stern (1985), and the self as phenomenologically described by Husserl (1950/1973), a description that singles out what is essentially present in the experience of an animate organism. The striking complementarities between the two descriptive analyses show that the self is basically rooted in being a body, in animation, in kinesthesia, and in affectivity, an anchorage that recalls Freud's observation, 'The ego is first and foremost a bodily ego' (Freud, 1955, p. 26). Such anchorage furthermore brings to light certain affinities with the Buddhist notion of self as a construct (Kornfield, 2000; Goldstein and Kornfield, 1987; Thera, 1965) in that it makes evident a range of temporally enlightened aspects of self: being a body is a whole-life developmental reality, an ontogeny that spans the whole of life; kinesthesia is a matter of movement and is hence the experience of an inherently temporal qualitative dynamic; affec-tivity is dynamic: affective feelings move through bodies, moving them to move.

This is followed by Chapter 2 from the philosophers **Shaun Gallagher** from the USA, and **Dan Hutto** from Australia, and is entitled 'Narratives in embodied therapeutic practice: Getting the story straight'. It proposes an approach to embodied and narrative practice consistent with enactivist approaches to cognition. They conceive of intersubjective encounters in terms of non-representational embodied interactions, enhanced and supported by highly contextualised socio-cultural, narrative practice. They build on and integrate the enactivist approach developed in interaction theory (Gallagher, 2008; Gallagher and Hutto, 2008) and the narrative practice hypothesis (Hutto, 2008). As a result, they offer an alternative to individualist and intellectualist mainstream approaches to cognition and social cognition, reconceiving the status and importance of these practices in our capacities to relate to and understand others. They consider how this approach can contribute to therapeutic practices, looking at some existing practices, and suggesting some new avenues for diagnosis and treatment in a variety of psychotherapeutic contexts.

Jessica Acolin, a dance/movement therapist from the USA contributes Chapter 3 entitled 'Towards a clinical theory of embodiment: A model for the conceptualization and treatment of mental illness'. She proposes a clinical embodiment theory built upon phenomenological approaches of the lived body and findings from cognitive sciences. Embodiment research provides support for the clinical importance of nonverbal behaviours. Acolin's chapter builds upon research addressing the mind and body to propose a multi-dimensional model of health and illness as the foundation for a clinical theory of embodiment. The model's dimensions are Decision (Mind versus Body), Identity (Object versus Subject), and Focus (Internal versus External); the logic is to reach a balance and flexibility between the poles of each dimension. To illustrate the model, Acolin demonstrates its application to clinical treatment and discusses directions for further research.

Johannes Michalak, **Naomi Lyons** and **Thomas Heidenreich**, all from Germany, authored Chapter 4 called 'The evidence for basic assumptions of dance movement therapy and body psychotherapy related to findings from embodiment research'. Embodiment research as related to DMP and BP with reference to depressive disorders is presented in this chapter. Depression has a particular importance for the healthcare system as it is a mental disorder occurring in 4.4 per cent of the world's population, and accounting for the largest share in global disability and suicide deaths (World Health Organization, 2017). In contrast to the flourishing literature on brain mechanisms in depression, empirical research on the embodiment of depression is still relatively sparse. BP and DMP literature mostly presents qualitative descriptions of body posture and movement. At the same time, some indirect evidence for the significance of the body in depression comes from studies on processing emotional material in non-clinical populations. These studies have shown that the processing of emotionally negative and positive material can be influenced by bodily manipulations. The authors' conclusion is that the body is highly relevant in mindfulness-based treatment approaches, but that future research is needed in this field to understand the role of the movement, dance and body in depression.

Finally, to close this section **Jennifer Tantia**, a somatic psychotherapist and dance/movement therapist from the USA, writes on 'Having a body and moving your body: Distinguishing somatic psychotherapy from dance/movement therapy' in Chapter 5. She points out that embodied psychotherapy practices honour the cultivation of corporeal awareness as an integral part of emotional health. Somatic psychotherapy (or body psychotherapy) and dance/movement therapy (or dance movement psychotherapy) both focus on awareness and integration of embodied experience in the psychotherapeutic process, and, although seemingly interchangeable, distinct essential characteristics separate the two. This chapter builds on the original critical analysis (Tantia, 2016) that focuses on their similarities, and in this chapter, she explains the differences between them in terms of how each discipline attends to embodied experience through the lens of having a body (somatic psychotherapy) and moving one's body (dance/movement therapy), as well as their independent contributions to the larger field of psychotherapy.

References

Freud, S. (1955). *The Ego and the Id* (*Standard Edition of the Complete Psychological Works of Sigmund Freud*, Vol. 19). London: Hogarth. (Original work published 1923)

Gallagher, S. (2008). Direct perception in the intersubjective context. *Consciousness and Cognition, 17*(2), 535–543.

Gallagher, S., and Hutto, D. (2008). Understanding others through primary interaction and narrative practice. In J. Zlatev, T. Racine, C. Sinha, and E. Itkonen (Eds.), *The Shared Mind: Perspectives on Intersubjectivity* (pp. 17–38). Amsterdam: John Benjamins.

Goldstein, J., and Kornfield J. (1987). *Seeking the Heart of Wisdom: The Path of Insight Meditation*. Boston, MA: Shambhala Publications.

Husserl, E. (1973). *Cartesian Meditations*. (D. Cairns, Trans.). The Hague: Martinus Nijhoff. (Original work published 1950)

Hutto, D. D. (2008). *Folk Psychological Narratives: The Sociocultural Basis of Understanding Reasons*. Cambridge, MA: MIT Press.

Kornfield, J. (2000). *After the Ecstasy, the Laundry*. New York: Bantam Books.

Stern, D. N. (1985). *The Interpersonal World of the Infant*. New York: Basic Books.

Tantia, J. (2016). The interface between somatic psychotherapy and dance/movement therapy: A critical analysis. *Body, Movement and Dance in Psychotherapy, 11*(2–3), 181–196.

Thera, N. (1965). *The Heart of Buddhist Meditation*. York Beach, ME: Samuel Weiser.

World Health Organization. (2017). *Depression and Other Common. Mental Disorders: Global Health Estimates*. Geneva: World Health Organization.

1

ESSENTIAL DIMENSIONS
OF BEING A BODY

Maxine Sheets-Johnstone

'[T]he intrinsic motivation to order one's universe is an imperative of mental life. And the infant has the overall capacity to do so, in large part by identifying the invariants (the islands of consistency) that gradually provide organization to experience. In addition to this general motivation and capacity, the infant needs specific capacities to identify the invariants that seem most crucial in specifying a sense of a core self. Let us look closely at the four crucial invariants.'

(Stern, 1985, p. 76)

'The Body is, as Body, filled with the soul through and through. Each movement of the Body is full of soul, the coming and going, the standing and sitting, the walking and dancing, etc. Likewise, so is every human performance, every human production.'

(Husserl, 1989, p. 252)

Introduction

When we look at human life from beginning to end, and indeed look at all animate forms of life from beginning to end, we see movement. Animation is not simply a matter of being alive. It is a matter of movement. Eating, playing, searching, mating, fighting, stretching, crouching, and so on—even holding still—are essentially differentiated forms of animation that are analyzable in terms of differentiated qualitative dynamics. Moreover, animate forms of life are moved to move; that is, they are affectively motivated, most basically, to approach or to avoid. From this perspective, it is not just more reasonable to speak and write of mindful bodies rather than embodied minds, but more accurate. Indeed, evolution is a matter not of minds but of morphologies, specifically, morphologies in motion engaged in synergies of meaningful movement on behalf of their survival. The current attachment to embodiments of all kinds—not just embodied minds, but embodied self, embodied subjectivity, embodied language, even embodied movement (!)—is deflective; it straightaway packages an integral aspect of animate life that warrants proper elucidation. As pointed out elsewhere,

One finds the term 'embodiment' in all its forms to be, on the one hand, a lexical band-aid that covers over a 250-year-old still suppurating wound and, on the other hand, a linguistic implant that plumps up facets of humanness by giving them a body. It removes all thought of animation, i.e., of being a living body, from the scene of discussion and thus passes over recognition of animation as foundational to the discussion itself.

(Sheets-Johnstone, 2010, p. 122; see also, for example,
Sheets-Johnstone, 1999, p. 359/exp. 2nd ed. 2011b, pp. 310–311,
453, 496, 2009, 2011a, 2015)

In what follows, I begin by considering an ontogenetic account of animation, notably that of infant psychiatrist and clinical psychologist Daniel Stern, and a phenomenological account of animation, notably that of Husserl. The two accounts, one empirical, the other phenomenological, are complementary, and as we will see, their complementarity extends to psychoanalytic observations of Jung and to Buddhist observations of ordained monks.

I: Stern's analysis of the core self

Stern's perspicuous delineation of the core self attests to his extensive, keenly observant and meticulously researched studies of infants. The delineation is based in particular on four different kinds of infant self-experience, which Stern discusses in 'The Nature of an Organized Sense of Self', a section of his chapter on 'The Sense of a Core Self: I. Self versus Other' (Stern, 1985, pp. 70–72). The four-fold experiences are in effect the sine qua non of an organized sense of self: they constitute the core self. What is clearly of moment in these experiences—self-agency, self-coherence, self-affectivity, and self-history—is the *dynamic* nature of self. Self is not a thing, not a spatial entity, and certainly not something that needs to be embodied. On the contrary, the self-experiences that Stern describes are quintessentially experiences of a *tactile-kinesthetic/affective body*. More precisely still, they are experiences not simply of a moving body, but a body that is preeminently *affectively moved to move* and that is *volitionally capable of moving or not moving*. In short, though Stern does not describe these self-experiences as such, tactility, kinesthesia and affectivity are clearly at the root of the core self.

The three dynamically felt bodily modalities are differentially evident in the way Stern describes the four kinds of core-self experience. He pinpoints 'self-agency' in terms of volition, that is self-generated action, and in the realization of consequential relationships—'when you shut your eyes it gets dark' (Stern, 1985, p. 71). He pinpoints 'self-coherence' in terms of a non-fragmented wholeness, whether moving or still (ibid.). He pinpoints 'self-affectivity' in terms of 'patterned inner qualities of feeling' (ibid.) that are interwoven with and inform other experiences of self. He pinpoints 'self-history' in terms of a continuing flow of experience from past to present and a sense of 'regularities' therein (ibid.). In short, the core self is unmistakably dynamic in nature and is essentially grounded in the tactile-kinesthetic/affective body. Its dynamic nature becomes all the more unmistakable when Stern goes on to dissociate the sense of a core self from a construct of any kind. He states,

> A crucial term here is 'sense of', as distinct from 'concept of' or 'knowledge of' or 'awareness of' a self or other. The emphasis is on the palpable experiential realities of substance, action, sensation, affect, and time. Sense of self is not a cognitive construct. It is an experiential integration (ibid.).

Though Stern specifies 'substance', 'action', and 'sensation' as 'palpable experiential realities', it is evident from his descriptions that 'The Nature of an Organized Sense of Self' is anchored in a dynamically moving body. A brief vindication of particular word replacements—tactility for substance, movement for action, and dynamics for sensation—can easily draw first on Aristotle's insights into the sense modality of touch. In essence, Aristotle observes that 'without touch it is impossible for an animal to be' (435b17–18). He gives a number of detailed reasons for the existential preeminence of this sense modality, basically and most notably that 'without touch it is impossible to have any other sense' (435a13–14), that 'every body that has soul in it must . . . be capable of touch' (435a14), that 'touch is as it were a mean between all tangible qualities' (435a22–23), and that 'the loss of this one sense alone must bring about the death of an animal' (435b4–5). He explicitly states furthermore that the uniqueness of touch 'explains . . . why excesses of the other sensible objects, i.e., excess of color, sound, and smell, destroys not the animal but only the organs of the sense' (435b8–10) . . . whereas excess in tangible qualities, e.g., heat, cold, or hardness, destroys the animal itself' (435b14–15). We might also note that since living bodies are always in touch with something, the sense modality of touch is readily recognizable experientially and thereby warrants being given its due.

A further living reality of touch, specifically in relation to movement, goes unmentioned in Aristotle's otherwise keen observations. When we bend an elbow or knee, for example, or stoop to pick up an object, one body part touches another body part. The jointed anatomy of many forms of animate life, but particularly of humans whose skin is covered neither with fur nor feathers, makes tactile self-reflexivity in the context of self-movement a natural built-in of everyday movement. While clothes may mute the experience of self-reflexive tactile contact, the pivotal importance of tactile experiences in moving can hardly be denied. When in learning a new skill, for example, one is told to bend more this way or that, or to open one's arms to a further degree, or to bring one's leg further back in preparation for a kick, tactile pressures are in turn increased or decreased and one's movement is in turn spatially altered. The significance of tactile self-reflexivity can be of specific moment in psychotherapeutic contexts in which patient awarenesses may be directed to habitual postures, ones that, for example, may dramatize a constricted sense of self by way of a constricted tactile self-reflexivity, as when a patient's arms are consistently folded across his or her chest, a constricted sense that might be reinforced by tensely rigid folded arms.

As to replacing movement for action and dynamics for sensation, it is obvious that 'action' packages real-life, real-time movement into nameable 'doings' of one kind and another and ignores the distinctive qualitative dynamics of movement in a way not dissimilar from the way in which embodiments package real-life, real-time dimensions of animate being. *Action* packages movement into running, for example, or eating, or hammering, or even turning around or picking up dropped keys. In so doing, it bypasses the fact that in each instance, the movement unfolds a distinctive qualitative dynamic, a qualitative dynamic that can be parsed in terms of its particular spatial, temporal, and energic structure, a parsing that gives insight into the intricate ways in which the movement flows forth dynamically, including how it begins and how it ends. In brief, by simply putting a label on a certain 'doing', the word *action* gives no hint, much less insight, into the qualitative dynamics that constitute the doing and its qualitative nature from beginning to end. In effect, *action* effectively bars awareness of the myriad ways in which a movement can qualitatively flow forth. One can walk hesitantly, for example, quickly, determinedly, lethargically, openly, sneakily, and so on, and so on, and furthermore, in dynamic congruity with such kinetic possibilities, walk joyfully, dejectedly, fearfully, angrily, with wonder, with curiosity, and so on, and so on, being motivated by untold other affective surges.

As for dynamics over sensation, it is—or should be—clearly evident that *the experience* of running, or eating, or hammering, or turning around, or picking up one's keys is not like an itch or a flash of light or a felt shove. A sensation is temporally punctual and spatially pointillist. The experience of running is not a sensation or even a multitude of sensations, but a particular *kinesthetically felt dynamic.* Any time we care to pay attention to it, there it is. Indeed, as neuro-scientist Marc Jeannerod points out, 'There are no reliable methods for suppressing kinesthetic information arising during the execution of a movement" (Jeannerod, 2006, p. 56). "Information" terminology aside, especially in the context not of position or posture but of movement, Jeannerod's declarative finding speaks reams about the foundational ongoing reality and significance of kinesthesia. Moving bodies create and at the same time constitute a kinesthetically felt dynamic.

Stern's specification of the sense of self as the 'experiential integration' of four invariants may be specified phenomenologically as the experientially integrated dimensions of the '*uniquely* singled out' animate organism that is my animate organism (Husserl, 1973, p. 97). There is, in fact, a ready-made correspondence between Stern's account of a core self that distinguishes self from other and Husserl's 'sphere of ownness' that distinguishes what is personal from all that is alien, the word *ownness* having no reference to something *possessed*, but referring in a precisely analogous way to Stern's distinction of self and other.[1]

II: Husserl's analysis of 'my *animate organism*'

Husserl distinguishes five dimensions within the personal sphere: 'fields of sensation', 'I govern', a repertoire of 'I cans', 'self-reflexivity with respect to organs of sense and objects of sense', and 'psychophysical unity' (Husserl, 1973, pp. 97–98). He specifies this personal sphere of experience in terms of a distinctive living phenomenon, namely, an 'animate organism' that is '*uniquely* singled out' within Nature as 'my *animate organism*' (ibid., p. 97).[2] Fields of sensation constitute a 'field of warmth and coldness', a field of light and dark, and so on. 'I govern' is a matter of being the animate organism who '"*rule[s] and govern[s]*" immediately', governing particularly in each of its "organs"', as when '[t]ouching kinesthetically, I perceive "with" my hands'. 'I cans' refer to abilities, for example, 'I can push, thrust, and so forth'. 'Self-reflexivity' means that '*I* experience (or can experience) all of Nature, including my own animate organism, which therefore in the process is reflexively related to itself. That becomes possible because I can perceive one hand 'by means of the other'. 'Psychophysical unity' describes the unity of animate organism and psyche or 'personal Ego' which anchors the living reality of self and world (ibid., p. 97).[3] Though recognized and specified from a different perspective, this anchoring personal ego might be seen as fleshing out Freud's observation: 'The ego is first and foremost a bodily ego' (Freud, 1955, p. 26).

Experiential specifications of Husserl coincide with those of Stern regardless of their difference in naming. Agency and 'I govern', for example, home in on the same self-experience, as do agency and 'I cans'. Self-coherence and self-reflexivity are inherently related in that a non-fragmented wholeness underlies the reality of both. While Stern's 'inner qualities of feeling' (p. 71) and temporal flow go unmentioned in Husserl's specifications, they are prominent elsewhere in Husserl's writings, 'inner qualities of feeling' in his consistent references to 'affect and action' (Husserl, 1989, 2001), temporal flow in his painstaking elucidations of transcendental subjectivity and internal time consciousness (Husserl, 1964, 1970, 1977). What is furthermore of foundational significance is that each of Husserl's five dimensions originates in tactile-kinesthetic/affective experience, precisely as does Stern's (1985) core self. We can see this even more closely in terms of Stern's affirmation that 'In order for the infant to have any formed sense of self, there must ultimately be some organization that is sensed as a reference point. *The first such organization concerns the body*: its coherence, its actions, its inner feeling states, and the memory of all these' (Stern, 1985, p. 46; italics added). With respect to this 'first such bodily organization', a repertoire of 'I cans' corresponds to 'coherence' as well as 'actions' the former insofar as Husserl recognizes a build-up of abilities, a history of learning on the basis of experience, precisely as in his seminal observation, '*I move precedes I do and I can*' (Husserl, 1989; italics added). The affective/tactile-kinesthetic body is indeed foundational throughout insofar as 'actions' are propelled by felt dispositions, urges, motivations, and the like, and are themselves experienced kinesthetically and tactilely, the latter as in kicking, when the knee flexes and the back of the lower leg touches the back of the thigh. Notable too is the fact that 'psychophysical unity' corresponds to all four dimensions of the core self that is similarly, the locus of meaningful actions, of intentionalities that consistently play off my movings and doings, comings and goings, hesitancies and rushings, curiosities and wonderings, and more. In sum, the five characteristics that Husserl says '[bring] to light my animate organism', bring to light, and in the most foundational sense, my tactile-kinesthetic/affective body, precisely as do Stern's dimensions of the core self. Clearly, when we juxtapose Husserl's specification of self-experience that differentiates what is strictly personal from what is alien or other, hence experience akin to what Stern describes as 'sense of self' as distinct from sense of other, we find basic animate complementarities.

III: Jungian and Buddhist perspectives on the self

Stern's core self and Husserl's '*uniquely* singled out animate organism' have an affinity with Jung's analysis of symbols of self and his perspective on the intimate relationship of psyche and matter. Jung states 'Since psyche and matter are contained in one and the same world, and moreover are in continuous contact with one another and ultimately rest on irrepresentable, transcendental factors, it is not only possible but fairly probable, even, that psyche and matter are two different aspects of one and the same thing' (Jung, 1969, p. 125). While Jung's analysis and perspective have a broader scope—they are not concerned with basic aspects of the self but with psychoanalytic factors with respect to the self—they remain firmly anchored in the body and reverberate in living realities of being a body. With respect to symbols of self, Jung writes,

> The symbols of the self arise in the depths of the body and they express its materiality every bit as much as the structure of the perceiving consciousness. The symbol is thus a living body, *corpus et anima*. The deeper 'layers' of the psyche lose their individual uniqueness as they retreat farther and farther into darkness. 'Lower down', that is to say as they approach the autonomous functional systems, they become increasingly collective until they are universalized and extinguished in the body's materiality, i.e., in chemical substances. The body's carbon is simply carbon. Hence 'at bottom' the psyche is simply 'world' . . . The more archaic and 'deeper', that is the more *physiological*, the symbol is, the more collective and universal, the more 'material' it is. The more abstract, differentiated, and specific it is, the more its nature approximates to conscious uniqueness and individuality, the more it sloughs off its universal character.
>
> *(Jung, 1968b, 2nd ed., p. 173)*

Symbols of self are thus clearly not a construct but an expression of living bodies, an expression that at its deepest level is a reflection of a common humanity: the symbol, in Jung's terms, is an archetypal image. Of particular significance are Jung's probing comments on the relationship of archetype to instinct. He writes, for example, 'The fact that all the psychic processes accessible to our observation and experience are somehow bound to an organic substrate indicates that they are articulated with the life of the organism as a whole and therefore partake of its dynamism, in other words, they must have a share in its instincts or be in a certain sense the results of the action of those instincts' (Jung, 1969, p. 90). At a later point, he reflects, 'It is very probable that the archetypes, as instincts, possess a specific energy which cannot be taken away from them in the long run' (ibid., p. 129, note 124). Such an energy relationship is part and parcel of the inherent relationship, that is, the natural conjunction of psyche and matter.

That the natural conjunction of psyche and matter in the living world leads Jung to consider them as being of a piece, a singular piece, is significant in that his perspective runs counter to the common Cartesian distinction of mind and body as two absolutely different 'substances', a distinction that indeed runs counter to the evolution of animate forms of life. Animate forms of life move, and in different ways and to different degrees, are aware of their own movement. Jung does not develop his perspective in this direction, but it is surely evident that *kinesthesia* plays a central, even pivotal role in the natural conjunction of psyche and matter as does its forerunner *proprioception* in the form of an awareness of deformations and stress.[4]

Jung's comments about emotion also tie in with Stern's 'inner qualities of feeling'. With respect to archetypes, he comments, 'It would be an unpardonable sin of omission were one to overlook the *feeling-value* of the archetype. This is extremely important both theoretically and therapeutically' (Jung, 1969, p. 119). He goes on to give an example of natives he met in equatorial east Africa whose morning movement ritual at sunrise was not explicitly understood by them, that is, whose meaning they could not explicitly state, but whose meaning Jung relates to Westerners' Christmas tree ritual: 'The behaviour of the Elgonyi certainly strikes us as exceedingly primitive, but we forget that the educated Westerner behaves no differently. What the meaning of the Christmas-tree might be our forefathers knew even less than ourselves, and it is only quite recently that we have bothered to find out at all' (ibid., pp. 119–120).[5]

Jung's keen observation about the nature of emotions is of further significance with respect to the spontaneity of 'inner qualities of feeling'. Jung points out that emotion 'is not an activity of the individual but something that happens to him' (Jung, 1968a, 2nd ed., pp. 8–9). He does not analyse the nature of that happening, but it is surely of moment to ask, 'what is the nature of that happening?' Careful phenomenological analysis shows that the happening is clearly a bodily happening, a dynamic happening that is qualitatively distinct in the way that it moves through the body and moves the individual to move, or to stay still. The answer is significant in light of common talk about emotions as *states* of being. The further one moves from the body, whether on psychotherapeutic grounds or in a quest to understand the nature of human life, the further one moves from real-life, real-time human experience. Liabilities ensue, including the liability of focusing exclusive attention on the brain (the elevated human one, of course) in the absence of a whole-body nervous system. In many instances, including high profile ones, experiential ascriptions are made to brains. Thus we read, 'If you see the back of a person's head, the brain infers that there is a face on the front of it' (Crick and Koch, 1992, p. 153); 'In my view, emotional feelings represent only one category of affects that brains experience' (Panksepp, 2005, p. 162); 'An object's image varies with distance, yet the brain can ascertain its true size' (Zeki, 1992, p. 69). A much older ascription is significant in succinctly epitomizing the liabilities of living in a brain-tethered world: 'Nonhuman animals have brains capable of cooperative hunting' (Harding, 1975, p. 255), as if brains are out there hunting in concert on the savannah.[6]

Vipassana Buddhist teachings warrant attention in this context of recognizing the dynamics of bodily life and being true to the truths of experience. As Buddhist monk and clinical psychologist Jack Kornfield observes, 'When we listen to our bodies, our bodily wisdom grows. We can feel the body's urge to move and honor its cycles of rest, we can meditate and dance, we can respect its need for solitude, we can allow its lively senses, and we can know its pleasures and limitations. 'Instead of fearing our body, its losses and strange vulnerability, we honor it' (Kornfield, 2000, p. 188). Joseph Goldstein points out, 'While it is true that there is no enduring entity, no unchanging self that can be called "I," it is also quite obvious that each of us is a uniquely changing and recognizable pattern of elements' (Goldstein and Kornfield, 1987, p. 112). In particular, when we cultivate certain feelings, they grow stronger and thus easily arise again. As Goldstein comments, 'We tend not to pay attention to this conditioning factor of our experience, thinking instead that once an experience has passed it is gone without reside or result. That would be like dropping a stone in water without creating any ripples' (ibid.). His experiential insights accord with Stern's 'experiential integration' and Husserl's 'personal sphere'. Though not specified in such terms, it is clear that the changing 'pattern of elements' (the flux of experience) are anchored in the fact that being a body is a dynamic whole-life developmental reality, an ontogeny that spans the whole of life. Such anchorage in movement and change coincides with Aristotle's perspicuous observation that 'Nature is a principle of motion and change. We must therefore see that we understand what motion is; for if it were unknown, nature too would be unknown' (200b12–14). It coincides further with Husserl's perspicuous observation that 'consciousness of the world . . . is in constant motion' (Husserl, 1970). The anchorage thus also makes evident questionable if not deflective and even false concepts and formulations of self, notably, the concept of self as 'embodied' (e.g., Gallagher, 2005; Gallagher and Zahavi, 2012), the concept of self-tethered to ownership (Gallagher and Zahavi, 2012; Zahavi, 1999), and the concept of self as a basically spatial entity whose solidity precludes bona fide recognition of the dynamics of movement and affectivity and the realities of ontogenetic temporal change (ibid.).

Conclusion

In sum, living realities of being a body are integral to veridical conceptions of self, conceptions that are true to the truths of experience. Because they specify essential dimensions of being a body and illuminate these dimensions in first-person experience, they are essential aspects of psychotherapeutic practices that are rooted not in language but in movement. Movement indeed forms the 'I' that moves before the 'I' that moves forms movement, which is to say that movement is our mother tongue. That existential reality resonates with Jung's therapeutic advice: '[L]earn your theories as well as you can but put them aside when you touch the miracle of the living soul' (Jung, 1999, p. 22). The living soul is a Body. As Husserl affirms, 'The Body is, as Body, filled with the soul through and through. Each movement of the Body is full of soul, the coming and going, the standing and sitting, the walking and dancing'. Moreover, as Kornfield (2000) affirms, the living soul is a source of wisdom: 'When we listen to our bodies, our bodily wisdom grows' (ibid., p. 188). Clearly, the living soul is anchored in the tactile-kinesthetic/affective body and is thus a matter of movement and of feelings that move the body to move. Bodily wisdom, in effect, grows in listening to kinesthesia and affectivity.

Notes

1 It is of critical importance to emphasize that Husserl's sphere of ownness refers not to possession but to a foundational 'hereness'. Husserl wrote of the 'zero point of orientation' as an always present bodily hereness in relation to a thereness. In what follows, I consider the 'zero point' *tout court*, namely, an always present bodily hereness, what might be termed *an existential hereness*. Though one might relate this always present bodily hereness to a self and go on from there to speak of self-reference or self-affection, such terms would mislead us: they make an ontological entity, a self, out of a construct. The construct is largely linguistic, even an outgrowth of the linguistic practice of 'referring' to 'oneself', 'myself', 'yourself', 'our-selves', 'themselves', 'herself', 'himself'. What this common practice implicitly claims is not just a 'self', but a self that is 'mine', or 'yours', and so on, in short, a self that is 'owned' by someone. Ownership is thus a built-in of linguistic selves. When we compare this ontological-linguistic entity with infant psychiatrist

and clinical psychologist Daniel Stern's closely detailed account of the 'core self', we not only appreciate its falseness, but are led to a highly instructive developmental 'sense of self'.

2 See note #1 above regarding hereness as opposed to possession.

3 Being only briefly identified, the characteristics are incompletely analyzed, both in themselves and, most importantly as a composite whole. Although one may certainly find references to, and fuller discussions of each of the characteristics in other Husserlian texts, they are not fleshed in the present context as the integrally-related structural units of wholly personal experience that Husserl identifies them to be. Indeed, Husserl explicitly states with respect to the intentionalities of self-constitution that 'admittedly we have not investigated them in these meditations. They belong to a distinct stratum and are the theme of vast investigations into which we did not and could not enter' (Husserl, 1973, p. 110; for a further discussion, see Sheets-Johnstone, 1999, p. 99).

4 'Sense organs capable of registering continuously deformation (changes in length) and stress (tensions, decompressions) in the body, which can arise from the animal's own movements or may be due to its weight or other external mechanical forces' (Lissman, 1950, p. 35; quoted in Mill, 1976, p. xvi). In a word, proprioceptive sensitivity is *continuous*. Not only is a creature's surface in contact continuously with other surfaces in the environment, whether it is moving or whether it is still, but its own conformations continuously change in the course of moving.

5 Jung proceeds to point out that 'The archetype is pure, unvitiated nature, and it is nature that causes man to utter words and perform actions whose meaning is unconscious to him, so unconscious that he no longer gives it a thought' (1969, p. 120).

6 Perhaps the most outlandish if not egregious of all is a Teaching Company advertisement on behalf of a course taught by a neuroscientist. The course, titled 'How Your Brain Works', is described as follows: 'Everything you hear, feel, see, and think is controlled by your brain. It allows you to cope masterfully with your everyday environment and is capable of producing breathtaking athletic feats, sublime works of art, and profound scientific insights. But its most amazing achievement may be that it can understand itself' (Teaching Company, 2014, p. 3).

References

Crick, F. and Koch, C. (1992). 'The problem of consciousness'. *Scientific American*, 267(3), 153–159.

Freud, S. (1955). *The Ego and the Id* (*Standard Edition of the Complete Psychological Works of Sigmund Freud*, Vol. 19). London: Hogarth. (Original work published 1923)

Gallagher, S. (2005). *How the body shapes the mind*. Oxford: Clarendon Press/Oxford University Press.

Gallagher, S. and Zahavi, D. (2012). *The phenomenological mind* (2nd ed.). London: Routledge.

Goldstein, J. and Kornfield, J. (1987). *Seeking the heart of wisdom*. Boston: Shambhala.

Harding, Robert S. O. (1975). 'Meat-eating and hunting in baboons'. In R. Tuttle (ed.) *Socioecology and psychology of primates* (pp. 245–257). The Hague: Mouton Publishers.

Husserl, E. (1964). *The phenomenology of internal time-consciousness* (J. S. Churchill, Trans. and M. Heidegger, ed.). Bloomington: Indiana University Press.

Husserl, E. (1970). *The crisis of European sciences and transcendental phenomenology* (D. Carr, Trans.). Evanston: Northwestern University Press.

Husserl, E. (1973). *Cartesian meditations* (D. Cairns, Trans.). The Hague: Martinus Nijhoff. (Original work published 1950)

Husserl, E. (1977). *Phenomenological psychology* (J. Scanlon, Trans.). The Hague: Martinus Nijhoff.

Husserl, E. (1989). *Ideas pertaining to a pure phenomenology and to a phenomenological philosophy, Ideas II* (R. Rojcewicz and A. Schuwer, Trans.). Dordrecht: Kluwer Academic. (Original work published 1952)

Husserl, E. (2001). *Analyses concerning passive and active synthesis* (A. Steinbock, Trans.). Dordrecht: Kluwer Academic. (Original work published 1920)

Jeannerod, M. (2006). *Motor cognition: What actions tell the self*. Oxford: Oxford University Press.

Jung, C. G. (1968a). *Aion: Researches into the phenomenology of the self* (R. F. C. Hull, Trans.). Princeton: Princeton University Press.

Jung, C. G. (1968b). *The archetypes and the collective unconscious* (R. F. C. Hull, Trans.). Princeton: Princeton University Press.

Jung, C. G. (1969). *On the nature of the psyche* (R. F. C. Hull, Trans.). Princeton: Princeton University Press.

Jung, C. G. (1999). Contributions to analytical psychology. *Self and Society*, 27(1), 22.

Kornfield, J. (2000). *After the ecstasy, the laundry*. New York: Bantam Books.

Lissman, H. W. (1950). Proprioceptors. In *Physiological mechanisms in animal behaviour (Symposia of the Society for Experimental Biology)* (Vol. 4, pp. 34–59). New York: Academic Press.

Mill, P. J. (ed.). (1976). *Structure and function of proprioceptors in the invertebrates.* London: Chapman and Hall.

Panksepp, J. (2005). On the embodied nature of core emotional affects. *Journal of Consciousness Studies*, 12 (8–10) (Special Issue on Emotion Experience, ed. Giovanna Colmbetti & Evan Thompson), pp. 158–184.

Teaching Company (2014). Advertisement. *Science News.*

Sheets-Johnstone, M. (1999). Rethinking Husserl's fifth meditation. *Philosophy Today* (Suppl.), 45, 99–106.

Sheets-Johnstone, M. (2009). Animation: The fundamental, properly descriptive, and essential concept. *Continental Philosophy Review*, 42, 375–400.

Sheets-Johnstone, M. (2010). Kinesthetic experience: Understanding movement inside and out. *Body, Movement and Dance in Psychotherapy*, 5(2), 111–127.

Sheets-Johnstone, M. (2011a). *Embodied minds or mindful bodies? A question of fundamental, inherently related aspects of animation.* Guest Lecture in conjunction with Alumni Achievement Award, School of Education, Department of Dance, University of Wisconsin, Madison, 29 April 2011. [Published in *Subjectivity* (December 2011), vol. 4/4, 451–496.]

Sheets-Johnstone, M. (2011b). *The primacy of movement* (2nd ed.). Amsterdam/Philadelphia: John Benjamins. (Original work published 1999)

Sheets-Johnstone, M. (2015). Embodiment on trial. *Continental Philosophy Review*, 48(1), 23–39.

Stern, D. N. (1985). *The interpersonal world of the infant.* New York: Basic Books.

Zahavi, D. (1999). *Self-awareness and alterity: A phenomenological investigation.* Evanston, IL: Northwestern University Press.

Zeki, S. (1992). The visual image in mind and brain. *Scientific American*, 267(3): 69–76.

2

NARRATIVES IN EMBODIED THERAPEUTIC PRACTICE

Getting the story straight

Shaun Gallagher and Daniel D. Hutto

Introduction

In discussions of narrative practices and the narrative self, the concept of narrative itself often goes undefined. When one looks for a working definition of narrative, one encounters a multiplicity of definitions, some of which push the concept of narrative or narrative structure widely to include non-linguistic expression or proto-narrative performances. Thus, for example, Jerome Bruner writes: 'Narrative structure is even inherent in the praxis of social interaction before it achieves linguistic expression' (1990, p. 77; also see e.g., Halliday, 1978).

Along this line, the concept of 'body narrative', not in the sense of a narrative about a body (as in e.g., Charon, 2006; Ling and Liu, 2008; Scholz, 2000) but in the sense of the body generating narrative through its movement, can be found in discussions of body psychotherapy (BP). Christine Caldwell (2014), for example, defines such narratives as 'nonverbal narratives . . . the body telling its stories on its own nonlinear and nonverbal terms' (p. 89). She explains, 'conscious body movements generate a fluid, nonverbal narration of self and identity no less important than the verbal stories we may tell' (ibid.). There are two ways that one might understand the concept of a body narrative in this context.

First, body and dance movement psychotherapists often employ techniques that call for the patient to enact a narrative through bodily movement or dance. In this way the patient tells a story by engaging in movement, similar to the way a mime would be telling a story (in a conscious, somewhat reflective way), or the way a dancer might enact a particular story through expressive movement. On this understanding, bodily movement tells a story, or as Caldwell puts it, the body tells a story 'on its own terms, through expressive movement'. Citing Koch, Holland, Hengstler and van Knippenberg (2009), Caldwell (2017, pp. 61–62) indicates that, 'the deliberateness of sensorimotor processing as well as the commitment to the emotional and relational accuracy of movement can restore this feeling of self-authorship'.

A second way to think of body narrative is to think that the body 'on its own terms' tells a story that is already embedded in its way of moving, and that a narrative structure is inherent in its movement.[1]

For example, Richard Erskine (2014, p. 25), in his psychotherapeutic practice, 'focuses on the body and the unconscious stories requiring resolution'. He understands the body as keeping 'unconscious "score" of emotional and physiological memories' (ibid., p. 22), and as storing experiences of a pre-symbolic, implicit, and relational kind – that have never been narrated by conventional means but for which there is, nevertheless, 'an emotionally laden story waiting to be told' (ibid., p. 22). BP, on Erskine's view, provides the means and methods of bringing to light the 'emotion filled story embedded in the body' (ibid., p. 25). Thus, he says of his clients:

> They say they have no memories of being younger than ten or twelve years of age yet they describe having anxiety attacks, bouts of depression or loneliness, digestive prob-lems, back aches, or like me, the tensions in their shoulders and neck. Each of these emotional and physical symptoms may be the memories – often the only memories – of despairing loss, neglect, or traumatic events. These significant memories are expressed in our affect and through our bodily movements and gestures.
>
> *(Erskine, 2014, p. 22)*

Much of this story about body narratives, however, remains undeveloped. For example, it is not always clear from such accounts how movement produces meaning, how the intersubjective context of therapist and patient contributes to this productive performance, and what principles guide the interpretation process within the therapeutic setting.

In the following we are concerned about this second way of understanding the notion of body narrative. Specifically, we argue against the idea that bodily movement constitutes a nar-rative or has an inherent narrative structure. One issue concerns how the structure of bodily movement relates to linguistic narrative. One might think that bodily expression reinforces or supplements linguistic narratives in the way that gestures supplement (add new meaning to) verbal language (McNeill, 2008). Thus, Rucinska and Reijmers (2014, p. 39) suggest that in play therapy,

> the action of playing [. . .] counters the tendency to focus exclusively on the meanings of words and narratives, text and discourse. Instead, playing adds and reinforces the narratives, allowing new perceptions and meanings to be created through the use of objects and interaction with the therapist. That is because playing should allow mutual creation of meanings to a greater extent than mere speaking as it incorporates non-verbal communication, and so, has more degrees of freedom in how to interpret it. When therapist and client play with objects, words, [verbal] narratives, text and discourse are less important as the playing takes over their role. The meanings get 'offloaded' to the objects one is playing with, and through staying in the play discourse, a new dimension to narrating the problems emerges.

This is a view than can be easily endorsed, especially the important point that the meaning emerges through the intersubjective interaction of client and therapist. But on this view bodily movement and expression have a different structure to narrative, and this is precisely what allows it to add to meaning, and to motivate new dimensions to be explored by narrative.

To make some progress on these issues and on understanding the therapeutic relevance of both bodily movement and narrative, we will consider definitions of narrative, and specifically the relation between the structure of bodily movement and narrative structure, from three dif-ferent disciplinary perspectives – developmental psychology, embodied and enactive cognitive science, and semiotics. We will argue that although embodied activity is structured in a way that naturally lends itself to narration, and that it is no accident that our most faithful narratives about such activity should replicate or reflect that structure, the structure of embodied activity itself is not essentially or already narrative in nature. Moreover, the existence of a structure in embodied activity that is ripe for narration falls short of what is needed for securing the idea that bodies *actually* tell their own stories. Finally, we propose an alternative way of understanding what goes on in such therapy, replacing the notion of body narratives with the concept of structured, embodied activity – activity that is ripe for, and benefits from, narration in therapeutic contexts.

Ontogenesis, movement and meaning

Some developmental psychologists contend that embodied narratives are part of our lives from very early on and are even implicit in neonatal movement. If this were true it would lend support to the idea that embodied activity has its own inherent narrative structure. Delafield-Butt and Trevarthen (2015), for example, look for the origins of narrative and find them in 'the innate sensorimotor intelligence of a hypermobile human body' (p. 1). The kind of movement from which narrative originates, they argue, can be traced to the intentional (planned) movements of the prenatal (midterm) fetus. This kind of movement is continuous with postnatal, structured movement in which we can identify distal goals and social meaning. Such movements are further shaped in 'early proto-conversations and collaborative play of infants and talk of children and adults' (p. 1). The structure in such processes, they propose, is fourfold, and temporal, involving introduction, development, climax and resolution (Figure 2.1). Accordingly, the serial 'organization of single, non-verbal actions into complex projects of expressive and explorative sense-making become conventional meanings and explanations with propositional narrative power' (p. 1).

As Delafield-Butt and Trevarthen (2015) suggest, this kind of structured movement shares the same 'vitality dynamics' of play in infancy (Stern, 2010, *passim*) involving bodily arousal and points of focused intensity (Trevarthen and Delafield-Butt, 2013), reflected also in heart rate, respiration rate, affective responses and expressive movements to convey felt meaning. 'Within these dynamic emotional events, relations between objects and participants, their properties, motivation and character, can become placed and named in 'artificial', learned and conventional language' (Delafield-Butt and Trevarthen, 2015, p. 2). These dynamics, at least at first and importantly, are embedded in intersubjective interactions, and only in such contexts can we speak of meaningful engagement – a meaning that emerges in the interaction itself (De Jaegher, Di Paolo and Gallagher, 2010).

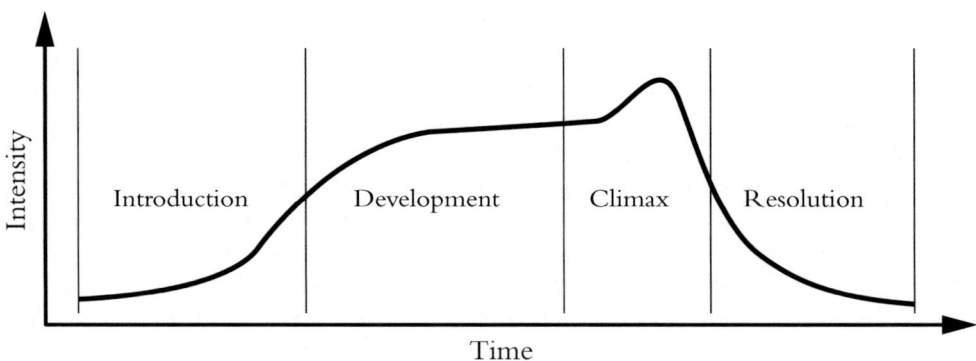

Figure 2.1 Intensity contour of impulses to move in a pattern over four phases

A good example of this can be found in the emergence of pointing behaviour in the nine-month-old infant. If we follow Vygotsky's (1986) analysis, a spontaneous reaching movement by the infant for an object not within reach becomes an expressive movement of pointing only if a caregiver is present to interpret it as such. The reach begins as instrumental, but in the presence of the other it becomes expressive, and this is reinforced for the infant by the action of the caregiver, who moves the object to within reach, or gives the object to the infant. Through ongoing practice and repetition, the infant's reach takes on the interpreted meaning – pointing for a desired object – for the infant herself. A kind of meaning emerges from movement, a movement that forms an instrumental action with a goal, and, perceived as such in the intersubjective context, becomes a request for help. This expressive action can be the beginning of a set of interactions of infants and caregivers that develops beyond any instrumental goal into the structure of, for example, a playful interaction. One can easily put such events into a verbal narrative – 'The baby really enjoyed playing with that toy; she let me know when she wanted to play with it; but after a while she threw it to the ground and was done with it'. Thus, Delafield-Butt and Trevarthen propose, emergence into verbal form is helped along by 'the collaborative narratives of sound and gesture in pre-verbal proto-conversations' (2015, p. 2).

Why think that the structure of movement or action is narrative in nature? Arguably because a similar four-fold structure is found in semiotic accounts of narrative, which identify the four stages as: contract; competence; performance and sanction. These stages are taken to constitute the canonical structure of all narratives in semiotics (Greimas, 1970; Martin and Ringham, 2000, pp. 31–32; Paolucci, 2016).

We think the order of things is important, however. First, developmental studies show that we learn to form linguistic narratives through interactions with others – specifically when caregivers elicit accounts of just-past actions or events and when, as young children around two or three years, we appropriate the narratives of others for our own stories (Bruner, 1996; Legerstee, 2005; Nelson, 2003b; Reddy, 2008, 2012; Trevarthen, 2013). Second, the contours of our narratives are shaped by the structures of the actions and events they recount. Primarily, we narrate our actions and the actions of others. If we think that narrative not only reflects on action, but that it is generated out of action, then it seems possible to say that *narrative derives its structure from action*. Actions take time to unfold; they have a beginning, they develop, they accomplish a goal, and they conclude. That is a structure that narratives must reflect if they are going to capture what Bruner (1990) calls the landscape of action. We note, however, that this does not mean that actions have a narrative structure; we propose that the derivation goes the other way.

Narrative may start to emerge from pretend play, typically when engaging with others, where the creation of such narratives is 'accompanied by – rather than [achieved] solely through – language' (Nelson, 2003a, p. 28). In early pretend play, the language that goes along with the play process is not narrative itself but is performative vocalization. The mother takes the toy car moving it in a forward action and says 'Zoom, zoom, zoom'. She is not providing a narrative about the car, she is pretending to play with the car. The child then takes a turn. The vocalization, and gradually the words, become part of the narrative structure that captures the pretend action. The mother says, 'The car goes zoom'. She is now on the way to giving a narrative about the car. Later she says, addressing the child, 'You played so nicely with the car this afternoon, didn't you?' The mother is leading the child into a kind of narrative. Later the child says, 'I play with car'. The child is beginning to narrate his action. Even without the proto-conversation, intentional, goal-directed actions have structure. They exhibit 'initiation toward the goal, progression with fast rhythmic timing of corrective maneuvers keeping the movement on track, and final climactic contact with its object, as a unit of meaning-making that tests and confirms a knowledge of expectations' (Delafield-Butt and Trevarthen, 2015, p. 3).

Narrative comes to reflect that structure of action as it represents the action. In this sense, narrative structure derives from action structure.

Narrating action

Richard Menary (2008) cautions against taking narratives as abstract processes disconnected from embodied experience. He cites Kerby (1993) and Hutto (2006) who describe embodied experiences as reflecting a pre-narrative or narrative-ready quality. While Menary acknowledges the importance of narratives and draws a connecting line between the actions of embodied agents and the narratives that depict them, he also insists on drawing another, orthogonal line that demarcates pre-narrative embodied activity from the domain of the properly narrative. This demarcation reflects the difference between two senses of self – one as an embodied experiencer that acts in the world and another sense of self as endowed with narrative capacities, able to reflect on and give an account of his or her own actions, and the actions of others. Menary's worry is that we make narrative do too much work, if we think that narratives in some sense structure our actions. In this respect, however, he is resisting the idea that in every case our intentional significant actions are reflectively guided by our narrative conception of who we are, as proposed by Velleman (2006), Mackenzie (2007) and others. On this view, '[n]arratives do not simply report sequences of events or actions. By explaining the causal connections between the events or actions they recount, they give shape and coherence to our lives, or at least to the various sequences that make up our lives . . .' (Mackenzie, 2007, pp. 268–269). Menary wants to safeguard the idea that most of our actions remain pre-reflective skillful accomplishments that do not require reflective guidance. In this respect, he wants to resist reading narrative structure back into pre-narrative action. Our actions are not necessarily or primarily transcribed by narrative.

Menary also rejects the idea that our actions are implicitly structured by narrative, an idea he attributes to Marya Schechtman (1996, 2011). This is the idea that narratives that reflect norms and customs, as well as personal experiences, start to inform our behavior without our being aware of it. Narratives in some sense would implicitly impose structure on actions, bestowing coherency and meaning where there was none. In contrast, for Menary, pre-narrative actions are neither incoherent nor meaningless to begin with, and do not require the imposition of narrative structure to make them coherent and meaningful.

Strawson (2004) too worries about the claim that all of our structured actions have a narrative character. He holds that the narrativist view becomes trivially true – as a kind of unhelpful and uninformative stipulation – if it is held, for example, that 'making coffee is a Narrative that involves Narrativity, because you have to think ahead, do things in the right order' (Strawson, 2004, p. 439). In holding that our actions are not inherently or primarily narrative in character, Menary (2008) avoids Strawson's charge of triviality.

Menary's conception of the embodied, acting self is consistent with the idea that narrative can repeat or replicate the structure of action. 'Our embodied experiences are ready to be exploited in a narrative of those experiences. Narrative arises from a sequence of bodily experiences, perceptions and actions in a quite natural manner' (Menary, 2008, p. 75). He cites Mark Slors' (1998) idea that movement is narratable because of its sequential structure, perceived by the agent as he is engaged in action. Narrative is anchored in this pre-narrative (pre-reflective, non-representational) structure. 'Narratives arise directly from the lived experience of the embodied subject and these narratives can be embellished and reflected upon if we need to find a meaningful form or structure in that sequence of experiences' (Menary, 2008, p. 76).

Thus, Menary's view offers guidance on where to draw lines between actions and narratives, and how to read the developmental accounts: 'It is not narratives that shape experiences [or actions] but, rather, experiences [or actions] that structure narratives. Experiences [and actions] are the sequence of events that give structure and content to narratives . . . the temporal ordering, the structure is already there in our lived, bodily experience' (Menary, 2008, p. 79).

Narratologists, also, have been much concerned with trying to define what narratives are, and to give: '. . . a principled account of what makes a text, discourse, film or other artifact a narrative. Such an account would help clarify what distinguishes a narrative from an exchange of greetings, a recipe for salad dressing, or a railway timetable' (Herman, 2007, p. 4; see Cobley, 2014; Ryan, 2007).

Minimally, narratives are taken to be complex representations that describe or depict a particular series of events or happenings – happenings that are meaningfully related over time in ways that cannot be captured in purely logical or formal terms (see Lamarque, 2004, p. 394). Gregory Currie (2010) offers a conservative proposal for distinguishing narratives from other kinds of artifact; he holds that narratives do not occur just anywhere in nature. Rather narratives are a special kind of representational artifact. They are products of a particular kind of labour: 'story-makers make stories' (Currie, 2010, p. 3). In a similar vein, Cobley (2014, pp. 2–8) also understands narratives to be essentially representational creations – creations that involve the selective arrangement and ordering of discursive signs of some sort.

The advantage of conceiving of narratives as representational artifacts with specific storytelling functions is that it wards off any concern that the notion of narrative is so loose that narratives wind up being found simply everywhere. To hold the latter view is to endorse pan-narrativism; that is, the idea that all things – the world in-itself, human lives – are, at root, narrative in nature. Pan-narrativism arguably stretches the concept of narrative so widely and elastically as to make it trivial or vacuous; it would include any and all activities or performances, and indeed all happenings of any sort. Holding that narratives are representational artifacts produced for special communicative functions provides a ready-made prophylactic that protects against an unattractive pan-narrativism.

Peter Goldie offered a more liberal view of narratives. Goldie's account does not insist that all narratives are artifacts or that they must have an essentially communicative function. Instead he maintains that, 'a narrative or story is something that can be told or narrated or *just thought through in narrative thinking*' (2012, p. 2). Elaborating on the idea of narrative thinking he tells us that it 'involves not text or discourse, but another kind of representation: thought' (p. 3). Goldie's (2012) view, although less restrictive, is not so lax as to be at risk of pan-narrativism. Thus, for Goldie (2012, p. 6), it is always the case that, 'a narrative is distinct from what it is a narrative of'. He thereby respects the distinction between 'representation and what is represented' (2012, p. 4), and draws a clear line between narratives and what they narrate.

Goldie does insist that narratives are always and everywhere representational. It is not the case, however, that representational thought features in most of what we do and experience. Specifically, most of our structured actions do not require representational (or narrative) content (Chemero, 2011; Gallagher, 2017; Hutto and Myin, 2017; Thompson, 2007). Consequently, if bodily activities and movements do not involve intrinsic representational processes, they cannot embed narratives or tell stories of their own.

The reason that actions might appear to have a narrative structure is that, as we have suggested, the contours of our narratives naturally conform to the structures of actions and the events they narrate. Well-crafted narratives capture the most salient features of the sequence of happenings they describe, and it turns out that the happenings we are most interested in describing are our own actions and the actions of others, and the dramas that surround them. As Herman (2007, p. 11) notes, 'narrative prototypically roots itself in the lived, felt experience of human and human-like agents interacting in an ongoing way with their cohorts and surrounding environment'.

Since these dramas naturally unfold in particular sequences of actions and events occurring at a spatio-temporal scale at which we ordinarily witness things happening, it is easy to see how narratives draw on the pre-existing structure of action, as in the example above: 'The baby really enjoyed playing with that toy; she let me know when she wanted to play with it; but after a while she threw it to the ground and was done with it'. Action structure gets built upon, but predates the structure built by narrative. The narratives we tell about events, can tap into the dramatic structure of action and depict it more or less faithfully. But there is no reason to think that such structure is already inherently narrative in nature in any stronger sense than that it lends itself and is ripe for narration.

In the next and final section we examine whether structured embodied activity – and not body narratives *per se* – might be doing the required work in body and dance movement psychotherapy.

Narrating the body in therapy

Engaging in narrative practices, those that involve giving accounts rich in storied content, has been shown to correlate positively with mental health. Numerous studies suggest that people 'who are able to narrate the emotional events of their lives in more self-reflective ways, show better physical and psychological health' (Fivush et al. 2010, p. 46; see also Fivush et al. 2003, 2010). Furthermore, individuals whose narratives include more causal explanatory language (words such as 'because', 'thus', and 'understand') and more emotional language (the inclusion of both positive and negative emotion words) subsequently show lower anxiety, lower depression, a higher sense of well-being, and higher immune system functioning than individuals who use less of this kind of language (Fivush and McDermott Sales, 2006, p. 126).

These studies focus on explicit reflective narratives – narratives that we are able to formulate either retrospectively or prospectively in regard to our actions. Two questions are relevant to this process. First, if we reflectively impose a particular narrative on our actions, is it important that it fits the structure that is already intrinsic to the action? Second, are the structures of embodied actions always obvious and apparent, or do we need to do some work in order to discover them?

In response to the question about there being a good fit between our reflective, explicit, linguistic narratives and our embodied actions, on the one hand research suggests that choice of a narrative, but not necessarily its accuracy, is important to our well-being. 'How we remember the stressful events of our lives has an impact on our ability to cope' (Fivush and McDermott Sales, 2006, p. 125; McDermott Sales et al. 2005), but this doesn't mean that we need to remember them with detailed accuracy. More important is a forward-looking basis for dealing better with other, similar stressful future happenings. On the other hand, if one thinks that authenticity is valuable, then formulating a narrative that is consistent with the broad outlines of our actions seems important.

If, for the sake of authenticity, it is important for a narrative to be consistent with the original action structure, the fact that in some cases our actions may be informed by forces or effects that remain unconscious, makes consistency and authenticity more difficult. Part of the work of psychotherapy, then, may be to discover the forces hidden in the structure of our embodied actions, and to explicate those forces in narratives that reflect them without distortion.

If we accept this, or some variation of this account, then what is the nature of the work that needs to be done in psychotherapy? As described by Helen Payne (2006), for example, body-related and creative movement psychotherapy may be based on a movement dialogue between therapist and patient. The therapist may move and posture to reflect or mirror the patient's movement patterns (see e.g., Koch et al. 2015), which may allow the patient to gain a perspective on her own movement, and for the therapist to grasp the significance of the patient's movement and emotional state via a form of interaffectivity (Fuchs and Koch, 2014). The therapist may also engage with, and respond to, the patient's emotional expression as manifested in their movements, with the aim of creating a non-verbal communion – a form of kinaesthetic intersubjectivity (Samaritter and Payne, 2013).

The non-verbal, or minimally verbal 'conversation' in this interaction is a case of 'coordination-with' (Fuchs and De Jaegher, 2009, p. 471) that goes beyond individual unidirectional embodied actions, therapist to patient. Coordination-with involves coordination or attunement between patient and therapist who give and take as they engage in a variety of creative bodily expressions, including gaze direction, positioning, utterances and intonations, gestures, facial expressions, hands-on or other physical intentional interactions, leading to a mutual enactive coupling in instances of joint attention and joint action. Allowing or helping the body to move in different ways and bringing some of the unconscious effects to light can then open the possibilities of re-narrating or forming new, alternative life narratives. The aim of such a psychotherapy is the establishment of self-authorship, or the appropriation of the parts of self-narrative that come from others.

This is where a proper understanding of the structure of action comes into play. As we noted, Delafield-Butt and Trevarthen (2015) identify a four-fold structure: introduction, development, climax and resolution. A similar four-fold structure is found in semiotic accounts of narrative and action: contract, competence, performance, and sanction (Greimas, 1970; Martin and Ringham, 2000; Paolucci, 2016). To understand this structure, and to show how it reflects, and gets reflected in embodied actions, we think it best to translate it into terms related to enactivist approaches to embodied cognition:

- Introduction or contract: taken as an affordance – that which presents itself as a viable action in any particular (physical or intersubjective or problematic) situation.
- Development or competence: what the actor is capable of, in terms that can be defined by skill, interest and intention.
- Climax or performance: the actual doing of the action.
- Resolution or sanction: the resulting situation that can be judged or evaluated, by oneself or others – a point that can transition into narrative.

One can typically work backwards from an evaluation of the resulting situation to ask, in the doing of the action, whether something was revealed, or something went wrong, or the skill, interest or intention was misaligned with the situation – a misalignment of agent and affordance. When the action is part of an interaction with others (where the affordance may be a social one), the details are more complex.[2]

This intersubjective interaction that takes place in body-related and creative movement psychotherapy, the dialogue between therapist and patient, the 'coordination-with' described above, may be then expressed or formulated in a linguistic narrative as a reiteration of the interaction that has just occurred (Panhofer, 2011). Morag (2016), for example, stresses the need for the therapist to recognize the importance of what gets added to our memory of specific past events when we narrate such events much later on using conceptual and descriptive resources that were unavailable at the time the target memory was formed. She readily admits, 'the relation between the memory and the emotional symptom lends itself to the kind of storytelling familiar from everyday life and the therapeutic setting' (Morag, 2016, p. 126). Nevertheless, given that she denies that emotions come with 'subtitles' in the form of conceptual contents, she is sensitive to the fact that 'When we remember what we did, or what other people did, we may also rethink, redescribe and refeel the past' (Hacking, 1995, p. 249).

The action itself, as well as the reiteration, can inform the therapist's clinical reasoning process, *in situ*, with the patient (Gallagher and Payne, 2014). The way the patient moves with the therapist, or does not move, will inform the therapist and help her to assess the way forward for the patient; or indeed, in the movement process, the patient may find his/her own way forward, or may lead the therapist to a co-assessment. The interactive movement can allow the patient's story to unfold more deeply. The experiences of both the therapist and the patient (feelings, sensations, thoughts, images, expressed in bits of narrative) may inform clinical judgment and promote understanding for both of them.

On the four-fold scheme outlined above, the action may begin with an affordance presented by the therapist herself, as part of the therapeutic situation. Given the skill, interest and intention of the patient in engaging with the therapist, as well as the skills of the therapist, a performance follows, and the resulting situation can be judged or evaluated, by the therapist or by the therapist and patient together. In this regard, the structure of the action includes the resolution, which forms a new affordance to continue into further interaction.

In this kind of therapeutic interaction with individuals who are presenting with socio-emotional disorders, the therapist can identify disruptions in prospective timing and in the affective integration of motor intentions.[3] Why should this work as therapy? As Delafield-Butt and Trevarthen (2015) suggest,

> episodes of dramatic or more aroused action, of speaking in conversation . . . appear to be essential in the emotional regulation of all forms of movement and to all forms of inter-subjective co-creation of meaning in dyadic states of human consciousness. . . . They make predictable patterns of engagement, and lead to mutual 'sympathetic' involvement in vocal and motor expressions of changes in feeling.
>
> *(p. 8)*

The sharing of movements reveals more than the individual agent can discover her-/himself; such movements, and their affective and self-related dimensions, can be restructured in the continuing development of narrative and action. In this respect, narration complements the embodied activities and engagements by adding something new and quite important into the psychotherapeutic mix.

In the final analysis, it seems possible to understand the complementary roles played by embodied engagements and narration and how they work together to build upon and add to the existing resources of clients and practitioners of body or dance movement psychotherapies without embracing the idea that there is a pre-existing narrative embedded in the body that requires interpretation. Embodied activity can invite and encourage narration without it being the case that an embodied form of psychotherapy uncovers and gives voice to a pre-existing body narrative. We maintain that accepting this conclusion makes better sense of the practice of body and dance movement psychotherapies and the important role that narratives have to play in those practices even if, as we contend, bodies do not auto-generate or tell any narratives of their own.

Acknowledgements

SG's research on this project was supported by the Humboldt Foundation's Anneliese Maier Research Award.

Notes

1 This view may derive from psychoanalytic or postmodern traditions where theorists sometimes talk about reading the body in the way one might read a text or reading meaning that is inscribed in the surface behavior of the body (Brain, 2002).
2 Indeed, such interactions may require the kind of detailed microanalysis found in Goodwin (2000). The notion of intersubjective alignment itself is defined in different ways by different authors. Some researchers equate it with simple matching, imitation or entrainment and distinguish it from other more intentional coordination processes (e.g., Rothwell, Shalin and Romigh, 2017); others define it as more than mimicry, and as including more complex forms of coupling (Tollefsen, Dale and Paxton, 2013). It is clear from the research on conversational analysis and communicative interaction, however, that there is a broad range of embodied and ecological processes integrated into such events, and that different circumstances (e.g., how structured or unstructured the immediate environment might be) and different intentions elicit different dynamical balances among these processes.
3 Recent research on Autism Spectrum Disorders (ASDs) has shown characteristic disruptions in basic sensory-motor/proprioceptive processes (Brincker and Torres, 2013; Gallagher and Varga, 2015; Torres, 2013). Thus, in subjects with ASD, one would expect to find 'errors in sensorimotor capacity to efficiently enact desired intentions . . . regularly thwarting success, creating distress and isolation, and consequent social and emotional compensations' (Delafield-Butt and Trevarthen, 2015, p. 12; see Trevarthen et al. 2006).

References

Brain, J. (2002). Unsettling body image: 'Anorexic body narratives and the materialization of the body imaginary'. *Feminist Theory*, 3(2), 151–168.
Brincker, M. and Torres, E. B. (2013). Noise from the periphery in autism. *Frontiers in Integrative Neuroscience*, 7, 34. doi:10.3389/fnint.2013.00034
Bruner, J. S. (1990). *Acts of meaning*. Cambridge, MA: Harvard University Press.
Bruner, J. S. (1996). *The culture of education*. Cambridge, MA: Harvard University Press.
Caldwell, C. (2014). Mindfulness and bodyfulness: A new paradigm. *Journal of Contemplative Inquiry*, 1, 77–96.
Caldwell, C. (2017). Conscious movement sequencing: The core of the dance/movement therapy experience. In H. Payne (ed.), *Essentials of dance movement psychotherapy: International perspectives on theory, research, and practice* (pp. 53–66). London: Routledge.
Charon, R. (2006). The self-telling body. *Narrative Inquiry*, 16(1), 191–200.
Chemero, A. (2011). *Radical embodied cognitive science*. Cambridge, MA: MIT Press.
Cobley, P. (2014). *Narrative*. London: Routledge.
Currie, G. (2010). *Narratives and narrators: A philosophy of stories*. Oxford: Oxford University Press.
De Jaegher, H., Di Paolo, E. and Gallagher, S. (2010). Can social interaction constitute social cognition? *Trends in Cognitive Science*, 14, 441–447.
Delafield-Butt, J. T. and Trevarthen, C. (2015). The ontogenesis of narrative: From moving to meaning. *Frontiers in Psychology*, 6, 1157. doi:10.3389/fpsyg.2015.01157
Erskine, R. G. (2014). Nonverbal stories: The body in psychotherapy. *International Journal of Integrative Psychotherapy*, 5(1), 21–33.
Fivush, R., Berlin, L., Sales, J. M., Mennuti-Washburn, J. and Cassidy, J. (2003). Functions of parent–child reminiscing across negative events. *Memory*, 11, 179–192.
Fivush, R., Bohanek, J. G. and Zaman, W. (2010). Personal and intergenerational narratives in relation to adolescents' well-being. In T. Habermas (ed.), *The development of autobiographical reasoning in adolescence and beyond. New directions for child and adolescent development, 131* (pp. 45–57). San Francisco, CA: Jossey-Bass.
Fivush, R. and McDermott Sales, J. (2006). Coping, attachment, and mother-child narratives of stressful events. *Merrill-Palmer Quarterly*, 52(1), 125–150.
Fuchs, T. and De Jaegher, H. (2009). Enactive intersubjectivity: Participatory sense-making and mutual incorporation. *Phenomenology and the Cognitive Sciences*, 8, 465–486.
Fuchs, T. and Koch, S. C. (2014). Embodied affectivity: On moving and being moved. *Frontiers in Psychology*, 5, 508.

Gallagher, S. (2017). *Enactivist interventions: Rethinking the mind.* Oxford: Oxford University Press.

Gallagher S. and Payne, H. (2014). The role of embodiment and intersubjectivity in clinical reasoning. *Body, Movement and Dance in Psychotherapy*, 10(1): 68–78.

Gallagher, S. and Varga, S. (2015). Conceptual issues in autism spectrum disorders. *Current Opinion in Psychiatry*, 28(2), 127–132.

Goldie, P. (2012). *The mess inside: Narrative, emotion and the mind.* Oxford: Oxford University Press.

Goodwin, C. (2000). Action and embodiment within situated human interaction. *Journal of Pragmatics*, 32(10), 1489–1522.

Greimas, A. J. (1970). *Du Sens II. Essais sémiotiques.* Paris: Seuil

Hacking, I. (1995). *Rewriting the soul: Multiple personality and the sciences of memory.* Princeton, NJ: Princeton University Press.

Halliday, M. A. K. (1978). Meaning and the construction of reality in early childhood. In J. H. Pick, Jr. and E. Saltzman (eds.), *Psychological modes of perceiving and processing information* (pp. 67–98). Hillsdale, NJ: Erlbaum.

Herman, D. (2007). Introduction. In D. Herman (ed.), *The Cambridge companion to narrative.* Cambridge: Cambridge University Press.

Hutto, D. (2006). Narrative practice and understanding reasons: Reply to Gallagher'. In R. Menary (ed.), *Radical enactivism.* Amsterdam: John Benjamins.

Hutto, D. D. and Myin, E. (2017). *Evolving enactivism.* Cambridge, MA: MIT Press.

Kerby, P. (1993). *Narrative and the self.* Bloomington, IN: Indiana University Press.

Koch, S., Holland, R., Hengstler, M. and van Knippenberg, A. (2009). Body locomotion as regulatory process. *Association for Psychological Science*, 20(5), 549–550.

Koch, S. C., Mehl, L., Sobanski, E., Sieber, M. and Fuchs, T. (2015). Fixing the mirrors: A feasibility study of the effects of dance movement therapy on young adults with autism spectrum disorder. *Autism*, 19(3), 338–350.

Lamarque, P. (2004). On not expecting too much from narrative. *Mind and Language*, 19(4), 393–408.

Legerstee, M. (2005). *Infants' sense of people: Precursors to a theory of mind.* Cambridge: Cambridge University Press.

Ling, Y. R. and Liu, L. H. (2008). Body narrative in western modernist literature. *Journal of Southwest University (Social Sciences Edition)*, 3, 34.

Mackenzie, C. (2007). Bare personhood? Velleman on selfhood. *Philosophical Explorations*, 10(3), 263–281.

McDermott Sales, J., Fivush, R., Parker J. and Bahrick, L. (2005). Stressing memory: Long-term relations among children's stress, recall and psychological outcome following Hurricane Andrew. *Journal of Cognition and Development*, 6(4), 529–545.

McNeill, D. (2008). *Gesture and thought.* Chicago: University of Chicago Press.

Martin, B. and Ringham, F. (2000). *Dictionary of semiotics.* London: Bloomsbury Publishing.

Menary, R. (2008). Embodied narratives. *Journal of Consciousness Studies*, 15(6), 63–84.

Morag, T. (2016). *Emotion, imagination and the limits of reason.* London: Routledge.

Nelson, K. (2003a). Narrative and the emergence of a consciousness of self. In G. D. Fireman, T. E. J. McVay and O. Flanagan (eds.), *Narrative and consciousness* (pp. 17–36). Oxford: Oxford University Press.

Nelson, K. (2003b). Self and social functions: Individual autobiographical memory and collective narrative. *Memory*, 11(2), 125–136.

Panhofer, H. (2011). Languaged and non-languaged ways of knowing. *British Journal of Guidance and Counselling*, 39, 455–470.

Paolucci, C. (2016). *Narrative practices and semiotics.* Philosophy Colloquium. University of Memphis, 21 October.

Payne, H. (ed.). (2006). *Dance movement therapy: Theory, research and practice.* London: Routledge.

Reddy, V. (2008). *How infants know minds.* Cambridge, MA: Harvard University Press.

Reddy, V. (2012). Moving others matters. In A. Foolen, U. M. Lüdtke, T. P. Racine and J. Zlatev (eds.), *Moving ourselves, moving others: Motion and emotion in intersubjectivity, consciousness and language* (pp. 139–163). Amsterdam: John Benjamins.

Rothwell, C. D., Shalin, V. L., and Romigh, G. D. (2017). Quantitative models of human-human conversational grounding processes [Private Circulation via Research Gate].

Rucinska, Z. and Reijmers, E. (2014). Between philosophy and therapy: Understanding systemic play therapy through embodied and enactive cognition (EEC). *InterAction*, 6, 37–52.

Ryan, M.-L. (2007). Toward a definition of narrative. In D. Herman (ed.), *The Cambridge companion to narrative.* Cambridge: Cambridge University Press.

Samaritter, R. and Payne, H. (2013). Kinaesthetic intersubjectivity: A dance informed contribution to self–other relatedness and shared experience in nonverbal psychotherapy with an example from Autism. *Arts in Psychotherapy*, 40, 143–150.

Schechtman, M. (1996). *The constitution of selves*. Ithaca, NY: Cornell University Press.

Schechtman, M. (2011). The narrative self. In S. Gallagher (ed.), *The Oxford handbook of the self* (pp. 394–416). Oxford: Oxford University Press.

Scholz, S. (2000). *Body narratives: Writing the nation and fashioning the subject in early modern England*. London: Palgrave Macmillan.

Slors, M. V. P. (1998). Two conceptions of psychological continuity. *Philosophical Explorations*, 1(1), 59–78.

Stern, D. N. (2010). *Forms of vitality*. Oxford: Oxford University Press.

Strawson, G. (2004). Against narrativity. *Ratio*, 17(4), 428–542.

Thompson, E. (2007). *Mind in life: Biology, phenomenology, and the sciences of mind*. Cambridge, MA: Harvard University Press.

Tollefsen, D. P., Dale, R. and Paxton, A. (2013). Alignment, transactive memory, and collective cognitive systems. *Review of Philosophy and Psychology*, 4(1), 49–64.

Torres, E. B. (2013). A typical signatures of motor variability found in an individual with ASD. *Neurocase*, 19, 150–165.

Trevarthen, C. (2013). Born for art, and the joyful companionship of fiction. In D. Narvaez, J. Panksepp, A. Schore and T. Gleason (eds.), *Evolution, early experience and human development: From research to practice and policy* (pp. 202–218). New York: Oxford University Press.

Trevarthen, C., Aitken, K. J., Nagy, E., Delafield-Butt, J. T. and Vandekerckhove, M. (2006). Collaborative regulations of vitality in early childhood: Stress in intimate relationships and postnatal psychopathology. In D. Cicchetti and D. J. Cohen (eds.), *Developmental psychopathology* (pp. 65–126). New York: John Wiley and Sons.

Trevarthen, C. and Delafield-Butt, J. T. (2013). Biology of shared meaning and language development: Regulating the life of narratives. In M. Legerstee, D. Haley and M. Bornstein (eds.), *The infant mind: Origins of the social brain* (pp. 167–199). New York: Guilford Press.

Velleman, J. D. (2006). *Self to self: Selected essays*. New York: Cambridge University Press.

Vygotsky, L. S. (1986). *Thought and language*. Cambridge, MA: MIT Press.

3

TOWARDS A CLINICAL THEORY OF EMBODIMENT

A model for the conceptualization and treatment of mental illness

Jessica Acolin

Introduction

Surrounded by increasingly sophisticated diagnostic tools and interventions, many clinicians have forgotten one crucial factor: the individual. While many agree that healing is dependent upon a patient's motivation and behaviour (in adherence to medication or clinical homework), current diagnoses and medical language depersonalize the experience. A person is more than a list of symptoms; they are the lived *experience* of those symptoms, and their lived experience is what will determine their motivation and behaviour. In order to treat mental illness, clinical practitioners need tools and language for connecting with, assessing, and intervening at the level of a patient's lived experience.

Thus far, such an approach has been relegated to the realm of 'clinical judgment'; that is, a hazily defined realm of subjective evaluations that varies according to practitioner and patient. This is borne from necessity and efficacy: necessity, due to the dearth of research or tools to standardize such important judgments [for a notable exception, see Pallagrosi, Picardi, and Biondi (2013)]; and efficacy, as clinicians instinctually have access to sophisticated, fast, and at times unconscious evaluations of nonverbal cues and behaviour that may supersede the information accessible through existing standardized diagnostic tools.

Such unconscious evaluations are largely based on nonverbal cues such as movement, facial expressions, postural changes, or tone of voice. Such evaluations, rather than being subjective and unreliable, are increasingly being shown to be important, reliable, and measurable in the laboratory environment. Embodiment researchers from diverse academic backgrounds are beginning to illustrate this connection between the verbal and the nonverbal, the unconscious and the conscious, and the mind and the body. This body of work supports the clinical importance of 'subjective' clinical judgments and may, in time, show how such evaluations are as important as, if not more important than, existing symptom checklists.

Nevertheless, the development of standardized tools based on embodiment research would advance mental health practice and encourage additional research to understand and improve existing clinical judgment and interventions. Thus, it is beneficial for researchers, clinicians, and patients alike to integrate embodiment research gained in the labs with clinical expertise gained through practice. The formulation of such a model of health, illness, and change—in short, a clinical theory of embodiment—would guide future research, inform current clinical interventions, and ultimately move individuals more effectively from illness to health. This chapter outlines such a practical model for clinicians as a foundation for such a clinical theory of embodiment.

Background

Embodiment research illustrates how embodiment and the mind-body connection are important in cognition, social interaction, emotional regulation, and self-expression. Here, embodiment is defined as the dynamic interaction between mental and physical states that comprise individual experience. This definition is raised in opposition to out-dated models of human behaviour based on Cartesian dualism, which treats the mind and its processes, such as cognition, logic, judgment, preference, and personality as both separate from and more important than the body and physical sensations. While Cartesian dualism continues to guide certain branches of research and practice, particularly the 'hard' sciences which encourage purely cognitive interventions, embodiment researchers are showing that the mind-body connection is central to a full understanding of human experience.

Cognition, for instance, long touted as the epitome of the human brain overcoming limitations of the physical body, is embodied. Language comprehension engages the sensorimotor cortex; comprehending a word such as 'cinnamon' automatically involves sensory processing (Pulvermüller, 1999, 2013).

Thinking about complex social concepts such as age can elicit unconscious bodily responses such as slower gait (Bargh, Chen, and Burrows, 1996). Abstract concepts of time elicit gentle sways forward for the future and backwards for the past (Miles, Nind, and Macrae, 2010). Thus, cognition, or what has been considered disembodied 'thinking', is not as separate from the body as previously believed.

Similarly, social judgments such as threat, friendliness, and intimacy are embodied. Individuals have been shown to judge a neutral stranger as more generous and caring when holding a warm versus cold beverage (Williams and Bargh, 2008). Individuals with positive evaluations of a demographic group (the elderly) unconsciously mimicked their movement patterns (slower gait) (Cesario, Plaks, and Higgins, 2006). Social psychology research increasingly illustrates the myriad ways in which social interactions and behaviour are embodied (Niedenthal, Barsalou, Winkielman, Krauth-Gruber, and Ric, 2005).

The advice to 'take a step back' when agitated is more than an expression; physically stepping backwards has been shown to improve cognitive control (Koch, Holland, Hengstler, and Knippenberg, 2009). Deep breathing, sometimes called 'belly breathing', has been shown to regulate emotional arousal without additional cognitive intervention (Benson and Klipper, 1992). Depression and sadness manifest in downward gaze and slower gait (Meier and Robinson, 2004, 2006; Michalak et al., 2009). In these and other ways, human experience is being increasingly understood as embodied.

A significant challenge is the search for a language to consistently describe the body-based variables being studied. Here, two systems of movement analysis and notation used by dance researchers and dance/movement therapists are valuable. Laban Movement Analysis (LMA), provides a vocabulary that describes movement behaviour based on body position, movement quality, and relationship to space (Dell, 1970). The Kestenberg Movement Profile (KMP) adds criteria for observing rhythms and patterns of motion (Kestenberg-Amighi, Loman, Lewis, and Sossin, 1999). When used by trained movement analysts, these two languages provide a comprehensive, objective, and efficient system of observing and categorizing nonverbal behaviour.

This movement vocabulary captures relationships between psychological phenomena and the mechanics of movement (such as pace, tension, or direction) as well as the *quality* of movement

(Koch, 2014). Movement quality and patterns play an important role in connecting nonverbal behaviour to mental functions and may provide much-needed order to the overwhelming variety of variables currently studied by embodiment researchers.

Phenomenological theory reminds us to pay attention, not only to external observations, but also to the individual's lived experience. The importance of embodied experience lies in the meaning it holds for the individual, regardless of whether it was observed via neuroimaging, lab measurements, or in the clinical session room. This phenomenological approach invites greater introspection on the part of the observer of personal biases and movement. Defining and standardizing such a clinical approach represents a new and exciting direction (Pallagrosi et al., 2014) and will contribute to a greater respect for the opinions, experiences, and interpretations of both patient and clinician.

Fuchs (2010) outlines a phenomenological account of psychopathology which categorizes mental illness by disturbances in the patient's lived, embodied experiences. In this account, schizophrenia is defined by an overwhelming sense of disembodiment, or a broken connection between cognition and bodily self-awareness. Depression is characterized by an inescapable sense of confinement to the lived body, which Fuchs refers to as hyperembodiment and a falling back in or out of time. Fuchs categorizes the experience of mental illness based upon disturbances in balanced embodiment: the balance between the subject and the object body, the immediate and the narrative self, and the mental processes and physical sensations.

Advances in neuroscience support this understanding of mental illness as rooted in the individual lived experience. Trauma researchers increasingly show how the plethora of symptoms currently associated with attention deficit hyperactivity disorder, oppositional defiant disorder, obsessive compulsive disorder, panic disorder, generalized anxiety disorder, bipolar disorder, borderline personality disorder, and others can be traced to fundamental physical reactions associated with survival and body regulation (Soma, 2016). Anxiety, for instance, results from the body remaining in a hyper-aroused state in preparation to respond to threats; this bodily state is then interpreted by the individual as fear, even when no immediate threat is present. Anxious behaviour follows. The individual's lived experience of their physical state, thus, is important in understanding how to clinically intervene.

Emphasizing balance, functional adaptability, and in-the-moment observation, rather than unilateral increase or decrease of symptoms, or analysis of past or future experiences, reflects ancient Eastern philosophies and underlies approaches such as dialectical behaviour therapy, dance/movement therapy, and trauma-informed yoga (Levy, 2005; Linehan, 1993; van der Kolk, 2014). In these models, health is not defined by a static maintenance of a desired state but rather by the ability of an individual to move and self-regulate as a situation requires. Acknowledging that life experiences and stressors are varied and require different solutions, such therapies focus on enhancing an individual's access to many functional states and empowering the individual to access varied skills and strategies as needed. From this body of research, theory, and practice, a clinical theory of embodiment begins to emerge.

Towards a clinical theory of embodiment

Several key conclusions can be drawn from the literature that provide the foundation for a clinical theory of embodiment. First, it becomes clear that humans are embodied beings who understand and interact with the world around them via the dynamic relationship between mind and body. In addition, this mind-body connection is complex and is involved in anything from language acquisition to abstract concept comprehension; in fact, in view of its complex nature and high inter-subject variability, the task of merely describing embodiment from an external observer's perspective may seem daunting.

Nevertheless, humans are embodied. Their individual lived, embodied experiences are essential to understanding their distress and, in turn, to ameliorating it. Thus, a shift in focus from the external observation of symptoms and behaviours to the individual's lived and embodied experiences provide an important direction forward for clinical intervention. It is the individual's interpretation of symptoms, the interplay of their mind with their lived body, which is of key clinical significance.

This approach emphasizes the individual's lived experience in the present, or what is called the 'here and now'. It focuses on how past experiences (all simultaneously) manifest themselves in current body experiences, which acknowledges the importance of formative memories (Fuchs, 2012) while providing an immediate avenue for intervention. Thus, assessments and interventions are designed to be immediate and to be implemented in the present, in the session room, rather than as homework or as analysis of past memories.

Next, the theoretical emphasis on balance and flexibility in coping with the environment, rather than a static or unilateral focus on symptoms, offers a widely applicable clinical approach that empowers the patient in the long term and better meets the needs of individuals living in a dynamic world. A clinical theory founded on *balance* serves both clinicians and patients by acknowledging the multifaceted nature of individuals and normalizing temporary fluctuations in behaviour while allowing for varied capabilities.

Finally, a standardized tool for assessing and diagnosing an individual's lived experience in order to best design interventions is both important and possible. Observation approaches of body movement such as LMA and the KMP, alongside phenomenological theories of psychopathology, provide the rudimentary structure for such a tool.

A clinical model

The model presented in this chapter identifies three axes of embodiment, each of which is important in its own right but can be maladaptive when taken too extremely or rigidly. Though an individual may, at different times, fall in different places on each axis, the clinical goal is for the individual to find balance in order to regularly adapt to changing needs and desires.

The first axis addresses how an individual experiences, understands, and makes decisions. Does the individual rely primarily on thoughts, logic, and reasoning (mental processes) or on intuition, sensory experience, and feeling (body processes)? For instance, two individuals both have the same experience of walking by the beach. One who relies primarily on mental processes may explain tides, measure temperature, and categorize marine biology. One who relies primarily on physical processes may focus on the warm sand, crashing waves, and the smell of saltwater. Neither approach is better than the other. Cognitive processes are necessary in problem solving, while physical sensations are important in intimate relationships. A well-balanced individual can access both forms of processing and is able to adjust according to environmental and situational demands. However, inflexibility or too strong a preference in one direction results in maladaptive behaviours. This axis is called the decision access, with Mind at one pole and Body at the other.

The second axis focuses on an individual's identity, or how they see themselves. Are they defined by their own perceptions, judgments, and expectations—or those of others? The latter is called an objectified body, where the individual sees themselves (and their bodies) from an external point of view, sometimes even as objects to be manipulated or controlled. Such a body may feel contorted and confined by excessive demands and judgments (Fuchs, 2010; Serlin, 1996). The former is referred to as a subject or lived body, and it is one that is guided by internal sensations such as pleasure, pain, and instinct. Again, both the object and subject body are important for optimal functioning. Awareness of social expectations and exerting conscious control over our bodies and lives are the hallmark of civil society. Yet, access to internal experiences and desires are important for immediate threat detection, pleasurable enjoyment, and social attunement. Thus, a balance and flexibility of movement between the two poles is necessary. This axis is called the identity access with Object at one pole and Subject at the other.

The third axis brings attention to where an individual directs their focus. Is the individual turned inward, noticing only their own thoughts and feelings and ruminating on the past or future? Or is the individual turned outward, seeing and reacting to the world around them and living in present sensations? The former is crucial to successful problem solving and conscious decision-making. However, an individual stuck in internalized focus can become anxious, dissociated, or paralyzed by inactivity. Engagement with the outside world underlies initiation, action, and since humans are fundamentally social beings, emotional regulation (Homann, 2010). Again, balance and flexibility on this axis leads to a well-functioning and adjusted individual. This axis is called the focus access, with Inner at one pole and Outer at the other.

This model is graphically illustrated below and can be used to assess both an individual's capacity and their current state. What an individual has access to determines the range within which they can move at the present time; one therapeutic goal can be to increase the individual's capacities through skill-building and practice. An individual's current state can be marked within the model; the therapeutic goal may then be to assist the individual in accessing greater balance. Such representation both of an individual's capabilities and current state provides the practitioner with a practical tool for here-and-now assessment and intervention to help an individual achieve greater balance and flexibility.

This model of health, illness, and adaptive functioning prizes balanced access to both poles and flexibility. As stated above, no individual pole is sufficient in isolation; each is necessary in certain instances. Thus, balance on all three axes is important to healthy functioning. Flexibility is the ability to move between poles as needed. Environmental demands are varied and ever changing.

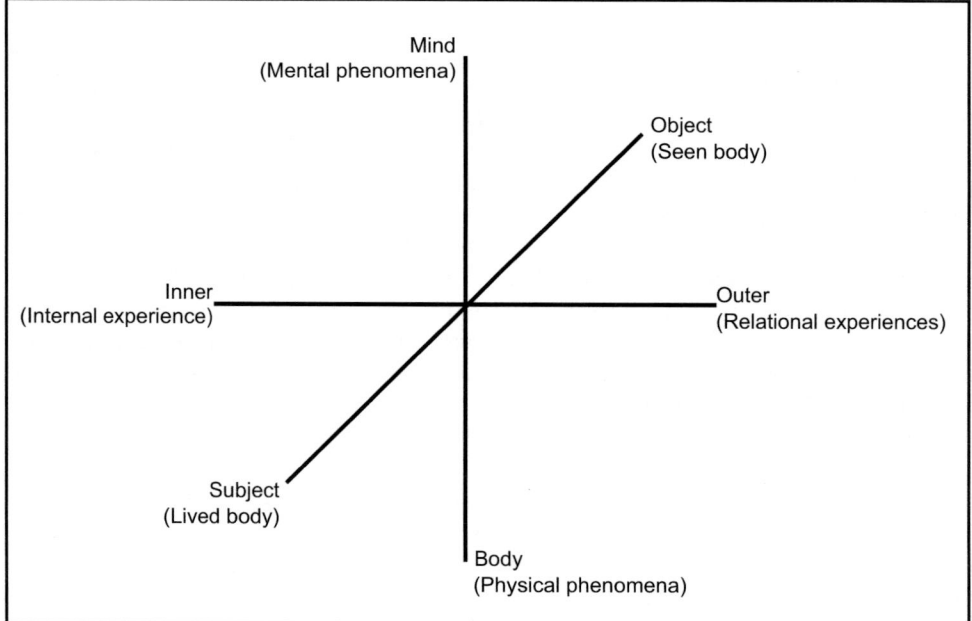

Figure 3.1   A clinical model of embodiment

The facility with which an individual has access to each pole contributes to their ease of inter-acting effectively with any challenges they may face. Thus, the therapeutic goal is to achieve greater balance and flexibility, rather than to unilaterally increase individual capacities. Figure 3.1 illustrates a clinical model of embodiment.

Case study: Applying the clinical model of embodiment for conceptualization

Schizophrenia

Currently, schizophrenia is characterized in the American Diagnostic and Statistical Manual of Mental Disorders (DSM) 5 *by psychotic symptoms (hallucinations or delusions), disorganization, and negative symptoms such as flat affect and lack of motivation.*

Imagine the experience of such an individual. Internal thoughts and feelings are so strong that they partly constitute reality, creating a tyranny of the mind. There is little connection to the outside world; reassurances from others feel threatening, less 'real' than the world their mind has trapped them in. Body sensations are foreign and dangerous, and touch feels alien or threatening. The body is held in rigid defence, muscles tensed in preparation for danger, pleasurable sensations ignored. The physical body is forced to suc-cumb to the mind's control. Such individuals often present with disorganized movement patterns (Davis, 1997), giving the observer the sense that their limbs are separate from their torso and their body parts have been cobbled together from incompatible sources.

This is a thought experiment, an attempt to imagine the lived experience of schizophrenia. However, in engaging in the exercise, it becomes clear how an individual with schizophrenia may be conceptualized through this clinical model of embodiment. Fuchs (2010) describes schizophrenia as a disorder of disembod-iment, and this is consistent with the conceptualization provided by this model.

First, on the Decision axis, the individual with schizophrenia is guided primarily by the Mind. Delusions and hallucinations are faulty interpretations by the mind of thoughts, feelings, and body sen-sations. The individual does have access, at the extremes, to both mental and physical processes; what is lacking is any connection between the two. The result is a disorganized method of decision-making shaped simultaneously by body sensations and mental interpretations, while lacking a bridge, or any integration, of the two.

The individual is represented in Figure 3.2:

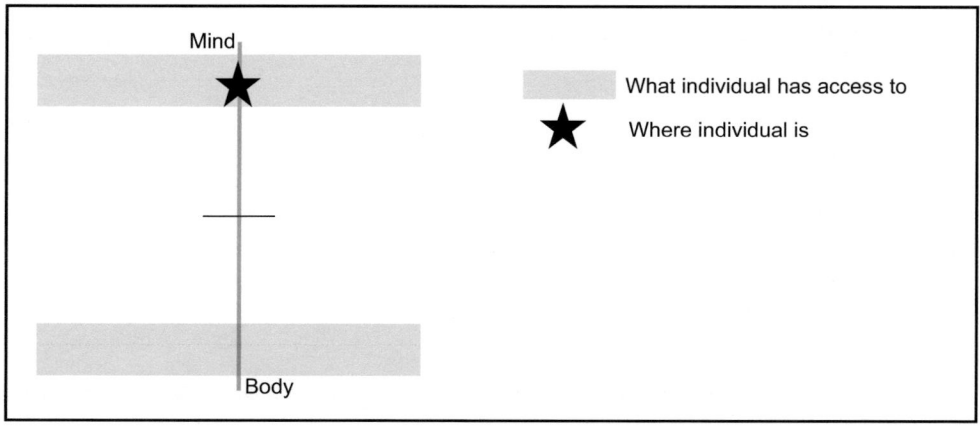

Figure 3.2   Decision axis in schizophrenia

On the second axis, Identity, the schizophrenic body is one that is controlled, confined, and fought. Muscles are held rigidly in defence against any subjective feelings, as if the individual is at war with their own body. The individual sees themselves as separate from their body, and the possibility of subjective experience can be threatening. The individual is thus represented as in Figure 3.3 below:

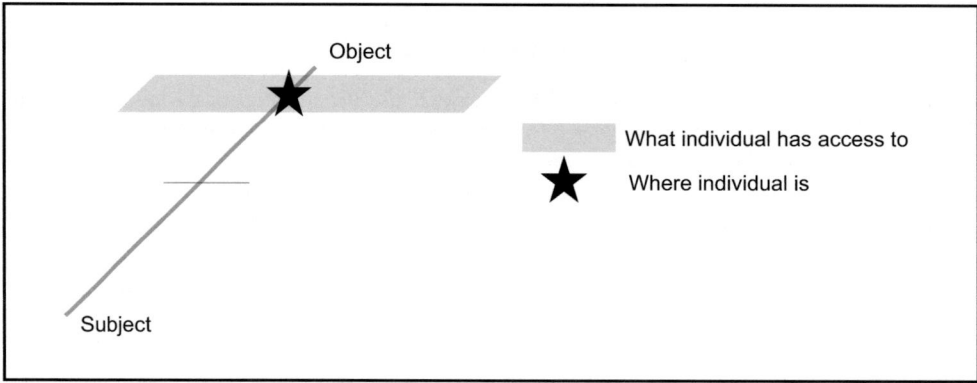

Figure 3.3   Identity axis in schizophrenia

Finally, the individual is trapped in an internal world; connection to or comprehension of others is limited as in Figure 3.4.

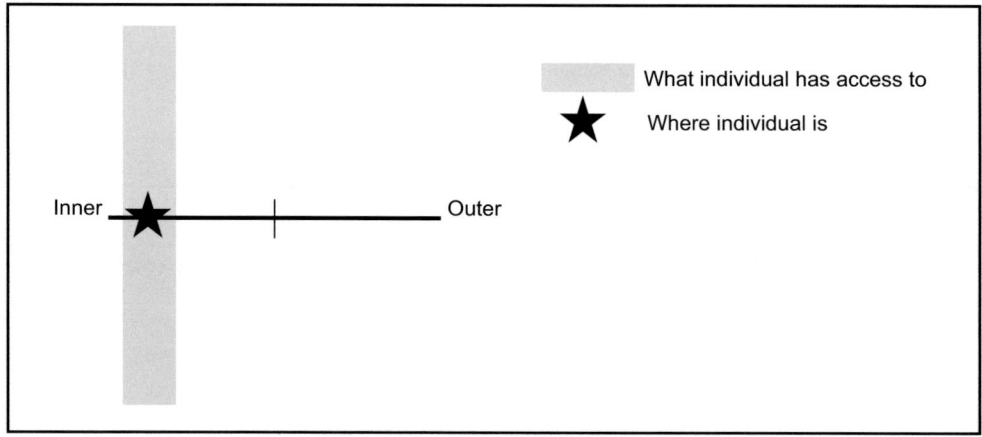

Figure 3.4   Focus axis in schizophrenia

The disembodiment referenced by Fuchs thus appears on all three axes, placing the individual in the top left quadrant of the model as in Figure 3.5.

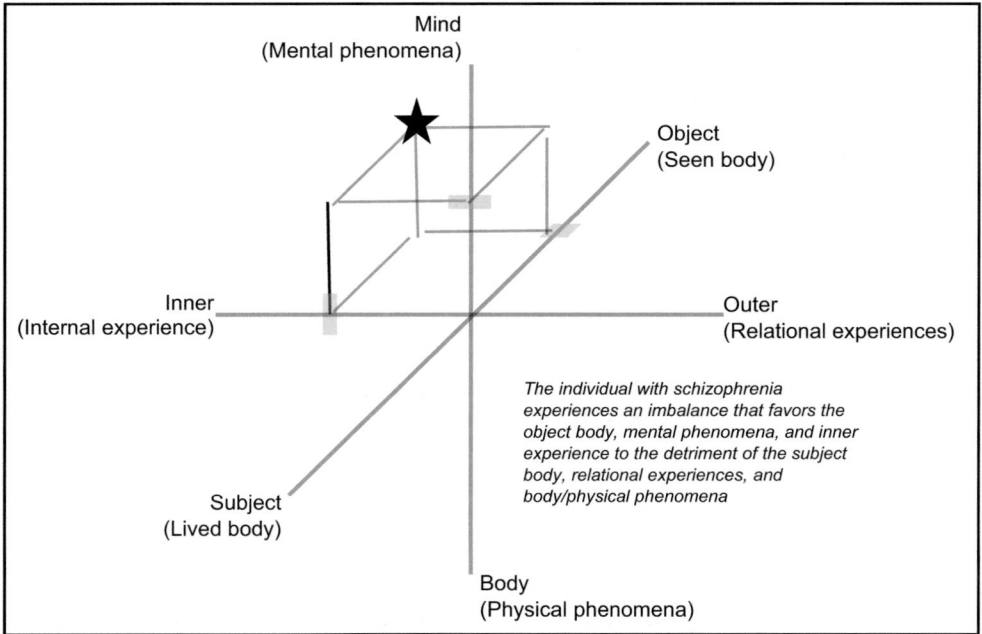

Mind
(Mental phenomena)

Object
(Seen body)

Inner
(Internal experience)

Outer
(Relational experiences)

The individual with schizophrenia experiences an imbalance that favors the object body, mental phenomena, and inner experience to the detriment of the subject body, relational experiences, and body/physical phenomena

Subject
(Lived body)

Body
(Physical phenomena)

Figure 3.5   Schizophrenia conceptualization

Applying the clinical model of embodiment: Clinical interventions

When selecting clinical interventions, two kinds of information are important: what is the goal? And what options or resources are available? The proposed model provides direction on both questions.

First, the goal for any individual is to bring balance and improve flexibility. Thus, it is relevant to ask: What does the individual currently have access to, and what capacities need to be strengthened?

Individuals who have unipolar strength, such as having access to Mind but not Body or Subject but not Object, need to gain access to the opposite pole. Their current abilities provide the entry into treatment, while what they lack provides the direction. For instance, individuals high on the Mind (thinking) axis may benefit from body awareness and sensory interventions such as yoga, massage, somatic experiencing, progressive muscle relaxation, and guided body scans. However, these body-based interventions may best be introduced through cognitive reasoning, step-by-step explanations and rationales for effectiveness. Conversely, individuals high on the Body (feeling) axis may benefit from development of cognitive analyses as offered by cognitive therapies. Such individuals may respond best if these cognitive therapies are presented first in terms of body sensations, and therapists may teach such individuals cognitive strategies for examining body sensations.

In both cases, while the Mind or the Body provide the entry into treatment, the end goal is to increase capacity at both poles and to encourage flexible movement. As illustrated by embodiment research, a body-based intervention has ramifications for mental processes of cognition, judgment, and social interaction. Similarly, cognitive interventions can impact physical processes such as regulating heart rate and blood pressure. Again, mind and body are intimately connected, and each of the three axes exist in dynamic relationship with each other.

In selecting the intervention, it remains important for the clinician to consider the individual's unique state and background. Is a lack of balance due, not to a lack of capacity, but rather to a recent traumatic event that has cut off access to it? Dissociation, for instance, is a common reaction to severe trauma and can translate into an avoidance of the Body/Physical Phenomena and Lived Body/Body as Subject poles of the model. However, the momentary loss of the capacity to access these poles is different from a case where the individual, for biological or early childhood trauma reasons, never gained it. Disability, developmental delay, and biological limitations may all influence the individual's lived experience and must be taken into account.

Case study: Applying the clinical model of embodiment for clinical interventions

Schizophrenia

An individual with schizophrenia may be conceptualized as follows in Figure 3.6.

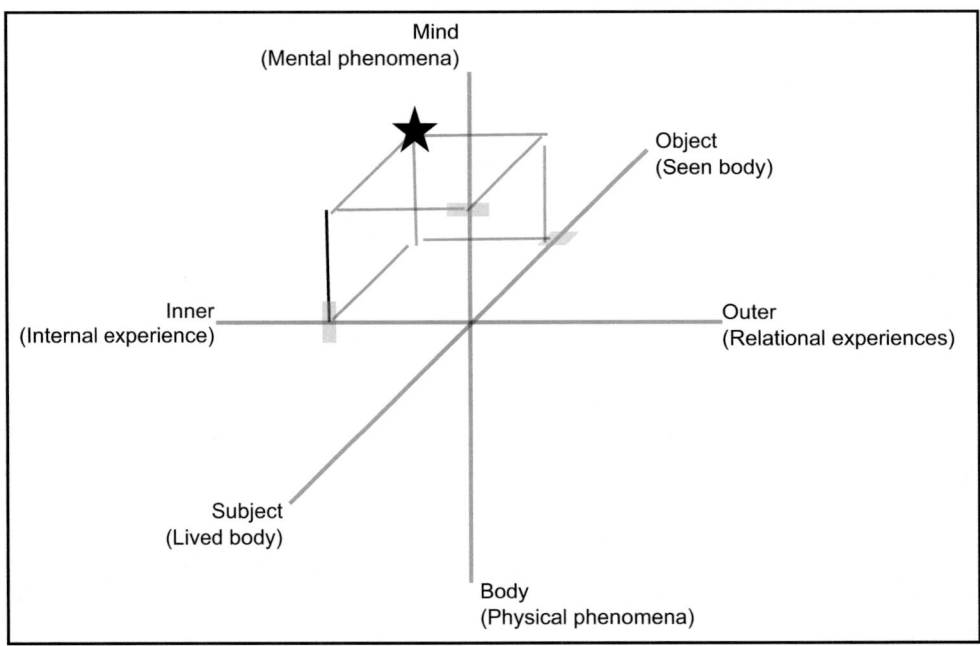

Figure 3.6 Schizophrenia conceptualization

This is an individual who is imbalanced, with limited access to the poles of Outer and Subject, and inflexible, with little ability to move between the extremes. The first step, then, would be to build the individual's capacity to access a complete range of embodiment experiences. Interventions to increase access to the Outer world may include the dance/movement therapy technique of mirroring, where a therapist coaxes the individual into the intersubjective space through the matching of movements and movement quality, or dance/movement therapy groups, where the individual is placed in a space with others and encouraged to interact through the use of music, rhythm, props, and games. Interventions to increase awareness of the Subject body may include progressive muscle relaxation, focusing on the breath, and guided body scans.

It is possible that the individual's limited capacities are related to chemical imbalances in the brain and body. A lack of proprioceptive ability, which may translate to a lack of ability to experience the Subject body, may be the result of biological abnormalities. In such cases, administration of pharmacological interventions may be necessary.

As the individual's capacity to access a wider range increases, the focus of therapeutic interventions shifts to address their ability to flexibly move between poles as the environment requires. Structured and mindful movement styles such as yoga may encourage integration of Mind and Body. Social dances, such as ballroom or Latin dancing, encourage both Inner and Outer focus, as the individual learns to balance their own impulses with cues given by their partner. Finally, practicing movement in a mirrored studio space allows the individual to practice experiencing the Subject body while being simultaneously aware of the Object body, or the body the individual observes in the mirror.

In this manner, the proposed framework provides direction for designing therapeutic interventions to help an individual achieve better balance and increased capacity for interacting with the environment.

Discussion

This chapter outlined the beginnings of a clinical theory of embodiment. The framework presented offers a method of understanding mental illness as existing on a multi-dimensional continuum and defines health in terms of balance and flexibility, rather than symptomology or traits. It provides a structure for categorizing a broad range of mental illness and for selecting clinical interventions based on the individual's needs. It also brings attention to the lived experience of the individual, as opposed to diagnostic criteria identified by an outside observer and highlights the importance of the here-and-now in clinical work.

This approach carries a number of benefits. First, by drawing from advances in phenomenological theory and current embodiment research, it is positioned at the forefront of research. It questions the assumption that psychiatric illness is a purely 'mental' phenomenon, an assumption that has been challenged by empirical data illustrating the substantial connection between the mind and the body. In addition, building this bridge between psychology and embodiment provides a basis for explaining phenomena such as the effectiveness of psychiatric medication and the use of body-based methods in treating mental illness. In sum, a clinical theory grounded upon embodiment most accurately reflects the latest developments in the understanding and treatment of mental illness and incorporating current research into one clinical theory provides an invaluable tool for clinicians and researchers.

Second, an approach that values the lived experience of individuals and places the choice of intervention in the hands of the individual both normalizes the range of human experience and empowers individuals to take control of their own treatment. Current diagnostic trends and societal stereotypes stigmatize mental illness, leaving those suffering from mental illness feeling ashamed, broken, or fundamentally different from others. Distinguishing between those who are 'normal' and those with mental illness creates a sense of other-ness that may leave those with diagnoses feeling helpless, incapable of reaching normalcy, while discouraging those without diagnoses from seeking treatment. The clinical theory of embodiment presented in this chapter places both mental illness and mental health on one continuum, illustrating how one can move between illness and health due to imbalance or rigidity. It offers a way for understanding how mental illness may be caused and, consequently, how it may be cured.

Third, this approach provides a language to bridge the gap between clinical language and alternative treatment methods such as yoga, meditation, dance, and the creative arts. Thus far, these treatment methods have been shown to be effective in outcome studies (eg. Koch, Kunz, Lykou, and Cruz, 2013).

However, the mechanisms by which they are effective and how they relate to mental illness remain a mystery. The proposed clinical theory includes potential mechanisms that may explain effectiveness. For instance, a treatment such as dance/movement therapy groups may work by bridging Inner and Outer experiences, as the individual simultaneously experiences internal body sensations while being seen and interacting with other members. A treatment such as yoga encourages integration of Mind and Body, as individuals are encouraged simultaneously to be mindful of their movement and to concentrate on physical sensations to achieve various poses. Thus, the proposed clinical theory offers a language to begin to explain the relationship between alternative therapies and mental health.

Finally, embracing this new approach, one grounded on embodiment and lived experiences, organizes current research while highlighting a research agenda for future investigation. Existing research can be categorized according to which continuum of health and illness it addresses. In this way, previously unrelated research and methods can be compared and integrated. Results need no longer be isolated according to field (such as social psychology versus cognitive science) or diagnosis (such as depression, trauma, or attention deficit hyperactivity disorder) but can be analysed in relation to each other and to their connection to embodied understandings of health and illness. Applying this lens of analysis may, in turn, further elucidate these complex categories and point the way towards future research questions. Each category and continuum presented in this chapter is preliminary and, thus far, very broadly defined. Much can be done to further clarify what is meant by Body/Mind, Inner/Outer, and Subject/Object. A clinical theory of embodiment thus provides the foundation both for understanding current research and lighting the way for future investigation.

It must be noted that an embodied clinical theory, based on lived experiences and the connection between mind and body, differs fundamentally from other diagnostic tools such as the DSM 5. The theoretical orientations of phenomenology, which emphasizes subjectivity and lived experience, may not be compatible with post-positivism, which emphasizes objectivity and external observation (Mertens, 2010). These differences play out in fundamental issues such as the definition of health and illness, whether or not there is one 'right' diagnosis, what training or professional role is required for the ability to give a diagnosis, and how to measure the efficacy of an intervention. Thus far, the majority of mental health treatment has spawned from the theoretical orientation of post-positivism. Phenomenological approaches, as proposed in this chapter, are gaining support from clinical practitioners but remain on the sidelines. Acknowledging this fundamental difference and contributing to a body of knowledge grounded in phenomenology and embodiment can only strengthen the dialogue between these two theoretical orientations and, in turn, increase our understanding and ability to treat mental illness.

Conclusion

Embodiment research and phenomenological theory provide the foundation for a clinical theory based on the mind-body connection and individual lived experiences. The disconnection between current clinical practice, which is grounded primarily in a disembodied conceptualization of mental illness and in an external observation of symptoms, and growing research, theory, and clinical evidence on the importance of embodied approaches, highlights the need for the development of such a theory. The proposed theory includes a framework on which individuals may be conceptualized and on which interventions can be based. This framework envisions mental illness and health as falling on a continuum and values balance and flexibility over unilateral improvement of symptoms. It identifies three axes—Decision, Identity, and Focus—on which an individual may be situated. The proposed clinical theory and associated framework represent a significant departure from current post-positivist diagnostic language and provides a structure upon which current research may be organized, empirical data may be analysed, and future research may be guided.

References

Bargh, J. A., Chen, M., and Burrows, L. (1996). Automaticity of social behavior: Direct effects of trait construct and stereotype activation on action. *Journal of Personality and Social Psychology, 71*(2), 230–244.

Benson, H., and Klipper, M. Z. (1992). *The relaxation response.* New York, NY: HarperCollins.

Cesario, J., Plaks, J. E., and Higgins, E. T. (2006). Automatic social behavior as motivated preparation to interact. *Journal of Personality and Social Psychology, 90*(6), 893–910.

Davis, M. (1997). *Guide to movement analysis methods. Part 2: Movement Psychodiagnostic Inventory* (Unpublished manual). Available from Martha Davis.

Dell, C. (1970). *Primer for movement description using effort/shape* (2nd ed.). New York, NY: Dance Notation Bureau Press.

Fuchs, T. (2010). Phenomenology and psychopathology. In D. Schmicking and S. Gallagher (Eds.), *Handbook of phenomenology and cognitive science* (pp. 547–573). Dordrecht, Netherlands: Springer Science + Business Media B.V.

Fuchs, T. (2012). The phenomenology of body memory. In S. Koch, T. Fuchs, M. Summa, and C. Müller (Eds.), *Body memory, metaphor, and movement* (pp. 9–22). Philadelphia, PA: John Benjamins Publishing Company.

Homann, K. B. (2010). Embodied concepts of neurobiology in dance/movement therapy practice. *American Journal of Dance Therapy, 32,* 80–99.

Kestenberg-Amighi, J., Loman, S., Lewis, P., and Sossin, K. M. (1999). *The meaning of movement: Developmental and clinical perspectives of the Kestenberg Movement Profile.* New York, NY: Brunner-Routledge.

Koch, S., Holland, R. W., Hengstler, M., and van Knippenberg, A. (2009). Body locomotion as regulatory process: Stepping backward enhances cognitive control. *Psychological Science, 20*(5), 549–550.

Koch, S., Kunz, T., Lykou, S., and Cruz, R. (2013). Effects of dance movement therapy and dance on health-related psychological outcomes: A meta-analysis. *The Arts in Psychotherapy, 41*(1), 46–64.

Koch, S. C. (2014). Rhythm is it: Effects of dynamic body feedback on affect, attitudes and cognition. *Frontiers in Psychology, 5,* 537.

Levy, F. (2005). *Dance movement therapy: A healing art.* Reston, VA: AHERF.

Linehan, M. M. (1993). *Skills training manual for treating borderline personality disorder.* New York, NY: Guilford.

Meier, B. P., and Robinson, M. D. (2004). Why the sunny side is up: Associations between affect and vertical position. *Psychological Science, 15*(4), 243–247.

Meier, B. P., and Robinson, M. D. (2006). Does "feeling down" mean seeing down? Depressive symptoms and vertical selective attention. *Journal of Research in Personality, 40*(4), 451–461.

Mertens, D. M. (2010). *Research and evaluation in education and psychology: Integrating diversity with quantitative, qualitative, and mixed methods* (3rd ed.). Thousand Oaks, CA: Sage Publications.

Michalak, J., Troje, N. J., Fischer, J., Vollmar, P., Heidenrech, T., and Schulte, D. (2009). Embodiment of sadness and depression: Gait patterns associated with dysphoric mood. *Psychosomatic Medicine, 71,* 580–587.

Miles, L. K., Nind, L. K., and Macrae, C. N. (2010). Moving through time. *Psychological Science, 21*(2), 222–223.

Niedenthal, P. M., Barsalou, L. W., Winkielman, P., Krauth-Gruber, S., and Ric, F. (2005). Embodiment in attitudes, social perception, and emotion. *Personality and Social Psychology Review, 9*(3), 184–211.

Pallagrosi, M. F. L., Picardi, A., and Biondi, M. (2014). Assessing clinician's subjective experience during interaction with patients. *Psychopathology, 47,* 111–118.

Pulvermüller, F. (1999). Words in the brain's language. *Behavioral and Brain Sciences, 22*(2), 253–279.

Pulvermüller, F. (2013). How neurons make meaning: Brain mechanisms for embodied and abstract-symbolic semantics. *Trends in Cognitive Sciences, 17*(9), 458–470.

Serlin, I. A. (1996). Kinesthetic imaging. *Journal of Humanistic Psychology, 36*(2), 25–33.

Soma, C. (2016). *Advanced mind-body interventions.* Harrisburg, PA: The National Institute of Trauma and Loss in Children.

van der Kolk, B. (2014). *The body keeps the score: Brain, mind, and body in the healing of trauma.* New York, NY: Penguin Books.

Williams, L. E., and Bargh, J. A. (2008). Experiencing physical warmth promotes interpersonal warmth. *Science, 322*(5901), 606–607.

4

THE EVIDENCE FOR BASIC ASSUMPTIONS OF DANCE MOVEMENT THERAPY AND BODY PSYCHOTHERAPY RELATED TO FINDINGS FROM EMBODIMENT RESEARCH

Johannes Michalak, Naomi Lyons and Thomas Heidenreich

Introduction

Body psychotherapy (BP) is defined as the treatment of mental illness or suffering with bodily and verbal methods (Büntig, 1992, p. 179) while Dance Movement Therapy (DMT) is the psychotherapeutic use of movement in terms of a process that fosters emotional and bodily integration (Trautmann-Voigt, 2003). These were established in psychotherapeutic care for mental disorders long before psychotropic drugs revolutionised their treatment (Boadella, 2002). However, the lack of emphasis on the empirical evidence base for BP right from the beginning may have been one reason why the dissemination of BP has been limited.

Looking at the contents of this book, it becomes obvious that there is a huge diversity in theories and methods ranging from ideas about the treatment of specific disorders to applying specific methods for a wide range of human problems. Even though the lack of a unifying approach that could be studied empirically led to a shortage of randomised controlled trials, in recent years there has been a growing interest in the question of evidence for DMT and BP (Geuter, 2015; Koch et al., 2014; Röhricht, 2009, 2014; Strassel, Cherkin, Steuten, Sherman, and Vrijhoef, 2011).

Röhricht (2009, 2014) and other authors (Acolin, 2016; Geuter, 2015; Tantia, 2015) formulate theoretical and practical assumptions that underlie different schools of BP and DMT focusing on their similarities in order to facilitate the process of providing empirical evidence. Some similarities are obvious, such as the assumption that there is an interaction between body, emotion and cognition. This assumption of BP, although popular in psychotherapy in general since William James (1884), goes beyond the general views on the involvement of the body as held in verbal psychotherapy. BP assumes that the body has a primary role in the development and maintenance of psychological disorders. Still, psychological research has only recently started to investigate the assumptions of BP with experimental methods that allow inferences about the causal mechanisms involved. In the past decade, embodiment research has emerged as an interdisciplinary field, focusing especially on the complex interactions between bodily, cognitive and emotional processes (Niedenthal, 2007). So far, embodiment research has mainly focused on psychological processes in healthy individuals. To further investigate this basic assumption of BP research has to focus on the population that is targeted by therapy, i.e. individuals with mental disorders.

In this chapter, we will present findings from embodiment research related to depressive disorders. Depression has a particular importance for the healthcare system as it is a mental disorder occurring in 4.4 per cent of the world's population, and accounting for the largest share in global disability and suicide deaths (World Health Organization, 2017). In contrast to the flourishing literature on brain mechanisms in depression, empirical research on the embodiment of depression is still relatively sparse. Yet there is growing interest in treating depression with BP/DMT and a first manual for depression has been presented (Röhricht, Papadopoulos, and Priebe, 2013). The literature on BP mostly presents qualitative descriptions of body posture and movement. At the same time, some indirect evidence for the significance of the body in depression comes from studies on processing emotional material in non-clinical populations. These studies have shown that the processing of emotionally negative and positive material can be influenced by bodily manipulations (e.g. Riskind and Gotay, 1982).

The purpose of this chapter is to present potential overlaps between embodiment research and assumptions held in DMT and BP. The idea of this chapter is not to give an exhaustive review of the BP/DMT literature but to use carefully selected examples that already show a link to psychological embodiment research. We will first give a brief introduction into embodiment research and then present three different basic assumptions of BP/DMT in the treatment of depression and its empirical support. In the final section of this chapter, we will review our conclusions from each subchapter.

Embodiment

As a reaction to the cognitive perspective in psychology, which restricted relevant processes of the mind to amodal cognition, some alternative approaches have been developed during the past decades. One important alternative is the growing field of research on embodiment. Embodiment expresses the notion that knowledge is grounded in bodily states and in the brain's modality-specific systems (for reviews see Niedenthal, 2007; Winkielman, Niedenthal, Wielgoz, Eelen, and Kavanagh, 2015). According to an embodied perspective, physical body position and movement can change the way people think, the conclusions they draw and the decisions they reach.

In emotion research, several theories stress the idea of embodiment (e.g. Damasio, 1994; Niedenthal, 2007; Teasdale and Barnard, 1993), proposing a complex reciprocal relationship between the bodily expression of emotion and the way in which emotional information is processed. As presented in the following sections the embodiment perspective can also be used to deepen our understanding of mental disorders and might be a useful framework for evaluating the evidence base of basic assumptions of BP and DMT.

Assumptions in embodied approaches to Body Psychotherapy and Dance Movement Therapy

Assumption 1: Body and mind are intertwined in depression

Body and dance movement psychotherapists assume that the connection between body and mind is essential for all mental processes. Thoughts, emotions, even memory, operate through a fundamental interconnection between the bodily states and the brain. Therefore, this assumption goes beyond theories that state a mutual dependence between body, emotion and cognition and often see body sensations and changes as a by-product of therapeutically caused emotional and cognitive changes (Geuter, 2015, p. 3). With its focus on the bidirectionality or rather circularity of movement and cognitive-affective processes (Fuchs and Koch, 2014; Koch, 2017), BP/DMT assumes a holistic conception of the human being that relates to a unity of body, soul and mind that is not divided into its subunits in the therapeutic process (see also Acolin, 2016).

The notion of an integrative relationship between body and mind is further elaborated by the assumption that the movements of individuals with mental disorders show inflexible and bizarre habitual patterns (Bartenieff, 2014). Narrowing the focus to depression, phenomenologists describe the body of depressed individuals as heavy and solid, putting up resistance to the individual's inner impulses (Fuchs and Schlimme, 2009). In conclusion, BP/DMT practitioners assume that in depression the body becomes rigid and opaque, preventing the regular flow between individual and environment. In other words, a person with depression may feel as if walled in by his or her body, no longer able to engage in his or her environment. The restricted movement patterns of facial expressions and the whole body are broadened to help the client to regain his or her ability to contact the surroundings. This is done by introducing new and rarely used movement patterns, proposing that this results in many different physical and emotional changes (e.g. Bartenieff, 2014).

In order to present the empirical foundations of these assumptions, we will divide the following section into subsections. In a first step, findings from embodiment research on the general relationship between body and mind in depression will be discussed on the level of dynamic and static body states. Afterwards, we will present some preliminary evidence supporting the hypotheses that in depression inflexible movement patterns that might be linked to symptoms of depression can be made more adaptable through treatment.

Evidence for the interconnection on the level of dynamic body movements

Gait patterns

To be able to state that BP/DMT may have a potential role in the treatment of depression a clear link between body and emotion and cognition in depression needs to be shown. In addition to mere descriptions (Papadopolous and Röhricht, 2014, p. 174), several studies systematically analyzed gait patterns of depressed individuals (e.g. Lemke, Wendorff, Mieth, Buhl, and Linnemann, 2000; Sloman, Berridge, Homatidis, Hunter, and Duck, 1982; Sloman, Pierrynowski, Berridge, Tupling, and Flowers, 1987). In sum, these studies show that currently depressed individuals display reduced gait velocity, stride length, increased standing phase and gait cycle duration (Wendorff, Linnemann, and Lemke, 2002). Michalak et al. (2009) conducted a study that utilised methods allowing a three-dimensional analysis of the whole body during walking. They recorded gait patterns of 14 currently depressed inpatients and 14 matched never-depressed control participants with a high temporal and spatial resolution. As a result, depressed participants walked more slowly and showed smaller arm swings than healthy participants. Remarkably, in depressed patients a larger amplitude in lateral body sway was present than in never-depressed people. When a depressed patient approaches an observer, the observer might see pronounced swaying lateral movements of the upper body. Also, a depressed patient's gait was characterised by a slumped posture and reduced vertical up-and-down movements of the upper body.

In a second study, Michalak et al. (2009, Study 2) were able to show that in a non-clinical population similar gait patterns characterised sadness. In a within-subject design, sad and happy mood were induced in a sample of undergraduate students. Again, the analysis revealed that speed, arm swing, lateral body sway, posture of the upper body, and the amplitude of vertical movement of the upper body were discriminating features between happy and sad mood.

To further elaborate the relationship between gait and mood, Michalak, Troje, and Heidenreich (2010, 2011) examined whether formerly depressed patients with a high risk of relapse show similar gait patterns to those of currently depressed and sad individuals. It was proposed that deviant gait patterns might be a trait-marker of depression, apparent not only in currently, but also in formerly depressed individuals. They found that residues of deviant gait patterns could also be observed in the formerly depressed individuals. Specifically, the latter displayed reduced walking speed and reduced vertical movements of the upper body.

Support for an effect on gait patterns through training in body awareness comes from an uncontrolled study with 23 formerly depressed patients investigating gait after Mindfulness-based cognitive therapy (MBCT) (Michalak et al., 2010). MBCT is a structured group-based program developed for relapse prevention in depression (Segal, Williams, and Teasdale, 2012). It was shown that, in patients who were trained in mindful body awareness during MBCT, walking speed was increased and lateral body sway reduced. Moreover, a trend to normalization of vertical up-and-down gait dynamics was observed. Results give a first hint that body awareness, as it is targeted in MBCT, has an effect on movement patterns in depression.

To directly test whether changes in gait have effects on processes related to depression Michalak, Rohde, and Troje (2015) conducted an experimental study that investigated effects of gait manipulation on negative memory bias. In the memory-bias task participants are presented with words that are either of positive, negative or neutral valences. Depressed individuals show an increased recall of negative self-referential material, whereas non-depressed individuals recall positive material more often. In Michalak et al.'s (2015) study, 39 undergraduates were given computerised feedback that changed their walking style in a way that was either more depressed or happier than usual. The results showed that participants in the happy condition remembered more positive than negative words. By contrast, participants who adopted a depressed walking style showed a lower difference between positive and negative recalled words. This means that non-clinical individuals walking in a depressed way showed memory characteristics that resembled those of depressed individuals.

Head movement

Another dynamic aspect of the body that has been studied in embodiment research on depression is head movement. Rahona, Ruiz Fernández, Roke, Vázquez, and Hervás (2014) induced sad mood in 42 undergraduate students and afterwards showed them positively valenced pictures with two green dots that were aligned either vertically or horizontally. Instructions were to look from one dot to the other, simulating a nodding (vertically aligned dots) or a shaking (horizontally aligned dots) of the head. When participants were asked to shake their heads, the depressive mood was more stable in participants who had a higher initial depression score than when they were asked to nod.

In summary, the studies on gait patterns and head movements of depressed and formerly depressed individuals show that emotional processes and the motor system are closely interconnected. Moreover, they preliminarily indicate that motoric processes such as gait can be modified through body awareness training or feedback and that the modification of motoric processes can change depressed processes.

Evidence on the interconnection on the level of static body states: Sitting posture

Evidence from static body states comes from studies focusing on sitting posture (Riskind and Gotay, 1982; Veenstra, Schneider, and Koole, 2017). A study conducted on the effect of sitting posture on memory bias in depression illustrates an equally strong connection between body and emotion (Michalak, Mischnat, and Teismann, 2014) as in gait studies. In this experimental study, 30 depressed inpatients were randomly assigned to either a slumped or an upright sitting posture and presented with the memory-bias task described above. Participants sitting in a slumped position showed a depressive memory bias, remembering significantly more negative words than positive. However, this bias disappeared in the group of participants who were seated in an upright non-depressed posture. Results indicate that the body influences cognitive-emotional processes that are asserted to be crucial for the maintenance of depression.

Treatment of restricted movement patterns

Assuming that depressed individuals show inflexible or restricted movement patterns, BP/DMT propose that extension of the movement repertory changes emotional and cognitive experiencing. Hence, training an individual with depression to adopt new movements or posture styles might lead to a movement flexibilisation and more psychological well-being. Preliminary evidence for this assumption from the embodiment perspective comes from Michalak et al.'s (2014) study described above. Patients with depression show a slumped body posture associated with a memory bias for negative stimuli. When the patient's posture is altered in its sitting style – namely, sitting in an upright manner – effects on memory bias could be shown.

Further evidence for effects of changes in movement patterns on depression was obtained in a study by Koch, Morlinghaus, and Fuchs (2007). They assigned 31 currently depressed patients to one of the following three conditions: (1) *dance condition*: performing a traditional upbeat circle dance characterised by pronounced up-and-down movements, (2) *music condition*: listening to music without dancing and (3) *home trainer bike condition*: moving on a home trainer bike up to the same level of arousal as the dance group. Depression scores most strongly decreased, and vitality scores most strongly increased in the dance condition. Pure bodily arousal, as in the home trainer bike condition, did not affect depression and vitality scores as much. These results indicate that even short changes of movement patterns might causally influence depressive mood.

On a more basic level, results on exercise as a therapy method for depression can be discussed as well (for a review, see Cooney et al., 2013). Individuals with depression who are instructed to do regular exercises showed a reduction in symptomatology similar to that in cognitive psychotherapy (Cooney et al., 2013). Exercise is defined as a planned, structured and repetitive bodily movement that has the aim to improve or maintain physical fitness (American College of Sports Medicine, 2001). Even though mechanisms are not clear, it can be assumed that an increase in movement generally improves symptoms of depression.

Are body and mind intertwined in depression?

In sum, results discussed in this subchapter indicate a correlational relationship between body and mind in depression. However, it should be noted that it is not yet possible to firmly state that the body is a relevant causal factor in the development or maintenance of depression. Currently, there is only evidence from studies on short-term body manipulations on depression-related cognitive processes. Longitudinal studies on the effects of posture or movements on depressive symptoms are lacking. Moreover, it is not yet possible to state that broadening the movement repertoire of a client with depression is a causal mechanism for the effect of BP/DMT on depression. One important reason for this is the lack of BP/DMT studies on mediating mechanisms showing that changes in body movement and posture precede changes in symptomatology (for a discussion of methods to study mechanisms of change in psychotherapy, see Kazdin, 2007).

Assumption 2: There is reduced body awareness in depression

Body awareness is defined as an attentional focus on and awareness of internal body sensations (Mehling et al., 2009). It is often measured by interoceptive sensitivity, that is, the ability to perceive inner physical states of the body (Craig, 2002) such as the ability to accurately perceive one's heartbeat or gastric movement. Price and Thompson define body awareness as 'the ability to identify and experience inner sensations of the body [. . .] and the overall emotional/physiologic state of the body [. . .]. [It] also involves attending to bodily information in daily life, noticing bodily changes/responses to emotion and/or environment' (Price and Thompson, 2007, p. 947). Mehling et al. (2009), however, present body awareness as a conglomerate of proprioception and interoception.

Most BP and DMT schools assume that there is a reduction in body awareness in mental disorder or at least that an improvement in body awareness would lead a client to better come into contact with his or her emotions (Acolin, 2016; Tantia, 2015). In the following, we will first discuss whether research supports the assumption that in depression reduced body awareness can be found. Afterwards, the treatment of body awareness will be illuminated. In a last step, we will present a questionnaire designed to measure body awareness.

Reduced interoceptive sensitivity in depression

A lack of interoceptive sensitivity in depressed individuals has been observed in a number of empirical studies (for review see Harshaw, 2015) and acts as a foundation for many BP and DMT approaches as well as for mindfulness-based therapies and other contemplative interventions for depression (e.g. Geuter, 2015, p. 135; Segal et al., 2012). Terhaar, Viola, Bär, and Debener (2012) compared 16 depressed patients with 16 healthy controls using a heartbeat perception task that measures the accuracy in detecting one's heartbeat. This task is widely used to capture interoceptive sensitivity. Terhaar et al. (2012) could show that depressed patients showed significantly reduced heartbeat perception accuracy with an effect size of $d = 0.85$. However, studies addressing interoceptive sensitivity in depression are so far only correlational. More research with longitudinal study designs is needed to clarify whether the strong assumption of BP/DMT on the causal role of reduced interoceptive sensitivity in depression can be maintained.

Alexithymia in depression

Alexithymia is a construct developed by Sifneos (1973) referring to the inability to identify and describe one's feelings. It has been studied in a number of mental disorders including depression. A meta-analysis found that individuals with depression showed a medium correlation of alexithymia total score and depression ($r = 0.46$). Several studies have also directly demonstrated a close connection between alexithymia and interoceptive awareness (Herbert, Herbert, and Pollatos, 2011). Herbert et al. (2011) even suggest that interoceptive awareness might be a predictor for alexithymia as the ability of feeling one's bodily states might be a necessary precondition for feeling one's emotions.

In a study comparing healthy individuals with depressed patients, the neural correlates of alexithymia and interoceptive awareness were examined (Wiebking and Northoff, 2015). In healthy subjects a high association between higher alexithymia scores and an increase in insula and decrease in supragenual anterior cingulate cortex activity during a heartbeat perception task was found. In depressed subjects with high alexithymia scores the increase of insula activity could not be found. As insula activity is related to somatic and emotional awareness results were interpreted such that healthy subjects compensate for their high alexithymia with a stronger activation of the insula while depressed individuals are not able to compensate for high alexithymia.

In sum, there is a clear connection between depression and the inability to identify and describe one's emotions even though this correlation is not exclusively found for depression. Nevertheless, the causal factors of this relationship remain unknown. Preliminary evidence suggests a neural network that is similar for alexithymia and interoception and assumes that physical changes and the interoception of them are the first step to the feeling of emotions.

Theoretical reflections on the treatment of body awareness from body psychotherapy and dance movement therapy perspectives

In BP as well as in DMT, enriching body awareness is assumed to be the first step on the path to mental health (Acolin, 2016; Tantia, 2015). While learning to better sense their body, clients focus on experience in the here and now. Tantia (2015) argues that when an individual experiences his or her body or the surroundings through his or her body, self-knowledge is fostered. This self-knowledge might be especially important in depression for two different reasons.

Firstly, as the body plays a central role in emotions, mindfully coming into contact with one's body also means coming into contact with one's emotions. People with a history of depression often report that they become aware of their negative mood only after it has grown into a full-blown episode of depression. Correspondingly, improved body awareness might help people with emotional vulnerabilities to realise very early when dysfunctional emotional processes are escalating. Administering training that focuses on raising awareness of the body might assist formerly depressed individuals to be aware of subtle bodily signs of depressive mood. Increased body awareness might help them to react to signs of possible escalation with more awareness instead of acting out dysfunctional automatic reactions to their mood states (e.g. excessive rumination).

A slightly different aspect is emphasised by Fuchs and Schlimme (2009); they argue that psychological disorders such as depression affect a pre-reflective embodied sense of self. They postulate that in psychological disorders the person's being-in-the-world might be affected. From this perspective, mental disorders manifest themselves in particular disturbances of embodied existence, even if only in very basic 'existential feelings' (such as existential feelings of encapsulation). As BP/DMT might shape the awareness of existential feelings (i.e. the pre-reflective and mostly non-verbal sense of self as connected with the environment), it could be supposed that BP/DMT can help clients identify these subtle forms of disturbances at an earlier stage. For example, a person who comes into contact with his or her embodied self might sense a feeling of encapsulation on a concrete and embodied level. Moreover, through the experiential and lived contact with the body and its connection with the environment, BP/DMT might reduce tendencies towards such existential feelings of encapsulation.

In their manual for depression, Röhricht et al. (2013) describe addressing reduced self-awareness through increasing body awareness as the first component of the treatment. Depression is assumed to be a mental disorder that is realised in, and through the body, which makes it important to focus on the awareness of subtle body experiences.

Although there is no study investigating the causal relationship of interoceptive awareness training and symptomatology improvement in depression, there are a few studies analyzing this connection in healthy subjects. In a study with a total of 318 healthy participants, a contemplative training was applied for nine months (Bornemann and Singer, 2016). After six months including body awareness training, heartbeat perception accuracy improved as well as emotional awareness, defined as a low score of alexithymia. The results give a first hint that raising body awareness might be useful in depression because it improves interoceptive and emotional awareness.

A further study supporting the assumption of the relevance of body awareness in depression was conducted by Burg and Michalak (2011). They investigated the clinical relevance of maintaining contact with one's body while mindfully breathing. Specifically, the authors examined the associations between a mindful breathing exercise (MBE) and depression-related variables, namely rumination and depressive symptoms. In the MBE, participants were instructed to observe and sense their breathing for about 18 minutes and to return to their breathing whenever they lose the mindful sensation of it. Within this time period, participants were prompted at irregular intervals to indicate whether they have lost contact with their breathing as a result of mind-wandering. Moreover, participants were requested to indicate states of mindlessness every time they notice them on their own. The results showed that people who were more able to remain in contact with their body during breathing meditation reported less rumination and fewer depressive symptoms. Correspondingly, reduced rumination might be a mediator between improved body awareness and reduced depressive symptomatology. However, it should be noted that other causal interpretations of this correlational pattern are also possible. For example, it might be easier for non-ruminators to stay focused on their breathing.

Neurobiological correlates of body awareness improvement

Another string of research on the effect of mindfulness can be found in neurobiological studies. In a study with functional magnetic resonance imaging, Farb, Mayberg, Bean, McKeon, and Segel (2010) could show that mindfulness resulted in a greater right-lateralised recruitment, including visceral and somatosensory areas associated with body sensation after the induction of sadness. Specifically, during a dysphoric challenge they found reduced deactivation in the insula in participants of an eight-week mindfulness training compared to a wait-list control group. The reduced deactivation is claimed to be an indicator of increased interoceptive awareness in the mindfulness group. Moreover, they found an association between the greater somatic recruitment during evoked sadness and decreased depression scores. A similar study analyzed the density of gray matter before and after mindfulness training (Hölzel et al., 2011), showing that the density in the temporo-parietal junction and the cerebellum increased after training. The temporo-parietal junction is an area involved in the conscious experience of self and the embodiment processes. The cerebellum is involved in the regulation of movement as well as emotional processes. These two findings suggest that mindfulness training (which emphasises body awareness) increases neurological correlates of body awareness and partly that this heightened body awareness has beneficial effects on depression. Still, none of these studies was conducted on individuals with depression.

Measuring body awareness

In order to measure body awareness more directly, the Body Mindfulness Questionnaire was developed (BMQ, Burg et al., 2017). It comprises two factors: 'Experiencing Body Awareness' and 'Appreciating Body Awareness'. Results show moderate positive associations of the first factor with other mindfulness scales and negative correlations with clinical variables, such as perceived stress, neuroticism, rumination, as well as depressive symptoms.

In sum, from a neurobiological as well as from a behavioural stance the findings indicate that an increase in mindful body awareness reduces depressive symptomatology. Although more research is needed on causal mechanisms in individuals with depression, this supports the rationale of BP/DMT, which aim to ameliorate body awareness to improve psychological health.

Assumption 3: In depression negative feelings towards one's own body are present

A negative feeling related to one's own body can be found in depression when looking at research on body image, body-esteem or body satisfaction. Correspondingly, body and dance movement psychotherapists assume that fostering a positive feeling towards one's body is a powerful tool in treating depression (Röhricht et al., 2013). One way to reach a more positive feeling for one's body is to heighten positive experiences one makes through one's body. In this subchapter we will first present results that indicate a depressed individual's negative attitude towards his or her body. Afterwards, the possible path of experiencing positive affect through sensing one's body will be described.

Negative attitude towards one's body in depression

Among others, constructs related to the attitude towards one's body, such as body image, often function as an outcome variable in research on the effectiveness of BP/DMT in depression (Koch et al., 2014). Several studies have found dissatisfaction with one's own body in depression, suggesting that self-criticism is important in the attitude towards one's body (Baker, Williamson, and Sylve, 1995). Marsella, Shizuru, Brennan, and Kameoka (1981) administered a body-image satisfaction scale, showing that depressed respondents had higher levels of body-image dissatisfaction overall and across 17 different body areas than non-depressed controls. Moreover, in an experimental study on the effect of negative mood on body-image disturbance, Baker et al. (1995) were able to show that experimentally-induced negative mood stimulated dysfunctional body size estimation and body dysphoria in healthy women, which might be effective in depressive disorders as well.

In an attempt to highlight the importance of the appreciation of the body, the scale 'Appreciating Body Awareness' of the BMQ mentioned above measures an affectionate, openhearted and interested attention towards the body (Burg et al., 2017). It significantly (negatively) correlated with depression in college students suggesting not only that body image is disturbed in depression, but also that the appreciation of the body might be distorted as well.

In summary, it can be concluded that enhanced body dissatisfaction concerning body image can be found in depression. Nevertheless, to our knowledge, there are no studies that permit firm conclusions about a causal role of negative attitudes towards one's body for the development and maintenance of depressive disorders. Moreover, evidence is lacking on the effectiveness of embodied psychotherapy methods directly targeting body image in depression.

Positive affect through experiencing one's body in depression

BP/DMT postulates that experiencing the body can be a source of positive affect. Relevant experiences are not only related to one's body in a static way but to the movement of the body as well. A client can learn a sense of agency when moving and employing his or her body as a source of positive affect (Sheets-Johnstone, 2010). In mindfulness training this aspect can be found as well. It is assumed that besides the focus on coming into contact with avoided and negative emotional patterns, the body, if sensed in an aware and non-judgmental way, can be a valuable positive resource (Michalak, Burg, and Heidenreich, 2012a, 2012b).

Tentative evidence for the assumption that positive affect emerges through sensing one's body finds support in a study on the effect of MBCT (Geschwind, Peeters, Drukker, van Os, and Wichers, 2011). Participants with residual symptoms of depression stated their positive emotions and appraisal of pleasant activities in daily life for six days before and after the intervention period. Results showed that in the MBCT group a significant increase of positive emotions and appraisal of pleasant activities could be found. Although this study did not focus on the body as the source of increased positive emotions, it can be speculated that, since MBCT entails intensive training in body awareness, at least parts of the effects of MBCT on positive emotions might be mediated by the increased body contact. More direct evidence for the effects of MBCT on positive affect through experiencing one's body was observed in the study of Burg et al. (2017). In chronically depressed patients a significant increase in the 'Appreciating Body Awareness' scales of the BMQ was specific to MBCT but was not observed in the treatment as usual condition.

Conclusion

The aim of the present chapter was to link prominent assumptions held in BP/DMT to empirical findings from embodiment research in depression. As every school has different basic assumptions we have focused on three fundamental assumptions of BP and DMT and reviewed their empirical basis.

Overall, we found preliminary evidence supporting all three fundamental assumptions. Firstly, clinical studies have demonstrated that body and mind might be intertwined in depression (assumption 1). Secondly, there is evidence for diminished body awareness in depression (assumption 2) and, third, for the fact that depressed individuals show negative feelings towards their own body (assumption 3).

As do other authors investigating the evidence base of basic assumptions in DMT, we find that much of this research is correlational in nature and a strong empirical test of many of the basic assumptions of BP/DMT is lacking (Acolin, 2016). For example, there are no studies allowing unambiguous *causal* inferences on the role of dysfunctional or inflexible movement patterns or posture in the aetiology of depression. Longitudinal and experimental studies are needed to draw stronger conclusions on basic assumptions of BP/DMT. Moreover, there are only a few studies testing the specific effects of treatment components in BP/DMT beyond unspecific factors such as alliance, expectations, social components, music, physical training and others (Strassel et al., 2011). Exceptions are from two studies in DMT conducted by Koch et al. (2007) and Koch (2014) finding promising specific effects of dance and specific movement patterns. However, more component studies or research using mediational analysis are needed to elucidate the contribution of body interventions to the overall effect of BP/DMT. This lack of unequivocal causal evidence is also characteristic for assumptions 2 and 3, which we reviewed in this chapter. Moreover, there are other assumptions of BP/DMT, which we did not review in this chapter, within general an even more limited evidence base (for further information on such assumptions, especially in DMT, see Acolin, 2016). For example, many schools of BP/DMT conjecture that fostering emotional expression to enable the expression of suppressed negative impulses is an important way to improve psychological health in depression. This method has its roots in the psychodynamic therapy of depression that asserts a link between depressive mood and suppressed aggression

(Busch, Rudden, and Shapiro, 2004). In addition, many BP and DMT practitioners suppose that physical states have a symbolic meaning developed through early pre-verbal experiences that are held in affect-motoric schemes (Downing, 1996; Tantia, 2015). To our knowledge, there is no empirical evidence supporting these assumptions yet.

However, to make a balanced estimate of the evidence base of BP/DMT it should be noted that even in cognitive behavioural therapy (CBT), an approach with a keen focus on empirical evidence, some of the fundamental assumptions have so far not been unequivocally proven. For example, evidence for the fundamental assumption of CBT that cognitive change is the specific mechanism underlying CBT is far from conclusive (Wampold and Imel, 2015).

Consequently, there is a long way to go to rigorously test the fundamental assumptions of BP/DMT on aetiology models and mechanisms of change and to prove effectiveness. But it is a path worth following considering the potential that lies in the more systematic inclusion of the body as a resource for healing. Testing basic assumptions may help to more precisely shape the theory and the interventions of BP/DMT. Moreover, consolidating the evidence base of BP/DMT can be a driving force to improve the dissemination of these interventions.

References

Acolin, J. (2016). The mind-body connection in dance/movement therapy: Theory and empirical support. *American Journal of Dance Therapy, 38*, 311–333.

American College of Sports Medicine (2001). *ACSM's Resource Manual for Guidelines for Exercise Testing and Prescription* (Vol. 4). Lippincott, Williams and Wilkins.

Baker, J. D., Williamson, D. A., and Sylve, C. (1995). Body image disturbance, memory bias, and body dysphoria: Effects of negative mood induction. *Behavior Therapy, 26*, 747–759.

Bartenieff, I. (2014). Tanztherapie. In E. Wilke, G. Hölter, and H. G. Petzold (Eds.), *Tanztherapie – Theorie und Praxis* (pp. 203–226). Wiesbaden: Reichert Verlag.

Boadella, D. (2002). Die erweckung der sensibilität und die wiederentdeckung der motilität. Psychophysikalische synthese als grundlage der körperpsychotherapie: Das 100-jährige vermächtnis von Pierre Janet (1859–1947). *Psychotherapie Forum, 10*, 13–21.

Bornemann, B., and Singer, T. (2017). Taking time to feel our body: Steady increases in heartbeat perception accuracy and decreases in alexithymia over 9 months of contemplative mental training. *Psychophysiology, 54*(3), 469–482.

Büntig, W. (1992). Die entfaltung der beziehung in der körperpsychotherapie. In P. Buchheim et al. (Eds.), *Liebe und Psychotherapie. Der Körper in der Psychotherapie. Weiterbildungsforschung* (S. 172–188). Berlin, Heidelberg: Springer.

Burg, J. M., and Michalak, J. (2011). The healthy quality of mindful breathing: Associations with rumination and depression. *Cognitive Research and Therapy, 35*(2), 179–185.

Burg, J. M., Probst, T. H., Heidenreich, T., and Michalak, J. (2017). Development and psychometric evaluation of the Body Mindfulness Questionnaire. *Mindfulness, 8*(3), 807–818.

Busch, F. N., Rudden, M., and Shapiro, T. (2004). *Psychodynamic Treatment of Depression*. Washington, DC: American Psychiatric Association.

Cooney, G. M., Dwan, K., Greig, C. A., Lawlor, D. A., Rimer, J., Waugh, E. R. . . . Mead, G. E. (2013). Exercise for depression. *Cochrane Database for Systematic Reviews, 9*, CD004366.

Craig, A. D. (2002). How do you feel? Interoception: The sense of the physiological condition of the body. *Nature Reviews Neuroscience, 3*, 655–666.

Damasio, A. R. (1994). *Decartes' Error. Emotion, Reason, and the Human Brain*. New York, NY: Avon Books.

Downing, G. (1996). *Körper und Wort in der Psychotherapie.* [Body and Word in Psychotherapy]. München: Kösel.

Farb, N. A. S., Mayberg, H., Bean, J., McKeon, D., and Segel, Z. V. (2010). Minding one's emotions: Mindfulness training alters the neural expression of sadness. *Emotion, 10*, 25–33.

Fuchs, T., and Koch, S. C. (2014). Embodied affectivity: On moving and being moved. *Frontiers in Psychology, 5*, 508.

Fuchs, T., and Schlimme, J. E. (2009). Embodiment and psychopathology: A phenomenological perspective. *Current Opinion in Psychiatry, 22*, 570–575.

Geschwind, N., Peeters, F., Drukker, M., van Os, J., and Wichers, M. (2011). Mindfulness training increases momentary positive emotions and reward experience in adults vulnerable to depression: A randomized controlled trial. *Journal of Consulting and Clinical Psychology, 79*(5), 618–628.

Geuter, U. (2015). *Körperpsychotherapie – Grundriss einer Theorie für die Klinische Praxi* [Body Psychotherapy. Outlines of a Theory for Clinical Practice]. Berlin: Springer.

Harshaw, C. (2015). Interoceptive dysfunction: Toward an integrated framework for understanding somatic and affective disturbance in depression. *Psychological Bulletin, 141*(2), 311–363.

Herbert, B. M., Herbert, C., and Pollatos, O. (2011). On the relationship between interoceptive awareness and alexithymia: Is interoceptive awareness related to emotional awareness? *Journal of Personality, 79*(5), 1149–1175.

Hölzel, B. K., Carmody, J., Vangel, M., Congleton, C., Yerramsetti, S. M., Gard, T., and Lazar, S. W. (2011). Mindfulness practice leads to increases in regional brain gray matter density. *Psychiatry Research, 191*(1), 36–43.

James, W. (1884). What is an emotion? *Mind, 9*, 188–205.

Kazdin, A. E. (2007). Mediators and mechanisms of change in psychotherapy research. *Annual Reviews in Clinical Psychology, 3*, 1–27.

Koch, S. C. (2014). Rhythm is it: Effects of dynamic body feedback on affect and attitudes. *Frontiers in Psychology, 5*, 537. doi:10.3389/fpsyg.2014.00537

Koch, S. C. (2017). Arts and health: Active factors and a theory framework of embodied aesthetics. *The Arts in Psychotherapy, 54*, 85–91.

Koch, S. C., Morlinghaus, K., and Fuchs, T. (2007). The joy dance – Specific effects of a single dance intervention on psychiatric patients with depression. *The Arts in Psychotherapy, 34*, 340–349.

Koch, S., Kunz, T., Lykou, S., and Cruz, R. (2014). Effects of dance movement therapy and dance on health-related psychological outcomes: A meta-analysis. *The Arts in Psychotherapy, 41*, 46–64.

Lemke, M. R., Wendorff, T., Mieth, B., Buhl, K., and Linnemann, M. (2000). Spatiotemporal gait patterns during over ground locomotion in major depression compared with healthy controls. *Journal of Psychiatric Research, 34*, 277–283.

Marsella, A. J., Shizuru, L., Brennan, J., and Kameoka, V. (1981). Depression and body image satisfaction. *Journal of Cross-Cultural Psychology, 12*(3), 360–371.

Mehling, W. E., Gopisetty, V., Daubenmier, J., Price, C. J., Hecht, F. M., and Stewart, A. (2009). Body awareness: Construct and self-report measures. *PLoS ONE, 4*(5), e5614.

Michalak, J., Burg, J., and Heidenreich, T. (2012a). Don't forget your body: Mindfulness, embodiment, and the treatment of depression. *Mindfulness, 3*, 190–199.

Michalak, J., Burg, J. M., and Heidenreich, T. (2012b). Mindfulness, embodiment, and depression. In S. C. Koch, T. Fuchs, M. Summa, and C. Müller (Eds.), *Movement and Body Memory – Interdisciplinary Perspectives* (pp. 393–413). Amsterdam: John Benjamins.

Michalak, J., Mischnat, J., and Teismann, T. (2014). Sitting posture makes a difference – Embodiment effects of depressive memory bias. *Clinical Psychology and Psychotherapy, 21*, 519–524.

Michalak, J., Rohde, K., and Troje, N. F. (2015). How we walk affects what we remember: Gait modifications through biofeedback change negative affective memory bias. *Journal of Behavior Therapy and Experimental Psychiatry, 46*, 121–125.

Michalak, J., Troje, N. F., and Heidenreich, T. (2010). Embodied effects of mindfulness-based cognitive therapy. *Journal of Psychosomatic Research, 68*, 312–313.

Michalak, J., Troje, N., and Heidenreich, T. (2011). The effects of mindfulness-based cognitive therapy on depressive gait patterns. *Journal of Cognitive and Behavioral Psychotherapies, 11*, 13–27.

Michalak, J., Troje, N., Heidenreich, T., Fischer, J., Vollmar, P., and Schulte, D. (2009). The embodiment of sadness and depression – Gait patterns associated with dysphoric mood. *Psychosomatic Medicine, 71*, 580–587.

Niedenthal, P. M. (2007). Embodying emotion. *Science, 316*, 1002–1005.

Papadopoulos, N. L. R., and Röhricht, F. (2014). An investigation into the application and processes of manualized group body psychotherapy for depressive disorder in a clinical trial. *Body, Movement and Dance in Psychotherapy, 9*(3), 167–180.

Price, C. J., and Thompson, E. A. (2007). Measuring dimensions of body connection: Body awareness and bodily dissociation. *Journal of Alternative and Complementary Medicine, 13*(9), 945–953.

Rahona, J. J., Ruiz Fernández, S., Roke, B., Vázquez, C., and Hervás, G. (2014). Overt head movements moderate the effect of depressive symptoms on mood regulation. *Cognition and Emotion, 28*(7), 1328–1337.

Riskind, J. H., and Gotay, C. C. (1982). Physical posture: Could it have regulatory or feedback effects on motivation and emotion? *Motivation and Emotion, 6*(3), 273–298.

Röhricht, F. (2009). Body oriented psychotherapy. The state of the art in empirical research and evidence-based practice: A clinical perspective. *Body, Movement and Dance in Psychotherapy, 4*(2), 135–156.

Röhricht, F. (2014). Body psychotherapy for the treatment of severe mental disorders – An overview. *Body, Movement and Dance in Psychotherapy, 10*(1), 51–67.

Röhricht, F., Papadopoulos, N., and Priebe, S. (2013). An exploratory randomized controlled trial of body psychotherapy for patients with chronic depression. *Journal of Affective Disorders, 151*, 85–91.

Segal, Z. V., Williams, J. M. G., and Teasdale, J. D. (2012). *Mindfulness-Based Cognitive Therapy for Depression* (2nd edn.). New York, NY: Guilford Press.

Sheets-Johnstone, M. (2010). Kinesthetic experience: Understanding movement inside and out. *Body, Movement and Dance in Psychotherapy, 5*(2), 111–127.

Sifneos, P. E. (1973). The prevalence of "alexithymic" characteristic mechanisms in psychosomatic patients. *Psychotherapy and Psychosomatics, 21*, 133–136.

Sloman, L., Berridge, M., Homatidis, S., Hunter, D., and Duck, T. (1982). Gait patterns of depressed patients and normal subjects. *American Journal of Psychiatry, 139*, 94–97.

Sloman, L., Pierrynowski, M., Berridge, M., Tupling, S., and Flowers, J. (1987). Mood, depressive illness and gait patterns. *The Canadian Journal of Psychiatry, 32*, 190–193.

Strassel, J. K., Cherkin, D. C., Steuten, L., Sherman, K. J., and Vrijhoef, H. J. M. (2011). A systematic review of the evidence for the effectiveness of dance therapy. *Alternative Therapies, 17*(3), 50–59.

Tantia, J. F. (2015). The interface between somatic psychotherapy and dance/movement therapy: A critical analysis. *Body, Movement and Dance in Psychotherapy, 11*(2–3), 181–196.

Teasdale, J. D., and Barnard, P. J. (1993). *Affect, Cognition and Change: Remodelling Depressive Thought.* Hove: Lawrence Erlbaum Associates.

Terhaar, J., Viola, F. C., Bär, K.-J., and Debener, S. (2012). Heartbeat evoked potentials mirror altered body perception in depressed patients. *Clinical Neurophysiology, 123*(10), 1950–1957.

Trautmann-Voigt, S. (2003). Tanztherapie – Zum aktuellen Diskussionsstand in Deutschland [Dance Therapy – Current discussions in Germany]. *Psychotherapeut, 48*, 215–229.

Veenstra, L., Schneider, I. K., and Koole, S. L. (2017). Embodied mood regulation: The impact of body posture on mood recovery, negative thoughts, and mood-congruent recall. *Cognition and Emotion, 31*(7), 1361–1376.

Wampold, B. E., and Imel, Z. E. (2015). *The Great Psychotherapy Debate: The Evidence for What Makes Therapy Work.* New York, NY: Routlegde.

Wendorff, T., Linnemann, M., and Lemke, M. R. (2002). Lokomotion und depression [Locomotion and depression]. *Fortschritte der Neurologie, Psychiatrie, 70*, 289–296.

Wiebking, C., and Northoff, G. (2015). Neural activity during interoceptive awareness and its associations with alexithymia – An fMRI study in major depressive disorder and non-psychiatric controls. *Frontiers in Psychology, 6*, 589.

Winkielman, P., Niedenthal, P., Wielgoz, J., Eelen, J., and Kavanagh, L. C. (2015). Embodiment of cognition and emotion. In M. Mikulincewr and P. R. Shaver (Eds.), *APA Handbook of Personality and Social Psychology* (Vol. 1, pp. 151–175). Washington, DC: American Psychological Association.

World Health Organization. (2017). *Depression and Other Common Mental Disorders – Global Health Estimates.* Geneva: Author.

5

HAVING A BODY AND MOVING YOUR BODY

Distinguishing somatic psychotherapy[1] from dance/movement therapy[2]

Jennifer Tantia

Introduction

Our body is the place from which we live, breathe and respond to our world, and embodied experience is the very nature of human phenomenological existence. While cognition allows us to travel into the past (in memory or regrets) and the future (planning or worry), the body exists solely in the present moment. In this author's view, somatic psychotherapy (SP) and dance/movement therapy (DMT) are approaches to emotional health that recognise embodied experience as the evidential source of self-awareness, self-comportment and interpersonal intelligence. They also acknowledge elements of body awareness such as breathing, posture and gesture to identify and address emotional content. One might ask then, if they are so similar, why do they have different names, training, accreditations and different professional organisations, and would it be advantageous for a patient to seek out one over the other? Following the findings of Tsakiris, Longo, and Haggard (2010), that distinguish differences in neurological correlates between having a body and moving your body, this chapter, although not exhaustive in its analysis[3], will offer an overview of how the two disciplines animate the emerging paradigm of embodied knowledge in psychotherapy and identify the differences of each discipline's practice.

The problem with nonverbal phenomena

The fields of cognitive psychology (Lakoff and Johnson, 1999; Varela, Thompson, and Rosch, 2017), sociology (Ignatow, 2007), anthropology (Csordas, 1993) and neuroscience (Damasio, 2000; Porges, 2011) have recently recognised embodied experience as a necessity for emotional healing and interpersonal connection. However, this is not a new concept. As early as the 1920s body-oriented practitioners were seeking how embodied knowledge can facilitate psychological healing. In Europe, Charlotte Selver (Lowe and Laeng-Gilliatt, 2007) was developing Sensory Awareness while studying how body movement informs emotion with Elsa Gindler in Berlin (Heller, 2012). In the 1930s Wilhelm Reich, a student of Freud, was exploring how the body contributes to, or hinders, emotional health. Reich began to develop his own following, with both Alexander Lowen and John Pierrakos evolving their own practices based on Reich's original theory (Heller, 2012). Not long after, Fritz Perls moved from Europe to New York in 1946 to work with Reich following the Second World War (Kripal, 2007). Perls developed what is now known as Gestalt Therapy, a form of psychotherapy that involves a keen attention to embodiment (Clemmons, 2012; Frank, 2001; Kepner, 1999) as a means toward cultivating the 'here and now' (Yontef, 1969, pp. 33–34) experience in the psychotherapeutic setting.

Concurrently in the United States in the 1940s, dancer and dance teacher Marian Chace began to experiment with music and expressive movement as forms of communication with psychiatric patients at St. Elizabeth's Hospital in Washington, DC (Levy, 2006). Mary White-house, who was also a dancer and a Jungian analyst, developed a style of healing called 'moving in depth', today known as a form of dance/movement therapy called Authentic Movement. Influenced by the humanistic potential movement, led by Aldous Huxley (1932) and Abraham Maslow (1943), these pioneers began to meet in 1962 at a spiritual resort called the Esalen Institute in Big Sur, California, to explore their common perspectives on the healing effects of embodied awareness (Kripal, 2007).

These pioneers, in both the United States and in Europe, not only discussed their ideas but experimented with their therapeutic techniques on each other, and most of them were not writers or formal researchers. Their informal approach juxtaposed them from clinical researchers who conducted experiments that were reported in peer-reviewed journals. Stringent testing and formal publication of clinical research is still the gold standard for what is considered knowledge and therefore is favoured over experiential, practice-based evidence. Embodied psychotherapies remain out of mainstream visibility due to the lack of sufficient evidence-based research acknowledged by the scientific community as the way to engage with health service providers, although there exist several peer-reviewed journals in the field. Despite their empirical shortcomings, somatic psychotherapy and dance/movement therapy are beginning to gain recognition from traditional psychology researchers and psychotherapists, as SP and DMT researchers continue to publish in traditional peer-reviewed journals (Tantia, 2017, slides 10, 11) and leaders from outer fields are increasingly involved in keynote talks at SP/DMT conferences. This may be partly due to the newly emerging research-based doctoral programs in dance/movement therapy and somatics that have been developed in formal educational settings within the past 10 years.

Embodiment as a lived paradigm

Over a decade ago, sociologist Ignatow (2007) stated that culturally we are in a 'post cognitive revolution' (p. 116) that is beginning to embrace the psychological importance of embodied awareness. Sensation and emotion are intricately woven into a system of knowing that is direct, subjective and nonverbal, and can be experienced prior to meaning-making. Anthropologist Csordas (1993) introduces 'somatic modes of attention' (p. 138) as a paradigm shift in anthropological phenomenology. 'Somatic modes of attention are culturally elaborated ways of attending to and with one's body in surroundings that include the embodied presence of others' (p. 138). He further distinguishes the difference between attending to one's physical body from an embodied state of awareness: '. . . the body is a biological, material entity, while embodiment can be understood as an indeterminate methodological field defined by perceptual experience and the mode of presence and engagement in the world' (p. 135). Csordas' distinction between attention to and attention with the body reflects what somatic and dance/movement therapists have been practicing as a source of emotional knowledge in the psychotherapeutic process for decades.

Somatic psychotherapy and dance/movement therapy support embodiment as a living source of knowledge that provides information about an individual beyond what can be logistically determined (Bloom, 2006; Frank, 2001; Hervey, 2007; Kaylo, 2006; Koch and Fuchs, 2011).

In an earlier publication on mindfulness and dance/movement therapy for healing trauma (Tantia, 2014), the distinction is made that attention to one's embodied experience is part of the process of mindfulness (a practice within somatic psychotherapy), while attention *with* the body is the enlivened and spontaneous response to that attention, expressed as a full-bodied movement, a smile, or a meaningful gesture, often described in dance/movement therapy.

Developmental psychologists (The Boston Change Process Study Group, 2010; Stern, 1985, 2010) and affective neuroscience theorists (Damasio, 2000; Porges, 2011; Schore, 2007; van der Kolk, 1994) now acknowledge that beyond thought, nonverbal experience which is often considered to be symbolic, experiential, illogical and intuitive, is a valuable part of psychological health. 'It is derived from stored nonverbal representations, such as "images, feelings, physical sensations, metaphors"' (Schore, 2007, p. 11). Today it seems as if the concept of body and mind integration are arriving at a bottleneck in the road of human discovery. The ways in which the body creates, defines and expresses the mind creates a phenomenon of embodiment.

Defining embodiment

Physical sensations of flesh, muscle, bone and organs are distinct from the internal visceral perceptions of one's body. Both are parts of embodied experiences; the former may include proprioceptive and kinaesthetic senses (exteroceptive experience) whereas the latter is an interoceptive experience, and both are actualisations of emotional or cognitive experience. For instance, you may be wrinkling your forehead after reading the last sentence; a possibly embodied response to learning something new. Or, perhaps you felt a vague internal sense of excitement or settling somewhere within your torso that aligned with a feeling of validation from reading something that agreed with something that you implicitly already know. Our bodies provide a finite location and sensation for discovering what is happening in any given moment.

Phenomenologists Husserl and Heidegger began to explore the integration of 'being' one's body; a living, breathing movement of experience that is happening now (Reniers, 2012; Welton, 1999). Additionally, Merleau-Ponty (1945/2008) contended that experience, action and language, among other things, are characterised through embodiment. Hanna extended these theories further, and created the term 'Somatics' (Hanna, 1986, p. 4). He defined the difference between body and soma; the former being the physical body and the latter a holistic aggregate of human experience:

> Somatics is the field which studies the soma; namely the body as perceived from within by first-person perception. When a human being is observed from the outside, i.e. from a third-person viewpoint – the phenomenon of a human body is perceived.
>
> *(ibid.)*

Additionally, contemporary embodiment theorists Koch and Fuchs (2011) contend that experience within the body is not just situated cognition, where 'knowing is inseparable from doing', but that embodied attention can produce information that can be felt without physical action, and that there are both subjective and objective perspectives of one's body:

> Some researchers have claimed that embodiment approaches are merely part of the recent research tradition of situated cognition. This argumentation ignores the fact that the body is a special category: It is the only 'object' that we can perceive from the inside as well as from the outside.
>
> *(Koch and Fuchs, 2011, p. 276)*

Their perspective of perceiving from the inside describes being able to stay with an experience as it is without having to move. This is prevalent in somatic psychotherapy that fosters attention to interoceptive experience without questioning its value or determining its meaning. Anderson (2002) makes a similar distinction regarding embodiment when she suggests asking not what the body feels like, as in physical sensation, but what the body is experiencing at a given moment, 'Embodiment is not commensurate with our physical senses' (ibid., p. 44). Embodiment involves facets of experience that are more than thinking about the body but includes both sensation and emotion that culminates in conglomerate knowing. Dance/movement therapist Kaylo (2006) describes the difference between consciousness and the embodied experience of consciousness. She writes, 'Consciousness is understood as a process of making meaning of one's existence, and the body is seen as the nexus, or gestalt, within which that meaning-making happens' (Kaylo, 2006, p. 5). In embodied psychotherapy practices, there is an innate moment of embodied self-awareness that precedes expression of the feeling through movement.

One area of therapeutic practice where the interoceptive experience is followed by movement expression is in embodied trauma treatment. Trauma theorists contend that subconscious information is stored in the nervous system (Ogden and Fisher, 2015; Porges, 2011; van der Kolk, 1994). Since symptoms often present in random and unpredictable sensations, images and emotions (as in flashbacks), the body is clearly a vehicle for inquiry to address and negotiate such memories, often known as 'body memory' (Koch, Caldwell, and Fuchs, 2013; Koch, Fuchs, Summa, and Müller, 2012). This is a valuable advancement in psychotherapy treatment and would benefit from a comparative analysis with other verbal-oriented treatment options. Embodied psychotherapy practices are part of the emerging paradigm shift toward inclusion of nonverbal awareness as part of psychotherapeutic healing.

Theoretical similarities in somatic psychotherapy and dance/movement therapy

Somatic psychotherapy (SP) and dance/movement therapy (DMT) share similar philosophical and theoretical foundations (Payne, Warnecke, Karkou, and Westland, 2016; Steckler, 2016; Tantia, 2016). For example, both have theoretical bases such as psychoanalysis, while practice for many has developed in a primarily relational, more humanistic angle of present-moment awareness. Both disciplines generally integrate principles from developmental psychology (Frank and La Barre, 2011; Tortora, 2005), while others maintain a base in Eastern philosophy (Adler, 2004; Musicant, 2007; Weiss, 2009).

In addition to integrating traditional psychology theories, further facets create a theoretical scaffold that makes them particularly embodied disciplines. 'Both SP and DMT are based in the psychophysiological philosophy that embodied awareness is the prima facie of self-knowledge, and that healing happens through experience' (Tantia, 2016, p. 184). In the same article, five over-arching principles were offered: (a) that the soma is the very essence of self-referencing, (b) postures and movement have symbolic meaning, (c) there is value in implicit memory and it is uncovered through embodied awareness, (d) repressed emotions and memory are held in the musculature and can be identified and released and (e) touch may be a healing element in practice (Tantia, 2016, p. 184).

Payne et al. (2016) add that the relationship with the therapist is one of the primary healing elements in embodied psychotherapy practice. Somatic psychotherapist Mark Ludwig described further facets of somatic psychology (incidentally also shared by dance/movement therapy) such as:

(a) a theory of the unconscious as an important dimension of motivation, behaviour and affect and as embedded in the body in the implicit action systems, (b) an approach to emotion that places affective experience at the heart of personality development and that sees emotion as fundamentally somato-psychological, (c) a developmental model that understands that we are differently organised organismically at different points of life experience and so we have different resources for adaptation/regulation/and integration of experience (M. Ludwig, personal communication, December 26, 2012).

These principles necessitate embodied awareness as part of the process for retrieving unconscious knowledge that can then emerge into consciousness through the body, and heal parts of the psyche that are otherwise hidden from awareness. However, SP and DMT each have distinct foundational practices that sets one apart from the other.

Having a body versus moving your body

Similarly to the ways in which Gallagher (2005) has distinguished the difference between body schema (how one perceives oneself from within), and body image (how one views oneself as an 'object' from a distant place beyond the body), neuroscience has observed neurological activity in the brain that distinguishes the difference between having a body and moving your body (Tsakiris et al., 2010). They contend, 'They are qualitatively different experiences, triggered by different inputs, and recruiting distinct brain networks' (Tsakiris et al., 2010, p. 2740). The authors also support the embodied psychotherapy theory that awareness and development of one's body is a potential indicator for how one relates emotionally to their environment. Furthermore, they found differing neurological correlates between having a body (the experience of body ownership) from moving your body (that produces a sense of agency). 'The observed pattern suggests that the sense of agency is underpinned by different brain areas from those related to the sense of body-ownership' (Tsakiris et al., 2010, p. 2744).

Further distinctions between SP and DMT show that each discipline has different intentions, practices and goals. Whereas SP focuses on the adaptations of biological energetic patterns within the client's body sensation as a source of emotional awareness, DMT prioritises movement as emotional experience that is expressed creatively and aesthetically within the therapeutic process. A second delineation is that SP focuses primarily on interoceptive intelligence (attention to breathing, sensation, visceral movement) inside the body, developing intrapersonal knowledge, while dance/movement therapy relies primarily on exteroceptive (also identified as kinesthetic) movement expression of the body in relation to others. Phenomenologically speaking, SP emphasises the individual as the subjective self-reference that allows the client to locate themselves via embodied experience, while DMT stresses the intersubjective other, or me as separate from another.

Somatic psychotherapy: Having a body

Perhaps the most identifying characteristic of SP is the way attention is given to the body. In treatment, attention to the body produces a sense of 'having', or 'owning', one's body; a natural phenomenon of health for a living human being. By bringing attention to one's own awareness of present moment experience of pain, vitality, urges and even the awareness of a vague, unclear sense of something that is not yet identifiable, is a process of self-knowledge. Sensations provide a gateway for emotional awareness that might be described with sensori-emotional words such as *gurgling, throbbing, zinging and flowing*. In a somatic sense, these words can be used to describe a physical sensation that is intricately connected with an emotion. Once the psychosomatic connection is made, memories tend to arise in relation to an embodied experience and meaning can begin to emerge from the whole experience.

Somatic psychotherapy practice attends to interoceptive experience to bring unconscious material to consciousness so that it can be renegotiated and healed. While attending to the body through a 'bottom up' process (Ogden, Minton, and Pain, 2006), beginning clients will state that they feel 'silly' or that, 'I don't know why I am saying this, but . . .' which is an indicator that the client is identifying something within themselves that exists, but does not yet have meaning. Once they begin to trust their experience, they begin to own a greater sense of themselves; thus, having a sense of body ownership. Body ownership is a part of self-recognition and locating oneself as an individual in the world. Self-recognition includes both recognition of one's body and of one's actions (van den Bos and Jeannerod, 2002) and therefore spans both the way one perceives oneself, as well as how one perceives themselves in relation to their world and with others. 'Body-ownership involves a psychophysiological baseline, linked to activation of the brain's default mode network' (Tsakiris et al., 2010, p. 2740). My body is an integral identification of 'me' in a way that other objects are not. The phenomenal body is the sensorial location of the consummate 'I' when one points to one's own physical manifestation of self as the place where consciousness and reality meet.

Perhaps the bedrock of SP practice came from philosopher and psychotherapist Eugene Gendlin who codified a process for attending to embodied awareness in a practice called Focusing. This was developed in the 1950s and 1960s during a research study on schizophrenia with Carl Rogers (Gendlin, 1967). Focusing is a process of bringing attention to the body in a way that brings forth information that may have been previously unconscious. Gendlin coined the term 'felt sense' (1981, p. 10) to describe bodily experiences that arise in sensation but are somewhat independent of emotion. He describes a 'felt sense' in five ways: '(1) it is felt rather than thought, (2) it occurs in present time, (3) it is directly experienced in the body, (4) it guides conceptualisation and (5) it is implicitly meaningful' (Gendlin, 1981, p. 10).

During Focusing, the therapist invites the client, or 'focuser', to check in with his or her embodied experience. When a sensation, image, colour, texture or other identification emerges, whether it is clear or not, the focuser states what it is, and the therapist reflects the client's words back to him or her. The client then checks in again with his or her internally felt experience to see if the words match what his or her felt sense is communicating. If the feeling of the words is not quite right, the focuser finds words that fit the feeling. This is repeated for as long as necessary to help the client to transfer from a vague sensation to clarity, defined as a 'felt shift' in which the client feels a change in his or her felt sense. This shift is a sign of healing and felt as an improved sense of self. Finally, the feeling is made explicit and new insight or meaning-making becomes the byproduct of that shift.

Dance/movement therapy: Moving your body

Dance/movement therapy (DMT) is aligned with the kinaesthetic philosophy of Sheets-Johnstone (2015) and acknowledges that the body's natural tendency toward creative expression, joined with aesthetic experience, is an integral part of healing. In the United States it emerged from modern dance of the 1940s and values the creative and aesthetic expression of the body through sublimated movement as part of healing (Bruno, 1990; Lewis, 1993). In the UK, DMT emerged in the 1950s from employing Laban creative dance in occupational therapy and later from occupational therapists/school teachers specialised in Laban dance, many of whom were trained by Laban and in Laban Movement Analysis and practicing in mental health or special education, respectively (Payne, 2006). Beyond mastering the task of honing body positions as in dance training, attending to the aesthetic experience of one's moving body, culminates in a sense of aliveness (pleasurable or not) through proprioceptive experience by both the mover and onlooker (Vukadinović and Marković, 2012). As Payne (2004) also expresses, 'It is a craft: a hybrid comprised of the theory and practice of psychological therapy and dance' (p. 3). The purpose of the therapy is not to create a work of art, nor does it necessitate that the client has training or proficiency in dancing. Instead, it provides an emotionally safe place for the client to explore/cultivate spontaneity and creativity in a way that develops a sense of self in relation to another. One figure of thought in DMT practice is that when the body moves more freely, the mind will follow (Steckler, 2016).

Probably the most inspirational description of dance/movement therapy comes from Espenak, when she wrote that the goals of DMT include, 'Stimulation and release of feelings . . communication and contact . . reduction of anxiety . . . experience of joy . . response to rhythm' (Espenak, 1981, pp. 7–11). These five goals, written 30 years ago speak to the foundational spirit of dance/movement therapy, and describe how the work seeks to recover original vitality from within an individual, rather than focusing on their pathology. This approach offers the potential for a patient to experience the expression of their enlivened response to their world. Bruno (1990) offers a perspective on the importance of creativity in DMT when she stated, 'Allowing the self to be recast in movement, sharing it with another without altering that expression to fit the expectations, provides the psyche with an opportunity to do its own unique transformative work towards wholeness' (p. 111).

Developmentally, movement not only helps to create cognition (Piaget, 1969/2000), but it is our first and therefore most important experience of 'Self' in relation to others in the world, and the first way we learn about our world. The chronological epistemological development of all humans, their learning on all fronts, is first through movement, prior to the execution of language. In other words, 'infants are not pre-linguistic, as is commonly declared; on the contrary, language is post-kinetic' (Sheets-Johnstone, 2005, p. 50). Infant development researchers have further proposed that movement creates interpersonal capacities (Sossin and Berkelein, 2006; Stern, 1985; Trevarthen, 2004). Sometimes when patients are struggling to develop their ego, a more structured approach is necessary. Specific interventions include attention to rhythm, space and shapes that the client makes, while indulging aesthetic expression and creativity (Tantia, 2016). In DMT, a client can begin to define who they are by finding themselves in relation to another. From a neuroscience perspective, Tsirkiris et al. (2010) support:

> Moreover, the relationship between my body and 'me' is quite different from the relation between my body and other people (Descartes, 1637/1998). In contrast, the feeling that I can move and control my body is called the sense of agency.
>
> *(p. 2740)*

Dance and creative movement in a psychotherapeutic setting also helps an individual to create boundaries and feel one's own sense of self as separate from another. In practice, several styles of dance/movement therapy are acknowledged as sources of structure for an individual (Evans, in Levy, 2006) and in group form (Espenak, 1981; Levy, 2006).

One of the more particular identifying aspects of group DMT is the formation of a circle. In dance history, the circle had significance for inclusion, community and therapeutically, the design offers a potentially safe space for all members of the group to be in an even participatory state with each other, omitting a hierarchy. 'Moving in concert in a circle – as in any and all spatial forms – involves not simply an awareness of the movement of others but a sensitive attunement to their qualitative dynamics' (Sheets-Johnstone, 2015, p. xxvii). While in a circle, each participant can see each other while they move together, either in synchrony or separately. Often, dance/movement therapists will mirror clients – moving in a similar way to that of the client with the intention of attaining a non-verbal attunement with the client. This non-verbal attunement also happens naturally and unconsciously among clients in a group and naturally between people in life. Gallese (2003) suggests that mirror neurons are responsible for that which dance/movement therapists call attunement, and they are the neuro-correlates of empathy. While moving/dancing together, mirroring helps clients to not only see each other, but to feel each other without physical touch. By moving with another, the client can find themselves, either as being joined in their movement (and therefore not feeling alone) or feeling a defined sense of separateness and individuation. Gallese's conclusion, 'Action is therefore a suitable candidate principle enabling social bonds to be initially established' (2003, p. 174) supports this intervention. As a result of moving together, mirroring, feeling included and developing the agency to support others in a group is summed up by Sheets-Johnstone who offers, 'What is a sign of life in our assessment of others, however, is experientially a feeling of aliveness for oneself, or at least potentially so' (Sheets-Johnstone, 2005, p. 3). The experience of joy and acceptance of humanness is one of the inevitable results of DMT practice.

Conclusion

The body is a living breathing organismic source of human intelligence that is a constant sympathetic reflection of the mind's complexity. Biological energetic patterns provide unconscious information regarding an individual's emotional health as well as their interaction with the environment. SP and DMT are unique disciplines within what are referred to in this volume as 'Embodied Perspectives in Psychotherapy'. They have similar theoretical bases, although with differing approaches and clinical goals, and together they form a new paradigm of theory and practice for the psychotherapy community. Having a body, or working with the intrapersonal nature of one's experience, is different from moving one's body, and yet each is dependent on the other. After delineating their processes, one might consider that the two may fall on a continuum of healing that begins with interior self-knowledge as it stands in the present moment and ends with expression outward into the world. Embodied psychotherapy practices invite a natural discovery of a present-moment experience that brings forth the awareness and expression of unconscious information that was not previously available through words, and therefore provide a valuable process to traditional psychotherapy approaches. Awareness of what is already happening in one's body (as in somatic psychotherapy) followed by feeling the desire to express what is being felt, and finally the action of expression (as in dance/movement therapy), provide a continuum of healing through the body that is essential to emotional health.

Notes

1 This is the term used to describe body psychotherapy in the United States.
2 This is the way dance movement psychotherapy is written in the United States.
3 Please see the special journal issue of *Body, Movement and Dance in Psychotherapy,* 2016, Vol. 11, issue 2–3 for more complete correlational analyses between the two disciplines.

References

Adler, J. (2004). *Offering from the Conscious Body*. Rochester, VT: Inner Traditions.
Anderson, R. (2002, Autumn/Winter). Embodied writing: Presencing the body in somatic research, part I. *Somatics, 13*(4), 40–44.
Bloom, K. (2006). *The Embodied Self*. London: Karnac.
Boston Change Process Study Group, The, Bruschweiler-Stern, N., Harrison, A. M., Lyons-Ruth, K., Morgan, A. C., Nahum, J. P., . . . Tronick, E. Z. (2010). *Change in Psychotherapy: A Unifying Paradigm*. New York: Norton.
Bruno, C. (1990). Maintaining a concept of the dance in dance/movement therapy. *American Journal of Dance Therapy, 12*(2), 101–113.

Clemmons, M. C. (2012). The interactive field: Gestalt therapy as an embodied relational dialogue. In T. B. Levine (Ed.), *Gestalt Therapy: Advances in Theory and Practice* (pp. 39–48). New York: Routledge.

Csordas, T. (1993). Somatic modes of attention. *Cultural Anthropology, 8*(2), 135–156.

Damasio, A. (2000). Subcortical and cortical brain activity during the feeling of self-generated emotions. *Nature Neuroscience, 3*, 1049–1056.

Descartes, R. (1998). *Discourse on Methods.* Indianapolis, IN: Hackett Publishing. (Original work published 1637)

Espenak, L. (1981). *Dance Therapy.* Springfield, IL: Charles C. Thomas.

Frank, R. (2001). *Body of Awareness: A Somatic and Developmental Approach to Psychotherapy.* Cambridge, MA: Gestalt Press.

Frank, R., and La Barre, F. (2011). *The First Year and the Rest of Your Life.* New York: Taylor and Francis.

Gallagher, S. (2005). *How the Body Shapes the Mind.* New York: Oxford University Press.

Gallese, V. (2003). The roots of empathy: The shared manifold hypothesis and the neural basis of intersubjectivity. *Psychopathology, 36*, 171–180.

Gendlin, E. T. (1967). Therapeutic procedures in dealing with schizophrenics. In C. R. Rogers (Ed.), *The Therapeutic Relationship and Its Impact. A Study of Psychotherapy with Schizophrenics* (pp. 369–400). Madison: University of Wisconsin.

Gendlin, E. T. (1981). *Focusing.* New York: Bantam.

Hanna, T. (1986, Spring/Summer). What is Somatics? *Somatics, 5*(4), 4.

Heller, M. (2012). *Body Psychotherapy: History, Concepts and Methods.* London: Norton.

Hervey, L. W. (2007). Embodied ethical decision-making. *American Journal of Dance Therapy, 29*(2), 91–108.

Huxley, A. (1932). *Brave New World.* New York: Harper and Brothers.

Ignatow, G. (2007). Theories of embodied knowledge: New directions for cultural and cognitive sociology. *Journal for the Theory of Social Behavior, 37*(2), 115–135.

Kaylo, J. (2006, Winter). The body in phenomenology and movement observation. *E-motion, 19*(17), 5–11.

Koch, S., and Fuchs, T. (2011). Embodied arts therapies. *The Arts in Psychotherapy, 38*, 276–280.

Koch, S., Caldwell, C., and Fuchs, T. (2013). On body memory and embodied therapies. *Body, Movement and Dance in Psychotherapy, 8*(2), 82–94.

Koch, S., Fuchs, T., Summa, M., and Müller, C. (2012). *Body, Memory, Metaphor and Movement.* Philadelphia, PA: John Benjamins.

Kepner, J. I. (1999). *Body Process: A Gestalt Approach to Working with the Body in Psychotherapy.* New York: Routledge.

Kripal, J. (2007). *Esalen: The Religion of No Religion.* London: University of Chicago.

Lakoff, G., and Johnson, M. (1999). *Philosophy in the Flesh: The Embodied Mind and Its Challenge to Western Thought.* New York: Basic Books.

Levy, F. (2006). *Dance/Movement Therapy: A Healing Art.* Reston, VA: The American Alliance for Health, Physical Education, Recreation, and Dance.

Lewis, P. (1993). *Creative Transformation: The Healing Power of the Arts.* London: Chiron.

Lowe, R., and Laeng-Gilliatt, S. (Eds.) (2007). *Reclaiming Vitality and Presence: Sensory Awareness as a Practice for Life. The Works of C. Selver.* Berkeley: North Atlantic Books.

Maslow, A. (1943). A theory of human motivation. *Psychological Review, 50*(4), 370–396.

Merleau-Ponty, M. (2008). *Phenomenology of Perception* (11th printing). New York: Routledge. (Original work published 1945)

Musicant, S. (2007). Authentic movement in clinical work. In P. Pallaro (Ed.), *Authentic Movement: Moving the Body, Moving the Self, Being Moved: A Collection of Essays Volume Two.* Philadelphia, PA: Jessica Kingsley Publishers.

Ogden, P., and Fisher, J. (2015). *Sensorimotor Psychotherapy: Interventions for Trauma and Attachment.* New York: Norton.

Ogden, P., Minton, K., and Pain, C. (2006). *Trauma and the Body: A Sensorimotor Approach to Psychotherapy.* New York: Norton.

Payne, H. (2004). Introduction: Embodiment in action. In H. Payne (Ed.), *Dance Movement Therapy: Theory, Research and Practice.* London: Routledge.

Payne, H. (2006). *Creative Movement and Dance in Groupwork.* Oxon: Speechmark.

Payne, H., Warnecke, T., Karkou, V., and Westland, G. (2016). A comparative analysis of body psychotherapy and dance movement psychotherapy from a European perspective. *Body, Movement and Dance in Psychotherapy, 11*(2–3), 144–166.

Piaget, J. (2000). *The Psychology of the Child.* New York: Basic Books. (Original work published 1969)

Porges, S. (2011). *The Polyvagal Theory: Neurophysiological Foundations of Emotions, Attachment, Communication, and Self-Regulation.* New York: Norton.

Reniers, G. M. (2012). Understanding the differences between Husserl's (descriptive) and Heidegger's (interpretive) phenomenological research. *Journal of Nursing Care, 1*(5), 119.

Schore, A. N. (2007). Psychoanalytic research: Progress and process. Developmental affective neuroscience and clinical practice. *Psychologist-Psychoanalyst, 27*(3), 6–13. (Summer: Official publication of division 39 of the American Psychological Association).

Sheets-Johnstone, M. (2005). Man has always danced: Forays into an art largely forgotten by philosophers. *Contemporary Aesthetics, 2*(1). Retrieved from www.contempaesthetics.org/newvolume/pages/article.php?articleID=273

Sheets-Johnstone, M. (2015). *The Phenomenology of Dance* (5th Anniversary ed.). Philadelphia, PA: Temple University Press.

Sossin, M., and Berkelein, S. (2006). Nonverbal transmission of stress between parent and young child: Considerations and psychotherapeutic implications of a study of affective movement patterns. *Journal of Infant, Child and Adolescent Psychotherapy, 5*(1), 46–69.

Steckler, L. (2016). The holographic body: The use of movement in body psychotherapy. *Body, Movement and Dance in Psychotherapy, 11*(2–3), 167–180.

Stern, D. (1985). *Interpersonal World of the Infant.* New York: Basic Books.

Stern, D. (2010). *Forms of Vitality: Exploring Dynamic Experience in Psychology and the Arts.* New York: Oxford University Press.

Tantia, J. F. (2014). Mindfulness and dance/movement therapy for treating trauma. In L. Rappaport (Ed.), *Mindfulness in the Creative Arts Therapies* (pp. 96–107). London: Jessica Kingsley.

Tantia, J. F. (2016). The interface between somatic psychotherapy and dance/movement therapy: A critical analysis. *Body, Movement and Dance in Psychotherapy, 11*(2–3), 181–196.

Tantia, J. F. (2017, September 18). *Dance/Movement Therapy Research: Current Trends and Possibilities.* Washington, DC: Invited panel speaker, Creative Forces Healing Arts Network, National Endowment for the Arts.

Tortora, S. (2005). *The Dancing Dialogue: Using the Communicative Power of Movement with Young Children.* Baltimore: Brookers.

Trevarthen, C. (2004). Learning about ourselves, from children: Why a growing human brain needs interesting companions? In *Annual Report-Hokkaido University Research and Clinical Center for Child Development* (pp. 9–44). Sapporo, Japan: Graduate School of Education, Hokkaido University.

Tsakiris, M., Longo, M., and Haggard, P. (2010). Having a body versus moving your body: Neural signatures of agency and body-ownership. *Neuropsychologia, 48*, 2740–2749.

van den Bos, E., and Jeannerod, M. (2002). Sense of body and sense of action both contribute to self-recognition. *Cognition, 85*, 177–187.

van der Kolk, B. (1994). The body keeps the score: Memory and the evolving psychobiology of posttraumatic stress. *Harvard Review of Psychiatry, 1*(5), 253–265.

Varela, F., Thompson, E., and Rosch, E. (2017). *The Embodied Mind: Cognitive Science and Human Experience.* Cambridge, MA: MIT Press.

Vukadinović, M., and Marković, S. (2012). Aesthetic experience of dance performances. *Psyhologija, 45*(1), 23–41.

Weiss, H. (2009). The use of mindfulness in psychodynamic and body oriented psychotherapy. *Body, Movement and Dance in Psychotherapy, 4*(1), 5–16.

Welton, D. (1999). *The Body: Classic and Contemporary Readings.* Oxford: Blackwell.

Yontef, D. (1969). *Awareness, Dialogue and Process.* New York: Gestalt Journal Press.

SECTION II

Theory and practice in dance movement psychotherapy

Introduction

This second section focuses on dance movement psychotherapy (DMP) research and practice, including most recent theory developments and connections to interdisciplinary embodiment research.

The section starts with Chapter 6 'A developmental taxonomy of interaction modalities in dance movement therapy', by **Marianne Eberhard-Kaechele**, from Germany, who describes the developmental foundations of mirroring modalities in movement. The chapter is a step in DMT theory development and points to the existentiality of reciprocity and being seen as we grow up. Eberhard-Kaechele provides a differentiated overview on how mirroring in movement successively develops and is the ground of our human capacity to be in healthy contact with each other. First described by Marian Chace, it was a clinical intuition regarding the use of mirroring which is today confirmed and elaborated by research on embodiment, neurobiology, and social, emotional, and cognitive infant development. The chapter presents a taxonomy of interaction modalities in accordance with developmental theories. The taxonomy is an aid for diagnostics and intervention planning to support the motor, cognitive, emotional, and social development of those in need.

Chapter 7 takes us to the method of Authentic Movement. **Tina Stromsted**, an American DMT, who has been in the authentic movement practice for more than 30 years, describes the method and its importance for the questions of seeing and being seen. She introduces the important role of the gaze in the method and relates the witnessing practice to neuroscience and cultural studies. Authentic Movement is about being seen, being heard, and being received for who we are. If these human needs have been neglected or have been difficult in development, they can be supported by the authentic movement practice of moving and witnessing.

Annette Schwalbe, a DMP from the UK and Kenya, in Chapter 8 subsequently introduces an important method of body image work: Body Mapping as developed in South Africa in the work with persons living with HIV. She lays out the method and applies it to women in times of transition in Kenya as well as in the UK. Body Maps are life-size creations that start with a person being traced around her whole body on paper. The drawings are then individually coloured paying attention to how body parts feel and are related to, rather than how the body appears. The work is transdisciplinary and includes elements of art therapy and poetry therapy. It is also partly based on the witnessing practice of authentic movement.

Next is Chapter 9 by **Diana Cheney**, a UK DMP, who highlights the topic of gravity and relates it to the development of the self in DMP. The baby is born into a world with laws of gravity, which are first explored in the horizontal, then in the vertical and finally in the sagittal plane. The chapter focuses on the relationship the infant establishes with gravity and the development of the (body) self and others can facilitate the infant's relationship with gravity. On the basis of developmental movement patterns, object-relations, and psychoanalytic theories, as well as notes from two years of infant observation, personal observations, and clinical materials, the chapter outlines our relationship with gravity, the relation between gravity and (body) self-development, and the use of the concept of gravity in clinical contexts through a case vignette.

Rosemarie Samaritter, from the Netherlands, in Chapter 10 provides an overview on resilience and how to build resilience through the shared practice of DMT. In her chapter, she describes resilience as a dynamic adaptive capacity of the human living system serving the purpose to adapt to the challenges of a changing environment. Building resilience supports the treatment of mental illness by moving clients from stagnation to vital adaptivity. Arts-based practices, such as DMT can contribute to the development of resilience. Core themes of dance are discussed for their therapeutic value and their potential contribution to strengthen a person's capacities to recover from stress, illness, trauma, or psychopathology.

Dance/movement therapist **Susan Imus**, from the US, in Chapter 11 describes a unique movement-based program of suicide prevention in the Chicago area. Suicide is a major health concern in the US and around the world. The Making Connections Suicide Prevention Program is an approach to suicide prevention that incorporates theory and practice from dance/movement therapy. Protective factors (resilience) as defined in public health are highlighted throughout the Gatekeeper Training programme by teaching an embodied approach to life skills development in feeling identification, tension reduction, affect regulation, and empathy building. The new model of *Movement Thinking Strategies* is presented to assist the community at large to observe, understand, and respond to the needs of its members.

In Chapter 12 is the prevalent topic of work with survivors of war, torture, and relational trauma offered by **Amber Gray**, an American dance/movement therapist with extensive experience in working with trauma survivors around the globe. These include in areas of war and civil war such as Syria and in areas of crises such as after the earthquake in Haiti. She presents DMT as a framework for restoring and healing trauma and exemplifies her arguments with a case study, emphasizing the resource-based approach of DMT to support traumatized clients in restoring meaning and their place of belonging in the world.

Dance movement therapist **Silvie Garnero**, from France, introduces a case-based approach to transgenerational trauma and more generally nonverbal trauma narrative in Chapter 13. This chapter summarises the work with a girl who suffers from the effects of transgenerational Holocaust trauma. The creative process as embodied in the dance experience and the issue of body-to-body transmission of the trauma is explored. The central question of emotions is linked with body memory and expressiveness. Forming body narratives is described as particularly relevant in the care of trauma patients by the author.

In Chapter 14 an account of integral dance movement therapy is delivered by **Alexander Girshon** and **Ekaterina Karatygina**, from Russia. The authors describe psychological re-sources in integral dance and dance movement therapy in four clusters: Pleasure, Engagement, Power, and Meaning. The article introduces the psychological resources model, which the authors use in DMT, based on Ken Wilber's transpersonal approach with the three major perspectives of subjective (I-resources), intersubjective (I–You- or I–We resources), and objective resources (I and material resources). Supported by research findings from positive psychology,

'Pleasure', 'Engagement', 'Power', and 'Meaning' have been identified as central 'I-resources'. The chapter focuses on these resources and the practical side of working with them.

Suzi Tortora and **Jennifer Whitley**, from the US, provide Chapter 15 on mother–son transgenerational transmission of eating issues using a co-treatment method. They present a case study, based on a multifaceted treatment using the *Ways of Seeing* DMT treatment approach by Tortora in 2012, addressing transgenerational transmission of family trauma. The development of eating issues originated in the parent–infant relationship and continued into the child's elementary years. The use of careful observation of nonverbal behavior during experiential parts of the sessions, thoughtful attention to the underlying themes of the conversations with the mother, and storylines created by the child, enabled the transgenerational themes to emerge and be processed. The *Ways of Seeing* framework includes three core elements: A co-treatment with each DMT working separately with the parent and child; a specific sequence of multi-arts activities using body awareness, drawing, dance-play, and storytelling to integrate the experiences on a body-mind-emotional continuum; and the coordination of the treatment plans between the co-therapists through regularly scheduled meetings, with attention to the therapists' embodied countertransference experience for optimal treatment.

In Chapter 16 entitled 'The BodyMind Approach and people affected by medically unexplained symptoms/somatic symptom disorder', **Helen Payne**, a researcher and practitioner in DMP from the UK, describes The BodyMind Approach™ designed specifically for patients with medically unexplained symptoms (MUS), and provides patient profiles and treatment examples. MUS are a global issue, consisting of persistent medical conditions for which doctors find no organic explanations, for example, fibromyalgia, irritable bowel syndrome, chronic fatigue, etc.; under these conditions patients usually visit their doctors frequently, yet no effective pathway for support is available. Payne describes what the DMP-based BodyMind Approach™ can do to facilitate patients to self-manage and reduce their suffering from MUS.

Chapter 17 is a contribution from **Haguit Ehrenfreund**, from Switzerland, who provides a psychodynamic account on the disruption of the psychosomatic balance, and asks, whether this is psychopathology. In her chapter, she aims to theorize the disturbance of the psychosomatic balance as a disorder of the body-mind relation. With clinical illustrations of patients with eating disorders, she demonstrates the power of transition via the body and its movement and sensations to the thinking processes. The chapter conceptualizes dance movement psychotherapy as a psychosomatic treatment practice, using psychoanalytical theory of mental disorders. Finally, a technique for working towards body-mind awareness, in order to exemplify its therapeutic use is presented.

In Chapter 18 three DMTs **Teresa Bas (Spain), Diana Fischman (Argentina)**, and **Rosa Mª Rodríguez (Spain)** describe their private practices with neurotic, now termed high-functioning patients. They point out particularities and differences from working with other patient groups, and explain how a DMT observes processes and changes, and plans interventions. The chapter employs a relational, enactive, and embodied approach in DMT, a form of psychotherapy that aims at body-mind integration, integration of implicit and explicit communication, and linking of verbal and non-verbal language. Psychotherapeutic processes with normal neurotics capable of reflecting on themselves are described as evolving and multi-layered dancing dialogues between patient and psychotherapist. Layers include movement exploration and words, primary processes of experience and secondary processes of reflection, psychodynamic concepts and the use of movement analysis, evoking images or metaphors, and embodying them through dance and body awareness techniques.

Miyuki Kaji, from Japan, in Chapter 19 offers an interesting insight into dance/movement therapy in Japan. She particularly addresses healing through the Japanese traditional performing art of 'Noh', considered representative of Japanese ways of expression and views of the body. DMT was introduced to Japan in the 1980s. Ways of expression, physical skills, and a concept of the body that is unique to Japanese culture have been incorporated into Japanese DMT methods. A case described in this chapter provides an example of Japanese style DMT, which holds a similarity to Noh training.

Rainbow (Tin) Ho, a DMT researcher and practitioner from Hong Kong, addresses, in Chapter 20, the embodiment of space in psychotherapy, related to issues of self and others. Space is a physical concept that usually refers to the three-dimensional geometric occupancy an object or a person can fill in. Although space usually is physical, there is also psychological space in the context of psychotherapy, spiritual space in Eastern philosophy, and social relations in all cultures. In dance/movement therapy, the physical spaces inside and outside the body are usually the entry points for dealing with issues related to the person and the person's relationships with others and the world based on the premise of the interconnectedness of the mind and body. In a psychotherapeutic context, the awareness of space outside the body and its relationship to the self, with the consideration of culture, reveals patterns of personal boundaries and social relationships. The author describes how an individual can develop his or her own identity and healthy relationships with others, if appropriate space can be maintained.

Iris Bräuninger, a researcher and practitioner in DMT from Switzerland and **Radwa Said Abdelazim Elfeqi**, from Egypt contribute Chapter 21, which is a fascinating chapter entitled 'From the Alps to the Pyramids: Swiss and Egyptian perspectives on dance movement therapy', and describes basic traditions of DMT in their countries. Furthermore, it highlights Egyptian and Swiss perspectives on DMT, embodiment and professional situations in two different cultural contexts with regards to education, recognition, employment opportunities, and challenges regarding practice and research. The discrepancy between developing a practice of DMT in the Middle East, particularly in Egypt, compared to one in Europe, particularly in Switzerland, is examined. The link from the pyramids to the alps originated when Radwa Elfeqi invited Iris Bräuninger to present at the XIII World Congress of Psychiatry's first symposium on the Creative Arts Therapies in Psychiatry in Cairo 2005.

6

A DEVELOPMENTAL TAXONOMY OF INTERACTION MODALITIES IN DANCE MOVEMENT THERAPY

Marianne Eberhard-Kaechele

Introduction: Embodiment, mirroring, and development

Embodiment is the concept that the sensing and moving body, embedded in the biological, psychological, and cultural environment plays an important role in cognition (Gibbs, 2005). Infant research (Bråten, 2006) has long proven that social cognition – the ability to perceive and interpret the intentions, wishes and feelings of oneself and others – occurs on a bodily level before infants have a mental concept of their own or others' minds. As Gibbs puts it: 'The emotional states of others are not something that infants must simulate or infer, but something that is directly perceived in the movement and experience of other's behaviour' (2005, p. 234). The idea of mentalising as a purely mental act, which occurs in the detached mind of the individual is giving way to an embodied and enacted perspective, in which mutual interactions of persons lead to shared meaning-making and reciprocal influence upon one another (Shai and Fonagy, 2013). Such embodied knowledge of how to relate to others is not replaced by later symbolic language-based forms of interaction, but rather remains influential over the lifespan (Fuchs and De Jaegher, 2010).

During early socio-emotional development, contingent, and imitative parent–child interactions of an optimal midrange (rather than too perfect or too constant interactions) serve many functions (Beebe, 2014). These include the development of secure attachment, the sensitisation of the infant to his/her internal affect states and their regulation, leading to the development of emotional self-awareness and self-control (Gergely, Koós, and Watson, 2010). The modern view on the mechanism of change in the development of social cognition is the opportunity for and quality of interactions with others (de Haan, De Jaegher, Fuchs, & Mayer, 2011). Working in an embodied way, as they intuitively did, it is not surprising that dance movement therapists in their clinical work with severely disturbed populations discovered the power of contingent and imitative interactions, i.e. mirroring, to treat mental illness.

Mirroring in dance movement psychotherapy

The history of the use of mirroring techniques in dance movement psychotherapy (DMP) is briefly described for a better understanding of the method. In the 1930s and 1940s, the American dance therapist Marian Chace applied dance as medium of treatment for psychiatric patients, actively engaging in movement interactions with her patients (Chaiklin and Schmais, 1979). One of the most important techniques of intervention used by Chace was, that which she called 'picking up': the multimodal reflection of the emotions and intentions of her patients, by means of her own movements, voice, speech, props, music and the spontaneous complex interventions, which she offered (Sandel, 1993). Chace's goals for 'picking up' were attracting the attention of withdrawn persons, engaging patients in basic communication, facilitating self-acceptance, externalising emotions, intensifying expression, expanding the symbolic expressive repertoire, accessing memories important for the understanding of feelings, and finally integrating physical activity, emotional experience and verbal reflection (Chaiklin and Schmais, 1979). Trudi Schoop also documented her use of 'picking up' or 'following' the movement of patients since the 1950s for similar purposes (1974, p. 169). Payne (1992, p. 63) spoke of 'joining' to name the therapist's movement with the patient in this sense. Today, DMP research confirms effects such as the experience of empathy, feeling seen and accepted, feeling connected with the therapist, and group cohesion (Rova, 2017).

Dance therapists often refer to this approach as mirroring, but because mirroring is usually interpreted as the full body reproduction of the movement shape, quality, and experience of another person this term entails the risk of oversimplifying Chace's concept (Sandel, 1993). Sandel (1993) suggests using the term 'empathic reflection' to better describe the variety of interactions and reactions involved in the Chacian approach, only one of which may be mirroring in the above-mentioned sense. Sandel's argumentation is appropriate for the description of therapeutic interventions. However, for a general description of interpersonal movement interaction, empathic reflection proves to be a one-sided term, regarding only the behaviour of the therapist. To generally describe interaction that may be performed reciprocally by patient and therapist, or between patients, a different terminology is necessary and will be the subject of this chapter.

Processes of affect attunement and trust building through picking up and reflecting movement by the therapist were also key concepts of Kestenberg, a psychoanalyst who worked together with dance therapists in the 1960s to develop a nonverbal technique of diagnostics and treatment, the Kestenberg Movement Profile (KMP). Rather than using the term mirroring, she differentiated between attunement to the dynamics of tension flow patterns of another person as a means of establishing empathy, and adjustment to the flow of changes in body shape and weight transference of another person as a means of establishing trust. According to Kestenberg Amighi and Sossin (1999), the focus of the KMP has been primarily intrapersonal, exploring the dynamics and structure within an individual, and only secondarily concerned with communication. By comparing two profiles, areas of accord and conflict between individuals could be analysed, but beyond the terms 'attunement', 'adjustment', and 'clashing', interactions have no further KMP terminology.

Examples of DMP literature and research dealing with the further delineation of modalities are Fraenkel (1983) who differentiated synchrony and echoing (deferred imitation in Table 6.1) and Payne (1992) who showed clinical applications of shadowing (parallel mirroring in Table 6.1), echoing, mirroring, and cross-modal mirroring in voice and verbal commentary.

The discovery of mirror neurons through neurobiological research by Gallese, Fadiga, Fogassi, and Rizzolatti (1996) expanded the perspective on mirroring in DMP to include the child picking up the movement of the parent, or the client/patient picking up the movement of the therapist, to improve empathy and other mental health issues. Mirror neurons serve, for example, the function of coordinating motor interactions with other people through anticipation of their movement and intentions or developing trust and empathy through the ability to neurologically reproduce the experience of what others are feeling in one's own mind (Bauer, 2005). Successful mirroring experiences contain phases of attunement and of differentiation and strengthen a

Table 6.1 Developmental taxonomy of mirroring modalities in DMP (see also Eberhard-Kaechele, 2009; 2012)

No.	Modality	Characteristics of movement and affect regulation	Cognitive development
1	initiating, continuing, terminating	The ability to begin, continue and end intending or attending processes (e.g., gazing towards something, keeping it in view, diverting one's gaze). Primary self-efficacy and pre-requisites for self/other regulation, and the repair of interactional ruptures.	Discovering contingency, self-discovery, causal thinking emphasizing movement origins. From birth on.
2	coordinating		
2a	synchronising (medial or oceanic mirroring)	Totally simultaneous movement between partners or play with controllable objects. Interpersonal transcendence, or unilateral dominance and submission, or a sign of non-personal perception of people as inanimate objects.	'Perfect' contingency, self-exploring, taking control. From 1 month on.
2b	alternating	Turn-taking, using repetition, phrasing and rhythm to facilitate reciprocal anticipation of turns. Congruent action as a means of self/other identification and primary intersubjectivity.	Congruency. Acknowledging intentions and being acknowledged. 2–3 months.
3	concordant mirroring		
3a	modal, autocentric mirroring (in-phase)	Mirroring in the literal sense, from the perspective of the responder, along a common axis of movement. The same mode of expression is used as the initiator. Primary intersubjectivity, testing contingency, affect attunement, learning from others, and sense of agency.	High level but not perfect contingency, exploring the social world. 2 months on.
3b	cross-modal mirroring	Dynamic/shape is mirrored by voice, another expressive medium or another body part. Facilitation of exploration, affect attunement.	Medium level contingency, exploring the environment. 4–9 months.
3c	parallel mirroring	Side by side = solidarity, one behind the other = support or leading and following. Joint attention toward a third entity. Shared interest. Social referencing. Secondary intersubjectivity, triangulation.	Joint attention, teleological/goal oriented thought. 9–12 months.
3d	altercentric mirroring	Each participant has their own axis of movement, virtual rotation of the movement, using the same side of the body in asymmetrical movements. Precursor of intersubjectivity.	Perspective taking, differentiation of perspectives. 14 months on.
3e	counter-moving (anti-phase)	Anti-phasic coordination of cyclic movements, e.g. open-close vs. close-open, forward-backward vs. backward-forward. Expresses differentiation.	Differentiation of perspectives, of self–other, of ingroup and outgroup.

(Continued)

Table 6.1 (Continued)

No.	Modality	Characteristics of movement and affect regulation	Cognitive development
3f	deferred imitating	Imitating with a time lag, retention and recall of movement, memory development, identification processes. Replacing one object with another in the recreation of a situation marks the beginning of symbolization and the pretend modality.	Recognition of others by movement, 2 months. Deferred imitating across contexts and intentional thought (part I): mental causality, 14 months. Symbolisation, 18 months.
4	completing developing	A goal-oriented movement of the other which is incomplete or faulty is completed or further developed by the partner. Integration of memory (knowing what the complete movement would be) and altercentric perspective (inferring what the other plans to do, would enjoy).	Memory for intentions inferring plans, desires. 18 months on.
5	contrasting	The main intention of the movement is reversed, e.g. speed: quick vs. slow, shape: round vs. jagged, direction: up vs. down etc. Ambivalent: doing the opposite serves differentiation, while the common theme/the friction serves connection.	Conceptual thought: e.g. opposites, forms, directions, positions. Intentional thought (part II): differentiation of self/other beliefs. 2 years.
6a	varying	Simultaneously maintaining contact and serving individuation and expansion of abilities. Self-regulation of affects through "tuning" the dynamics/forms of movement. Adaption to various situations. Forming the expression of a partner through encouragement or discouragement.	Precursor: Adaptivity at 9 months. Representational thought, value judgements, 3–4 years.
6b	marked varying	Differentiation of one's own and others affects. Regulation of arousal through mild and possibly humorous exaggeration or containment. Externalisation of affects in play or artistic activity, un-coupled from the consequences of reality. 'Showing off' – presenting oneself to others for appreciation.	Precursor: 'showing off' at 6 months. Representational thought, pretend play with mental elements (feelings, intentions, beliefs), 3 years.
7	complementing	The partner's roles are interdependent and constitute one another, e.g. the carrier & the carried, the seeker & the sought-for, the chaser & the chased, the protector & the protected, the victim & the perpetrator etc. Integration of reality and fantasy, self/others abilities, regulation of other people's affects (comforting, provoking etc.).	Complete representations theory of mind, perspective-taking (part III): thinking about thinking, understanding deception. Reflecting mode of thought. 4–6 years.

Source: Table 6.1 is based on research by Fonagy et al. (2002); Grossmann/Grossmann (2005); Kestenberg Amighi et al. (1999); Kestenberg/Sossin (1979); Lewis Bernstein (1981); Mahler, Pine, and Bergman (1975); Metzloff/Moore (2006); Sandel (1993); Schore (2003); Sodian (2012); Stern (1985); Trevarthen (2006); and Winnicott (1971).

person's sense of self-efficacy. By contrast, disturbances of mirroring opportunities, such as when contingency is completely missing, or when contingency is too high, lead to disintegrated states of self, between autistic isolation and pathological fusion (Gallese, 2003). In healthy relating, phases in which partners move out of sync should punctuate phases of synchrony.

Although Chace had already pointed out this perspective of the patient's mirroring in 1952 (Chace, 1993), it gained wider attention with respect to empathy development through research on DMP such as Berrol (2006), Wengrower (2010), McGarry and Russo (2011), Behrends, Müller, and Dziobek (2012), and Koch, Mehl, Sobanski, Sieber, and Fuchs (2014). However, in this literature, the interactions were undifferentiated beyond modal and cross-modal mirroring (see Table 6.1).

A new take on mirroring: A taxonomy of mirroring modalities

Interaction is defined as the mutual or reciprocal action or influence of things or people on one another (Webster, 2017). In over 30 years of clinical practice, the author has observed a variety of patterns of interaction, which changed over the course of therapy, seemingly in relation to the acquisition of psycho-social competencies. Based on the writings of Chace, Kestenberg, and Lewis, and informed by neurobiological and infant research, this author sought to systematise these observations in a developmental order. Stern (1985) used the term mirroring to describe parent–child interaction in his research; and, like Chace and Sandel, he did not consider parental mirroring to be a single form of interaction, but rather as a concept which includes different processes that serve age-specific functions in development: such as, responsivity, regulation, attunement, validation and modification. In this vein, this chapter proposes using the term 'mirroring modalites' to refer to forms of interaction in which the movement of a person or group is picked up and reflected in some more or less modified way by another person or group. An overview of the modalities will be given in Table 6.1, followed by more detailed descriptions.

The following taxonomy of 14 mirroring modalities, in accordance with embodiment theory, mark developmental stages which simultaneously address motor, cognitive, emotional and social levels of functioning. Since human infants are astonishingly capable from birth, the order does not suggest that any one modality is only relevant in this phase of development, but rather that it is highlighted during the acquisition of an aspect of social cognition and affect regulation. Table 6.1 has been structured according to these affinities and the ages named in the right column refer to the age at which this modality is highlighted, while mentioning earlier precursors.

In Table 6.1, the modalities are formulated as verbs rather than nominalisations, to emphasise their procedural nature. Table 6.1 begins with early, lower-order capacities and competencies and ends with higher-order achievements. Development in this model is cumulative rather than only a stage model of development, because lower-order competencies continue to be operational and supportive of higher order competencies throughout life (Bråten, 2013). The modalities are experienced mostly in dyads during infant development but can apply to any number of interacting individuals of any age. They can refer to many forms of expression besides dance movement, such a voice, speech, music, or art.

The following explanations are structured to first define the movement phenomenon, and then refer to the developmental function of the mirroring modality.

Initiating, continuing, terminating

Initiate means to cause or facilitate the beginning of a process or action (Merriam Webster, 2017; Oxford, 2017). To interact, a person must either become aware of a person directing attention at them (attending processes) or attract the attention of a person (intending processes). The human infant can respond to and initiate interaction less than an hour after birth (Kugiumutzakis, 1998; Meltzoff and Moore, 2006). Orientation reactions such as turning and gazing are hardwired, but after discovering contingency through feedback information, they are repeated for the pleasure of self-efficacy (Lichtenberg, Lachmann, and Fosshage, 2016). The term initiation can refer to a temporal aspect (who moves first?), an aspect of dominance (who leads the communal movement of partners?) or an aspect of innovation (whose movements are new or different?) (Lewis Bernstein, 1981). This modality is a primary form of self-efficacy and pre-requisite for self/other regulation, and the repair of interactional ruptures, which are commonplace in human interaction (Shai and Fonagy, 2013).

Initiating can take on the quality of a symbolic birth situation, in which case it touches on questions of the right to exist or feelings of worth (Will my movement be accepted?), questions of self-efficacy (Does my movement have any effect, and if so, what kind?), and on questions of identity (What is mine, what is the expression of others?). While an infant is naturally active and initiating, inadequate response such as excessive contingency or lack of contingency can severely inhibit the initiative of a person (Fonagy, Gergely, Jurist, and Target, 2002; Schore, 2003). Therefore, the therapist must find the appropriate relation between receptivity for the impulses of the patient, however small, on the one hand, and actively offering input on the other hand.

Continuing a joint movement is a means of maintaining a relationship. On an intrapersonal level, the ability to uphold a movement without the immediate participation of a caregiver is a result of retaining a representation of the partner. Severely depressed patients, for example, may be unable to continue a movement without the participation of a partner (Lewis Bernstein, 1981).

Terminating, putting an end to an interaction – for example through stillness, turning away spatially or setting a dynamic accent – is a crucial form of self- and other regulation (Lewis Bernstein, 1981). Studies of mothers with a borderline personality disorder show how they cannot tolerate their child averting its gaze and pursue it until the child resigns and presumably dissociates (Downing, 2004).

Coordination: Synchronising and alternating

Synchronising is the temporal matching of movement with high contingency. In natural interactions, synchrony is a phenomenon that comes and goes, lasting only a while before it dissolves in idiosyncratic movement of the partners.

Infant research has shown that we discern between self and not-self through the difference between perfect and incomplete contingency, in the comparison of one's own movements and the reaction of the world around us (Fonagy et al., 2002). For example, an infant recognises perfect contingency when she watches herself in a mirror or a live video recording. If given the choice, infants prefer the incomplete contingency of an attuned but individual reaction of a person or a toy. For only then can they develop a sense of agency, experience affective exchange and share communication (Fonagy et al., 2002). However, people who have hardly experienced mirroring in their early years have the tendency to completely give up their own movement and dissolve into the other, rather than enter an exchange with them. This modality can be termed medial or oceanic mirroring: the term 'medial' refers to the idea that the interactional partners do not experience themselves as separate entities but as dissolved in some medium (like water) or atmospheric conditions (like outer space) in which they experience unity. This feeling can only be achieved with very simple, symmetrical movements like bobbing, rocking, or breathing. Examples of medial experiences are the unity of a horse and rider, a dancing couple, or of a mass of people at a rock concert. In everyday meetings of people, the perfect contingency of medial mirroring is something that lasts only a few seconds.

Alternating occurs when partners take turns, initiating and following action. In this modality assertion and acceptance emerge as cooperative patterns. This modality is often, but not only related to vocal interaction, since simultaneous vocalising is not as easily discerned as visually perceived movement. Repetition, mimetic sympathy, phrasing, and rhythm all facilitate reciprocal anticipation of turns. Congruent action – staying true to one's own style – supports self/other identification and primary intersubjectivity (Trevarthen, 2006).

Concordance: Modal mirroring

Modal mirroring concerns the most exact fit between the initiated movement and the mirroring answer. Both parties use the same movement elements and the initiator feels a sense of agency and of being seen. On a neurobiological level, opiates are discharged to the brain, producing feelings of pleasure and bonding the partners to one another (Schore, 2003). During asymmetrical movements, we can observe that the partners share a common imaginary movement axis, each representing a half of the whole picture. When one person moves the right side of her body, the partner will move with the left side, as our reflection in a mirror would. Should one partner continuously take the lead, the atmosphere of a partial-object relationship will ensue, as can be observed in persons with self-alienation syndromes. If it is possible to alternate the leadership of the concordantly mirrored movement, the sense of a harmonious relationship between autonomous partners may result. Recently, Feninger-Schaal and Lotan (2017) found that adult mirroring behaviour could reveal embodied secure attachment or anxiety and avoidance.

Cross-modal mirroring is based upon the neurological connection between the senses, also known as synaesthetic perception. For example, a rising tone has an affinity to a rising line or a light source growing brighter, the vertical rising of the body and so forth. When we mirror cross-modally, we respond to the dynamic or the form of the movement but use a different sensory modality or part of the body than the initiator (Kestenberg and Sossin, 1979; Stern, 1985). Person A is attuned to the affect of person B, but signals her interpersonal differentiation using another medium. For example, a shaking movement of person B's hands may be mirrored by a head movement or a sound by person A. Performed in direct interaction, this modality emphasises the simultaneous connection and differentiation between the individuals, similarly to marked mirroring. When the mirroring person does not interact directly with the initiator, she can support the independent activity of the initiator, by cross-modally accompanying her from a certain distance.

Parallel mirroring requires both partners turn their attention and their movement in the same direction towards a goal outside of their dyad, in the sense of joint attention. Mirroring activity may pertain to the whole body or isolated parts, including facial expression. In the horizontal position next to one another this modality conveys an atmosphere of solidarity or support in the encounter with a third entity. This position can be particularly helpful for the regulation of troublesome affects during therapeutic processes, such as when patient and therapist look at photographs, drawings, letters, and other documents together, side by side, or during imaginative trauma exploration.

This modality facilitates the ability to play and explore. Ideally, a child may engage in its own interests and can see mirrored in the face of their caretakers that these also take an interest in the child's activity, without trying to interfere. In dysfunctional families, activities that are not directly related to the needs of the caretakers may be disregarded, suppressed, devalued, or intruded upon. When play in the presence of a caretaker involves emotional or physical entanglement, the development of a core self and feelings of individual importance and vitality are in jeopardy (Stern, 1985; Wöller, 2013).

Altercentric mirroring is the motor precursor of intersubjectivity and theory of mind, as this modality involves taking on the perspective of the other. In contrast to modal mirroring, here each partner has his own movement axis. Payne (1992) described this as joining. When positioned across from each other, the partners mirror movement alter(other)-centred in the way the initiator experiences it, not as a mirror would reflect it, so a movement to the right side of the body is also performed to the right by the mirroring partner. A slight differentiation ensues, as the movements seem to go in opposite directions to each other, when both move to their own right side. Both autocentricity and altercentricity coexist throughout the lifespan. The ability to approach things, situations, and relationships from both an external (altercentric) and a felt (autocentric) perspective is a hallmark of healthy child development (De Robertis, 2008).

Mirroring with counter-movement depends on the spatial orientation of the partners to each other in a repetitive movement like walking, rocking, stepping up and down, or opening and closing limbs. The movements of the partners are coordinated out of phase so that when one goes forward the other goes back, right instead of left, up when the other is down, etc. Counter-movement is a modality that emphasises interpersonal boundaries and distinction within the constraints of a social context (Miles, Griffiths, Richardson, and Macrae, 2010). This phase coincides with the epistemic perspective taking, in which children at 2 years of age can infer the visual perspective of another person (Sodian, 2012).

Deferred imitating is imitating with a time-lag of seconds or days. It requires and strengthens retention and recall of movement, memory development, and identification processes. An early form of deferred imitating is available at 2 months, when babies recognise a person by a movement pattern (Metzloff and Moore, 2006). This ability to capture an impression of another person leads to temporal object constancy. Intentional thought develops at 14 months, in which children become aware of inner, not externally visible causes of behaviour. They begin to reflect on why a goal is pursued, not just that and how it is done, and thus learn to consider the needs and beliefs of others (Sodian, 2012). Replacing one object with another in the recreation of a situation marks the beginning of symbolisation, and the pretend modality of mentalising. Symbol usage (i.e. thinking in words and images) allows the child to more fully experience the world of shared perceptual meanings. For better or worse, abstract conceptualisations like 'within me' and 'outside of me' can now come into being (De Robertis, 2008).

Completing or developing a goal-oriented movement of a partner which is incomplete or faulty is a sign of intersubjective understanding of others. Based on shared knowledge of a movement and its meaning, completing integrates memory (knowing what the complete movement would be) and altercentric perspective (inferring what the other plans to do, would enjoy) and has been found in children as young as 18 months (Trevarthen, 2006). In dance, poetry, or in song, we may enjoy giving a partner the first part of a phrase, waiting for them to complete the second part as a sign of connection.

Contrasting takes the main intention of the movement of a partner and does the opposite e.g. changing the speed from quick to slow, or the direction from up to down, etc. This coincides with the development of the ability to realise that oneself and others may have different intentions and play with this situation, at around 2 years of age. The relationship is ambivalent, as doing the opposite serves differentiation, while the common theme and the friction, the influence on the other through going against them serves connection. This is also a phase in which conceptual thought about opposites, forms, directions, and positions develops through movement experimentation (Sodian, 2012).

Varying is the alteration or embellishment of a given movement. New aspects of form or dynamics may be added, while a similarity to the original movement remains. The ambivalence of contrasting is dissolved in a synthesis of self and other input. This modality facilitates the building of identity beyond the phase of identification through the individual interpretation of inspiration gained from others. In cognitive development, as of about 4 years of age, the mentalistic self-image of believing that one's thoughts and feelings depict reality is replaced by a representational self-image. This means the person realises that their thinking is only a variation, perspective or image of reality that can be wrong and should change if found so (Sodian, 2012). This allows for the development of explicit intersubjectivity.

Marked varying or pronounced mirroring is a form of goal-oriented misattunement (Stern, 1985) which exaggerates the form or dynamic of the initiator's movement with an addition of humour or scepticism, showing that this emotion is seen, but not taken quite as seriously as by the initiator ('My, aren't you angry!'). This distinction between the person mirrored and the person mirroring confirms their interpersonal differentiation and strengthens the sense of agency of the initiator. The mirroring person serves a containing function by means of this modality, because she is less emotionally involved than the initiator, and so she can be a model for the regulation of intensity (Fonagy et al., 2002). In development, this phase involves imaginary play with emotions, intentions, and beliefs in role-play as of 3 years of age, enabling the person to practice dealing with such mental elements ('I am an angry bear who will eat you up!' 'Oh, I am so afraid!'). A precursor begins at 6 months in the self-conscious and other-conscious display of actions with social meaning, 'showing off' not only for personal relief or expression but to provoke an effect in the social environment (Trevarthen, 2006).

Complementary interaction concerns sequences of interaction in which the activities of partner A and B are different, yet depend on and complete each other, such as leading and following, holding and being held, chasing, and fleeing. They are called complementary. Complementary interaction is closely related to contrasting interaction but is more complex. The focus is not on movement qualities, as is the case with contrasting, but on the function of the movement. Furthermore, the partner's actions have a direct functional influence on one another in comparison to contrasting, in which the movements might take place in a functionally independent way. For example, in contrasting, partner A might hold herself upright, while partner B falls to the ground. In a complementary relationship, partner A would catch and hold partner B upright, while B lets herself fall into A's arms. They experience a functional dependency, and directly exert an influence upon one other.

Bateson (1972) differentiated between one-sided complementarity and reciprocal complementarity. In one-sided complementarity the roles are fixed, and the co-regulation of the partners may escalate ('the more you . . . the more I . . .') and fail. Reciprocal complementarity on the contrary, allows the partners to regulate the relationship by trading roles. They may integrate regressive and progressive aspects of the personality, which enables self-regulation.

Ideally, a person will encounter many different forms of complementary relationships and have opportunities to embody both sides of a complementary constellation. In this way they develop a complete representation of self and others, the ability to self-regulate, and a theory-of-mind, enabling intersubjective perspective-taking.

Applications in practice

For the use of the modalities in DMP practice, the following variations should be considered:

- Degree of body involvement: most modalities can be explored with isolated movement of body parts, including gaze activity (e.g. gazing towards something, keeping it in view, diverting one's gaze), full body movement or travelling through space.

- Number of participants: the modalities are experienced in dyads during infant development but can apply to any number of interacting individuals.
- Diagnostics and evaluation: clinicians might classify the spontaneous behaviour of patients or they might use the taxonomy as a test, offering patients different interaction modalities to discover their preferences, strengths and deficits. This allows them to understand the situation of the patient, and subsequently choose appropriate interventions to first support resources and second encourage development. Similarly, spontaneous or systematic classification of the interactions of the patient can serve to evaluate the progress of the patient.
- Interventions: the modalities can be viewed as a catalogue of fundamental skills that can be developed independently of the specific disturbance of the patient, by offering appropriate interventions. In contrast, individual modalities may be selected to help meet the challenges facing patients with a particular disorder, symptom, or problem. They are suitable for work with children and adults.

Critical aspects of therapeutic mirroring

In the course of DMP's development, problematic aspects of picking up patients' signals became apparent. Clinical observations are related to findings from infancy research and DMP research. Meltzoff and Moore (2006) describe the parent's intention to participate in exchanges with their offspring as selective, interpretive, and creative. On the one hand, they are an essential aspect of parental scaffolding (Vygotsky, 1978), a term referring to successive levels of temporary support, that help infants or adult learners reach higher levels of skill acquisition than they would be able to achieve on their own. Like physical scaffolding, the supportive strategies are gradually removed when no longer needed, as the parent or therapist gradually shifts more responsibility to the subject. However, the selective, interpretive side of parental/therapeutic participation can have negative effects on the child/patient. The same is true for sibling/co-patient interaction. Examples of such negative forms of mirroring are presented here.

- Under-attunement, or a receiver's echo with an unclear relationship to the expression of the sender may go unnoticed (Kalish, 1977; Wengrower, 2010). Too little attunement may lead to a limited spectrum of expression, depressive resignation and the feeling that certain affective states cannot be shared, or to over-achievement to attract attention (Stern, 1985).
- Over-attunement (Kestenberg and Sossin, 1979; Stern, 1985) or perfect contingency (Fonagy et al., 2002) lacks differentiation between the sender and the receiver of an emotional expression. This may be experienced as mocking or provocation (Chaiklin, 1975) or as impingement that sparks withdrawal (Kalish, 1977). In other cases, it may cause boredom (Fonagy et al., 2002) to the point of being experienced as abandonment if no input comes from the following partner (Romer, 1993). In a therapeutic context, over-attunement can be a sign of an over-identification of the therapist with her patient or the projection of the therapist's affect onto the patient. Without a reflective distance and stable interpersonal boundaries, the therapist offers no regulative abilities to the patient and affective processes may get out of control (Sandel, 1993).
- Selective attunement and misattunement are manipulative processes in which the receiver picks up certain affective or motoric qualities and neglects others or modifies the intensity of attunement (higher or lower than the sender), respectively (Stern, 1985). The receiver thus shapes the behaviour of the sender towards a predetermined goal of their own, neglecting the interests of the person to whom they are attuning. This stands in contrast to

attunement or varying, which is open regarding the outcome of the interaction and respects the interests of both interactional participants. Since human evolutionary development favoured social over individual needs, people are vulnerable to manipulation, which can lead to serious limitations of the affective and behaviour repertoire (Stern, 1985). Sandel (1993) also warns against the tendency of the dance therapist in group therapy to respond only to the highest energy level or to collude with avoidance tendencies in the group, due to her own anxiety.

- The mirroring of movements intended to express or achieve self–other differentiation or distancing undermines their function and may provoke anger or fear in the partner (Sandel, 1993). In such cases, the modality of contrasting or complementing would be more appropriate (see Table 6.1).
- Mirroring involuntary or uncertain movements in the context of somatic symptoms (such as the tremor in patients with Parkinson's) is experienced as ridicule. Similarly, picking up a movement that is tentative and not yet intended for the attention of others may make the mover feel ridiculed.
- Premature mirroring, expansion, or variation of the patients' movement may overwhelm the subject and disturb the stabilisation of competencies (Kestenberg & Robbins, 1975; Sandel, 1993).
- Secondary traumatisation or burnout can result if the therapist does not debrief, or 'empty their emotional container' and rejuvenate after prolonged or intense engagement with burdening states of others (Lewis, 1984). It is essential for therapists to be informed of these phenomena, to reflect on the causes of their occurrence in each situation, and if necessary to make corrections in procedures.

Professional implications

The taxonomy presented here emphasises the importance of embodied interaction and the interdependence between movement patterns and cognitive and emotional developmental milestones. The critical aspects show, that this interdependence opens the possibility for negative effects of parental and therapeutic interaction. This knowledge allows us to choose appropriate movement interventions to facilitate cognitive or emotional competencies and avoid treatment mistakes. Because of the wide interest in mirror neurons in science and medicine, and the reciprocal perspective, the use of the term mirroring has had a renaissance.

A professional issue facing any discipline in healthcare is to maintain a distinct profile of unique characteristics which make it an essential part of treatment. DMP is characterised by the use of embodied interaction, possibly nonverbal. The importance of nonverbal communication skills for psychotherapeutic practice is becoming more widely recognised and is increasingly included in the training of verbal psychotherapists (Foley and Gentile, 2010). While this trend leads to more acceptance of DMP, it also challenges DMP's uniqueness in its use of movement interaction. However, the depth and scope of skills taught in such a context are not comparable to those taught to dance movement therapists in training. The taxonomy presented in this chapter makes for a differentiated degree of expertise in DMP clear to interdisciplinary colleagues, which maintains the unique contribution DMP can make to healthcare services. This contribution is the differentiated and skilled ability to embody these interventions in a bio-psycho-socially integrated form, through dance movement. It is therefore essential, that the dance movement therapist is trained to engage herself on a kinaesthetic, acoustic, tactile, and visual level as a model or responder to the patient, and to be able to embody the various roles, which the mirroring modalities require.

References

Bateson, G. (1972). *Steps to an Ecology of Mind.* Chicago: University of Chicago Press.

Bauer, J. (2005). *Warum Ich fühle, was Du fühlst – Intuitive Kommunikation und das Geheimnis der Spiegelneurone* [Why I feel what You feel – Intuitive Communication and the Mystery of Mirror Neurons]. Hamburg: Hoffmann und Campe.

Beebe, B. (2014). My journey in infant research and psychoanalysis: Microanalysis, a social microscope. *Psychoanalytic Psychology, 31*(1), 4–25.

Behrends, A., Müller, S., and Dziobek, I. (2012). Moving in and out of synchrony: A concept for a new intervention fostering empathy through interactional movement and dance. *The Arts in Psychotherapy, 39*, 107–116.

Berrol, C. (2006). Neuroscience meets dance/movement therapy: Mirror neurons, the therapeutic process and empathy. *The Arts in Psychotherapy, 33*, 302–315.

Bråten, S. (Ed.) (2006). *Intersubjective Communication and Emotion in Early Ontogeny.* Cambridge: Cambridge University Press.

Bråten, S. (Ed.). (2013). *Roots and Collapse of Empathy.* Amsterdam: John Benjamins.

Chace, M. (1993). Opening doors through dance. In S. Sandel, S. Chaiklin, and A. Lohn (Eds.), *Foundations of Dance/Movement Therapy: The Life and Work of Marian Chace* (S. 199–203). Columbia, MD: The Marian Chace Memorial Fund of the American Dance Therapy Association. (Original work published 1952)

Chaiklin, S. (1975). Dance therapy. In S. Arieti (Ed.), *American Handbook of Psychiatry* (pp. 700–720). New York: Basic Books.

Chaiklin, S., and Schmais, C. (1979). The Chace approach to dance therapy. In P. Lewis Bernstein (Ed.), *Eight Theoretical Approaches in Dance-Movement Therapy* (pp. 15–30). Dubuque, IA: Kendall/Hunt.

de Haan, S., De Jaegher, H., Fuchs, T., and Mayer, A. (2011). Expanding perspectives: The interactive development of perspective-taking in early childhood. In W. Tschacher and C. Bergomi (Eds.), *The Implications of Embodiment* (pp. 129–150). Exeter: Imprint Academic.

De Robertis, E. (2008). *Humanzing Child Developmental Theory.* New York: iUniverse.

Downing, G. (2004). Emotion, body, and parent–infant interaction. In J. Nadel and D. Muir (Eds.), *Emotional Development: Recent Research Advances* (pp. 429–449). Oxford: Oxford University Press.

Eberhard-Kaechele, M. (2009). Von der ko-regulation zur selbstregulation: Spiegelungsphänomene in der tanz- und ausdruckstherapie [From co-regulation to self-regulation: Mirroring phenomena in dance-movement therapy]. In M. Thielen (Ed.), *Körper-Gefühl-Denken. Körperpsychotherapie und Selbstregulation* [Body-Feeling-Thought. Body Psychotherapy and Self-Regulation] (pp. 251–264). Gießen: Psychosozial.

Eberhard-Kaechele, M. (2012). Memory, metaphor, and mirroring in movement therapy with trauma patients. In S. Koch, T. Fuchs, M. Summa, and C. Müller (Eds.), *Body Memory, Metaphor and Movement* (pp. 267–287). Amsterdam: John Benjamins.

Feninger-Schaal, R., and Lotan, N. (2017). The embodiment of attachment: Directional and shaping movements in adult's mirror game. *The Arts in Psychotherapy, 53*, 55–63.

Foley, G. N., and Gentile, J. P. (2010). Nonverbal communication in psychotherapy. *Psychiatry, 7*(6), 38–44.

Fonagy, P., Gergely, G., Jurist, E. L., and Target, M. (2002). *Affect Regulation, Mentalisation, and the Development of the Self.* New York: Other Press.

Fraenkel, D. (1983). The relationship of empathy in movement to synchrony, echoing, and empathy in verbal interactions. *American Journal of Dance Therapy, 6*, 31–48.

Fuchs, T., and De Jaegher, H. (2010). Non-representational intersubjectivity. In T. Fuchs, H. Sattel, and P. Henningsen (Eds.), *The Embodied Self: Dimensions, Coherence and Disorders.* Stuttgart: Schattauer.

Gallese, V. (2003). The manifold nature of interpersonal relations: The quest for a common mechanism. In C. Frith and D. Wolpert (Eds.), *The Neuroscience of Social Interaction: Decoding, Imitating, and Influencing the Actions of Others* (pp. 159–182). Oxford: Oxford University Press.

Gallese, V., Fadiga, L., Fogassi, L., and Rizzolatti, G. (1996). Action recognition in the premotor cortex. *Brain, 119*(2), 593–609.

Gergely, G., Koós, O., and Watson, J. (2010). Contingent parental reactivity in early socio-emotional development. In T. Fuchs, H. Sattel, and P. Henningsen (Eds.), *The Embodied Self: Dimensions, Coherence and Disorders* (pp. 141–169). Stuttgart: Schattauer.

Gibbs, R. (2005). *Embodiment and Cognitive Science.* New York: Cambridge University Press.

Grossmann, K., and Grossmann, K. (2005). *Bindungen – Das Gefüge Psychischer Sicherheit* [Attachment – The Fabric of Psychological Security] (2nd ed.). Stuttgart: Klett-Cotta.

Kalish, B. (1977). Body movement therapy for autistic children. *Focus on Dance*, pp. 48–59.

Kestenberg, J. S., & Robbins, E. (1975). *Children and Parents: Psychoanalytic Studies in Development.* New York: Jason Aronson.

Kestenberg, J., and Sossin, M. (1979). *The Role of Movement Patterns in Development* (Vol. 2). New York: Dance Notation Bureau.

Kestenberg Amighi, J., Loman, S., Lewis, P., & Sossin, K. (1999). *The Meaning of Movement: Development and Clinical Perspectives of the Kestenberg Movement Profile.* New York: Brunner-Routledge.

Koch, S. C., Mehl, L., Sobanski, E., Sieber, M., and Fuchs, T. (2014). Fixing the mirrors: A feasibility study of the effects of dance movement therapy on young adults with autism spectrum disorder. *Autism, 19*(3), 338–350.

Kugiumutzakis, G. (1998). Neonatal imitation in the intersubjective companion space. In S. Bråten (Ed.), *Intersubjective Communication and Emotion in Early Ontogeny* (pp. 63–88). Cambridge: Cambridge University Press.

Lewis Bernstein, P. (1981). *Theory and Methods in Dance-Movement Therapy* (3rd Edition). Dubuque, IA: Kendall/Hunt.

Lewis, P. (1984). The somatic countertransference: The inner pas de deux. In P. Lewis (Ed.), *Theoretical Approaches in Dance-Movement Therapy* (Vol. 2, pp. 181–194). Dubuque, IA: Kendall/Hunt.

Lichtenberg, J., Lachmann, F., and Fosshage, J. (2016). *Self and Motivational Systems. Toward a Theory of Psychoanalytic Technique.* New York: Routledge.

Mahler, M., Pine, F., and Bergman, A. (1975). *The Psychological Birth of the Human Infant. Symbiosis and Individuation.* New York: Basic Books.

McGarry, L., and Russo, F. (2011). Mirroring in dance/movement therapy: Potential mechanisms behind empathy enhancement. *The Arts in Psychotherapy, 38*(3), 178–184.

Meltzoff, A., and Moore, M. K. (2006). Infant intersubjectivity: Broadening the dialogue to include imitation, identity and intention. In S. Bråten (Ed.), *Intersubjective Communication and Emotion in Early Ontogeny* (pp. 47–62). Cambridge: Cambridge University Press.

Miles, L., Griffiths, J., Richardson, M., and Macrae, C. (2010). Too late to coordinate: Contextual influences on behavioral synchrony. *European Journal of Social Psychology, 40*, 52–60.

Oxford. (2017). Retrieved November 12, 2017, from English Oxford Living Dictionaries https://en.oxforddictionaries.com

Payne, H. (1992). Shut in, shut out: Dance movement therapy with children and adolescents. In H. Payne (Ed.), *Dance Movement Therapy: Theory and Practice* (pp. 39–80). London: Routledge.

Romer, G. (1993). Choreographie der haltenden umwelt. [Choreography of the holding environment] In K. Hörmann (Hrsg.), *Tanztherapie [Dance Therapy]* (pp. 33–56). Göttingen: Verlag für Angewandte Psychologie.

Rova, M. (2017). Embodying kinaesthetic empathy through interdisciplinary practice-based research. *The Arts in Psychotherapy, 55*, 164–173.

Sandel, S. L. (1993). The process of empathetic reflection in dance therapy. In S. L. Sandel, S. Chaiklin, and A. Lohn (Eds.), *Foundations of Dance/Movement Therapy: The Life and Work of Marian Chace* (pp. 98–111). Columbia, MD: The Marian Chace Memorial Fund of the American Dance Therapy Association.

Schoop, T., and Mitchell, P. (1974). *Won't YOU Join the Dance? A Dancer's Essay into the Treatment of Psychosis.* Palo Alto, CA: Mayfield Publishing.

Schore, A. (2003). *Affect Regulation and the Repair of the Self.* New York: Norton.

Shai, D., and Fonagy, P. (2013). Beyond words: Parental embodied mentalizing and the parent–infant dance. In M. Mikulincer and P. Shaver (Eds.), *Mechanisms of Social Connection: From Brain to Group* (pp. 185–203). Washington, DC: American Psychological Association.

Sodian, B. (2012). Entwicklung des denkens [The development of cognition]. In W. Schneider and U. Lindenberger (Eds.), *Entwicklungspsychologie* [Developmental Psychology] (6th rev. ed., pp. 436–479). Weinheim: Beltz.

Stern, D. (1985). *The Interpersonal World of the Infant.* New York: Basic Books.

Trevarthen, C. (2006). The concept and foundations of infant intersubjectivity. In S. Bråten (Ed.), *Intersubjective Communication and Emotion in Early Ontogeny* (pp. 15–46). Cambridge: Cambridge University Press.

Vygotsky, L. (1978). Internalization of higher psychological functions. In M. Cole, V. John-Steiner, S. Scribner, and E. Soubermann (Eds.), *Mind in Society* (pp. 52–67). Cambridge, MA: Harvard University Press.

Webster, M. (2017). Retrieved November 12, 2017, from Merriam Webster Dictionary www.merriam-webster.com/.

Wengrower, H. (2010). I am here to move and dance with you. Dance movement therapy with children with autism syndrome disorder. In V. Karkou (Ed.), *Arts Therapies in Schools. Research and Practice* (pp. 179–197). London: Jessica Kingsley.

Winnicott, D. (1971). *Playing and Reality.* London: Penguin Books.

Wöller, W. (Hrsg.). (2013). *Trauma und Persönlichkeitsstörungen* [Trauma and Personality Disorders] (2nd ed.). Stuttgart: Schattauer.

7

WITNESSING PRACTICE

In the eyes of the beholder©

Tina Stromsted

Introduction

What does it mean to be *seen*, to be *heard*, and to be received for who we are? To experience ourselves as real people, and to belong? Promoting these experiences is at the core of witnessing practice. When such deeply human needs have not been met in a person's early development or have been thwarted or injured through subsequent life experiences, they can be fostered through the practice of moving and witnessing in Authentic Movement.

Authentic Movement

A form of dance/movement therapy, Authentic Movement was originated by pioneer dance therapist Mary Starks Whitehouse in California in the 1950s–1970s, and has continued to evolve and thrive in many parts of the world.[1] A modern dancer and dance teacher, Whitehouse sought to better understand the interrelationships between body, psyche, and spirit (Whitehouse, 1958/1999), and engaged in Jungian analysis followed by studies in Jungian depth-psychology in Zurich. Applying Jung's active imagination method (Chodorow, 1997, 2006; Jung, 1916/1957, 1928/1966, 1955/1970) to movement experience, she developed a way to support people in fostering self-awareness and accessing unconscious processes through embodied exploration. The practice allowed for the development of the authentic self, a greater sense of well-being, self-knowledge and a deepened connection with others and with life's sacred dimension. Embodiment is a felt sense of aliveness and well-being in the body, and an awareness of one's whole being in the present moment. Authentic Movement helps people re-inhabit their body through a natural process (Stromsted, 1995; Stromsted and Sieff, 2015).

In Authentic Movement practice, the mover/client closes her eyes, waits, and then, in the presence of her witness/therapist, moves in response to body-felt sensations, movement impulses, emotions, memories, dreams, and/or internal images. The opportunity to be 'seen' by a witness who is not *watching* or *observing* the mover, but rather *holding* her in a receptive, compassionate gaze – without interpretation or judgment – allows the mover to experience and to follow the immediacy of her own authentic experience safely. While teaching, I often say to my students that, in this practice, 'my body is my teacher, and I am the student who follows'. In this way, the mover can reconnect with her instinctual ground of being, discovering and transforming

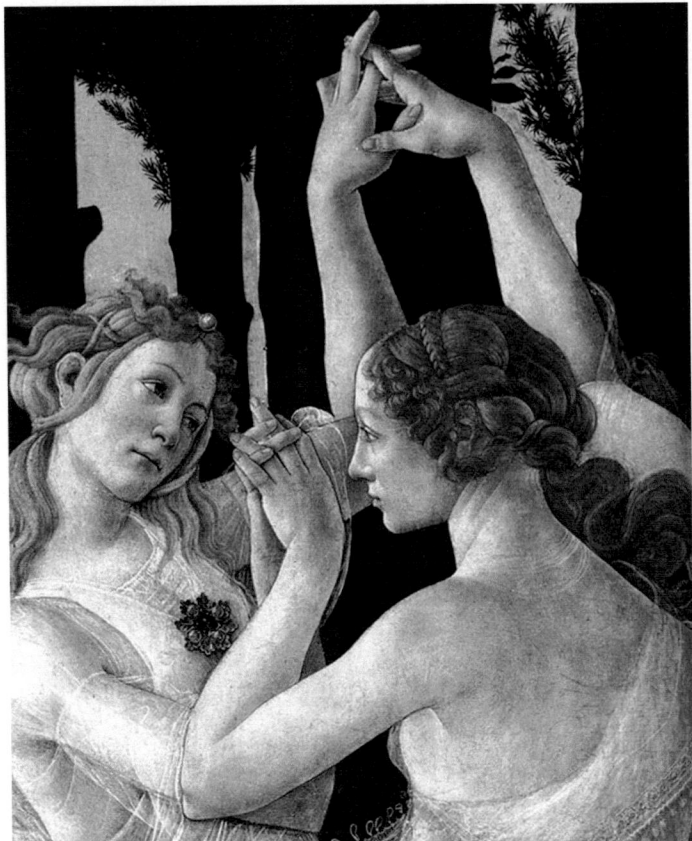

Figure 7.1 Sandro Botticelli, 'Primavera', ca. 1482

emotions and undeveloped capacities held in the body beneath the level of consciousness. During the mover's explorations, her witness sits to the side with her eyes open, bringing a sense of quiet warmth, receptive focus, and presence to the space. She also monitors the time allowed for the session and maintains an awareness of her own embodied experience.

Following the movement session, the mover often shares significant moments from her movement journey and receives verbal reflection from her witness if she wishes. Witnessing (W) language is rooted in describing movement literally, using the present tense to stay with the immediacy of the experience (Stromsted and Haze, 2007, p. 65). For example, 'I see your head bow down and a tear stream down your cheek; as I see this, I feel a release in my jaw and softening and warmth in my chest'. This language of neutral observation is used instead of interpretation, such as: 'I see you crying and bowing your head, so I imagine that you are ashamed'. Sometimes witnesses share images that come to them as well, though they are careful to own them as their own. This leaves the mover free to be curious about them, without needing to take them on. As such, witnessing represents a departure from the interpretive language that is often a part of psychotherapy. In this way, the mover remains the expert of her own experience, a democratic format that allows each to *be* in the other's presence.

Over the years, I have found that witnesses who are psychotherapists often make interpretations, as they have been trained to do in verbal psychotherapy, thinking that it was helpful to the mover. However, in some of these instances, the mover experiences a sense of being hurt, judged, or simply unseen following her movement, at a time when she is deeply vulnerable. I have often heard witnesses, with the best of intentions, unconsciously using evaluative language like 'You looked a little stiff', 'I wish you'd kept going with that', or even, 'You were absolutely beautiful!' This last sounds affirming, but it may leave the mover with the take-away message that she needs to be beautiful for her witnesses (Stromsted, 2015, p. 348). Thus, the witness needs to strip language down to its essential ingredients, stay true to the mover's personal metaphors, and acknowledge his or her own embodied experience as a witness, when asked. To this end, Janet Adler introduced the concept of 'percept language' adapted from her studies with psychologist John Weir (Haze and Stromsted, 1994/1999, p. 114). Using 'I' statements to own one's experience, this non-judgmental, non-interpretive way of speaking provides additional clarity, safety, and depth for movers and witnesses alike.

The seeds of Authentic Movement work began decades before Whitehouse developed a distinct method. In a journal entry, writing around 1924, Tina Keller, a patient of Jung's who later worked with his associate Toni Wolff (Keller, 1972; Keller-Jenny, 1982; Keller, in Swan, 2012; Oppikofer, 2015) describes her experience of moving in an analytic hour:

> When I was in analysis with Miss Toni Wolff, I often had the feeling that something in me hidden deep inside wanted to express itself; but I also knew that this 'something' had no words. As we were looking for another means of expression, I suddenly had the idea: 'I could dance it'. Miss Wolff encouraged me to try. The body sensation I felt was oppression; the image came that I was inside a stone and had to release myself from it to emerge as a separate, self-standing individual. The movements that grew out of the body sensations had the goal of my liberation from the stone just as the image had. It took a good deal of the hour. After a painful effort I stood there, liberated. This very freeing event was much more potent than the hours in which we only talked. This was a 'psychodrama' of an inner happening, or that which Jung had named 'active imagination'. Only here it was the body that took the active part.
>
> *(Keller, 1972, p. 22, translated by R. Oppikofer)*

Healing Movement has been practiced from the beginning of human history. Among traditional peoples, shamans allowed themselves to 'be moved' from an inner source, opening to a spirited upwelling of sensory and imaginal experiences to express themselves through dance (Eliade, 1964; Stromsted, 1995; Wosein 1974). Communities acted as collective witnesses, forming an outer circle to contain the dance, so that the dancer/Shaman could be free to deeply follow what was moving him or her from within. Authentic Movement occurs in a similar way, within a safe container provided by witnesses, though the emphasis is not on fostering trance states, but on the development of individual and collective consciousness. Also known as Active Imagination in Movement, the practice allows the mover to bring awareness to his embodied experience in the present moment, attending to it as it unfolds without agenda or plan. This supports the development of emotional intelligence as primal affects are experienced in the body, explored, brought to consciousness, and gradually integrated into a more whole personality. Genuine feelings emerge enhancing self-knowledge and connection, rather than being repressed, polished for 'political correctness', 'acted out' in the world, or turned inward in potentially self-destructive cognitions and behaviors. Over time this cultivates embodied presence and empathy – one's capacity to hold and receive the depths of another's experience. Simple in format, this approach allows for a range and depth of experience and is practiced in both individual and group settings.

The gaze

The mover–witness process has parallels to the process of child development. D.W. Winnicott, a child psychoanalyst and pediatrician, spoke of the importance of the mother's gaze for an integrated sense of self, a sense of 'being real'. Self-psychologist Heinz Kohut described this responsiveness as the 'gleam in the mother's eye' that gives the child a sense of being safe, secure and loved (Kohut, 1966, p. 251). The mother's face is the 'precursor of the mirror' (Winnicott, 1971, p. 111), reflecting her pleasure in her baby. When the baby sees his mother's loving expression, he feels lovable and good. Over time, as the baby sees himself in her 'mirror', he comes to see himself. As Winnicott says, 'When I look, I am seen, so I exist' (1971, p. 114).

But how does healing occur when the gaze has been distorted, or less than loving? Parents may not have received enough emotional containment and empathic mirroring themselves. When this is the case, they are thwarted in being able to embody their own genuineness, their own sense of goodness/enoughness, to mirror and pass down this sense of wholeness and goodness to their children. Kohut asserted that parents' failures in empathizing with their children – and their children's responses to these failures – were 'at the root of almost all psychopathology' (Nersessian and Kopff, 1996, p. 661).

Witnessing helps address this by providing a relational environment that can reflect the 'real self'. Crucial to the process of witnessing is the quality of the witness' gaze. Having a 'good enough' witness/therapist/mother-figure (Winnicott, 1971, p. 81) who is capable of containing the mover's experience makes it possible to explore unconscious material safely, within a 'free and sheltered space' (Kalff, 1980, p. 29). This allows for regression – which is necessary in order to access earlier developmental experiences – as well as exploration, expression, reintegration, and transformation. It also allows for new experiences, as the mover feels safe enough to leave the familiar shore and embark on a deeper journey. Over time, the experience of being held and mirrored by an attuned witness allows the mover to develop an 'inner witness' (Adler, 2003/2007, p. 25; Sager, 2015; Stromsted, 2009, p. 207), a capacity to pause, contain, and reflect on her own experience. This brings about a deeper sense of embodied awareness, emotional literacy, and discernment, an embodied wisdom that becomes a potent guide in the person's life.

The following example illustrates how the witness helps the mover explore painful emotions generated by childhood and adult relationships, integrating them into a more fully embodied sense of self:

> *'Elia,' the mover, has just gone through a wrenching breakup with her partner when she meets with her Authentic Movement peer group. At first, she walks aimlessly, meandering around the circle with her eyes closed. Sensing the warmth of a pool of light she comes to a standstill and begins to play with the material of the baggy white blouse she is wearing, swooping her arms up and away from her body in wide, vigorous arcs and figure eights. Gradually she comes to a pause, wraps her arms around her chest, and begins to sway.*
>
> *Following Elia's sharing of her experience in the circle, a witness says that at first she feels distraught as Elia walks in different directions throughout the space. Then, as Elia pauses and swings her arms the witness feels strength in her spine and torso, with a growing sense of warmth and comfort as Elia begins to sway. 'Throughout your movement I find myself very drawn to your feet', her witness recalls. Elia responds that it is affirming to hear the witness' experience, and that the attention to her feet helps bring her own awareness from her upper body down to her feet, helping her feel more grounded during a time of disorientation. A second witness shares that as Elia makes figure eights with her billowing blouse that an image of 'a sailboat with gusts of wind filling its big white sail' comes to her, 'moving as if lost at sea before finding its home harbor.' 'I feel really sad and unmoored at first', she says, 'then revitalized as you play with your shirt; and at*

peace when you come to a resting place at the end.' Elia nods and responds, 'Hearing your feelings and the image of the sail boat coming into harbor helps me find meaning in my movement. I feel seen at a really painful time in my journey. Now I can begin to find my way home.'

Following the movement session, Elia journals about her experience and remembers the anguish she felt when her mother left her father when she was five years old. Her breath releases and tears come, softening her jaw and her heart as a new sense of spaciousness and belonging emerge.

Here we see how sensation, movement, emotion, image, and memory come together generating an integrative, embodied experience in the safety of a contained space of conscious, compassionate witnesses.

Witnessing also helps mitigate the rise of narcissism, the 'me-first-and-most' character traits that a growing percentage of our population – including our world leaders – suffer from. One might even understand the rampant use of 'selfies' as a symptom of insufficient, inaccurate mirroring. Witnessing provides a safe container (*temenos*) from which the authentic self can emerge, from beneath the 'adapted' or socialized 'false self' (Winnicott, 1965, p. 140). This is increasingly important in today's world, where one's outer image must be manicured, managed, and 'branded', converting personhood into a commodity valued in terms of beauty, fame, or net worth, threatening to overshadow genuine feelings, experience, and meaningful relationships.

In an Authentic Movement group I facilitated in East Asia, a participant reported the following dream:

'I am alone on the top floor of a tall skyscraper; when I look out the window I tumble down toward the sidewalk below. Though I am terrified that I will die from the impact, I wake up before I land.' Afterward, I ask her if it would be okay for me to slowly mirror the movements I saw her do as she shared her dream. Her shoulders had been pulled in and raised up around her ears, her breath shallow, her eyes wide and her mouth turned down.

My mirroring gave her a sudden insight. 'It's as if I'm coming down from the tower of my head where I have been living, finding my way to earth. I didn't even know how much I lived there, until I was afraid of falling . . . But you are catching me now'. Ultimately, the witness was doing what the mover's own mother had not done: provide a safe container, mirror her feelings, and accept her body, so that she could inhabit it. 'When I was born, [my mother] was profoundly disappointed; while she was pregnant she went to a doctor and a shaman to get medicines, herbs and prayers to be sure I'd be a boy and has always been angry with me for being a girl. . . . I could feel my curves on the floor yesterday, and felt safe and accepted for who I am. Today is the first day that I can feel that I have a woman's body'. In this movement exploration and integrative dream sequence, we see a young woman 'descend' into her softening body. The process brought consciousness to her cellular experience. Her emotions opened, she began to grieve, and was joined by many other women in the workshop who resonated with her experience of being a woman in a culture in which women are to be accommodating and men tend to be more prized.

Witnessing practice can also be deeply moving and healing for the witnesses themselves. As a witness maintains an open, receptive presence she may be deeply touched by what she sees and senses, as her mover engages experiences that go to the deepest levels of human experience. Some years ago, a participant in a cancer recovery group asked me whether, in my own psychotherapy practice, *I* was the mover and my *client* the witness. When I looked surprised, she explained, 'I felt so deeply touched by witnessing my mover that it brought tears, and such warmth in my heart'. This sense of being profoundly moved by another's humanity is a feeling that I, too, have experienced on many occasions. 'When two strings of an instrument resonate . . . each is changed by the impact of the other' (Siegel, 2010, p. 54).

Contributions from neuroscience

What about the science behind the gaze? Advances in interpersonal neuroscience indicate that witnessing is supported by the mirror neuron system, among others. This system is thought to be the root of empathy, contributing to our capacity to 'resonate' with another (Cozolino, 2006, p. 187; Gallese, 2003). Mirror neurons 'fire' in the brain of a witness when she observes her mover performing an action that is familiar to her (Berrol, 2006; Damasio, 2010, p. 104). In this way, 'We pick up not only another person's movement but her emotional state and intentions as well' (van der Kolk, 2014, p. 59).

Though the witness may resonate with her mover's experience, she maintains a quality of stillness, containing the mover's response instead of enacting it in the moment. As she 'holds space' for her mover's experience and for her own, information from her body – particularly from the primitive, survival-oriented areas in the brain stem and limbic system – forge links and deeper levels of connectivity and integration with the higher cortical centers in the brain (the prefrontal cortex). This provides an opportunity to reflect on and bring language to what she is sensing and feeling. The process of pausing, breathing, and bringing sustained attention to one's own responses and 'knee-jerk' reactions quiets the limbic system, invokes the parasympathetic (rest/digest) nervous system, and supports insight, self-knowledge, and self-regulation.

The presence of an empathic witness also supports the mover in widening what psychiatrist and neuroscience author Daniel Siegel calls the 'affect window of tolerance' (Ogden and Fisher, 2015; Siegel, 2010, p. 252). Intolerable emotions can arise in the presence of others, as old relational issues surface. These are often accompanied by affects that weren't acceptable to one's parents, which resulted in shaming, abandonment, or abuse. Therefore, working with a safe witness can make it possible for the client to begin to tolerate a wider range of feelings – such as hate, rage, shame, contempt, disgust, grief, hope, and love – experience them safely in the body, become curious about them, and explore them in a relational context. This, in turn, helps to create trust, repair early wounding, and foster the development of healthy attachment and a capacity for more flexible, reciprocal relating. This is essential for self-care, for relating to others, and for preserving and fostering community (Homann, 2017; Keleman, 1985; Schore, 2012; Schore and Sieff, 2015; Siegel, 2010, p. 55; Wilkinson, 2010, p. 46).

Culture's body

Witnessing is not only important in the therapeutic process, but crucial for our development as human beings. It helps prepare us to become family members, friends, parents, workers, and world citizens. 'Having been seen' with all of our contradictions in the wholeness of our experience enables us to see others, including 'others' who are not like us: children at school, colleagues in work settings, partners/spouses, our own children, people on the street, citizens of other countries, those who have emigrated from other parts of the world, and those who were born in our own country but look different from us.

Authentic Movement practice is deeply shaped by different cultures, and yet opens to profoundly universal, archetypal experiences as well. For example, while teaching in Japan, I learned that direct eye contact is sometimes experienced as intrusive, and that bowing is the accustomed way to greet someone. I invited movers and witnesses to explore a soft gaze that included the face and shoulders of their partner, rather than focusing on the eyes. In groups in Argentina where there is a history of dictators, military juntas, and 'disappeared' people, movements expressing protective containment and discipline oscillated with those of smoldering wildness and the elegant intimacy of tango! Also notable was a deep capacity for reflectiveness, resilience, and passion in connection. Moving and witnessing in post-Apartheid South Africa affirmed the importance of re-connecting with their deeper cultural heritage, integrating more 'non-traditional' embodied approaches into contemporary verbal psychotherapy. My experience in these and other cultural settings has helped me gain a deeper appreciation for the diversity both in the mover, and in the projections, biases and new learnings possible in the 'eyes of the beholder'.

Conclusion: Witnessing and community

The body is home to the senses, feelings, thoughts, breath, memories, dreams, and all of life's experiences; it is the bedrock of who we are. Being 'in touch' with oneself is the root of empathy; without it, other people's feelings don't register in us, or do not matter. This creates an environment where one must live from 'image', a condition promulgated by consumerist culture. Being split off from our bodies also means being disconnected from others and from the world around us. This not only leads to a sense of alienation, both from ourselves and from others, but ultimately creates the conditions for unrestrained aggression, including bullying, shaming, and other acts of violence. Distorted, paranoid attempts to maintain boundaries between 'us' and 'them' become rigidly maintained for paranoid safety. This is like an autoimmune disease in the cultural body, which seeks to reject what could help it grow.

Today children and adults in industrialized cultures are learning to occupy themselves in isolation, and to work without time boundaries via the ever-available email, text, or tweet. In industrialized countries, children do much of their work on personal computers or iPads, rather than engaging in games that involve safe touch or physical proximity to others. In this setting, children now are learning to self-regulate through machines rather than learning to *co-regulate* in a healthy, reciprocal way with others. Adults are also profoundly impacted by their use of technology. Astonishingly, even the number of adults who are on their smartphones while having sex is on the rise (Porges, 2016). Though it's beyond the scope of this chapter, implications of this 'selfie culture' deserve more attention. We want to be seen, known, and accepted for who we are. It's a profoundly human need, as is contact and co-regulation through the intersubjective dance of relationship with others. These are among the reasons that witnessing is so relevant for contemporary practice.

A common side effect of trauma is to feel that we must do everything alone (Kalsched, 2013). This is a natural reaction to feeling endangered or neglected by others – including early caretakers – resulting in a profound lack of trust in our environment. Authentic Movement is an active, relational approach that helps repair attachment wounds, allowing us to rebuild trust in our own bodily responses, in others, and in our vital connection to the natural world and the cosmos. Shakespeare said the eyes are the windows to the soul. Witnessing practice invites us to 'see' with the heart and with all of our senses, a practice that transforms both the 'seer' and what is seen and helps make the world a better place.

Note

1 As a full history of witnessing practice is beyond the scope of this chapter I'd like to acknowledge the major contributions of three pioneering teachers of this approach: dance therapist Mary Starks Whitehouse, innovator of Authentic Movement, and two of her students, dance therapist and Jungian analyst Joan Chodorow and teacher of the Discipline of Authentic Movement, Janet Adler. Jungian analyst Marion Woodman has also deepened our understanding of the interrelationship of psyche and soma and the cultivation of embodied presence (Woodman, 1993). Their writings are rich with embodied descriptions, spirited inquiry, psychological insights, and more; I highly recommend them. Subsequent generations of practitioners have furthered moving and witnessing practice, including diverse perspectives

and applications in the arts, education, medical recovery, differing levels of physical abilities, diversity awareness, conflict mediation, mystical practice, and eco-psychology. Readers interested in learning more about the fundamentals of Authentic Movement are referred to Pallaro's excellent 1999 and 2007 collections. Further resources include: Corrigall, et al., 2006; Whatley, et al., 2015; the Authentic Movement Community Website; and others.

References

Adler, J. (2007). From autism to the discipline of authentic movement. In P. Pallaro (Ed.), *Authentic Movement: Moving the Body, Moving the Self, Being Moved: A Collection of Essays* (Vol. 2, pp. 24–31). Philadelphia, PA: Jessica Kingsley. (Original work published 2003)

Authentic Movement Community Website: www.authenticmovementcommunity.org/.

Berrol, C. (2006). Neuroscience meets dance/movement therapy: Mirror neurons, the therapeutic process and empathy. *The Arts in Psychotherapy, 33*, 302–315.

Chodorow, J. (Ed.). (1997). *Jung on Active Imagination*. Princeton, NJ: Princeton University Press.

Chodorow, J. (2006). Active imagination. In R. Papadopoulos (Ed.), *The Handbook of Jungian Psychology: Theory, Practice and Application* (pp. 215–243). London: Routledge.

Corrigall, J., Payne, H., and Wilkinson H. (Eds.). (2006). *About a Body: Working with the Embodied Mind in Psychotherapy*. New York: Routledge.

Cozolino, L. (2006). *The Neuroscience of Human Relationships: Attachment and the Developing Brain*. New York: W.W. Norton.

Damasio, A. (2010). *Self Comes to Mind: Constructing the Conscious Brain*. New York: Pantheon Books.

Eliade, M. (1964). *Shamanism: Archaic Techniques of Ecstasy*. Princeton, NJ: Princeton University Press.

Gallese, V. (2003). The roots of empathy: The shared manifold hypothesis and the neural basis of intersubjectivity. *Psychopathology, 36*, 171–180.

Haze, N., and Stromsted, T. (1999). An interview with Janet Adler. In P. Pallaro (Ed.), *Authentic Movement: Essays by Mary Starks Whitehouse, Janet Adler, and Joan Chodorow* (pp. 107–120). London: Jessica Kingsley Publishers. (Original work published 1994)

Homann, K. (2017). Dynamic equilibrium: Engaging neurophysiological intelligences through dance/movement therapy. In H. Payne (Ed.), *Essentials of Dance Movement Psychotherapy: International Perspectives on Theory, Research, and Practice*. London: Routledge.

Jung, C. G. (1957). *The Transcendent Function* (A. R. Pope, Trans.). Zurich: Privately printed booklet for the Student's Association, C. G. Jung Institute. (Original work published 1916)

Jung, C. G. (1966). The technique of differentiation between the ego and the figures of the unconscious. *Collected Works, 7*. Princeton, NJ: Princeton University Press. (Original work published 1928)

Jung, C. G. (1970). Mysterium coniunctionis. *Collected Works, 14*. Princeton, NJ: Princeton University Press. (Original work published 1955)

Kalff, D. (1980). *Sandplay*. Santa Monica: Sigo Press.

Kalsched, D. (2013). *Trauma and the Soul: A Psychospiritual Approach to Human Development and Its Interruption*. New York: Routledge.

Keleman, S. (1985). *Emotional Anatomy: The Structure of Experience*. Berkeley, CA: Center Press.

Keller, T. (1972). IV. Körperempfindung und bewegung in der psychotherapie [Chapter IV. Body awareness and movement in psychotherapy]. In *Wege inneren Wachstums: Aus Meinen Erinnerungen an C. G. Jung* [Pathways to Inner Growth from my Memories of C. G. Jung] (pp. 22–27). Erlenbach ZH, Switzerland: Bircher-Benner Verlag.

Keller-Jenny, T. (1982). Beginnings of active imagination: Analysis with C.G. Jung and Toni Wolff, 1915–1928. In J. Hillman (Ed.) *Spring Journal Books*, 279–294. New Orleans, LA.

Kohut, H. (1966). Forms and transformations of narcissism. *Journal of the American Psychoanalytic Association, 14*, 243–272.

Nersessian, E., and Kopff, R. (1996). *Textbook of Psychoanalysis*. Washington, DC: American Psychiatric Press.

Ogden, P., and Fisher, J. (2015). *Sensorimotor Psychotherapy: Interventions for Trauma and Attachment*. New York: W.W. Norton.

Oppikofer, R. (2015). Tina Keller – Her fascinating life and creative work inspired by the psychology of C. G. Jung. *Jung Journal of Culture and Psyche, 9*(1), 56–62.

Pallaro, P. (Ed.). (1999). *Authentic Movement: Essays by Mary Starks Whitehouse, Janet Adler, and Joan Chodorow*. London: Jessica Kingsley Publishers.

Pallaro, P. (Ed.). (2007). *Authentic Movement: Moving the Body, Moving the Self, Being Moved: A Collection of Essays* (Vol. 2). Philadelphia, PA: Jessica Kingsley.

Porges, S. W. (2016, April 22). *Connectedness as a biological imperative: Understanding the consequences of trauma, abuse, and chronic stress through the lens of the Polyvagal Theory.* Keynote lecture presented at the ADTA 51st National Dance Therapy Conference, Bethesda, MD.

Sager, P. (2015). Journey of the inner witness: A path of development. *Journal of Dance and Somatic Practices: Authentic Movement: Defining the Field, 7*(2), 365–376.

Schore, A. N. (2012). *The Science of the Art of Psychotherapy.* New York: W.W. Norton.

Schore, A. N., and Sieff, D. (2015). On the same wave-length: How our emotional brain is shaped by human relationships. In D. Sieff (Ed.), *Understanding and Healing Emotional Trauma: Conversations with Pioneering Clinicians and Researchers* (pp. 11–136). London: Routledge.

Siegel, D. (2010). *The Mindful Therapist: A Clinician's Guide to Mindsight, and Neural Integration.* New York: W.W. Norton.

Stromsted, T. (1995). Re-inhabiting the female body. *Somatics: Journal of the Bodily Arts and Sciences, 10*(1), 18–27.

Stromsted, T. (2009). Authentic movement: A dance with the divine. *Body Movement and Dance in Psychotherapy Journal, 4*(3), 201–213.

Stromsted, T. (2015). Authentic movement and the evolution of soul's body® work. *Journal of Dance and Somatic Practices: Authentic Movement: Defining the Field, 7*(2), 339–357.

Stromsted, T., and Haze, N. (2007). The road in: Elements of the study and practice of authentic movement. In P. Pallaro (Ed.), *Authentic Movement: Moving the Body, Moving the Self, Being Moved: A Collection of Essays* (Vol. 2, pp. 56–68). Philadelphia, PA: Jessica Kingsley Publishers.

Stromsted, T., and Seiff, D. (2015). Dances of psyche and soma: Re-inhabiting the body in the wake of emotional trauma. In D. Sieff (Ed.), *Understanding and Healing Emotional Trauma: Conversations with Pioneering Clinicians and Researchers.* London: Routledge.

Swan, W. (2012). *The Memoir of Tina Keller-Jenny: A Lifelong Confrontation with the Psychology of C.G. Jung.* New Orleans, LA: Spring Journal Books.

van der Kolk, B. (2014). *The Body Keeps the Score: Brain, Mind, and Body in the Healing of Trauma.* New York: Viking.

Whatley, S., Bacon, J., Garrett, N., and Alexander, K. (2015). Editorial. *Journal of Dance and Somatic Practices: Special Issue on Authentic Movement, 7*(2), 205–216.

Whitehouse, M. (1999). The Tao of the body. In P. Pallaro (Ed.), *Authentic Movement: Essays by Mary Starks Whitehouse, Janet Adler, and Joan Chodorow* (pp. 41–50). Philadelphia, PA: Jessica Kingsley Publishers. (Original work published 1958)

Wilkinson, M. (2010). *Changing Minds in Therapy: Emotion, Attachment, Trauma, and Neurobiology.* New York: W.W. Norton.

Winnicott, D. W. (1965). Ego distortion in terms of true and false self. In *The Maturational Process and the Facilitating Environment: Studies in the Theory of Emotional Development* (pp. 140–157). London: The Hogarth Press and the Institute of Psycho-Analysis.

Winnicott, D. W. (1971). *Playing and Reality.* Oxford, UK: Routledge.

Woodman, M. (1993). *Conscious Femininity: Interviews with Marion Woodman.* Toronto, ON: Inner City Books.

Wosein, M.-G. (1974). *Sacred Dance, Encounter with the Gods.* London: Thames and Hudson.

8

SOMATIC BODY MAPPING WITH WOMEN DURING LIFE TRANSITIONS

Annette Schwalbe

Introduction

Body Maps are life-size creations that start with a person being traced around her whole body on paper or canvas. The resulting outline shapes the body-world that is then explored and visually expressed through a combination of body meditations, movement, ritual, mark making, drawing, painting, and sculpting. Tracing and mapping of the body is an ancient human practice and has been part of creative explorations in psychotherapy for a long time. A formal methodology, however, was only conceived in 2000 at Cape Town University, South Africa, in collaboration with women living with HIV/Aids (Solomon, 2008). The resulting body-mapping tool has since been adopted by researchers, artists, and creative arts therapists in a variety of settings worldwide (Crawford, 2010; Gastaldo, Magalhães, Carrasco, and Davy, 2011; Lu and Yuen, 2012; Lummis, 2015; Verhoest and Kamiru, 2016). This chapter will illustrate my particular application of the South African methodology and its development into a therapeutic and somatic approach to working with women during life transitions. It spans 10 years of practice in Kenya and the UK and highlights different influences from movement and somatic practices which have allowed me to increasingly 'flesh out' the original and mostly narrative and art therapy-based methodology.

The writing in this chapter is organised around a guiding interest in the connections between the organic body, the experienced body and the represented body on canvas. Throughout, embodiment is understood as a process in which neglected, unconscious, and dissociated aspects of being are brought into conscious and bodily felt presence.

Outline of beginnings: Between heaven and earth

The act of marking the outline of one's body in spiritual and social practices or simply for play is as old as human civilisation. In the Gargas cave of Aventignan, France, dozens of hand stencils line the rock wall. They date from about 27,000 years BC and are presumed to have been part of funeral and sacrificial ceremonies. Hands were laid on the stone and their shapes immortalised by blowing pigments over them, leaving a clearly defined outline. According to Van Beest Holle (1986), the stencils speak of a fundamental human longing to touch the mystery of existence and the worlds beyond.

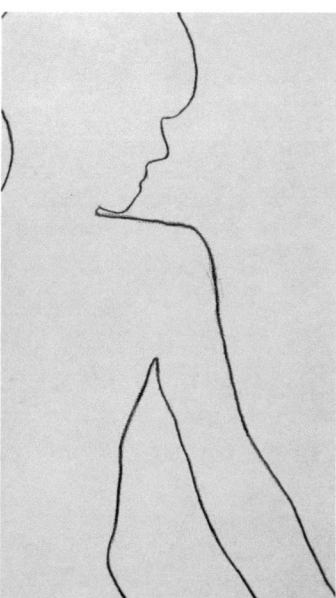

Figure 8.1   Annette Schwalbe (2016)

In our modern world, body tracing and printing is familiar to many children in and out of school. Whether on paper with paint, in sand with sticks and fingers, or in snow making 'snow angels', the pleasure of making and leaving one's own life size mark is the same. It touches something fundamentally confirming about being in this world and in our individually shaped body. To meet one's own outline is not unlike seeing one's shadow and can evoke feelings ranging from exhilarating to unnerving.

To meet the life size body outline of someone else is similarly impactful. In 2002 'Long Life', an exhibition of body maps by women living with HIV/Aids, opened at the South Africa National Gallery in Cape Town. It caused a storm of critical acclaim, public emotional response, and political debate. This was at a time when people with HIV/Aids had lived and died through decades of political denial, social stigma, and exclusion from life-prolonging treatment. With the beginning of a political change such treatment was now finally becoming available, and with the devastating extent of the epidemic increasingly visible people started to 'come out' as HIV positive. In this context, the body maps and stories on display were revolutionary. They provided a completely new perspective on living with HIV/Aids and seemed to emerge from a world of death, displaying a life force and palpable humanity that could not be ignored when standing face to face.

Putting the shunned on the map: South Africa

The body maps in the exhibition 'Long Life' had been created in a process developed by psychologist Jonathan Morgan and artist Jane Solomon together with the Bambanani women's group. Morgan (2004) describes body mapping as a participatory qualitative research tool and a process that draws on the therapeutic disciplines of art therapy, narrative therapy, and body work. The methodology involved a sequence of creative and reflective steps in which participants were

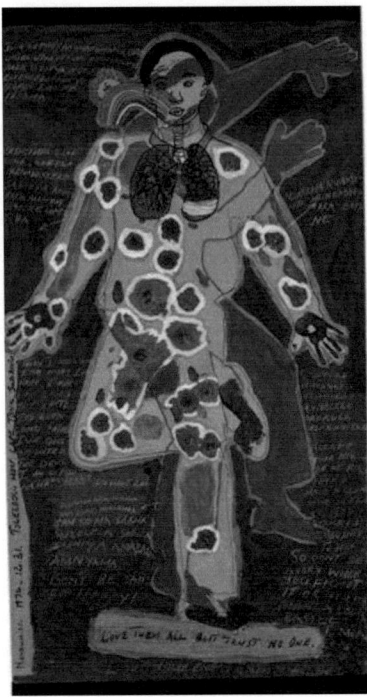

Figure 8.2   Body map by Nondumiso Hlwele, Cape Town 2002

traced around their whole body and then gradually filled the resulting body outline and the space around it with pictures, symbols, and words to represent the path that their bodies had taken through life. This included physical marks (e.g. scars and stretch marks), body parts/areas of emotional significance (e.g. hands and womb), current states of well-being and illness, and visions of the future. The painting of the maps took place in a group setting and was interwoven with personal storytelling, discussions, and guided visualisation.

The overall emphasis was celebratory and life-enhancing and represented a clear departure from previous creative tools that Morgan and his team had developed for the documentation of personal memories as a preparation for death and legacy to one's own children. Body Mapping, on the other hand, was a preparation for starting again, finding new life. Not by pushing the suffering away but by giving it colour, shape, and word alongside what each woman treasured and loved about herself and her life. Body Mapping recognised the importance of a positive outlook in maintaining a healthy immune system and enabled participants to mark their resources and map out their path ahead.

As Victoria, one of the Bambanani women, put it: 'When I look at this picture I can see what I am and what I'm not, and what I believe in and what I don't. I can see that my finger is missing, and I have HIV, but also that I'm strong, very strong' (Morgan, 2004, p. 56).

Apart from self-reflection and motivation body mapping also served the purpose of communicating not just with one's own children, but with the family and community at large. Participants used the final art works to start conversations about HIV/Aids and tell others that they were HIV positive. This 'disclosure' was a crucial step in finding new life as most people were used to suffering in silence and under cover for fear of the very real possibility of being demonised and rejected. Being colourful, life affirming and full of personal symbolism the body maps helped break this silence in a more playful way. They made it safer to broach the subject and allowed its creator to reveal their personal truths at their own pace. When taken further, body maps also contributed to awareness-raising through exhibition during community events, festivals, and conferences. This possibility of 'going public' was an intrinsic part of the methodology and workshop participants were invited in a final step to write onto their maps a 'message to the world'.

Today, I do not follow the original step-by-step methodology anymore nor work in the context of South Africa at the turn of this century. However, the essence of mapping a lesser-known territory – that which has been rejected by self and society – is still core to how I work with women in the UK. For centuries in the Western world, the body has been dominated and objectified by the mind, the feminine relegated to the shadows and the natural world exploited. Body mapping in this context strives to put back on the personal and cultural map that which has been shunned and to give voice to a knowing and wisdom that is much needed beyond the creator's world. The collective message to the world remains the same: see, listen and learn from us!

Painting the living and dreaming body: Kenya

Wisdom of the living body

In 2004 I moved to Kenya with my family. Working as a dance movement psychotherapist in Nairobi I joined visual artist Verhoest (2016) in facilitating body mapping workshops, community projects and international events with women, men, and children living with HIV/Aids. Xavier had been trained by Morgan (2004) and my particular interest in the body mapping methodology was to further tap into body wisdom, here understood as an instinctual, felt and often not yet fully conscious knowing in the body (Stromsted, 2001). Changing the original body

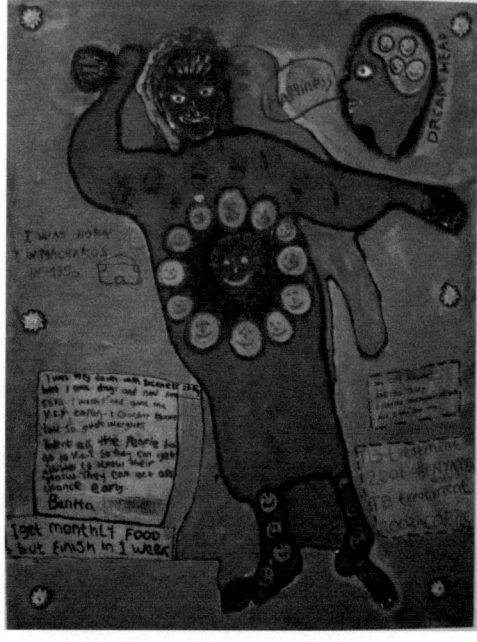

Figure 8.3 Body map by Berita Mutua, Nairobi 2005

mapping format of weekly group meetings to a 5-day long workshop created a sense of retreat which allowed for deep exploration. Each workshop became an invitation not just to speak out but also to listen to the felt-body; to hear what our flesh and blood has to say. For this we gave time and space for rest and incorporated a number of interactive exercises in which participants used touch to sense their own bodies, connect with others and experience being cared for, held and supported. Inspired by Olsen's work in Experiential Anatomy (1998, 2002) and Brook's approach to Sensory Awareness (1974) participants were enabled to perceive the body from the inside and nurture a felt sense of aliveness:

> The mere fact that one comes to the other quietly and without overt manipulation is normally very moving to the person touched. He feels cared for and respected. And the one who touches, if he is really present in what he does, is apt to feel something of the wonder of conscious contact with the involuntary, subtle movement of living tissue . . . an exchange of vitality occurs simply because we are all alive and give off energy and have the senses and consciousness to perceive aliveness.
>
> *(Brooks, 1974, pp. 103–104)*

This sensory focus was applied to the key steps of the body mapping process. For example, in order to make the initial body outline on canvas, participants found their position through a process of receiving touch, sensing their contours and moving in response to those sensations into a position on the canvas that *felt* right rather than what *looked* right. Once settled, they would be traced around by a partner, which is another opportunity to feel the gentle touch by the other as he or she slowly moved the crayon around one's body. Filling the outline with a background colour was likened to painting the inside walls of one's home – a deliberate antidote to the medical picture of their bodies as the battlefield of HIV/Aids. The making of hand and foot prints as marks of identity became an act of honouring as participants helped each other to apply paint to palms and soles, often with much hilarity as the cool paint and the bristles of the brush touched the sensitive skin.

Expressions of the dreaming body

Central to each workshop was the development of two key symbols: a Symbol of Difficulty and a Symbol of Strength. Body meditations – a combination of body scan, self-touch, and breath awareness – were incorporated in order to locate and experience the difficulty, often the impact of the HIV virus, and one's life-sustaining force in the body. Finding colour, shape, and word for those experiences were part of building the symbols that were eventually painted on the body map. This linking of bodily experience with visual expression was inspired by Jung's technique of Active Imagination (Chodorow, 1997) and based on the understanding that 'our moving, living body is intelligent, and our thinking arises through material physical sources as surely as it may seem to move beyond them' (Fraleigh, 2000, p. 57). Mindell (1982) coined the term DreamBody for what 'hovers between body sensation and mythical visualisation' (ibid., p. 8), the spirit that animates both:

> In practice, work on the dreambody depends on its mode of expression. Sometimes it appears as the psyche in dream form, sometimes as matter in body motions; sometimes as synchronicities or accidents. In any given session dreambody processes oscillate between psyche and matter.
>
> *(ibid., p. 54)*

This is where body mapping becomes not just a way of recording and communicating experience but a creative process in which healing can take place and new direction can be found. The forth and back between the living, felt-body and the represented body on the map opens the space for a transformative spirit to enter. In such moments, the role of the workshop facilitator ceases to be one of guidance as the guiding power of this spirit or energy is beyond human agency. Instead, the presence of a witness is called for who can perceive, mentally record, and, if needed, recall and reflect back what has happened.

The following extract is based on what I witnessed during a body mapping workshop in the township of Korogocho, Nairobi:

> *Berita, the elder in the group, finds her symbol of strength in a dream. Half way through the body meditation she falls asleep and dreams that she is walking on a path back to the house in the village where she was born. Her house has got a vegetable garden, and she is healed and strong. Normally very quiet, Berita immediately shares her dream with the group as she wakes up at the end of the exercise. With some help she draws a head next to her own head on the body map. She calls it her dream head that speaks to her of happiness.*
>
> *Some-time later, while everybody is busy on the floor and bent over their canvases and paintings with much concentration, one of the women, her baby in her arms, suddenly starts singing. It is a traditional song of rebirth in a very old language the literal meaning long-lost. It is a song that is sung during rites of passage such as marriage or birth of a child. Now she sings it in honour of Berita's dream. Other women join in and they rise with their voices to dance in-between the others painting on the floor.*
>
> *This is the middle day of the overall workshop and it leaves me in awe. Something is born in the midst of the group and with it not only the paintings but also gestures, movements and simple activities take on a symbolic, even sacred character. I remember yesterday's washing of paint-covered hands and feet, two women bending in front of every participant and pouring water over skin. Today, canvases are being carried out of the room and into the sun to dry. Like shrouds they are taken out of darkness to let their brilliant colours shine. Later, they are brought back in to be stored for the night. The workshop space empties and fills again as if following a natural cause.*
>
> *Six months later, Berita tells me that instead of walking home to her place of birth like in her dream, some relatives from her home village had decided to come and visit her in Korogocho – a first after many years of estrangement. This reconnection came after they had seen her on TV in a report on the Nairobi Art for Action Festival in which Berita had shown her body map and told her story in the lead-up to World Aids Day, 1st December 2005.*

Authentic witnessing

Today, my facilitation style still rests on the intent to witness that which animates and moves the body from a source that seemingly lies beneath the physical and sometimes beyond the individual. This kind of witnessing is based on my ongoing practice of Authentic Movement as developed by Adler (2002) and personally experienced through the teachings of Stromsted (2015) and Hartley (2001). During the body mapping process, it means that I am present to the detail of observable changes in participants' movements, be it spontaneous gestures while sharing with the group, shifting positions during body meditations or a particular energy, rhythm, or pace in which a mark is made on the body map. Whilst witnessing I also make a mental note of what sensations, feelings, images and thoughts are stirred in me, knowing well that this might be different from the participant's personal experience. If she shares her experience and welcomes feedback I might offer to reflect back what I have witnessed. At such times I speak in the present tense and stay with simple observations in order to bring the remembered alive and allow each woman to make meaning herself. If helpful I might also share some of my own experience in order to affirm or complement a woman's experience with an aspect of which she might be unaware. By owning my interpretation of the experience, I steer away from analysis and labelling of bodily experience, movement, or artistic expression. Ultimately, each woman remains the expert reader of her own body and map.

Awakening the cyclical and emergent body: UK

New research into feminine embodiment (Ardagh, 2011) and cellular memory of pre- and perinatal experience (Gyllenhaal and Gyllenhaal, 2016) has further influenced my approach to body mapping since returning to the UK in 2009. Concepts of a woman's womb as her embodied seat of creativity (Northrup, 1994/2009) and concepts of rebirthing as a process of resolving womb and birth related trauma (Noble, 1993) have led to a womb-like reshaping of the body mapping set-up. The creative process now follows a cyclical rhythm and includes additional elements of ritual that engage with experiences of incarnation at and before birth. Participation in weekend intensives is limited to an intimate circle of maximum six women and enhanced by a deliberately luxurious setting with red and orange rugs, cushions, sheepskins, soft blankets, and cosy lighting. The aim is to provide safety, comfort and pleasure for the timider voices of the body to come to the fore and speak from places hidden and often shamed.

The cyclical body in body mapping

Inspired by explorations of the menstrual cycle and the four natural seasons as experienced in the UK the body mapping intensives are now offered as a cycle of seasonally themed weekends

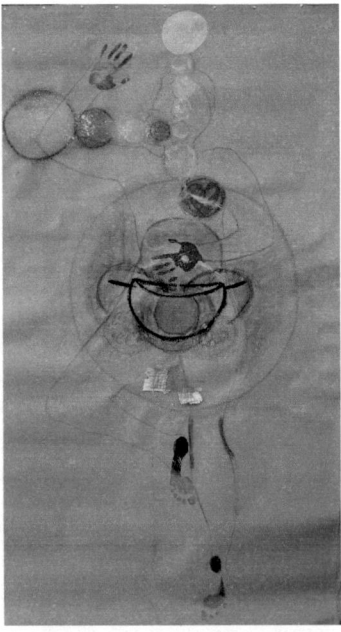

Figure 8.4 'Stir it up' by Ruth Love, Bristol 2015

each of which can be attended separately. Themes such as Nurturing New Life Within (Spring), Coming to Full Bloom (Summer), and Gathering Riches for the Winter to Come (Autumn and Winter) allude to the creative and psychological dynamics that Pope (2009) calls a woman's 'elemental intelligence' (ibid., p. 4). According to her, the different stages of the menstrual cycle are a mirror of the coming and going of the natural seasons. As such, it is an innate feminine compass to navigate life's challenges from an embodied, interconnected and co-creative rather than controlling place. It fosters an acceptance and active engagement with changes in the body and in life:

> The menstrual cycle is . . . a template for psychological and spiritual evolution, an innate intelligence that works, guides and matures you. A repeating rhythm you can't control, the cycle is your training ground for coming to know and love this elemental intelligence.
>
> *(Pope, 2009, p. 4)*

In the opening movement exploration of each intensive participants are guided to resonate with the seasonal theme and locate themselves in what they know about their bodily cycles, be they menstrual, energetic or otherwise. This initial connection is then spoken to and in the circle collectively woven into the thematic canopy under which the women enter the body mapping process. Love (2015), a participant whose body map is depicted in the picture above (Figure 8.4) speaks to her experience in her poem 'stir it up' which was shown alongside her body map at the group exhibition 'Seasons of a Woman' in Bristol, UK, in 2015:

> This power is buried deep in the girdle of my hips,
> in the sacred grove of my womb,
> I have been searching for a way
> to reach it, touch it, for years, yet,
> now I have caught a glimpse of the bloody depths,
> reached in and stirred the cauldron up
> it frightens me. so much potential is there,
> can I really let it out?

The body mapping creative cycle

Following the opening circle, the creative body mapping process starts with the first body meditation. 'Meditation' thereby connotes a mindful, curious, and receptive meeting of one's body world. Whilst in the past this had been framed as two contrasting explorations of 'a difficulty in one's life' and 'one's inner strength' I have come to fully trust that the body will respond to what has been spoken in the circle in just the way that is needed. As a result, the invitation now is non-binary: to '[b]e open to the messages and mysteries of your body and its symptoms. Be eager to listen and slow to judge' (Northrup, 1994/2009, p. 54). Such letting go of control requires a safe physical and conceptual container as well as a clear sequence of engagement.

Each woman is guided to set up her own comfortable place with cushions and blankets, a mini womb space mirroring the larger workshop setting. In line with the concept of mapping, the ensuing body meditation is accompanied by my narrative, that likens the body to an inner landscape that can be sunk into, travelled and discovered. Participants are guided to attend to one or two places in their body that call them through a particular sensation or an absence of sensation.

Stillness, movement, and self-touch support 'getting to know' these places and patience allows for textures, shapes, colours, and intuitive images to come into view. The shift from sensing to inner seeing lays the ground for the later mark making and facilitates the gradual re-surfacing from the inner landscape to outer seeing when opening the eyes.

As the creative cycle continues participants are guided to cast their eyes over the art materials on display. In order to maintain a felt connection with what has been experienced and seen inside a choice of materials are offered that are not only visually compelling but also appealing to the senses and linked to the natural season at the time. This comprises paint, crayons, and pastels; fabrics and leather of different textures; beads, clay, charcoal, stones, shells, bones, feathers, leaves, petals, seeds, moss, bark, roots, seaweed, and anything else I might have gathered in 'the land out there'. Participants spontaneously choose what to work with and either draw, paint, or sculpt. Only when the artistic marking of the experience is completed do we return to speaking, sharing, and reflecting, thereby completing the core creative cycle of body mapping.

This cycle of speaking – sensing – seeing – marking – speaking is repeated several times throughout the body mapping process. At the beginning of the intensive, however, it has particular significance and serves each woman to find the starting point of her track of exploration. The first artwork is like the seed that is later planted into the ground of her body map. Like a seed, it already contains all that will unfold. Brought forth from the woman's inner land, it connects her past, present, and future in a way that is relevant at that particular moment in time.

Sackey (2015), a participant and contributor to Seasons of a Woman describes the creative unfolding of her inner bodily landscape in 'Transfiguration':

> Every fingerprint of paint became a new discovery of who I am, as did every colour, every texture and every curve. My hair felt like a mane of power untamed, released and free. I could feel my energy moving, shifting around, even dancing around inside my body. I felt vibrant within and I understood why I wasn't afraid. I was, in fact, excited. My life was changing shape but so was I.

Birth of a new sense of self

Most women attend body mapping intensives during a time of transition in their lives and with a longing to explore who they are right now and who they are becoming. What prompts participants can be natural transitions such as becoming a mother or entering menopause; deliberate changes such as ending a relationship or changing career; or unexpected life events such as illness, loss of work, or death of a loved one. These are prime times for past wounding to re-surface as well as untapped potential to be released. Whilst the repetition of the creative cycle described above provides the safety and containment needed to process both, an additional process has recently been developed that supports the birth of a new sense of self. It is a collective ritual designed by each woman in preparation for coming onto her map and being traced around her body. At this point in the process, having moved through the initial creative cycle and found her thematic and artistic starting point, her map is still a blank canvas, cut to size but yet unmarked.

One at a time and in conversation with me she intuitively comes up with key movements and 'ingredients' that she would like to be part of her transition from 'off the map' to 'on the map'. This can be an extended journey through space or a simple step, begun from any position she chooses. She is also encouraged to enlist as much support as she wishes from the group: This can be touch, mere physical presence or witnessing, specific movements or gestures, sounds, or words. This is then tried out with the group, double-checked, and reworked until the sequence and important details are clear to everyone and exactly as the woman wishes. Only then do we 'go live' and perform the ritual, which usually takes a few minutes, followed by spontaneous movement, shifting, and resting on the canvas until she has found her position and feels ready to be traced.

The emergent body

This arrival and 'coming into shape' on a yet unchartered ground touches something primal. It echoes with our original coming into human body: our incarnation at the time of conception; our first human contact during implantation in our mother's womb; our development through the various embryonic and foetal stages; and our coming into the world 'out there' at birth. Research in pre- and perinatal psychology shows that:

> "[I]n any particular moment, who we are and who we think we are is layered upon our cellular history and the early cellular responses that led to our most basic bio-logic functions. The early human cells, like primitive or simple organisms they were, grew and survived and learned while engaging in challenges and transitions marked by chemical and cellular processes. When challenges occur, transitions are faced, and successes achieved in our experiences as children or adults, we feel an intensity of life. Stimulating experiences translate into emotions and thoughts that echo our primal experiences: desire, hunger, hope, fear, struggle, and success—all of which are elements of myth.
>
> *(Terry, 2013, p. 282)*

In the ritual journey onto the body map these 'elements of myth' come into play through gestures, movements, path ways, pace, flow, contact with others, sounds, props, shapes, shifts, position, and colour(s) chosen for the outline and the words spoken to describe the experience of the ritual. Whilst many of these elements are chosen deliberately, some emerge spontaneously as the ritual takes place. This mix of control and surprise allows each woman to actively participate in the Creation Myth of her emergent being imprinted on the canvas. As the echoes of her primal past present themselves she chooses how she brings them into outline on her body map. Since this is done with the caring and midwife-like support of the other women her creative rebirth also counteracts some of the collective experiences of women in our Western society that still controls, commoditises, shames, and medicalises the female body right from our beginnings in the womb.

The aim of body mapping as practised today is aligned with Northrup's vision, to fall in love with our blood and flesh (Northrup, 1994/2009, p. xxiii). For this to happen we need to gently and compassionately bring back into our conscious, tangible, and vibrant body those aspects of ourselves that we have not yet felt safe to be in, or return to, this world: that which we have left behind, blanked from our minds, frozen in our bodies, and neglected in our souls – in this lifetime or for generations. In the body mapping process, the retrieval can be done with pleasure: pleasure in our feminine body with no other aim but to satisfy our own desire to be more fully who we are. Workshop and Seasons of a Woman exhibition participant Greenland (2015) speaks to this in her body map poem 'Love Story':

> I find you floating in the heavens,
> You are free and peaceful

But alone,
Without boundaries or ground.

I fear for you,
Lest you should float forever or disintegrate.
And you fear the earth,
And the harshness of life.

Carefully and deliberately
I mark your boundaries.
And others help
And with touch and with love
We coax your corporeal body
Preparing for your arrival.

You arrive.
And I go under your skin,
Trace the constellations of your body,
Hear the pounding of your heart,
Feel the warmth of your hands in mine.
And with my breath I give life to you while you fill my lungs with air.

Conclusion

At the end of each woman's body mapping process lies new ground charted: visible on her map and felt inside her body. This new embodied image of self is the result of a careful forth and back between experience and creative expression within the bounds of her physical being and at the moment of transiting from one phase in her life into another. As this chapter has shown, the particular combination and sequencing of group exchange, movement, touch, body meditation, ritual, drawing, painting, and sculpting have changed and evolved over the years. What remains throughout, however, is the effect that body mapping has: to restore life force to aspects of being that had been lost. This is beautifully expressed in the ending of the already featured body map story 'stir it up' by Love (2015):

now face to face with myself,
I look myself in the eye,
in the womb,
in the heart,
and am so achingly terrified
and so overcome with love
that tears fall down my cheeks.
this woman, this creation is me, a me
I don't, can't
see and yet I'm there, always.
I have unleashed myself, broken through
my walls, and leapt out, onto a page

to be seen, to be remembered,
to be looked at and pondered over,
to be greeted, like an old friend who
I haven't seen in years.

Acknowledgements

I would like to honour all the women with whom I have worked and body-mapped together over all those years. To partake in your cultures, communities, and moments of renewal has fundamentally shaped me as a woman and practitioner. I also honour all men who were part of the body mapping work in Kenya and deeply treasure my collaboration with Xavier Verhoest, Thomas Mboya, and Shabu Mwangi during that time. Thank you for your lasting friendship and inspiration.

References

Adler, J. (2002). *Offering from the Conscious Body: The Discipline of Authentic Movement.* Rochester, VT: Inner Traditions.

Ardagh, C. G. (2011). *Embodying the Feminine* [Adobe Digital Editions version]. Retrieved November 3, 2013, from http://awakeningwomen.com/embodying-the-feminine-life-lessons-and-practices-for-awakening-women/.

Brooks, C. (1974). *Sensory Awareness – The Rediscovery of Experiencing.* New York: The Viking Press.

Chodorow, J. (1997). *Jung on Active Imagination.* Princeton, NJ: Princeton University Press.

Crawford, A. (2010). If 'The Body Keeps the Score': Mapping the dissociated body in trauma narrative, intervention, and theory. *University of Toronto Quarterly, 79*(2), 702–719.

Fraleigh, S. (2000). Consciousness matters. *Dance Research Journal, 32*(1), 54–62.

Gastaldo, D., Magalhães, L., Carrasco, C., and Davy, C. (2012). *Body-Map Storytelling as Research: Methodological Considerations for Telling the Stories of Undocumented Workers Through Body Mapping.* Retrieved July 21, 2014, from www.migrationhealth.ca/undocumented-workers-ontario/body-mapping

Greenland, C. (2015). *A Love Story.* Retrieved September 19, 2016, from www.annetteschwalbe.co.uk/2015/05/seasons-of-a-woman-may-body-map/.

Gyllenhaal, S. (producer), and Gyllenhaal, M. K. (director). (2016). *In Utero* [Motion picture]. Los Angeles, CA: MRB Productions and Upstream Cinema.

Hartley, L. (2001). *Servants of the Sacred Dream – Rebirthing the Deep Feminine.* Essex: Elmdon Books.

Love, R. (2015). *Stir It Up.* Retrieved September 19, 2015, from www.annetteschwalbe.co.uk/2015/03/seasons-of-a-woman-march-body-map/.

Lu, L., and Yuen, F. (2012). Journey woman: Art therapy in a decolonizing framework of practice. *The Arts in Psychotherapy, 39*(3), 192–200.

Lummis, C. (2015). *Therapeutic Body Mapping* (Unpublished doctoral dissertation). Mount Mary University, Milwaukee, WI.

Mindell, A. (1982). *Dreambody – The Body's Role in Revealing the Self.* London: Routledge and Kegan Paul.

Morgan, J. (2004). *Long Life: Positive HIV Stories.* Cape Town: Double Storey.

Noble, E. (1993). *Primal Connections.* New York: Fireside.

Northrup, C. (2009). *Women's Bodies, Women's Wisdom.* London: Piatkus. (Original work published 1994)

Olsen, A. (1998). *Body Stories – A Guide to Experiential Anatomy.* New York: Station Hill Opening/Barrytown.

Olsen, A. (2002). *Body and Earth – An Experiential Guide.* New England: Middlebury College Press.

Pope, A. (2009). *The Woman's Quest.* Retrieved April 15, 2012, from www.redschool.net.

Sackey, N. (2015). *Transfiguration.* Retrieved September 19, 2015, from www.annetteschwalbe.co.uk/2014/10/seasons-of-a-woman-october-body-map/.

Solomon, J. (2008). *Living with "X": A Body-mapping Journey in the Time of HIV and AIDS. 27. Facilitator's Guide.* Retrieved May 12, 2015, from www.comminit.com/?q=africa/node/284318.

Stromsted, T. (2001). Re-inhabiting the female body – Authentic movement as a gateway to transformation. *The Arts in Psychotherapy, 28*, 39–55.

Stromsted, T. (2015). Authentic movement and the evolution of Soul's body work. *Journal of Dance and Somatic Practices, 7*(2), 339–357.

Terry, K. (2013). Implantation journey: The original human myth (Part I). *Journal of Prenatal and Perinatal Psychology and Health, 27*(3), 276–288.

Van Beest Holle, G. (Ed.) (1986). *Holle World Cultural History: The First High Cultures* (translated from German). Baden-Baden: Holle Verlag.

Verhoest, X., and Kamiru, W. W. (2016). *Who I Am, Who We Are: An Art Project on Kenyan Identity.* Nairobi: Kuona Trust.

9

GRAVITY AND THE DEVELOPMENT OF THE (BODY) SELF IN DANCE MOVEMENT PSYCHOTHERAPY

Diana Cheney

Introduction

Although there is no one agreed definition for the concept of 'Self' within the psychotherapeutic milieu, the role of the body in the structuring of the Self has been more or less widely neglected. A historical and philosophical body–mind dualism resulted in the splitting of theories: the body and verbal psychotherapies apparently stand on different sides.

Recent psychotherapeutic trends have started using the concept of 'embodiment' seemingly in an attempt to repair a concept of Self that has been theoretically divided. From a phenomenological perspective, however, the mind is never detached from the body. The non-verbal aspects of experience and communication specific to the early years do not disappear to be replaced with the verbal and reflective function of later stages. Instead, thoughts and symbolic representation are always associated with the body and actions, which in turn are related to early experiences including the early primary relationship (Fonagy and Target, 2007).

From this perspective, the Self is always embodied with the different areas of one's experience weaved into each other. My question in the consulting room is not 'is this individual embodied?' as this question presupposes other conditions than the 'natural' state of being embodied. My aim is to explore the elements that will bring to light the degrees of difficulty in the (body) self-concept and how they can be manifested in pathologies associated to one's sense of (body) self. Dissociation is an extreme example of such pathology consisting of the individual's attempt to split the sense of self from the body.

In order to emphasise the individual as an embodied entity, I will use the term '(body) self' or body (self) when referring to the individual's 'self'. This chapter will focus on the function of gravity in the developing (body) self within the context of the infant's primary relationships.

Pollack (2008), an object-relations psychoanalyst, affirms that 'object-relations are the organizing context on the mental level, corresponding to the physiological function of gravity' (p. 493). Pollack brings to the fore the importance of gravity by situating it on the same level of importance as human relationships in the development of the (body) self.

This chapter will follow a progression from the first contact with gravity, to coming into vertical. Then I will explore the importance of playing with gravity and end with a reflection on gravity in psychotherapy. I will use some observations and reflections from a 2-year infant observation, personal observations, as well as some clinical material.

First contact with gravity

The force of gravity attracts objects towards the centre of the earth and other physical objects. This inevitably puts us in physical contact with our surroundings. It is in the simultaneity of contact of our bodies with surfaces or in the tension between the body and the pull of gravity, that our sense of weight, substance and agency is discovered.

In utero, the amniotic liquid reduces the effects of gravity on the foetus' body. Nevertheless, the baby moves and is moved by the mother's movements which are directly related and dependent on her gravitational context. Bainbridge-Cohen's developmental movement patterns (cited in Hartley, 1989) suggest that the baby's body parts are initially organized around the navel with no concrete awareness of directions and probably no awareness of inside, outside, and how their limbs are, or can be, linked together.

When born, the infant's body weight, through the first contact with the earth's gravity, will be experienced for the first time. In Rachel Rose's (2015) *Everything and more*, a video installation shown in the exhibition *Infinite Mix: Contemporary Sound and Image*, US astronaut David Wolf narrates his experience of being in space and talks about his sensory disorientation on his return from space: gravity was felt to be too heavy, his ears felt heavy, his wrist watch felt like an iron ball, and when he tilted his head to the right he felt as if his body accelerated to the left. David Wolf described a sense of disintegration in his embodied experience, and we can only extrapolate to the world of the infant and imagine her experience when in contact with a new gravitational reality outside of her mother's womb. Of course, the experience of a newborn starts from a state of under-integration that requires the parents' handling and holding (Winnicott, 1960b) if the infant is to develop a satisfactory level of self-organization.

It is proposed here that the repetitive and rhythmical movements of the holding, up and down, side to side, that parents perform as they envelop their newborns in their arms in an attempt to soothe them, are a response of the parents' 'thinking body', as in Bion's alpha function (Bion, 1962), to soothe the infant's under-integrated state. Some movements and sensations that might have been experienced inside the womb are recreated while offering at the same time some rudimentary experience of one's weight being moved in space as a way to introducing and transitioning to the new gravitational reality.

Due to their lack of body cohesion the infant spends much of her early life in the horizontal position both when in their cot and in their parents' arms. The intimate relationship that is established between mother and infant when breastfeeding also happens horizontally with the mother introducing verticality especially after breastfeeding to help release trapped wind.

In the system of Laban movement analysis weight is related to the three-dimensional bodily substance. Winnicott (1960b) states that holding is 'a three-dimensional or space relationship with time gradually added' (p. 589). When we think of the infant's (body) self's three-dimensionality we think of flesh, body boundaries and internal linkages that are developed via the enveloping of the infant's body, but also through the 'complementary gravity-based data coming from inside the body via the proprioceptive and kinaesthetic systems' (Pollack, 2008, p. 493). The infant's movements seem random and indiscriminate at first. As she engages in the spinal developmental movement patterns characterized by the yield/push and reach/pull patterns (Hackney, 2002), one can observe an increasing exploration of different body parts and engagement with pushing with the legs and reaching with the hands.

At 5 weeks baby Caroline, an infant I observed for 2 years, pushed her baby carrier with her legs resulting in her body moving upwards. At 2 months and 2 weeks she seemed to realize that when she moved her legs in excitement the little toys hanging in her baby carrier moved. When the toys stopped she would move her legs again. At 4 months and 2 weeks Caroline lifted her hands in front of her, opening and closing them slowly and touching each hand with the other hand. She seemed to have discovered that she was the one who was opening and closing her hands. These first explorations of gravity with different body parts initiate thoughts and reflective awareness in the baby. In this way, gravity provides organizing physiological responses that will function as organizers of one's sense of (body) self, who is also an agent in the environment. Stern (1985) refers to 'self-agency' as part of a sense of a relational 'core self'. In this example, Caroline became aware of being the performer of her actions and thereby having an impact in the world and also producing a response from others.

I observed baby Caroline's early yield/push and push/pull patterns within the context of a relationship highlighting the three-dimensionality that was co-created in the dyad. At 16 weeks Caroline and her mother engaged in lively bodily interactions with various affective and (body) self links happening at the same time. Caroline lay down on her back on her mother's lap and pushed her feet against mother's hands in excitement. Recognizing Caroline's need to push, mother used her hands as a resistance for Caroline to exert pressure and consequently move away. The contact on the surface of Caroline's back with another surface (mother's legs) provided the necessary bond to make the push possible, with her centre being activated and her different body parts connected as a consequence. Pushing against a resistant surface, the infant becomes aware of her weight and bodily substance, which allows for a sense of an (em)bodied self to emerge.

Although the mother's body offered some resistance for Caroline to push against it did not accurately reflect back to Caroline's body her real weight and substance since her mother's body absorbed part of Caroline's weight. In order to discover and create her separate sense of (body) self, Caroline would need to engage with gravity in the world separate from her mother.

The 'thirdness' of gravity

The thirdness of gravity is first expressed in the space that exists between mother and infant and is connected to the child but also to the mother. But there may be occasions when the caregiver cannot, for their own and very often unconscious reasons, open a space for thirdness. One of the most important acquisitions of human evolution was coming into verticality. It allowed the expansion of the human's view and perspective of the world but also freed the human's hands allowing for an immense creative potential to develop. Ontogenetically, the baby's early experiences of contact with the external world happen on the horizontal plane. Verticality is progressively achieved as the infant prepares for changes in levels from lying down to upright. The baby discovers gradually that she has the capacity to establish connections with the external world as well as getting away from it (Hackney, 2002).

Propelling into gravity thus entails moving away from the horizontal plane that has characterized her primary dependency on her mother. Reflecting on baby Caroline, she started rejecting horizontality more assertively at six months when she was weaned. Possibly the horizontal position evoked a connection with the breast but cut her off from the environment with which she wished to actively engage. Verticality would support her overcome the loss of the breast but also facilitate accessing the world.

The relationship that the infant establishes with gravity can be thought to possess qualities of thirdness. In addition, the role it plays in the creation of space between mother and baby and it also contributes to the multiplication of relationships with others, objects, space and time. This influences the constitution of the individual's sense of (body) self.

Benjamin (2004) affirms that the true and functional third is one that is shared and that facilitates symbolic functioning. Benjamin suggests that 'the primary parent must create the space of thirdness by being able to hold in tension her subjectivity/desire/awareness and the needs of the child' (Benjamin, 2004, p. 13). In Caroline's case, whose developmental progression was thought about by careful parents, there seemed to be a period in which some ambivalence about Caroline's rapid growth might possibly have been present in the family. Caroline and mother found themselves involved in body play, often in one place, and Caroline's engagement with gravity and verticality was somewhat delayed. She had not, for example, been able to roll over to her tummy. When at 8 months she once managed to roll to her tummy she looked very scared. She could not lift her head and cried. She was then turned back over and did not attempt to turn again. Pushing her body weight into verticality appeared difficult.

Despite this, Caroline also desired to establish her own omnipotent relationship with gravity that all her family members shared. At 1 year and 1 month old she could not crawl and her eyes and her upper body seemed to thrust into space to where all her family members gathered momentarily. I could sense her frustration of not being able to meet with them. However, when mother tried to encourage Caroline to walk, at 1 year and 2 months, Caroline appeared to feel very insecure and scared when she tried to balance in the upright position. Haag (2000) refers to Bick's idea that the early ego is 'formed conjointly by the mother-and-the-infant-in-the-family' (p. 15). I wondered if Caroline's lack of engagement with gravity was reflective of an unavailability of the *third* in the family's mind, as well as a learned over-reliance on her mother's body. Caroline, the youngest of three lively children, needed to negotiate the physical and metaphorical space in her family in order to grow up as a subject with agency and desire.

Benjamin (1995) speaks of a pre-oedipal father that can be symbolized by anyone other than the mother adult, regardless of gender. This other offers a point of identification as a 'like subject [that] makes the child imaginatively able to represent the desire for the world outside' (Benjamin, 1995, p. 57). It is the adult who is capacitated to understand the baby's needs and, as Winnicott (1960a) affirmed, 'to meet the infant's gesture' (p. 145).

Caroline had previously rejected her father, possibly resisting separation from her mother, which could also be attributed to a lack of trust in her (body) self, perhaps due to reduced exploration of gravity. But a shift in the family dynamics contributed to the resolution of Caroline's impasse. As her mother reengaged with her own autonomy through work and social activities her father became more present during the observation sessions and took it upon himself to support Caroline engage with gravity more actively. With his help she took the up of gravity with much bravery and at 1 year and 6 months she walked without the support of hands for the first time.

Playing with gravity: Separation and individuation

Bodily interactions and play involving gravity between the child and the parents follow a progression that appears to start with very early soothing movements up and down and that develop as the baby matures into larger up and down movements. At times, the parent holds the baby up in the air while vocalising and mirroring the excitement that the baby seems to feel. Then the baby is brought down, sometimes gently and sometimes accelerating to stop with an assertive safe holding of the infant. The movement up and down stimulates on one hand the experience of the infant's (body) self, i.e. her weight when she comes down and lands in her parent's arms. On the other hand, it offers the infant the opportunity to experience reliance and safety in a gravitational reality that they are only starting to be acquainted with.

Winnicott (1960b) thought that the illusion of omnipotence while the baby is absolutely dependent on the mother is essential for the beginning of the development of the infant's (body) self and emotional health. The parent tells the baby when lifting her up 'How big you are! Bigger than me!' to then bring her down back to the reality of her 'small' and dependent condition.

This play serves thus transitional functions touching on the theme of closeness and separation often lived in the fear of falling forever just before sleeping or in dreams. Possible recollections of birth and death anxieties related to earlier states, as well as fear that mother might literally and metaphorically drop the baby, can be re-enacted and worked through via this play. In the author's practice, some children have used 'falling' as a way to encourage a physical holding response from the therapist. For example, one child would climb onto a table and fall so that the therapist would stop his fall. It is proposed that these children were both trying to discover their sense of weight and substance as internal structure by using gravity but also to test whether someone would be able to hold their literal and metaphorical weight.

A higher degree of risk is progressively introduced in the variations of the early play with gravity: when pretending that the child is an aeroplane or when the child is thrown up in the air and held up with great energy as gravity brings the child down. The child experiences a strong omnipotent other to which she not only has access to but who also makes her, through identification (Benjamin, 1995), feel all-powerful. Interestingly, this kind of play, from toddlerhood onwards, has been observed by the author many times and usually performed by people of stronger stature. These were mainly male. Music (2011) notes that in Western cultures fathers relate to their children with more physical stimulation. During separation/individuation the father is invested with idealized attributes that not only are essential to (body) self but also to sexual development (Benjamin, 1995). This continues as the child enters the overstimulating oedipal movement that both girls and boys go through, with the up of verticality facilitating further differentiation and confrontation with the limits of the child's omnipotence.

As I walked with a friend, his 5-year-old son climbed a wall, inhaled, lifted his hand and announced that he was all powerful. His father, validating the boy's need for omnipotence (possibly in his identification and/or desire to overpower his father) confirmed in a playful way his power, smiling and vocalizing, as the child exhibited proudly his strong muscles and movements. But a few minutes after this expression of heightened grandiosity the boy tripped and fell. Omnipotence was replaced by what felt to be shame and humiliation imposed by the limits of the relationship between his own body (self) and gravity.

His father, well attuned to his child, picked him up back to his feet and comforted him. The boy, still embarrassed, hid his face from me, an onlooker. As I grew in my spine, inviting him to reconnect with some aspects of the previous feeling, he started running and playing with a more balanced view of the up and down of gravity and of his own body (self).

Benjamin (1995) highlights the polarization of the oedipal period as it is still structured in our culture: male and female, good and bad, and I would add, horizontal and vertical, and 'down' and 'up' of gravity. Following Benjamin's (1988) idea that the classical Oedipus Complex attributes to the father the role of rescuing the child from the mother's regressive pull, one can see how the 'down' of gravity can be in the same polarized way attributed to the mother and the 'up' to the father.

It is of interest that further exploration of gravity towards greater autonomy and self-agency seem to indicate, as observed in life long personal and professional situations,[1] that boys continue to explore gravity in the direction 'up' while girls may take less risks 'up' engaging in more sophisticated play in the horizontal plane. Music (2011) affirms that in the West, girls tend to engage more verbally in symbolic play related to nurturing while boys are more active.

In fact, more often than not boys seem to climb walls, trees and even roofs to then jump down just to find out that one survives the fall. Are they only revisiting earlier stages of development with a degree of control that they didn't experience before? Are they practicing gender and sexual potency inevitably embedded in their muscles and sexual organs, the penis growing into gravity when erect? Are they practicing cultural and biological expectations of 'going up' reflecting the gender divide often translated, in boys' cases, by what Benjamin (1995) thought to be a repudiation of the mother and consequent identification with the father?

Benjamin (1995) explains that the father represents, traditionally, the subject of desire and agent in the world and that father tends to reject the girls' attempts at identifying with him. The girls are then left to identify with the mother, traditionally seen as a more passive entity, based on her gender difference. According to Benjamin (1995) the complementary divide between genders, also reflected in how we think and engage with gravity, can be overcome in the post-oedipal form by 'sustaining the tension between contrasting elements so that they remain potentially available rather than forbidden and the oscillation between them can be pleasurable rather than dangerous' (Benjamin, 1995, p. 73).

A game prevalent among girls is spinning, which happens in the horizontal plane while spinning round the vertical axis. The child makes herself lose control and get out of balance just to discover over and over again that being out of control is only a moment that will end and that falling is not forever. The ground is there to hold her and she finds that she too has the capacity to stand on her 2 feet. Sexual exploration may also be a component of this play. She makes herself lose control and gives in to the excitement of her sexual organs that hold the horizontal bed in which life is conceived and nurtured to existence. This play may reflect the girls attempt at integrating her agency and sense of desire in a more controlled way than boys. She practices how to be in control of her losing control, possibly of her sexuality and the pleasure that she gets from it.

Verbal language presents us with symbolic expressions of the social hierarchy related to gravity. 'Going up the ladder', 'moving up in a job or financial position', are symbolic expressions of a developmental phase in which going up into verticality is connected to desirable autonomy and independence. On the other hand, 'feeling down', 'reaching the bottom' and 'low mood' are expressions connected to the 'down' of verticality and intimately related to the need for nurture, support and therefore dependency. These are, however, aspects that are increasingly vilified in our culture, not only historically as the traditional Oedipus complex shows, but also politically, economically and consequently socially. The up of verticality needs to be intertwined with the down of verticality. It is by inhabiting both the 'down' and 'up' of gravity that we let go of omnipotence. After the 'up' we need the 'down' to rest and recover, mirroring the rehearsal of life and death, in which after taking up gravity we surrender to it, as we approach our death journey.

Gravity in psychotherapy

Probably for most people the experience of psychotherapy has been verbal. Some might have chosen to sit down while others might have reclined on the couch. The horizontal position in psychoanalysis is thought, classically, to reduce the patient's defence mechanisms to encourage regression and provide easier access to fantasies and unconscious memories from early life.

Friedberg and Linn (2012), conducted interesting research of the use of the couch in psychoanalysis and psychoanalytic psychotherapy. They refer to psychoanalyst Goldberg's findings that the couch prevented engagement with conflicting feelings and thoughts related to independence, safety, shame and so on. Furthermore, early attachment needs may require visual contact, as well as other non-verbal forms of connection which have been much explored by infant researchers. Sitting down offers the possibility to see and to be seen, and therefore to not only be found but also to find the other in their corporeal realities, deepening in this way the intersubjective experience.

What these two different accounts of the horizontal and vertical position seem to reflect is that both have something to offer and both, if used in isolation, can present limitations. It is no wonder that many psychoanalytic psychotherapists have both a chair and couch in their consulting-rooms.

In movement psychotherapy, however, both verbal and non-verbal expressions are considered and all planes of the (body) self-organization can be explored through movement. Movement psychotherapy offers the possibility to re-live embodied relational experiences and to integrate new (body) self-experiences that result from the intercorporeal encounter.

The following example describes a brief reflection on some aspects related to gravity from a patient's treatment that lasted one year and two months.

Case example: Silvia

Silvia suffered from anorexia and she was 17 years old when we met. There seemed to be in Silvia a polarized view of the 'up' and 'down' of gravity. The fourth child of a mature couple, her siblings had left home when she was born, and her parents divorced when she was 10 years old.

Initially, Silvia sat on a chair in front of me. Her back did not touch the back of her chair and her body tensed as if stretched up to avoid an imminent fall or collapse.

If I suggested that she could touch the objects available for exploration there was an intensification of her fearful facial expression and bodily tension as if she feared that I might punish her. She told me that she did not remember playing much as a child and that she did not like mess. She also remembered a time in which she tended to lean on the walls and furniture, actions that resulted in reprimands by mum. All in all, Silvia didn't remember much physical contact, except when she sat on her mum's lap on busy public transport.

Silvia appeared to feel her spontaneous gesture, which Winnicott (1960a) saw as the source of the 'True Self' (ibid., p. 145), to be wrong and bad. Adding to this, there seemed to have been a very difficult dynamic with her mother when she went through periods of depression with overt aggressive incursions towards Silvia. Not having someone to protect her, Silvia eventually yielded to the comfort of food and became overweight. In an attempt to control her weight, she engaged in anorexic rituals that led to hospitalization.

I thought of Silvia's reluctance to lean onto the chair and to engage with objects as a reflection of Silvia's fear of her desire to surrender to the 'down' of gravity which might have represented both the desired but forbidding nurturing mother and the sexual impulses of her adolescent body (self). She appeared to fear that she might lose control and collapse into the horizontal to never come to vertical again and remained vertical inhabiting a 'false body' (Orbach, 2002, p. 129) that not only has not been recognized in her spontaneity and sexuality but also that had been attacked and punished.

When she eventually started exploring the floor horizontality I noticed that she did not quite yield into the ground. Silvia thought that her mother found her needs too much to bear and there was as a sense of feeling anxious as if her weight was too heavy and damaging. That she was too heavy was Silvia's biggest fear which was later translated into her body image.

Further explorations consisted of movement caricatures of what she recognized as her need to remain vertical and in control, never losing composure. Progressively, she was able to explore her deep fears of being out of control and unable to hold herself vertically by letting her weight collapse to the force of gravity. With time a more integrated version of these two polarized aspects of herself started emerging. She bounced, span and rolled on the floor, explored the weight of different body parts, leaned on the wall and the big exercise ball. And, Silvia also threw the big exercise ball at me using strong weight. The thought I might not be able to catch the ball created a lot of anxiety as this would mean that she was too heavy and too damaging.

Once, she sat on the exercise ball and played with getting out of balance. She discovered that she could regain equilibrium by using her feet and her core muscles, giving her movement a sense of freedom but also safety. Silvia seemed to have found that yielding to her weight was contained within the limits of a containing structure, her own body; a sense of body (self) found in the containing structure of the therapeutic alliance.

Conclusion

This chapter focused on how horizontality and the 'down' of gravity characterized the infant's early life, in which a relationship of closeness and dependency in mother is at its peak. It emphasised how verticality is to be achieved and how gravity functions as a *third*, further opening the space between the infant and mother and into the world. It then looked at how development of the relationship with (up) gravity is facilitated by the father and its relation to the oedipal situation. Finally, a reflection on gravity in psychotherapy brought to life the clinical relevance of gravity in the construction of the (body) self.

Note

1 To counteract unhelpful generalizations it would be interesting to make a formal study on how boys and girls explore gravity, especially in an era of great change in traditional gender roles and parenting, greater cultural influences and high technological advancement.

References

Bion, W. R. (1962) The Psycho-Analytic Study of Thinking. *International Journal of Psychoanalysis*, 43, 306–310.

Benjamin, J. (1988) *The Bonds of Love*. New York: Pantheon Books.

——. (1995) *Like Subjects, Love Objects: Essays on Recognition and Sexual Difference*. New York: Yale University.

——. (2004) Beyond Doer and Done To: An Intersubjective View of Thirdness. *Psychoanalytic Quarterly*, 73, 5–46.

Fonagy, P. and Target, M. (2007) The Rooting of the Mind in the Body: New Links Between Attachment Theory and Psychoanalytic Thought. *Journal of the American Psychoanalytic Association*, 55(2), 411–456.

Friedberg, A. and Linn, L. (2012) The Couch as Icon. *Psychoanalytic Review*, 99(1), 35–62.

Haag, G. (2000) In the Footsteps of Frances Tustin: Further Reflections on the Construction of the Body-Ego. *Infant Observation: International Journal of Infant Observation and Its Applications*, 3(3), 7–22.

Hackney, P. (2002) *Making Connections: Total Body Integration through Bartenieff Fundamentals*. London: Routledge.

Hartley, L. (1989) *Wisdom of the Body Moving: An Introduction to Body-Mind Centering*. Berkeley, CA: North Atlantic Books.

Music, G. (2011) *Nurturing Natures: Attachment and Children's Emotional Sociocultural and Brain Development*. Hove: Psychology Press.

Orbach, S. (2002) The False Self and the False Body. In B. Kahr (ed.) *The Legacy of Winnicott: Essays on Infant and Child Mental Health* (pp. 124–134). London: Karnac.

Pollack, T. (2008) The 'Body-Container' A New Perspective on the 'Body-Ego'. *International Journal of Psycho-Analysis*, 90(3), 487–506.

Rose, R. (2015) *Everything and More*. [Video installation]. London: Southbank Centre, The Store.

Stern, D. (1985) The Interpersonal World of the Infant: A View from Psychoanalysis and Developmental Psychology. New York: Basic Books.

Winnicott, D. R. (1960a) Ego Distortion in Terms of True and False Self. In: *The Maturational Processes and the Facilitating Environment* (pp. 140–152). London: Hogarth Press (1965).

——. (1960b) The Theory of the Parent–infant Relationship. *International Journal of Psycho-Analysis*, 41, 585–595.

10

DANCE MOVEMENT THERAPY

Building resilience from shared movement experiences

Rosemarie Samaritter

Introduction

Resilience has been the focus of (mental) health research for many years. Recent publications consider resilience an important factor for positive mental health (Huber et al., 2016). New developmental phases, life events, social and political events throughout life hold a manifold of challenges for the individual to adapt to changing life situations and to recover from threat or crises. The dynamic equilibrium of adaptive psychosomatic structures may be disorganised by the sensory overload caused by overwhelming life events. The living system's capacity to rebalance into adaptive responsivity may be suppressed or even put on hold. Dance movement therapy (DMT) seeks to develop and restore a responsive embodiment in the present moment (Pylvänäinen, 2010). Embodiment here is considered an *a priori* of the human condition (Koch and Fuchs, 2011; Sheets-Johnstone, 1999). With the body being the locus of our existence, sensations from the body provide us with a sense of self and with traces from lived experiences (Gendlin, 1997), while expressions from the lived body connect us with others and the world around (Schmais, 1985). The chapter will present five core themes that together contribute to the specific character of dance as socio-cultural practice. Interventions in DMT seem to cover these dance informed themes in the therapeutic setting. A thematic overview will show examples from the DMT literature on the therapeutic application of dance-based interventions and will discuss how DMT in a broad variety of populations seems to contribute to resilience by strengthening healthy potentials rather than focussing on negative symptoms or pathological traits.

Resilience: An exploration

Psychology research has focussed on resilience since the 1950s, when developmental psychologists began to study the impact of significant life experiences on the psychological development of a child. Werner and Smith (1992), two American psychologists, followed children born in 1955 on the Hawaiian island Kauai in a large cohort study for over 40 years. They observed that children who experienced similar life-threatening events seemed to recover from these experiences in different ways. Resilience seemed to emerge even in fragile life situations as long as a child experienced sufficient shelter, emotional acceptance and respect. Resilience hence was no longer considered only an individual's inherited strength, but also considered to be dependent on the specific life circumstances.

Garmezy (1987) broadened the perspective with a more developmental dimension when framing resilience as depending on the unfolding of personal and social constellations throughout life. The developing interplay of individual capacities, early family bonding and social embeddedness in community structures contributes to the individual's resilience over (life) time. Bonanno (2004) coined the term 'potentially traumatic events' (PTEs) (p. 20), to indicate that an event in itself may not necessarily lead to a traumatic experience, but that the response to an event may depend on a person's specific constellation of individual and social protective factors.

Peterson and Seligman (1987) found that a person's explanatory style also could influence the level of impact of a threatening event. People who recognised the *external* elements that lead to *one specific* event and saw it as limited to a specific time frame, seemed to be more successful in recovering from severely threatening events than people who did not have these characteristics, but instead felt that the adversity was an ongoing, overall disaster. Hence, resilience here was not only understood as a personal capacity that was sensitive to context, maturation and development, but was also seen as being sensitive to the individual's interpretive activity, to a person's ability to integrate events in the personal history and build meaning within the personal context and act from there.

Summarising these contributions, resilience seems to be best described as a multi-layered interplay of a living system's adaptive capacities that are informed by hereditary, developmental and biographical qualities. The dynamic interaction of the individual's capacities to cope with challenges or burdening life experiences (Wagnild and Young, 1993) and of the responsive interpretation and agency build throughout development (Luthar, Cicchetti, and Becker, 2000), their social embeddedness, individual strengths, coping strategies and ability to form life narratives contribute to a somato–psycho–socio–cultural understanding that interprets resilience as a flexible and responsive agency towards life events. This capacity may change throughout life and is informed and built on by life events (Masten, 2007). A healthy, resilient condition is characterised by the individual's capacity to reconnect to somatic resources and mobilise the organism towards a vital, that is a constantly rebalancing equilibrium, and to (re-)connect with nurturing self–other relationships. This condition enables people to move (on) after threatening events and to regain social and cultural embeddedness after loss.

When resilience breaks down

When the heaviness of events is too powerful, adjustments to the changing affordances of a life situation may be disturbed. This may be the effect of a single moment of disaster or the cumulative effect of long-term malign experiences, both will influence the hormonal balances in stress regulation. Continuously increased levels of stress hormones have shown to have an impact on the functional patterns of neurotransmitters (Groc, Choquet, and Chaouloff, 2008). These changes will affect the connectivity between lower and higher brain regions, signals from the experiential level will no longer be processed towards cortical regulation, which will leave the living system in a continuous state of arousal (Ogden, Pain, and Fisher, 2006). Corresponding with these processes, a person may dissociate from proprioceptive sensations coming from the body to cope with traumatic overload of experiences. Patients with early traumatic experiences have described that their body parts did not feel connected or that they did not feel their body at all (Mills and Daniluk, 2002). Organs and brain functions will suffer allostatic overload (McEwen, 1998), which may lead to somatic responses as seen in medically unexplained somatic complaints. The living systems, i.e. the individual's creative recovery from threatening events will no longer occur as a spontaneous impulse. The individual's capacity to integrate experiences into life narratives turns into scattered partitioning. Social and interactional capacities to connect to significant others or resources are no longer accessible, which will lead to isolation.

Dance as marker of vital life experiences

In many cultures, significant life experiences are expressed accompanied by dance (Sachs, 1933/1984). People share and mark specific life events with expressive, rhythmic or ritualised movements that are situated in a specific context, i.e. the theatre, the village market, the street. One might think here for example of line dances that are used during wedding celebrations in many European cultures or street dance battles that follow a specific structure of improvisations in the group circle.

Dancers come to experience an embodied community in feeling the shared dance kinaesthetically and engaging in interpersonal rhythmic synchronisations. Seeing and being seen, moving and being moved contribute to both the mover's and the observer's experience of mutual engagement with one another and leave traces in their body's memory (Koch, Fuchs, Summa, and Müller, 2012), which are wired in sensorimotor neuronal patterns (Grezes, Adenis, Pouga, and Armony, 2013).

Folk dances as well as social dances serve social ritual and interpersonal attunement. They allow for expression of emotions and social role or identity as for example seen in Argentine tango or classical ballet. Throughout cultures dances combine the reception and expression of artistic engagement. Playful improvisations bring up new material and choreographies may tell the story of the maker. Transmission of dances from generation to generation build cultural heritage and collective memory.

Dance always goes along with a somatosensory activation. Vital somatic functions like heartbeat and breathing are energised by the heightened movement action, the senses are awakened while actively following other dancers' movements in space and adjusting to them, listening to the music and finding synchronising movement patterns. Memory is activated in recapitulating specific dance rhythms or spatial patterns. In all these dimensions dance has a vitalising effect on the participants (Leseho and Maxwell, 2010).

Thus, we find that dancing invites spontaneous somatic rhythmical and interpersonal synchronisation and supports emotional release and social or cultural synchronisation. Dancing with others carries the individual through sequences of shared expressive articulation and supports the sharing of lived experiences (Sheets-Johnstone, 1999). The simultaneous emergence and presence of somatic, emotional, social and cultural animation may be best understood as an aesthetic involvement (Fraleigh, 1987). Immersing in dance individuals (re-)connect with an inward sensing yet vital expressive self. Dance therefore might be especially helpful to contribute to recovery when the living system's resilient adaptivity has been put on hold. The described facets of dance form the resources for dance movement therapy interventions. The following paragraph will give a brief introduction to DMT and will then explore the specific application of these dance informed structures for building resilience through DMT interventions.

Dance movement therapy

Dance movement therapy is a professional field with a large diversity of methods and applications. All styles of DMT have in common that they use movement and dance to address patients in their integrated body-mind-existence. In dance movement therapy literature, resilience had been pointed out as a goal of DMT intervention (Wengrower, 2015). Therapy outcome evaluations show that patients experience more capacity to vitally adapt to their life situation after DMT (Bräuninger, 2014).

Patients in mental healthcare may present with reduced vitality, numbed mood or static personality traits. DMT interventions are tailored to help patients to (re-)connect to body sensations and bring awareness to the changes that occur during dance and movement. From the systematic analysis of the patients' use of body, space and movement patterns, the therapist adjusts the movement interventions closely to the participant's movement capacities (Bartenieff, 1983). The aim of the DMT interventions is to invite the body back into the experience of being present, with active perception and readiness to act. The therapist will support the patient to recognise expressions of recovery and release by pointing out changes in breathing rhythms, changes in tension, changes in movement range or expression (Schmais, 1985).

As an expressive art form, dance allows for symbolisation of life experiences (Meekums, 2002). The therapy room may function as a safe place that allows for an aesthetic staging of the patient's experiential world. In some styles of DMT, patients will be supported to capture material from their movement explorations into tiny (re-)presentations or improvised choreographies that allow for securely framed emotional expression of body memories from past events (Caldwell, 2012). Sharing of symbolised expression and ritualised performance with a partner or a group generates experientially shared meaning-making. In either case dance is the propelling medium to connect inner and outer worlds. Movement in itself carries the sense of overcoming stagnation, and dance in particular may support emotional and social resilience by offering opportunities for emotional release, articulation and expression of shared vitality patterns and synchronisation to social and cultural patterns.

In the beginning of the DMT session, the attention of the patient is oriented towards the body, to bring it into awareness and prepare for physical activity (Hindi, 2012). Once the connection with the subjective body is established, the attention may be guided towards themes that come up from the perception of bodily feelings (Chodorow, 2013). The therapist will encourage the patient to share these feelings through expressive dance/movement and will empathetically engage with the patient's movement patterns. S/he will invite exploration of movement structures and deepening of the movement qualities to support articulation of the potential emotional content. This type of work can be found in movement circles but also in open improvisation or group formations (Fischman, 2017). The therapist will support the patient by skilfully composed interventions to find and follow personal movement impulses. S/he will invite kinaesthetic responses to social interactions, like attunement and assertiveness. Finally, after shared dance explorations, the therapist will guide the patient back into the subjective perception of their own body, reflecting on the potential contribution of the experience for a positive (body) memory. The body as experiential container (Payne, 2006) will carry these experiences into life situations outside the clinical setting.

Dance movement therapy: Building resilience through dance

The dance informed structures that have been described before may be helpful to specify the diversity of potentially effective elements in DMT. These structures can be summarised in five core themes of supporting:

1) kinaesthetic self-perception/embodiment
2) functioning of anatomical, visceral and neuropsychological systems

3)   non-verbal articulation and expression
4)   sensitivity to non-verbal self–other relatedness
5)   social and cultural synchronization.

The following paragraphs will review the individual themes for their clinical application in DMT and will assess their relevance for building resilience.

1.   Kinaesthetic self-perception

The dance movement therapist will actively support and invite attention to the dynamics of being present through the body. Perception during action is activated by focussing on the dynamic changes in movement quality (Tufnell and Crickmay, 1990). The body's functional processes may serve as a point of departure here, like the dynamics of breathing rhythms with the concomitant widening or narrowing of the body shape. The therapist will act with responsive interventions to mirror the participant's movement impulses which, as a consequence of traumatisation or psychopathology, are often cut off from direct perceptive awareness. Through the therapist's postural and movement responses, patients get a reflection of their personal movement material, which then can come into consciousness and will be accessible for further exploration (Best, 2010). The therapist may invite variations of the movement qualities, like making a movement very big or very small, moving very slowly or very fast. Through these movement experiments body sensitivity and body awareness are increased, and the patients will gain new connections to the body's potential for change and regulation. Sensing and regulating are anchored in the proprioceptive awareness of the body's condition (Ribeiro and Fonseca, 2011). In the regulation of the moving body, patients can experience ownership and agency of their own bodies, which may help to overcome victimization (Mills and Daniluk, 2002). New narratives may develop from that movement informed sense of self.

2.   Functioning of the body's anatomical, visceral and neurophysiological systems

The therapist will conduct the therapy session carefully towards somatic and emotional release. Intensive motor activity, as experienced during dance, may contribute to the regulation of arousal (van der Kolk, 2000). The physical processes of the moving body are challenged into dynamic adjustments to regain and sustain the equilibrium of the living system. The regulation of autonomous rhythmic functioning is directly related to polyvagal regulation in the limbic system (Porges, 2007). The somatic responses of the body's autonomous regulatory systems like heartbeat and breathing rhythms can serve as a monitor for the regulation of arousal and release (Hanna, 2006). There is a growing research interest to investigate the impact of vitalising dance movement experiences on the body's functioning on structural and molecular level. Changes of stress hormone levels, i.e. modulation of dopamine and serotonin, have been found in patients after DMT intervention (Quiroga Murcia, Bongard, and Kreutz, 2009). Reports from medical dance/movement therapy describe patients' relief of pain afterwards (Bradt, Shim, and Goodill, 2015). In traumatised patients, the homeostasis of the living system may have suffered severe destabilisation. Pain and physical complaints may follow from damaged tissue functionality caused by chronic hormonal over-activation as, for example, the impact of high cholesterol and cortisol levels on the functioning of the adrenal glands (McEwen, 1998). Intense physical activities like dancing challenge the body's regulatory systems and support the release of allostatic overload. Movement experiences also directly contribute to the neuronal networks on self–other recognition and also help to develop equilibrium at molecular and cellular levels by adjustment to challenging environments (Carney, Amy, Cuddy, and Yap, 2010). Rhythmic movement activities organise alignment patterns and movement efficacy. Flexibility has been shown to improve in participants with frail motor functioning (Duncan and Earhart, 2012). Balance and motor coordination contribute to the brain's regulatory functioning.

3. Articulation and expression of emotional content

In DMT the aim is to recuperate expressiveness of bodily contained emotional content (Harris, 2007). The therapist will support the articulation and expression of emotions by guiding the participant to explore the specific qualities of movement patterns (Stanton, 1992). S/he may offer symbolisations and metaphors as safe modes for the expression of overwhelming experiences (Samaritter, 2009). Energetic movement experiences help to overcome expressive stagnation and support vital expression of inner impulses and emotional release (Margariti et al., 2012) and have an effect on the patients' self-esteem and increase of positive emotional experiences (Koch, Morlinghaus, and Fuchs, 2007). Coming from threatening life situations, patients' fragile or hidden body self can unfold in the safe place of DMT and the holding of the therapeutic relationship. In DMT patients are supported to articulate inner sensations through movement and movement traces like sounds or drawings. The way in which the body is experienced may change by, and during, the movement process as the proprioceptive and exteroceptive impulses generated while moving inform the movers' self-perception. Body images build within the dynamic interaction of sensing and expressing the moving self.

In narrative movement structures the dance therapist may support patients to 'choreograph' their life story as a piece of dance or in little dance patterns. A choreographic structure for example may provide a holding frame for threatening experiences as it allows them to move in and out of the scene or to move towards a safe place or towards a positive memory (Samaritter and Maagdenberg, 2012). The emotional arousal or release can be regulated according to the personal capacities in the present moment (Stern, 2004) and the patients can experience agency about the biographical content of their stories (Noë, 2007). Bringing the emotional themes into movement may unfold experiential alternatives for the biographical stagnation and contribute to a beneficial emotional experience. Group members and therapist act as supportive environment during this process.

4. Sensitivity to non-verbal attunement and communication

Connecting to others through expressive movement may help to overcome pathological isolation. To support interpersonal rapport therapists will use mirroring interventions as interactive rebound. The therapist's movement responses contain and hold participant's personal impulses within the shared movement experiences. Within these shared movement patterns the movers experience themselves through the kinaesthetic sense as well as through visual or auditory movement traces. Any contribution to the shared movement activity will leave a direct perceptible trace. Hence, patients can immediately experience their potential and agency to regulate the relational attunement as well as the shared movement content.

Patients who have experienced attachment trauma often report an overwhelming feeling of loneliness to a degree that they are afraid of 'falling' out of the world. Movement circles (Chaiklin and Schmais, 1979) offer the individual patient the containment of a holding environment while s/he is dancing in the middle of the group circle. When taking the lead during movement circles the patient is anchored by the group, who accepts the leadership of one of them and allows for settling back into the connectedness with the group when leadership is passed to another group member. A psychological theme, like the aforementioned 'falling out of life' may also be articulated as a movement exploration in a partnered activity with 'leaning and being supported' or 'falling and being caught' as themes. The social embeddedness of all activities during DMT adds to interpersonal experiences, which may be a holding quality or the mutual co-creation of the shared movement activity.

5.   Social and cultural synchronization

Dance in all cultures and in all socio-cultural contexts is a shared practice. The younger generation learns about the culture of the society in which they live through participation in traditional dances. At the same time, they will contribute to the renewal of the community's rituals by inventing new dance forms.

Within this context traditional as well as other existing dance forms deliver the material for synchronization with the socio-cultural existence of patients (Dosamantes-Beaudry, 1999). Examples for these forms are found in African or Asian collective dance rituals (Harris, 2007), but also in ballroom and social dancing, like tango, or community and folk dances (Siapno, 2012).

The therapist may offer movement material that presents the patients with a biographical or historical situatedness. This contextual holding through culturally shared movement structures may serve as a 'home/secure base'. In the work with migrants who have been on the move, seeking refuge or shelter, the connection to cultural identity through movement may offer the connection not only to positive memories but also to a bodily perceived notion of belonging. The dance situation offers an opportunity to transfer this cultural belonging into the present environment and to integrate biographical material with movement patterns from the present cultural context (Gray, 2002). Also in fragile developmental phases the cultural embeddedness of certain movement themes may offer anchorage during shifting identity. For example, during adolescence, when the cultural counter movement of underground and street communities offer social holding for the drifting juvenile identity. Hence, participation in social and cultural dance forms may be considered a form of acculturation or socio-cultural synchronisation, integrating the individual into community and supporting shared identity.

Conclusion

From the discussion of a broad diversity of approaches we find that DMT may contribute to resilience by applying facets of five dance-related themes. DMT interventions support the patients' capacity to maintain adequate functioning at multiple levels during changing and, at times, physically challenging movement activities.

The therapeutic context is composed such as to afford specific experiential spaces for the patients for the exploration of their capacities to develop, recover, move and move on. From a movement perspective we may consider pathology as a person's disconnectedness from a bodily felt sense of self. DMT guides patients to attentively perceive and follow bodily sensations. Dance informed structures provide the space for the patients' unfolding experiential landscapes. The disclosure of the experiencing self in the benign therapeutic relationship supports a new, or newly connected, sense of self. In dance-informed structures the participant can practice the synthesis of experiences from life-history with experiences from the present environments.

Engaging all these existential layers simultaneously in the aesthetic space of dance-based interventions, DMT seems to be well suited to support patients to build resilience from a *corps vecu* (Merleau-Ponty, 1945/1962), and, in doing so, to reconnect to vital adaptivity in the present moment and build community through corporeal sharing with group members and/or therapist. These procedures seem to fit well in a saluto-genetic perspective to mental health (Friedli, 2009) that emphasises the multi-layered interplay of emotional, cognitive, somatic, social, ecological and cultural capital.

References

Bartenieff, I. (1983). *Body Movement – Coping with the Environment*. New York: Gordon and Breach.

Best, P. (2010). Observing interactions being shaped. In S. Bender (Ed.), *Movement Analysis of Interaction/ Bewegungsanalyse von Interaktionen* (pp. 241–257). Berlin: Logos.

Bonanno, G. A. (2004). Loss, trauma, and human resilience: Have we underestimated the human capacity to thrive after extremely aversive events? *American Psychologist, 59*(1), 20–28.

Bradt, J., Shim, M., and Goodill, W. (2015). Dance/movement therapy for improving psychological and physical outcomes in cancer patients. *Cochrane Database of Systematic Reviews, 1*, CD007103.

Bräuninger, I. (2014). Specific dance movement therapy interventions – Which are successful? An intervention and correlation study. *The Arts in Psychotherapy, 41*(5), 445–457.

Caldwell, C. (2012). Sensation, movement, and emotion. Explicit procedures for implicit memories. In S. Koch, T. Fuchs, M. Summa, and C. Müller (Eds.), *Body Memory, Metaphor and Movement* (pp. 255–266). Amsterdam: John Benjamins.

Carney, D. R., Amy, J. C., Cuddy, A. J. C., and Yap, A. J. (2010). Power posing: Brief nonverbal displays affect neuroendocrine levels and risk tolerance. *Psychological Science, 21*(10), 1363–1368.

Chaiklin, S., and Schmais, C. (1979). The Chace approach to dance therapy. In P. L. Bernstein (Ed.), *Eight Theoretical Approaches in Dance-Movement Therapy* (pp. 43–50). Dubuque, IA: Kendall/Hunt.

Chodorow, J. (2013). *Dance Therapy and Depth Psychology*. Reprint. London: Routledge

Dosamantes-Beaudry, I. (1999). Divergent cultural self construals: Implications for the practice of dance/ movement therapy. *The Arts in Psychotherapy, 26*(4), 225–231.

Duncan, R. P., and Earhart, G. M. (2012). Randomized controlled trial of community-based dancing to modify disease progression in Parkinsons disease. *Neurorehabilitation and Neural Repair, 26*(2), 132–143.

Fischman, D. I. (2017). Understanding group shaping. Transcontextual metapatterns in dance movement psychotherapy. *Body, Movement and Dance in Psychotherapy, 12*(2), 83–97.

Fraleigh, S. (1987). *Dance and the Lived Body. A Descriptive Aesthetics*. Pittsburgh, PA: University of Pittsburgh Press.

Friedli, L. (2009). *Mental Health, Resilience and Inequalities*. Copenhagen: World Health Organisation, Regional Office for Europe.

Garmezy, N. (1987). Stress, competence, and development: Continuities in the study of schizophrenic adults, children vulnerable to psychopathology, and the search for stress-resistant children. *American Journal of Orthopsychiatry, 57*(2), 159–174.

Gendlin, E. T. (1997). *Experiencing and the Creation of Meaning*. Evanston, IL: Northwestern University Press.

Gray, A. E. L. (2002). The Body as voice: Somatic psychology and dance/movement therapy with survivors of war and torture. *Connections, 3*(2), 2–4.

Grezes, J., Adenis, M. S., Pouga, L., and Armony, J. L. (2013). Self-relevance modulates brain responses to angry body expressions. *Cortex, 49*(8), 2210–2220.

Groc, L., Choquet, D., and Chaouloff, F. (2008). The stress hormone corticosterone conditions AMPAR surface trafficking and synaptic potentiation. *Nature Neuroscience, 11*(8), 868–870.

Hanna, J. L. (2006). *Dancing for Health: Conquering and Preventing Stress*. Lanham, MD: AltaMira Press.

Harris, D. A. (2007). Dance/movement therapy approaches to fostering resilience and recovery among African adolescent torture survivors. *Torture: Quarterly Journal on Rehabilitation of Torture Victims and Prevention of Torture, 17*(2), 134–155.

Hindi, F. S. (2012). How attention to interoception can inform dance/movement therapy. *American Journal of Dance Therapy, 34*(2), 129–140.

Huber, M., van Vliet, M., Giezenberg, M., Winkens, B., Heerkens, Y., Dagnelie, P. C., and Knottnerus, J. A. (2016). Towards a 'patient-centred' operationalisation of the new dynamic concept of health: A mixed methods study. *BMJ Open, 6*(1).

Koch, S. C., and Fuchs, T. (2011). Embodied arts therapies. *The Arts in Psychotherapy, 38,* 276–280.

Koch, S. C., Fuchs, T., Summa, M., and Müller, C. (Eds.). (2012). *Body Memory, Metaphor and Movement.* Amsterdam: John Benjamins.

Koch, S. C., Morlinghaus, K., and Fuchs, T. (2007). The joy dance: Specific effects of a single dance intervention on psychiatric patients with depression. *The Arts in Psychotherapy, 34,* 340–349.

Leseho, J., and Maxwell, L. R. (2010). Coming alive: Creative movement as a personal coping strategy on the path to healing and growth. *British Journal of Guidance and Counselling, 38*(1), 17–30.

Luthar, S. S., Cicchetti, D., and Becker, B. (2000). The construct of resilience: A critical evaluation and guidelines for future work. *Child Development, 71*(3), 543–562.

Margariti, A., Ktonas, P., Hondraki, P., Daskalopoulou, E., Kyriakopoulos, G., Economou, N.-T., . . ., Vaslamatzis, G. (2012). An application of the Primitive Expression form of dance therapy in a psychiatric population. *The Arts in Psychotherapy, 39*(2), 95–101.

Masten, A. S. (2007). Resilience in developing systems: Progress and promise as the fourth wave rises. *Developmental Psychopathology, 19*(3), 921–930.

McEwen, B. S. (1998). Stress, adaptation, and disease. Allostasis and allostatic load. *Annals of the New York Academy of Science, 840,* 33–44.

Meekums, B. (2002). *Dance Movement Therapy: A Creative Psychotherapeutic Approach.* London: Sage.

Merleau-Ponty, M. (1962). *Phenomenology of Perception* (C. Smith, Trans.). London: Routledge and Kegan Paul. (Original work published 1945)

Mills, L., and Daniluk, J. (2002). Her body speaks: The experience of dance therapy for women survivors of child sexual abuse. *Journal of Counseling and Development, 80*(1), 77–85.

Noë, A. (2007). Welten Verfügbar Machen [Making Worlds Accessible]. In S. Gehm, P. Husemann, and K. von Wileke (Eds.), *Wissen in Bewegung* [Knowing while Moving] (pp. 125–133). Bielefeld: [transcript].

Ogden, P., Pain, C., and Fisher, J. (2006). A sensorimotor approach to the treatment of trauma and dissociation. *Psychiatric Clinic North America, 29*(1), 263–279, xi–xii.

Payne, H. (2006). The body as container and expresser: Authentic movement groups in the development of well-being in our bodymindspirit. In J. Corrigall, H. Payne, and H. Wilkinson (Eds.), *About a Body: Working with the Embodied Mind in Psychotherapy* (pp. 162–180). London and New York: Routledge.

Peterson, C., and Seligman, M. E. P. (1987). Explanatory style and illness. *Journal of Personality, 55*(2), 237–265.

Porges, S. W. (2007). The polyvagal perspective. *Biological Psychology, 74*(2), 116–143.

Pylvänäinen, P. (2010). The dance/movement therapy group in a psychiatric outpatient clinic: Explorations in body image and interaction. *Body, Movement and Dance in Psychotherapy, 5*(3), 219–230.

Quiroga Murcia, C., Bongard, S., and Kreutz, G. (2009). Emotional and neurohumoral responses to dancing tango argentino. *Music and Medicine, 1*(1), 14.

Ribeiro, M., and Fonseca, A. (2011). The empathy and the structuring sharing modes of movement sequences in the improvisation of contemporary dance. *Research in Dance Education, 12*(2), 71–85.

Sachs, C. (1984). *Eine Weltgeschichte des Tanzes* [A World History of Dance]. Hildesheim, Zürich, and New York: Olms. (Original work published 1933)

Samaritter, R. (2009). The use of metaphors in dance movement therapy. *Body, Movement and Dance in Psychotherapy, 4*(1), 33–43.

Samaritter, R., and Maagdenberg, T. (2012). Bewogen levens. Nonverbale interventies in psychotherapie [Lives moved. Nonverbal interventions in psychotherapy]. *Tijdschrift cliëntgerichte psychotherapie/Journal for Client Centred Psychotherapy, 50*(4).

Schmais, C. (1985). Healing processes in group dance therapy. *American Journal of Dance Therapy, 8*(1), 17–36.

Sheets-Johnstone, M. (1999). *The Primacy of Movement.* Amsterdam: John Benjamins.

Siapno, J. (2012). Dance and martial arts in Timor Leste: The performance of resilience in a post-conflict environment. *Journal of Intercultural Studies, 33*(4), 427–443.

Stanton, K. (1992). Imagery and metaphor in group dance movement therapy. A psychiatric outpatient setting. In H. Payne (Ed.), *Dance Movement Therapy: Theory and Practice* (pp. 123–140). London: Routledge.

Stern, D. (2004). *The Present Moment in Psychotherapy and Everyday Life.* New York: W. W. Norton.

Tufnell, M., and Crickmay, C. (1990). *Body Space Image.* London: Dance Books.

van der Kolk, B. (2000). Posttraumatic stress disorder and the nature of trauma. *Dialogues in Clinical Neuroscience, 2*(1), 7–22.

Wagnild, G. M., and Young, H. M. (1993). Development and psychometric evaluation of the Resilience Scale. *Journal of Nursing Measurement, 1*(2), 165–178.

Wengrower, H. (2015). Widening our lens: The implications of resilience for the professional identity and practice of dance movement therapists. *Body, Movement and Dance in Psychotherapy, 10*(3), 153–168.

Werner, E. E., and Smith, R. S. (1992). *Overcoming the Odds.* Ithaca, NY: Cornell University Press.

11

INTERRUPTED RHYTHMS

Dance/movement therapy's contributions to suicide prevention

Susan D. Imus

Introduction

The Making Connections Suicide Prevention Program is a unique approach to suicide prevention that incorporates theory and practice from dance/movement therapy. Protective/resilience factors as defined in public health are highlighted throughout the gatekeeper programme by teaching an embodied approach to life skills development in feeling identification, tension reduction, affect regulation, and empathy building. A new model called Movement Thinking Strategies is presented to assist the community at large to observe, understand, and respond to the needs of others.

Suicide: A staggering problem

The definition of suicide according to the United States (US) Centers for Disease Control (CDC) is 'death caused by self-directed injurious behavior with the intent to die as a result of the behavior' (CDC, 2016, para 1). Over 800,000 people globally die by suicide each year (WHO.int, 2016, para 1). There were 45,000 deaths by suicide in the US in 2015 (CDC and Prevention, 2018, para 6). The US CDC (2014) have listed suicide as the tenth leading cause of death for people of all ages and ethnicities. Suicide is the second leading cause of death for ages 10–34 (ibid., 2014) demonstrating an increase from 2005 when it was the third leading cause of death for ages 10–24 (2014). It is the fourth leading cause of death for ages 35–54 (ibid., 2014) and the eighth leading cause of death for ages 55–64 (ibid., 2014).

While there are fewer overall attempts, the rate of attempt to completion is significantly greater for ages 64 and older (McCoy and Bass, 2013). In the US, 90–95 per cent of suicides are attributed to mental illness (Nock et al., 2008; Mann et al., 2005), and 'by 2020 mental health and substance use disorders will surpass all physical disease as a major cause of disability worldwide' (SAMHSA, 2018, para 2).

While progress toward reducing the national rate has been slow in the last 50 years, progress has been made in identifying related factors and methods for preventing suicide (Silverman, 2008). The National Action Alliance for Suicide Prevention, the National Strategy for Suicide Prevention, the Suicide Prevention Lifeline, the US Military Suicide Research Consortium, the Suicide Prevention Resource Center (2016) and their nine Strategic Initiatives are a few recent additions to the US infrastructure working to reverse suicide rates.

History of making connections

Another national building block is the Garrett Lee Smith Memorial Act, passed by the US Congress in 2004 to provide 9.3 million dollars to college and university campuses, state, and tribal initiatives combatting suicide. The grants are managed by the Substance Abuse and Mental Health Services Administration (SAMHSA), a federal branch of the US Department of Health and Human Services. Columbia College Chicago (CCC), a private urban arts and media institution of higher education, was in the first cohort of 22 nationwide campuses awarded the grant in the fall of 2005 through this legislation. CCC received this grant because of a shared initiative between the Dance/Movement Therapy and Counseling (DMTC) department and the Office of Student Life and Support. CCC was cited in their award letter as receiving this grant because of the DMTC department's unique embodied approach to suicide prevention.

The American Dance Therapy Association (ADTA, 2016) defines dance/movement therapy (DMT) as 'the psychotherapeutic use of movement to promote emotional, social, cognitive, and physical, integration of the individual' (ADTA, 2016, para 1). DMT is an embodied approach, and a way of knowing and understanding the world (Fischman, 2009) through the body and its movement, for health promotion, prevention, treatment, and research.

The DMTC department developed a workshop called the Making Connections Suicide Prevention Program (MC) in 2002 which was presented nationally in five states and internationally in Seoul, South Korea. The program reached approximately 4,000 participants between 2002 and 2016 and has been facilitated by 12 dance/movement therapists. It has evolved into a three-hour workshop that provides a variety of pedagogical approaches including lecture discussion, experiential learning, and participatory education (Kickbush, Pelikan, Apfel, and Tsouros, 2013). It has been presented to students, student leaders, faculty, staff, and administrators at colleges, universities, high schools, mental health organizations, and professional DMT conferences.

The unique curriculum includes current best practice in suicide prevention from across the country. It is known as gatekeeper training, which is defined as 'training of community and organizational leaders who have contact with potentially vulnerable populations. The gatekeepers are in positions to identify at-risk individuals and direct them to appropriate assessment and treatment' (Mann et al., 2005, p. 2067). Gatekeepers vary in different contexts. Primary care physicians in healthcare, student leaders, staff, and teachers in education are prime examples. MC appealed to student leaders in student organizations and residential advisors in dormitories across campus.

Estimates of the impact of different interventions on national suicide rates shows that the most promising interventions are physician education, means restriction, and gatekeeper education (2010). Research also indicates that multi-layered interventions of varying intensities afford the best protection for suicide. The Suicide Prevention Resource Centre's (2016) nine Strategic Initiatives take this into consideration and are as follows: 1. Identify and Assist, 2. Increase Help-Seeking, 3. Effective Care and Treatment, 4. Care Transition Linkages, 5. Respond to Crisis, 6. Post-vention, 7. Decrease Access to Means, 8. Life Skills and Resistance, and 9. Connectedness. The MC workshop addresses strategies 1, 2, 5, 8, and 9, with the primary emphasis on 8 (Life skills) and 9 (Connectedness).

The structure

Since 2005, Making Connections (MC) has operated on the belief that suicide prevention is a community responsibility. The mission of the programme is to 'make connections with yourself (intra-personally), with another (inter-personally), and with your community to prevent death by suicide' (Imus, Downey, Lengerich, and Brownholtz, 2014, p. 3). The programme teaches the participants to Observe, Understand, and Respond (OUR) to the signs of suicide, which include risk factors, warning signs, protective/resilience factors, and body awareness/signals.

MC reflects a shift in suicide prevention from a biomedical model towards a public health model. The biomedical model treats suicide as an individual problem. Dance/movement therapists and similarly trained allied health professionals in the US are traditionally educated in biomedical mental health approaches to treat suicidality. This includes individual assessment, diagnosis, intervention, and follow-up for symptoms through psychotherapy and medication prescribed by the patient's psychiatrist.

Experts in suicidology now believe that biomedical explanations of suicide limit best practice (Reed, 2008). A larger context involving community, needs to be included to effectively address suicide, specifically public health approaches. Public health is defined as 'the science of protecting and improving the health of families and communities through promotion of healthy lifestyles, research for disease and injury prevention, and detection and control of infectious diseases' (CDC, 2016). Primary prevention and collective health promotion are part of the answer. When the bar is raised for the entire community in creating better health, the incidence of suicide declines (Frohlich and Potvin, 1999).

SAMHSA's National Registry of Evidence-based Programs and Practices requires instruction in risk factors, warning signs, and protective/resilience factors for best practice in suicide prevention. These three subjects are covered through creative engagement during the MC workshop and detailed below.

Risk factors: Risk factors are 'stressful events, situations, and/or conditions that may increase one's likelihood of attempting or dying by suicide' (Coleman and O'Halloran, 2004, p. 21). Examples include having multiple suicide attempts, a detailed plan for suicide, access to lethal means, and friends or family members who have died by suicide. Risk factors do not predict immediate danger of suicide, but they may suggest that an individual may need additional concern or monitoring (ibid., 2004).

Warning signs: According to experts from the American Association of Suicidology (Rudd et al., 2006) warning signs should be presented in a hierarchical fashion:

- When you hear, say, or see any of these behaviours you must call the emergency number in the US 9–1–1 or seek immediate help from a mental health provider: someone threatening to hurt or kill themselves, someone looking for ways to kill themselves by seeking access to pills, weapons, or other means, and someone talking or writing about death, dying, or suicide (p. 259).
- Seek help by contacting a mental health professional or calling 1–800–273–TALK in the US for a referral should you witness, hear, or see anyone exhibiting any one of these behaviours: hopelessness, rage, anger, seeking revenge, acting reckless, or engaging in risky activities without thinking, feeling trapped, increasing alcohol or drug use, withdrawing from friends, family, and or society, anxiety, agitation, unable to sleep or sleeping all the time, dramatic changes in mood, no reason for living or sense of purpose in life (ibid., p. 259).

Protective/resilience factors: Protective factors are the 'positive conditions, personal, and social resources that promote resiliency and reduce the potential' for suicide as well as other high-risk behaviours (Coleman and O'Halloran, 2004, p. 23). Protective factors may include life skills, positive social support, good health, sobriety, self-worth, empathy, and a helpful, safe environment. The US Public Health Service (1999) also lists the following for protective factors: effective clinical care for mental, physical, and substance abuse disorders; easy access to a variety of clinical interventions and support for help seeking; support from ongoing medical and mental health-care relationships; cultural and religious beliefs that discourage suicide; and support instincts for self-preservation.

MC, unlike many programmes, does not teach risk factors and warning signs through lecture format as best practice indicates that lecture-discussion approaches to learning are too passive and must be combined with experiential approaches (Pasco, Wallack, Sartin, and Dayton, 2012). As such, lecture-discussion approaches are allocated the smallest amount of time in the MC programme and include the presentation of suicide demographics, myths, and community prevention resources via a 25-page programme manual.

MC adopts an experiential learning and participatory educational approach to teach risk factors, warning signs, and protective factors including creative engagement, movement thinking, skill building, embodiment exercises, and experiential role plays.

Creative engagement and role play

Role play has become not only accepted but expected as the norm for best practice, as evidenced in popular programmes such as Question, Persuade, and Refer and Acknowledge, Care and Tell (Burnette et al., 2015). The three role plays in MC are not pre-scripted. Part of the learning is through the creation of the script by the participants. They develop scripts in small groups and put together a scene that demonstrates a variety of risk factors, warning signs, and protective factors affiliated with three different levels of risk: low, high, and immediate. The DMT facilitator provides verbal and non-verbal coaching following the role plays. Creative engagement and role play allow the participants to create, write, direct, perform, and coach one another, enhancing ownership in the process. This fosters efficacy and reinforces the belief that suicide prevention is all OUR responsibility.

Life skills development in MC includes education in intrapersonal and interpersonal communication skills, feeling identification, active listening, tension reduction, affect regulation, and empathy building (Figure 11.1). Training is provided in observing and understanding both affective and behavioural symptoms as presented through body movement. At the onset of the

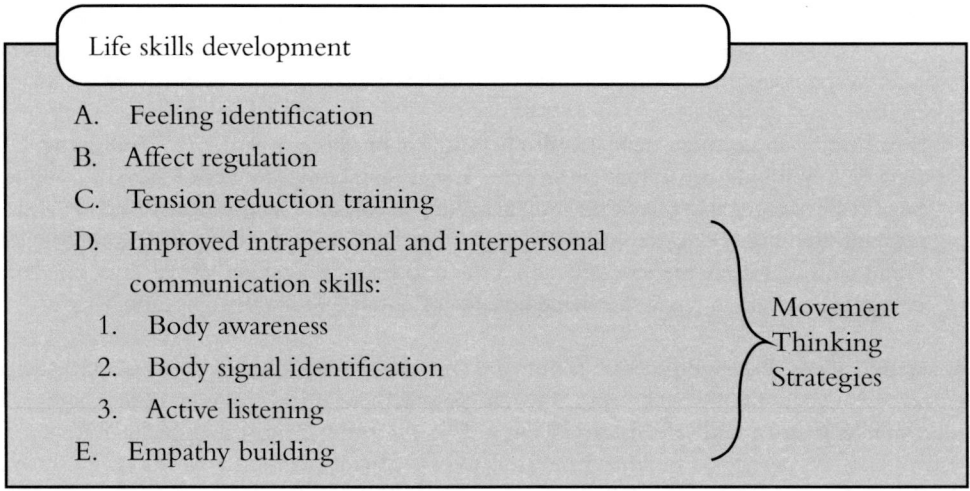

Life skills development

A. Feeling identification
B. Affect regulation
C. Tension reduction training
D. Improved intrapersonal and interpersonal communication skills:
　　1. Body awareness
　　2. Body signal identification
　　3. Active listening
E. Empathy building

Movement Thinking Strategies

Figure 11.1　Protective factors/life skills

workshop, participants are taught movement language that has been adapted from Laban Movement Analysis (Laban and Lawrence, 1947; White, 2009).

Intrapersonal communication

Body awareness: Participants are taught intrapersonal body awareness through movement exercises in energy identification, body-tension scanning, breath support, spatial centring, physical grounding, and tension regulation. These exercises focus primarily on internal body sensations and are labelled 'body awareness'. Mastery of these intrapersonal skills facilitates better interpersonal communication.

Body signals: Interpersonal communication skills are taught by applying intrapersonal body awareness to others. Participants observe and seek to understand another person's body signals as identified through shifts in energy including the motion factors of time, strength, space, tension, plus the body shape, facial expression, and focus. Participants identify with one another interpersonally through their similarities and differences as described in movement terms, for example 'We have less energy, so are moving slower and making no eye contact'. Facilitators constantly role model the movement language and its corresponding movement, creating coherency between what the body movement is communicating, and the mind is thinking and saying.

Active listening: Time is allocated for participants to share their personal stories about suicide. The facilitator de-limits the discussion of lethal means, assures no more than 20 minutes is spent in the talking circle, and models active listening skills. The importance of seeking mental health treatment in the community is emphasised, reducing stigma.

Tension reduction/affect regulation

A variety of dynamic relaxation exercises are presented: for example, Three-Dimensional Breathing (Bartenieff and Lewis, 1980), Progressive Muscular Relaxation (Jacobson, 1938), and Tai Chi exercises (Stone, 2009). Participants inwardly check in before and after each exercise to reinforce the power of the exercise in shifting/regulating their sensations, images, feelings, and thoughts.

Feeling identification

The facilitator verbally and non-verbally mirrors the feelings expressed in the talking circle and works on clarifying them with the participants. Natural discussions often include a description of the behaviour and affect of the person who died by suicide. This leads into a discussion of what the participants imagine a suffering person may have been feeling before they died. Hopelessness, loss, sadness, and anger are cited as the most frequently identified feelings by those who attempt suicide in adolescents and young adults (Mueller and Waas, 2002).

Empathy building

Once these words are identified, participants work in pairs (artists and sculptures) to embody the feelings. The sculpture partner is moulded into a body shape representative of a feeling selected by the artist and must hold the facial expression and focus, body tension, and body shape-posture while their partners try on all sculptures in the room. Artists must assist their sculpture-partner out of their body postures by finding recuperative movement to relieve them of the troubling body sensations. The partner's assistance in finding recuperative movement cannot be overlooked and provides insight into helping behaviours such as inquiry, direct assistance, and distraction. It also stresses the importance of the need for movement to assist in reducing the body tension that developed while holding the feeling postures. A discussion ensues about what partners observed, felt, imagined, thought, and sensed through their bodies to empathise, understand, and respond to each other. Identification of the embodied feelings are surprisingly easy for the group, and the participants develop efficacy through correct identification.

Movement thinking strategies

Movement Thinking Strategies (MTS) are a way of systematically teaching the community to develop intrapersonal and interpersonal communication skills for enhancing empathy. The term 'movement thinking' was coined by Rudolf Laban (1950) in the early twentieth century. Laban defined movement thinking in contrast to thinking in words:

> Movement thinking could be considered as a gathering of impressions of happenings in one's own mind for which nomenclature is lacking. This thinking does not, as thinking in words does, serve orientation in the external world, but rather it perfects man's orientation in his inner world in which impulses continually surge and seek an outlet.
>
> *(p. 17)*

MTS include teaching a person to develop a relationship through observing and understanding their personal movement experience and relating their experience to that of another's (Imus et al., 2014). Crucial to this strategy are the questions that are asked of oneself and others.

Observe
- Observe and make connections with Myself (intrapersonal) body awareness
- Observe and make connections with Another (interpersonal) body signals

Understand
- Nonverbally pick-up the shape, tension, focus, and affect of another
- SEE, SENSE, IMAGE, FEEL and THINK (Siegel, 2012) about their body signals
- Verbally ask what the person senses, images, feels and thinks (SIFT)
- Actively listen to their response and look for non-verbal and verbal discrepancies in their communication

Respond
- Tell a person who can make a difference
- Accompany the person when possible; walk with them to the counseling center on campus or in their community
- Provide community resources
- Call 911 in an emergency

Figure 11.2 Movement Thinking Strategies

The concept of SMIFT-ing, adapted from 'The Whole Brain Child Workbook' (Siegel and Bryson, 2015a), is one technique incorporated into MTS. For example, participants are asked what they sense, move, imagine, feel, and think (SMIFT) when their body is moving in this posture/shape, with this amount of tension, with this facial expression and focus, and with this amount of strength, use of space, and breath support. When they answer these questions, they can then use the discoveries to ask more informed questions of another person. They must actively listen to their verbal response and contrast and compare it with their body's non-verbal response to discover congruency between the verbal and non-verbal communication. Body awareness and body signal skills are interspersed throughout the training, but they are called MTS when combined with SMIFT-ing for understanding and responding (Figure 11.2).

Developing empathy is key in suicide prevention. According to Mueller and Waas (2002) '. . . prevention programs may be more effective when incorporating activities and information designed to increase empathic responding on the part of peers' (ibid., pp. 335–336). As previously indicated, empathy building, particularly using 'OUR' is the mission of MC (Imus et al., 2014, p. 5).

The integration of DMT methods, such as MTS, and other embodied exercises are what makes MC stand out among suicide prevention programmes. The combination is not only unique but beneficial in introducing community participants and suicidology experts to many important principles, methods, and techniques from DMT theory and practice that lend themselves to improving best practice in suicide prevention.

Dance/movement therapy principles and techniques

Dance is communication and Marian Chace, a 1940s founder of the DMT field in the US, stated this premise as the basis for her groundbreaking work (Chaiklin and Schmais, 1993). 'Dance therapy is a purposeful and knowledgeable use of expressive action as a potent means of direct communication' (ibid., p. 246). Neurobiologists today support this statement and have found 'more support for the idea that dance began as a form of representational communication' (Brown and Parsons, 2008, p. 83). Chace's followers in both the DMT field and in the MC workshop facilitation teach participants that their bodies and its movement/dance are in constant communication.

Discrepancies between verbal and non-verbal expression can help identify hidden meaning and facilitate more congruent communication. Chace (1961) stated that people do not often dare to express their emotions directly 'This would not matter so much if there were more frequent agreement between our verbal speech and our inadvertent body actions' (p. 326). During role play, participants are taught to reflect their emotions and question the role player if they notice discrepancies between the spoken word and their non-verbal dance.

DMT is experiential, action-oriented, and embodied learning, furthermore Fischman (2009) states that DMT is an enactive approach and explains this by citing Maturana (1987), 'We can only know by doing' (Fischman, 2009, p. 35). Meekums stated that, 'DMT respects the lived body as an active source of knowledge production' (Meekums, 2006, p. 169). As Payne (2004, p. 511) comments: 'It is about 'knowing (feeling) from the inside'. The body self-awareness exercises in MC introduce the process of knowing from the inside. This principle is reinforced throughout MC as skill development builds.

Sensations, images, feelings, and thoughts are readily accessible through movement and assist in linking the body-mind and the development of intrapersonal and interpersonal communication. Many people do not understand how to identify a body sensation from a feeling, image, or thought (Siegel and Bryson, 2015b). They may be confused with communicating inwardly (the personal) from outward communication (the social) (Capello, 2009; Karkou, 1992; Schmais, 1991). During MC training, through the dynamics of dance/movement, participants are taught a language to assist them in deepening their understanding namely body self-awareness, intrapersonal communication leading to body-signal awareness and interpersonal communication.

There is a reciprocal relationship between body and mind, whereby changing one's body can change one's mind (Karkou, 1992; Schoop and Mitchel, 1974; Stanton-Jones, 1992). As another founding DMT figure Trudi Schoop notes, 'If psychoanalysis brings about a change in the mental attitude there should be a corresponding physical change. If DMT brings about a change in the body's behaviour, there should be a corresponding change in the mind' (Schoop and Mitchel, 1974, p. 45). This principle is applied throughout MC. The facilitator frequently asks, 'If you want to change your mood how can you change your "dance?"' The emphasis on recuperative movement following embodied sculptures is one example of this. Tai Chi (Stone, 2009) exercises are taught following embodied sculptures to re-stabilise on a body level following the surfacing of the uncomfortable emotions like hopelessness and anger.

DMT is 'active interaction' (Karkou, 1992, p. 38) fostering adaptability and creative interventions by the facilitator and adaptive creative responses from the participants (Downey, 2016; Imus, 2012, 2016; Karkou, 2006; Levy, 2005). Although the DMT facilitator is doing prevention in MC, it is not uncommon for them to create an intervention. This occurred during one workshop when the MC facilitator adapted an exercise in the moment after observing that three participants were hesitant to close their eyes during a relaxation exercise. Instead, all participants were invited with eyes open to make 'fun-filled faces' as they alternated between tensing and releasing muscle groups. The cadence of the facilitator's voice matched the playfulness of the expressive exercise, which fostered the participants' creativity (Imus, 2012, 2016). A sense of safety returned to all, reinforcing social cohesion and a feeling of belonging essential to suicide prevention (Joiner, 2005). It also provided the opportunity to create and play, emphasising the importance of creativity and laughter as important life skills.

Dance/movement is simultaneously the assessment and intervention tool in DMT through a process called empathic reflection. Empathic reflection is a DMT foundational concept. Downey's (2016) phenomenological study 'demonstrated the use of empathic reflection as an assessment and evaluation tool, but most importantly as an inroad to efficiently and effectively developing and maintaining a therapeutic relationship' (ibid., p. 68). MTS are a low context method of teaching empathic reflection. The process simultaneously serves as informal assessment, intervention, and the development of a compassionate interpersonal connection.

Dance/movement changes one's biochemistry and promotes feelings of well-being (Berrol, 1992; Goodill, 2005; Homann, 2010; Svoboda, 2007) 'Biological factors most consistently correlated with suicidal behaviour involve disruptions in the functioning of the inhibitory neurotransmitter, serotonin. Persons who die by suicide have lower levels of serotonin metabolites in their cerebrospinal fluid' (Nock et al., 2008, p. 8). Conversely, it is known that dancing can elevate the 'mood-lifting neurotransmitter serotonin and norepinephrine' (Svoboda, 2007, para 3). This principle becomes evident at the onset of MC when participants report feeling immediately better following a dance/movement enactment of low and high energy. Participants are taught that they can feel better through dance.

Dance/movement is contagious and motivating through rhythmic group activity (Chaiklin and Schmais, 1993, Dosamantes-Alperson, 1979; Schoop and Mitchel, 1974). Neuroscientists Brown and Parsons (2008) have proven that there exists an 'unconscious entrainment' (p. 78) for humans to absentmindedly pick up a beat. Brown and Parsons noted, 'By far the most synchronized group practice, dance demands a type of interpersonal coordination in space and time that is almost nonexistent in other social contexts' (ibid., p. 78). We are motivated, even without conscious awareness, to join the dance of others. This bio-behavioural phenomenon lends itself to the power of DMT as prevention and intervention for anyone needing to connect, belong, increase socialization, and/or reduce isolation as rhythmic group activity is a core concept in all DMT practice (Chaiklin and Schmais, 1993; Schoop and Mitchel, 1974).

Evaluation

Formalized evaluation was required by all the Garret Lee Smith Campus Suicide Prevention Grant Program awardees. In total, 91 MC workshops were conducted between 2005 and 2008 with an attendance of 1,200 participants. Campus gatekeepers referred 298 people to on-campus resources in the Counseling Center and 550 people were referred to off-campus mental health providers, possibly indicating a decrease in stigma and an increase in help seeking behaviours on campus. A one to one correlation of the effect of MC workshops on help seeking behaviour was not conclusive due to a multiplicity of factors, including but not limited to a one-half hour didactic training called, Education and Empowerment in Suicide Prevention, and a safe-messaging campaign called the Suicide Prevention Stenciling Project that ran concurrently with MC.

Conclusion

Basic theory and principles from DMT can contribute to best practice in suicide prevention where experiential/action-oriented approaches like role modelling and resilience building are becoming more accepted. Observing body signals is key and working to understand these signals from our own body self-awareness, i.e. our experience of sensations, movement, images, feelings, and thoughts (SMIFT) is necessary. Asking difficult questions, actively listening, and ensuring that there is verbal and non-verbal congruence in communication is essential. The emphasis on protective/resilience factors in MC is also especially important as less emphasis has been placed on protective factors in many of the programmes approved for the National Registry of Evidence-based Programs, even though current research suggests balancing the emphasis between risk and protective factors (Nock et al., 2008).

During one of many SPRC trainings provided to the cohort of the first 22 campus-wide grantees (2005), a story from a survivor vividly portrayed the power of including body signal training in this work. A woman who lost her sister to death by suicide received a letter from her sister's co-worker 10 years after her passing. The co-worker had observed something unusual about the sister's non-verbal communication the day before her death when she saw her sitting alone in the cafeteria. The co-worker wrote she felt guilty that she had done nothing when she noticed the sister's unusual body posture, facial expression, and focus in the cafeteria. This woman had been signalling, but no one responded. Her normal rhythm was interrupted as evidenced through her isolated 'dance'.

Dance/movement therapists understand the power of body signals. Our job is to teach others about taking the time to observe, understand, and respond to one another's 'dance'. It is no longer the sole responsibility of the mental health practitioner meeting with an individual who has an identified problem. It is all OUR responsibility to create health in our communities. Dance/movement therapists can lead the way in an embodied approach to health promotion, prevention, treatment and research in suicidology.

Acknowledgements

Special thanks to Laura Downey, Shannon Lengerich, Bethany Brownholtz, Paul Holmquist, Katie Bellamy, and the Webinar Team of the American Dance Therapy Association. This work is dedicated to Shannon Hardy and her survivors.

References

American Association of Suicidology. (n.d.). *History of the American Association of Suicidology*. Retrieved from www.suicidology.org/about-aas/history.

American Dance Therapy Association. (2016). *FAQs*. Retrieved from https://adta.org/faqs/.

Bartenieff, I., and Lewis, D. (1980). *Body movement coping with the environment*. New York: Gordon and Breach Science Publishers.

Berrol, C. (2006). Neuroscience meets dance/movement therapy: Mirror neurons, the therapeutic process and empathy. *The Arts in Psychotherapy, 33*(4), 302–315.

Brown, S., and Parsons, L. (2008). The neuroscience of dance. *Scientific American, Inc.*, pp. 78–83.

Burnette, C., Ramchand, R. and Ayer, L. (2015). Gatekeeper training for suicide prevention. *Rand Health Quarterly*, July 15:5(1):16.

Capello, P. (2009). BASICS: An intra/interactional model of DMT with the adult psychiatric patient. In S. Chaiklin and H. Wengrower (Eds.), *The art and science of dance/movement therapy: Life is dance* (pp. 77–102). New York: Routledge.

Centers for Disease Control and Prevention. (2014). WISQARS. In *Leading cause of death report, all ages, both sexes*. Retrieved from www.cdc.gov/injury/wisqars/leadingcauses.html.

Centers for Disease Control and Prevention. (2016). *Injury prevention and control: Division of violence prevention*. Retrieved from www.cdc.gov/violenceprevention/suicide/definitions.html.

Centers for Disease Control and Prevention. (2018). *Trends in State suicide—United States, 1999–2016 and Circumstances contributing to suicide—27 States*. Retrieved from www.cdc.gov/mmwr/volumes/67/wr/mm6722a1.htm?s_cid=mm6722a1_x.

Chace, M. (1961). Our real lives are lived in rhythm and movement. In S. L. Sandel, S. Chaiklin, and A. Lohn. (Eds.). *Foundations of dance/movement therapy: The life and work of Marian Chace* (pp. 325–326). Columbia, MD: American Dance Therapy Association.

Chaiklin, S., and Lohn, A. (Eds.) (1993) *Foundations of dance/movement therapy: The life and work of Marian Chace* (pp. 77–81). Columbia, MD: American Dance Therapy Association.

Chaiklin, S., and Schmais, C. (1993). The Chace approach to dance therapy. In S. L. Sandel, S. Chaiklin, and A. Lohn (Eds.), *Foundations of dance/movement therapy: The life and work of Marian Chace* (pp. 77–81). Columbia, MD: American Dance Therapy Association.

Coleman, L., and O'Halloran, S. (2004). *Preventing youth suicide through gatekeeper training*. Augusta, ME: Medical Care Development, Inc.

Dosamantes-Alperson, E. (1979). Dance/movement therapy: An emerging profession. *Journal of Energy Medicine, 1*, 114–119.

Downey, L. M. (2016). *A phenomenological exploration of empathic reflection in dance/movement therapy* (Unpublished doctoral dissertation). Argosy University, Orange, CA.

Fischman, D. (2009). Therapeutic relationships and kinesthetic empathy. In S. Chaiklin and H. Wengrower (Eds.), *The art and science of dance/movement therapy* (pp. 33–53). New York: Routledge.

Frohlich, K. L., and Potvin, L. (1999). Health promotion through the lens of population health: Toward a salutogenic setting. *Critical Public Health, 9*(3), 211–219.

Goodill, S. W. (2005). *An introduction to medical dance/movement therapy*. London: Jessica Kingsley.

Homann, K. B. (2010). Embodied concepts of neurobiology in dance/movement therapy practice. *American Journal of Dance Therapy, 32*(2), 80–99.

Imus, S. D. (2012, October). *Dance/movement therapy's scope of practice in healthcare: Soaring to new heights*. Presented at the American Dance Therapy Association 47th Annual Conference, Albuqurque, NM.

Imus, S. D. (2016). *Re-generating DMT theory and practice*. Presented at the American Dance Therapy Association's 51st Annual Conference, Re-generation: Moving Pathways to Integration, Bethesda, MD.

Imus, S. D., Downey, L., Lengerich, S., and Brownholtz, B. (2014). *Making connections: A suicide prevention program* [Training manual]. Chicago, IL: Columbia College Chicago, Department of Creative Arts Therapies.

Jacobson, E. (1938). *Progressive relaxation.* Chicago, IL: University of Chicago Press.

Joiner, T. E. (2005). *Why people die by suicide.* Cambridge, MA: Harvard University Press.

Karkou, V. (1992). Dance movement therapy in the community: Group work with people with enduring mental health difficulties. In H. Payne (Ed.), *Dance movement therapy: Theory, research and practice* (2nd ed.). New York: Routledge.

Kickbush, I., Pelikan, J. M., Apfel, F., and Tsouros, A. D. (2013). *Health literacy: The solid facts.* Copenhagen, Denmark: World Health Organization Regional Office for Europe. Retrieved from www.euro.who.int/puberequest.

Laban, R. (1950). *Mastery of movement for the stage* (3rd ed.). Hampshire, UK: Dance Books.

Laban, R., and Lawrence, F. C. (1947). *Effort.* London: Macdonald & Evans.

Levy, F. (2005). *Dance movement therapy: A healing art-revised edition.* Reston, VA: American Alliance for Health, Physical Education, Recreation and Dance.

Mann, J., Apter, A., Bertolote, A., Beautrais, A., Currier, D., Haas, A., . . . Hendin, H. (2010). Suicide prevention strategies: A systematic review. *Journal of American Medical Association.* Retrieved from http://jama.ama.-assn.org/cgi/content/full294/16/2064.

Maturana, H. R., and Varela, F. J. (1987). *The tree of knowledge: The biological roots of human understanding.* Boston, MA: Shambhala Publications.

McCoy, K., and Bass, P., III. (2013). *Depression and suicide in old age.* Retrieved from everydayhealth.com/senior-health/depression-and-suicide.aspx.

Meekums, B. (2006). Embodiment in DMT training and practice. In H. Payne (Ed.), *Dance movement therapy theory, research and practice* (2nd ed.). New York: Routledge.

Mueller, M. A., and Waas, G. A. (2002). College students' perceptions of suicide: The role of empathy on attitudes, evaluation, and responsiveness. *Death Studies, 26,* 325–341.

Nock, M. K., Borges, G., Bromet, E. J., Cha, C. B., Kessler, R. C., and Lee, S. (2008). Suicide and suicidal behavior. *Epidemiologic Reviews, 30,* 133–154.

Pasco, S. Wallack, C., and Dayton, R. (2012). The impact of experiential exercises on communication and relational skills in a suicide prevention gatekeeper-training program for college resident advisors. *Journal of American College Health.* Retrieved from: www.tandfonline.com/doi/abs/10.1080/07448481.2011.623489.

Payne, H. (2004). Becoming a client, becoming a practitioner: Student narratives of a dance movement therapy group, *British Journal of Guidance and Counseling, 32*(4), 511–532.

Reed, J. (2008, May). *It takes a community.* Presented at Bridging the Divide: Suicide Prevention Summit, Denver, CO.

Rudd, M. D., Berman, A. L., Joiner, T. E., Nock, M. K., Silverman, M. M., Manddrusiak, M., . . . Witte, T. (2006). Warning signs for suicide: Theory, research, and clinical applications. *Suicide and Life-Threatening Behavior, 36*(3), 255–262.

Sandel, S. (1993). The process of empathic reflection in dance therapy. In S. L. Sandel, S. Chaiklin, and A. Lohn (Eds.), *Foundations of dance/movement therapy: The life and work of Marian Chace* (pp. 98–111). Columbia, MD: The Marian Chace Memorial Fund of the American Dance Therapy Association.

Schmais, C. (1991). *The journey of a dance therapy teacher: Capturing the essence of Chace.* Columbia, MD: Marian Chace Foundation of the American Dance Therapy Association.

Schoop, T., and Mitchel, P. (1974). *Won't you join the dance? A dancer's essay into the treatment of psychosis.* Palo Alto, CA: National Press.

Siegel, D. & Bryson, T. (2012). *The whole-brain child: 12 revolutionary strategies to nurture your child's developing mind.* New York: Bantam Books Trade Paperback.

Siegel, D., and Bryson, T. P. (2015a). *The whole-brain child: 12 revolutionary strategies to nurture your child's developing mind.* New York: Bantam Books.

Siegel, D., and Bryson, T. P. (2015b). *The whole-brain child workbook: Practical exercises, worksheets, and activities to nurture developing minds.* Eau Claire, WI: PESI Publishing and Media.

Silverman, M. (2008, January). *Cohort 1 Campus-wide Grantee Seminar,* Presented at SAMHSA's Suicide Prevention Annual Grantee Conference, Kansas City, MO.

Stanton-Jones, K. (1992). *An introduction to dance movement therapy in psychiatry.* New York, NY: Routledge.

Stone, J. (2009). *Tai chi chih: Joy through movement.* US: Good Karma Publishers.

Substance Abuse and Mental Health Services Administration. (2018). *Prevention of substance abuse and mental illness.* Retrieved from: www.samhsa.gov/prevention.

Suicide Prevention Resource Center. (2016). *A comprehensive approach to suicide prevention.* Retrieved from www.sprc.org/effective-prevention/comprehensive-approach.

Svoboda, E. (2007). *Dance therapy: Spin control: When the body swings the mind is swayed. Therapy on the dance floor.* Retrieved from www.psychologytoday.com/articles200703/dance-therapy- spin-control.

U.S. Public Health Service. (1999). *The Surgeon General's call to action to prevent suicide.* Washington, DC. Retrieved from https://profiles.nlm.niih.gov/ps/access/MMBBBH.pdf.

White, E. Q. (2009). Laban's movement theories: A dance/movement therapist's perspective. In S. Chaiklin and H. Wengrower (Eds.), *The art and science of dance/movement therapy* (pp. 218–236). New York: Routledge.

World Health Organization. (2016). *Preventing suicide—A community toolkit.* Retrieved from: www.who.int/mental_health/suicide-prevention/en/.

12

BODY AS VOICE

Restorative dance/movement psychotherapy with survivors of relational trauma

Amber Gray

Introduction

Exposure to traumatic events is life changing. Fifty years ago, survivors of trauma did not have a diagnosis to explain their suffering. The symptoms, or signs of distress, that occur when a body, or system, is held captive by fear or 'locked down' in terror, were observed but not adequately categorized or inclusive enough to aid survivors to have a context for their experiences of suffering. Today, the field of trauma has advanced, and we now know that those exposed to what seem like more frequent events on the planet, for example experiences of school shootings, wars, genocide, domestic violence, torture, natural disaster, terrorism, sadistic and ritual abuse, sudden loss, accidents, and all other manner of fear, provoke life changing events in which people are forever changed.

We do not 'recover' from trauma; we do not go back to being the same. This is not to suggest we do not continue our lives with enthusiasm and enjoyment; in fact, traumatic events can catalyze change and transformations of great meaning for survivors. To expect this as an outcome of treatment, however, can be unfair to survivors of extreme events who endure ongoing loss, isolation, and complex psychological and physical pain. We also do not release trauma; we now know that the shifts that occur in the moment of exposure are somatic (biological, physiological) and there are many body-based approaches that utilize the body's ability to discharge nervous system charge, or activation. This author suggests the healing occurring after life changing events, such as relational trauma, beg a restorative process, where we restore what aspects we can of a survivor's life in service of restoring a sense of belonging and meaning (see Figure 12.1). Approaches that remain solely cognitive, affective, or behavioral will not offer a thorough restorative process, because the imprint of fear is in the body.

Whether the exposure is violence, natural disaster, or an accident, we now know that the imprint of the fear response that occurs in the moment of exposure (i.e. the traumatic experience) is body-based. Current neuropsychiatric research endorses the use of non-verbal therapies for work with survivors of trauma, recognizing that trauma memories are implicit. Dance/movement therapy (DMT) acknowledges the body as central to human experience, and movement as a primary language, fundamental to our early communicational relationship with caregivers. Knowing that trauma changes the brain, recent scientific discoveries in interpersonal neurobiology and neuroplasticity promote mindfulness or contemplative practice, and movement, as

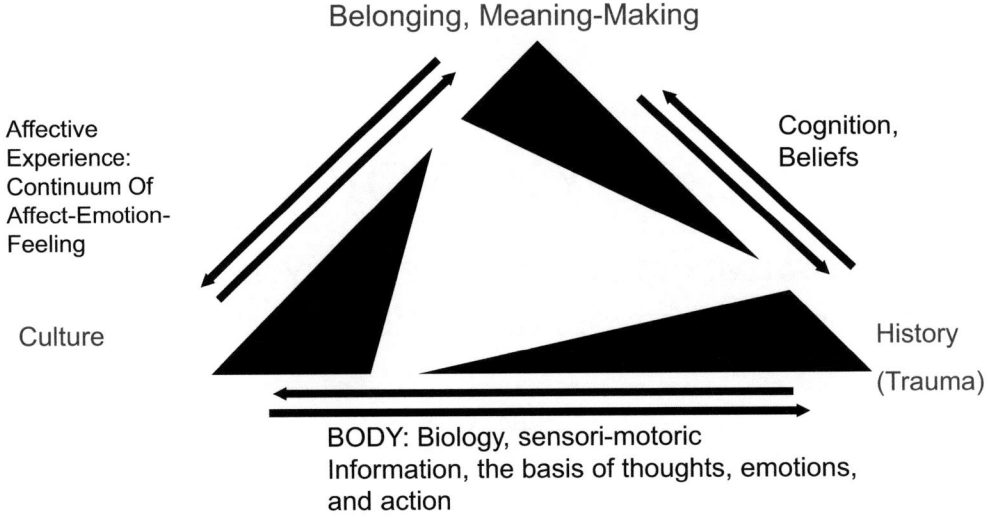

Figure 12.1 Human behaviour: Adjusting the framework for culture, context and the body

the most effective brain changers (Begley, 2007). Movement, as a primary language, and dance, as its creative expression, access the neurological underpinnings of all human thoughts, feelings, actions, and behaviors. DMT has a unique contribution to make in the growing convergence of science, theory, and clinical practice for trauma; the therapist's capacity and skill to promote interoceptive awareness and mindful movement, which are essential for healing, may promote our therapeutic approach as best or promising practice in the growing field of trauma. Relational trauma can literally force us to take a shape that is not our own; through work with posture, core support, effort shapes, rhythm, and sensori–motoric developmental sequences, the therapist can support traumatized clients to restore meaning and their place of belonging in the world. This chapter presents a framework, The 'Poto Mitan' Framework for Trauma and Resiliency (Gray, 2015a), and its clinical counterpart, Restorative Movement Psychotherapy (RTP), as a potential best practice approach to the restorative process with survivors of relational trauma.

Dance/movement therapy: A framework for restoration and healing

Dance/movement therapy is an integrative and holistic approach to psychotherapy. Founded in America by pioneer Marian Chace, who spent years working in the then back wards of St. Elizabeth's Hospital in Washington, DC, with severely psychotic patients for whom standard treatments did not help, Marian Chace (Chace, Sandel, and Chaiklin, 1993) continued to develop her work with veterans returning from the Second World War, whom other mental health professionals found challenging to treat. The inability to speak the horrors of war the soldiers had experienced made typical treatment almost obsolete, so Marian also worked with them, through movement and other forms of artistic expression, to process their traumatic exposures. DMT defined by the American Dance Therapy Association (ADTA) is 'Based on the empirically supported premise that the body, mind and spirit are interconnected' and as 'the psychotherapeutic use of movement to further the emotional, cognitive, physical and social integration of the individual' (ADTA, 2016). DMT has grown in application, theory and more recently, neuro-scientific endorsement as a best practice (ADTA, 2016). DMT is a convergence of developmental psychology, somatic psychology and creative arts therapies because of its emphasis on movement as a primary language, and its unique ability to access the creative process through the continuum of breath-movement-dance that is an inherent part of human expression. DMT recognizes that our primary relationships are initially non-verbal (Lewis, 1986) and that memories and self-identity are linked: 'Somatic material, unconscious material and conscious behaviour are stored in the body and are reflected in the breathing, posturing, and movement of an individual' (Lewis, 1986).

DMT merits recognition as a best practice for trauma treatment. Unlike other somatic approaches to trauma treatment, DMT does not solely focus on somatic awareness and/or verbal processing of both resource and trauma experience. DMT's developmental origins and capacity for working with an entire range of movement from simple breathing to creative expression offer clients a much bigger palette of options to move and heal from. DMT's are well trained in assessment and diagnostic skills that range from non-verbal observation of muscle tonus, energetic sequencing of movement; basic neurological actions and effort states to complete verbal and cognitive processing. Given the nature of traumatic memory and the now well-established classification of traumatization as a body-based state of fear DMT is a powerful approach for establishing resources and processing traumatic memories, towards the pathway of integration for the client. While casework, which is beyond the scope of this chapter, is the most direct means to demonstrate this claim, DMT emphasizes movement as a primary language combined with the aforementioned growing body of knowledge about the relationship between movement, attention, and neuroplasticity (Begley, 2007, p. 159). Thus, research on trauma, the brain and memory, and the very physiological nature of the trauma reaction at the moment of exposure, all converge to support DMT as perhaps the most comprehensive body and movement-based therapeutic approach for the treatment of trauma. Trauma treatment is not just about processing memories but about integrating life-changing experience in a holistic and meaningful way. This can only be done with the full engagement of the body and its primary language of movement.

Trauma and the body

The exposure to a dangerous or life-threatening event creates a fear (danger) or terror (life threat) reaction, and it is this reaction that creates traumatization. While the body itself may not distinguish between types of exposure (i.e. motor vehicle accident vs. rape), our minds, which Antonio Damasio (2005) describes as a function of brain and body, help us create meaning and determine the influence of these events on our life experience. What is important to understand is that trauma is not the event itself, it is the reaction [vs. the ability to respond, or pause and plan (McGonigal, 2013)] to an exposure: i.e., the act of terrorism, the violent sabotage or rape; the verbal abuse throughout childhood, the explosion, etc., and the amount of support that ensues, or not, that sets up an individual for traumatization. The root of the emotional overwhelm that is often how this reaction is described and remembered, is physiological. Figure 12.2 shows this set up.

Traumatization, for the purpose of this chapter, is not solely limited to a clinical diagnosis of Post Traumatic Stress Disorder (PTSD). Traumatization occurs when the fear or terror one experiences in that moment of exposure remains in the body; because the hormonal, neurological, bio-chemical, and functional changes that occur (van der Kolk, 2014) have not reset or returned to baseline. This is why trauma is not something from which we recover fully; if we manage to remain responsive in the moment of exposure, and have the appropriate support to heal, we may

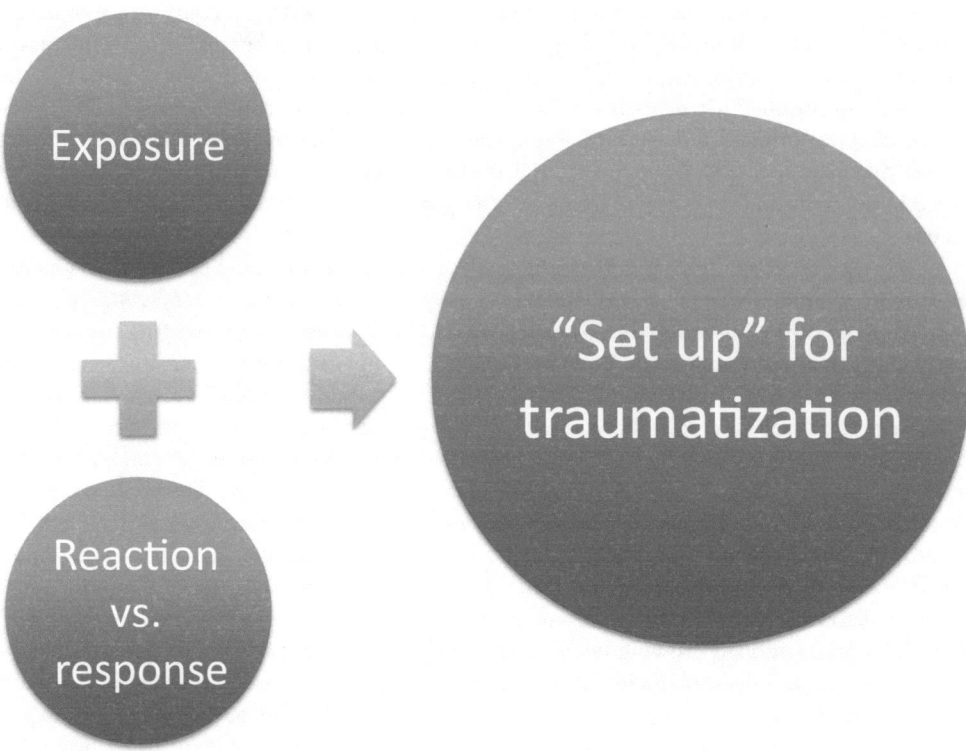

Figure 12.2 The trauma reaction

not be traumatized. However, for many survivors whose response was based on fear or terror, and who do not have access to whatever support they need to heal, be it spiritual, psychological, familial, communal, or otherwise, traumatization is likely, and the traumatization is a fear-based physiological state that is embodied.

Relational trauma

Recent years have seen increased theory and literature about types of trauma. Definitions range from primary and secondary trauma to intergenerational (Danieli, 1998) and historic trauma (Yellowhorse-Braveheart et al., 2011), betrayal trauma (Freyd, 2008), complex trauma (Courtois and Ford, 2013; Herman, 1992, 2015; Spinazzola et al., 2002), and more. An in-depth analysis of the types of trauma that are currently shared in the literature is beyond the scope of this chapter. Relational trauma, the subject of this chapter, has a unique complexity because relationship is so foundational to our humanity. From a developmental and a humanitarian perspective, safety precedes the trust that is essential to engage in meaningful relationship. When humans endure relational trauma, it can undermine the very basis of our humanity, of our sense of meaning and belonging. Relational trauma can be volitional or non-volitional, in terms of the relationship. Torture is a non-volitional relational trauma; domestic violence is volitional because the relationship is a chosen one. This is not to suggest that the abuse is volitional, rather that the relationship is volitional, which adds to the complexity of the traumatic experience and the suffering of the survivor.

Salter (1995) refines our understanding of relational trauma when she writes about the effect sadistic and non-sadistic abuse can have on victims; the very essence of sadistic abuse in the context of relational trauma is an exploitation of empathy. Ongoing research in, and theories about, mirror neurons and empathy (Buk, 2009; Iacoboni, 2009; Winters, 2008) contribute to our understanding that human beings are soft wired for empathy. It is something we are naturally inclined to develop (although not everyone does). Empathy is fundamental to our connection to other people. The exploitation of empathy by sadistic abusers adds to the complexity of the traumatization, and it is for these types of trauma that DMT is uniquely helpful.

DMT, like all good psychotherapies, utilizes empathy as a basis for our therapeutic rapport and connection to the client. Because of the inherently embodied nature of DMT, we may also be inclined in the direction of compassion, which is defined by Roshi Joan Halifax as 'empathy with action' (R. J. Halifax, personal communication, 2nd June, 2014). Tobey (H. Tobey, personal communication, 13th October, 2003) differentiates sympathy from empathy, and empathy from compassion, and this author describes her awareness of the potency of empathy not only to heal, but to disturb clients who suffered severe relational trauma (Gray, 2015b). Based on Tobey's work and the author's clinical experience, sympathy, which is defined as 'feeling sorry for another person' (Gray, 2015b, p. 32), is unhelpful in work with survivors of relational abuse because of the inherent power differential that has already undermined and distorted the basis of being human, and being in relationship, for that individual. Empowerment might always be a desired outcome of work with survivors of relational abuse.

Empathy is essential to the connection we feel for our clients and is essential in our embodied understanding of their clinical presentation. 'I feel your pain' (or, joy) might sum up an empathic response to a client's story. Tania Singer and colleagues have done research that pinpoints the areas of the brain that are activated when experienced meditators respond to stories of suffering. Empathy to another's suffering activates the pain related parts of the neural network associated with emotions but not sensorial experiences; it increases negative emotions (Singer, 2014, p. 1; Singer and Klimecki, 2013).

When these same experienced meditators practice compassion, which can be defined as the recognition of ones suffering or pain because I, or we, know my/our own and can see them as separate or unattached, the positive emotions increase and negative emotions decrease. We feel concern (not their pain), and feelings of love and warmth. It develops a strong motivation to help and lights up areas of the brain associated with reward, love and affiliation. This increases plasticity (Hanson and Mendius, 2009; Klimecki, Leiberg, Matthieu, and Singer, 2014; Singer, 2014).

Engaging with client survivors of relational trauma

Restorative Movement Psychotherapy (RMP) is the author's adaption of dance/movement therapy specifically for therapy with survivors of relational trauma. This framework has been developed, and is developing, ongoing, based on the authors work with survivors of human rights abuses who are displaced by war, torture, genocide, and terrorism. This work has also been influenced and informed by work with survivors of ritual abuse, child abuse and in disasters and other humanitarian contexts. The premise of RMP is that belonging and meaning-making (which sit at the apex of the triangle in Figure 12.1) are the ultimate clinical outcomes for those affected by relational trauma. Our sense of belonging is core to our connection to others, because it is a refraction of our connection to our self in our world. Current theories from neuroplasticity (Cozolino, 2014; Siegel, 2012) demonstrate how the plasticity of the brain is enhanced in relationship. Siegel refers to this in his definition of the brain as 'embodied and relational' (Siegel, 2013). It is through belonging that we can begin to create meaning out of our life experiences.

Many of the evidence-based therapies show results in positive clinical outcomes for specific symptomology, but do not necessarily take a more global approach i.e. measure significant changes in client lives. Changes such as restoration of intimacy, creating meaning out of suffering, a sense of safety in relationship and reduced isolation, are important in terms of any of our humanity. These more global consequences are often overlooked in mainstream clinical approaches and programs. Survivors of relational trauma, especially those displaced by war and violence, experience a sense of displacement and a loss of safety. Whether the displacement is from one's home country or land, or loss of a safe connection to one's own body, our place in the world is impacted by the experience of relational trauma.

The framework

RMP is based on the 'Poto Mitan' Framework for Trauma and Resiliency (Gray, 2015a). Poto Mitan translates as *Centerpost*, but its meaning in Haitian Creole is closely akin to 'The Center of All Things'. This name reflects the belief that for healing, or the restorative process, to occur one must return to one's own center. In Haitian tradition, healing ceremonies are marked by a Poto Mitan – sometimes visible, sometimes invisible – around which the community gathers to drum, sing, dance, and connect to one another and to spirit. The name of this framework reflects several movement therapies, such as DMT, Somatic Psychology, and Continuum Movement all of which have a unique ability to address all aspects of our humanness, from the most mundane to the most sublime. DMT is the core psychotherapy of this framework.

In the center of Figure 12.3 is belonging and meaning (which sit at the apex of the revised CBT triangle of Figure 12.1) reflecting the ultimate clinical outcomes, achievable only through a holistic and comprehensive approach to psychotherapy, in which DMT is uniquely positioned to provide. While amelioration of symptoms such as PTSD, depression, anxiety are important and hoped for outcomes of good therapy (often cited in evidence-based research), this research rarely offers insight into more global outcomes that may have meaning to the clients themselves, especially clients who come from more community or socio-centric cultures. The profoundly disruptive and heart-breaking experience of displacement, which may be the most defining feature of the refugee experience, by definition undermines our birthright sense of belonging and all that gives meaning to life. The arts, in all its forms, have a longer history as a source for healing, mourning, celebrating and marking life's passages than psychology or medicine.

The concentric circles placed out from the center illustrate RMP, a DMT-based approach to working with relational trauma across cultures. Its components-based format allows for the balance in structure, flexibility and adaptation that cross-cultural psychotherapy warrants. The concentric circles that surround the center progress outwardly and illustrate the components of the framework.

Closest to the center is a circle that illustrates the phases of this treatment approach. Complex trauma, a term coined originally by Herman (1992; 2015) and now endorsed and researched by many of the primary contributors to the field of traumatic stress research (Courtois and Ford, 2013; Spinazzola et al., 2002) was proposed as an alternative diagnosis to PTSD for the DSM-IV. While complex trauma did not become a diagnosis, theories, and research arising from the recognition that adult survivors of long-term child abuse and extreme interpersonal trauma, like torture and ritual abuse, who often present with significantly more chronic and complex symptomology, has made an impact on trauma treatment. For complex trauma, a phasic approach is the gold standard. While every theorist has their own interpretation of these phases, all of them begin with *Safety and Stabilization*.

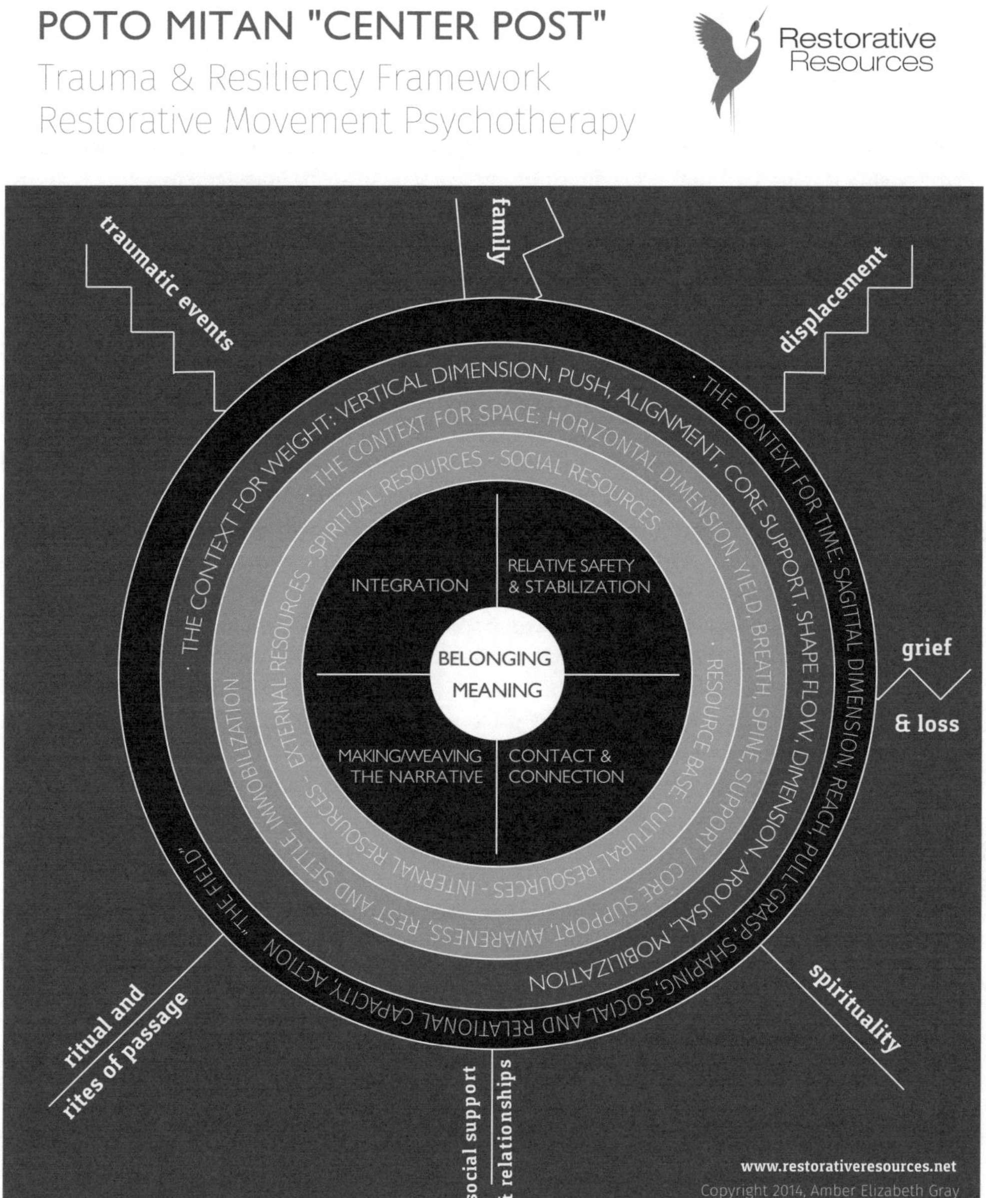

POTO MITAN "CENTER POST"
Trauma & Resiliency Framework
Restorative Movement Psychotherapy

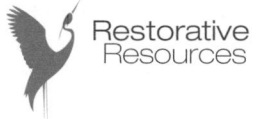

Restorative
Resources

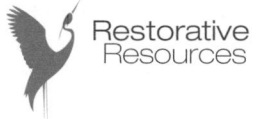

Figure 12.3 The Poto Mitan framework for trauma and resiliency

Relative Safety and Stabilization in this framework is therefore Phase 1, which describes the role of safety in any healing process. It has perhaps received the most current endorsement from Polyvagal Theory as crucial to psychological safety (Porges, 2011). Polyvagal-informed DMT and Polyvagal-informed Continuum Movement (CM) are subjects of several recent chapters (Gray, 2015a, c, 2018; Gray and Porges, 2017). The polyvagal theory emphasizes two neural circuits (ventral, or smart vagus and dorsal, or old vagus), and three responsive pathways (social engagement, mobilization, and immobilization) arising from five states: a) safety, which promotes social engagement; b) mobilization with fear; c) mobilization without fear; d) immobilization with fear; and e) immobilization without fear (Gray, 2018; Gray and Porges, 2017; Porges, 2011).

The fear-based states arise when our survival circuits are recruited, because we face danger (mobilization with fear, often known as fight or flight) or life threat (immobilization with fear/terror or shut down). In order to remain or promote a state of social engagement, safety is necessary. Safety, long appreciated as the base of Maslow's "hierarchy of needs" (1943, p. 376) is now demonstrated through current research as a physiological state that promotes our emotional and psychological sense of safety, and therefore ability to engage with the world.

St. Just (personal communication, 13th October, 2000) coined the term 'relative safety' to illuminate the reality that the world is never truly safe, and we are perhaps best described as being just safe enough. For survivors still living in violence, or for those so traumatized that their suffering is perpetual, relative safety is a more apt term. To suggest complete safety can be a set up. This is particularly true in any context where survivors are still at risk of exposure to traumatic events, for example, domestic violence, civil conflict, war, high-risk jobs, etc. Even for those survivors who are living in safe environments, until they can actually experience a sense of safety, even the smallest environmental cue can trigger a sense of danger. In this approach, relative safety and stabilization are embodied; RMP is one of the first body-based approaches to emphasize simple structured processes for stabilization that shift states effectively during both early phases in therapy, in resourcing work, or the traumatic processing that occurs when clients are adequately prepared to recall and process their traumatic histories. Psychological First Aid (2006) emphasizes stabilization early in the process and it is this author's clinical observation that establishing relative safety and stabilization is simultaneously the place we begin with new clients to build trust and rapport and is ongoing through the entire course of a patient's restorative process. Psychosocial education in this context is the normalizing trauma responses and assisting clients to understand the biological and physiologic basis of the stress response, or the basic frameworks of our theoretical foundations and clinical approaches. This together with resourcing are considered fundamental components of *Relative Safety and Stabilization* (Phase 1) in complex trauma treatment.

The remaining three phases vary from other phasic approaches to complex trauma. Many approaches to complex trauma follow Herman's (2015) framework, where Phase 2 is processing grief, loss and trauma, and Phase 3 is reconnection. *Contact and Connection*, described as Phase 2, proposes that prior to processing one's trauma history, making contact and connecting to one's own sense of self, broadly defined for socio-centric cultures that may include others, ancestors and even planets in sense of self, is essential. *Contact and Connection* are relational, and relationship is widely understood to heal, whether through the enhancement of neuroplasticity (Cozolino, 2014; Siegel, 2013, 2014) or through the comfort of togetherness. In Phase 2, therapists assist clients to connect to all levels of human experience: sensation and sensorimotoric information, perception, impulse to move and movement, the continuum of affect, and thoughts, cognitions, and beliefs (see Figure 12.3). Mystery, a more transpersonal perspective, is uniquely at both the base (source) and top (self-actualization) because DMT acknowledges all levels and dimensions of human experience, from physical to spiritual (ADTA, 2016). In the moment of exposure, the loss of safety that occurs spurs dissolution from our usual social engaged behaviors and interactions to behaviors arising from survival circuits. This dissolution can truncate the sequencing of energy that connects us through these various layers or levels of our humanness.

Weaving the Narrative is the *Meaning-Making* Phase 3 of therapy; this is when memories are processed. The establishment, through therapy, of relative safety, restoration and connection in self, and of self with other over time, provides the ground for this processing to occur and is also part of the processing. The restoration of these connections co-occurring with the establishment of resources, to increase relative safety and mastery of one's physiological or bodily responses (stabilization) prepares the client for the processing of trauma and loss. The strength of RMP for processing traumatic memory is the constant looping into the somatic or bodily experience of the memories, and exploration and sequencing to completion of sensations, micromovements and movements arising from the moment of exposure to physiological reactivity. Processing of trauma memories is bilateral and bi-directional in that we constantly connect thoughts and emotions to the sensations of the body, top down and bottom up, and we loop resource and trauma memories and experiences together to weave these experiences into the broader context of life experience and the client's entire life-line. It is referred to as the *River of Life* in this framework, which acknowledges the fluid nature of memory, in all circumstances, and especially for survivors of trauma whose time-space orientation has been altered.

Integration is the final Phase 4, and refers to a multi-dimensional integration: the integration of the brain (Siegel, 2013), referring to both old and new, or 'upstairs downstairs' (Siegel, 2012) and left and right brain and its ability to restore a narrative; the reduction of limbic reactivity when potential triggers present; the placement of traumatic experience in the context of one's life history; an ability to maintain mindfully present states and a sense of future, vs. being eternally stuck in the imprints of the past. In more practical terms, integration is the ability to take the change that occurs in therapy, the new neural pathways that movement is particularly beneficial for inspiring and incorporate them into one's daily life. Movement is what carves and creates new neural pathways (Perry, 2017); rest and settle, or sleep, states cement them into our mind, or consciousness.

These phases are not linear; like the rest of the framework that illustrates RMP, these phases are reference points for the restorative process. Early in therapy, we may focus almost exclusively on restoring relative safety and stability and fostering connection. As the restorative process continues, we weave all four phases together to process the aspects of clients' traumatic past with growing resources towards integration so that one can be present to participate and engage with life in the present moment.

Primary and secondary portals to embodiment

The primary and secondary portals to embodiment are pathways for these components to guide the restorative process. Simply stated, these are pathways that this author has observed are accessible to survivors of trauma in many different contexts. A mission of this framework is accessibility; many survivors of trauma remain in contexts where they cannot access any form of therapy or would not usually participate in psychotherapy due to cultural and spiritual beliefs that may offer other forms of healing as the norm. Stigmas about psychology and mental illness can make all mental health approaches less accessible in many settings. With the number of displaced peoples around the world at an all-time high (United Nations High Commissioner for Refugees, 2014) the need for straightforward approaches to any therapeutic process is essential. The use of this framework in an international humanitarian context merits its own chapter; for the purposes of this chapter, this framework has been developed through applied practice in United States-based clinics offering services to refugees and survivors of torture, as well as active conflict zones, complex humanitarian emergencies, and post-disaster contexts. The portals provide a direct pathway to somatic awareness (Hindi, 2012) a term which this author describes as combining embodied awareness (the feeling of experience, and our ability to interocept, or connect to our inner landscape) and conceptual awareness, which is our ability to describe, think about, evaluate or talk about inner experience.

Primary portals

Breath, spine, and weight are the primary portals to the embodiment in this framework, and space, time and rhythmicity are the secondary portals. Breath is a core influence on movement in Bartenieff Fundamentals because 'Movement rides on the flow of the breath' (Bartenieff and Lewis, 1980, p. 232). Breath is a well-known phenomenon around the world. From the very practical and necessary, autonomic act of breathing, to the more sublime and esoteric interpretations of the meaning of breath in many ancient traditions (such as Kundalini yoga) and more current breath-based practices [i.e. Holotropic Breath work (Grof and Grof, 2010)]; breath is a concept and an action that is globally understood. In many languages, breath and spirit are the same word (Prana in Hindi, Chi in Chinese, Pneuma in Greek). Breath is literally and metaphorically the wave we all ride into life, and ride out, when we die; it is the veil between worlds. As subtle as breath-based practices can seem, breath shifts our physiological state, which regulates our nervous system, faster than anything else (S. W. Porges, personal communication, 2nd October, 2008).

Many somatic therapies under-privilege the spine, which tends to remain in the domain of yogic movement practices and bodywork, such as osteopathy and chiropractic medicine. The spine is literally the backside of our mid-line. In fact, the physically invisible but ever-present mid-line, around which each body organizes in utero, together with the spine, is the physical embodiment of the Poto Mitan in this framework. In many ancient cultures and traditions, the spine was considered to be the axis mundi of our body, connecting us to heaven and earth. The spine is often considered only for its palpable presence in the very back of the body; the spine, as a structure, is enervated by all the major nerve systems in the body. The spinal cord is protected by the vertebral column known as the spine, and the front of the spine connects to respiration via the diaphragm, at T-12. Dance/movement therapy offers unique and well-developed theories about the role of the spine, and the sacrum, in maintaining physical and mental health. Blanche Evan and Liljan Espenak's pioneering work as founders of DMT includes theories, systems of assessment and intervention, and practices that focus on the spine as core to well-being. Evan (1992) considered the physiological health of the spine reflective of psychological health, and Espenak (2005) assessed client well-being through the wheel-like motion of the sacrum, at the base of the spine. Cottingham et al. (1988, p. 353) demonstrate the shifts in pelvic tilt can shift and promote vagal tone, which is one measure of a state of physiological health necessary to promote social engagement. Hindi (2012) describes the spine as a pathway for interoception; a 'corridor a corridor for sensory information to travel to the brain, making a pathway for unconscious interoceptive data to be brought into consciousness and processed' (2012, p. 135). More simply, this author has never encountered a person in any country or context that did not know what and where the spine is and did not have some relationship to its relevance to embodiment and to well-being.

Weight, which is the physical evidence of our presence, can seem more abstract to locate. However, a simple formula of finding points of physical contact between whatever surface one is lying, sitting or standing on, and the body, and sensing how much support is received, or not, through these points of contact, invites clients into a sense of their weight. It is also, of course, a measure of the ability to receive support, which relates to yield (Bainbridge Cohen, 2012). The LMA Effort states use weight, expressed on a continuum from strong to light, to assess effort in movement and action. Many survivors of relational trauma describe feeling very 'heavy', i.e. too weighted down, by the burdens of suffering they carry, or by sadness of loss. Likewise, 'lightness' has been associated with feeling empty in both positive and negative ways; it can also denote dissociative states. At times, a shift from heavy to more levity signals a restoration of embodiment; the reverse is true when one exists in chronic shut-down states, which are often expressed psychologically as dissociation. These shifts in sense of weight are cues that physiological state shifts have occurred; physiological state shifts are the foundation of emotional and psychological state shifts.

Secondary portals

The secondary portals to embodiment are so named because they tend to be processes that, while present in early phases of therapy, are usually more complex and more accessible to focus on later in treatment. Space is in the first concentric circle of the developmental process, and might be considered one of our earliest relationships, as we are in relationship to space in utero, and in the developmentally early horizontal dimension. Space, which in LMA is an effort that relates to our thinking and perceptual abilities and tendencies, is also literally that which we relate to through movement. We move through space. It is this therapist's observation over many years that many survivors of relational trauma whose exposure includes captivity (whether physical or psychological, such as being followed) have an altered and often very uncomfortable relationship to space. For some, it is simply terrifying to be in relationship to space. The kinesphere, our personal space bubble reflects our relationship to space and the environment around us. Konie (2011, p. 5) describing kinesphere from the perspective of Bartenieff Fundamentals, states the kinesphere is: 'The 3-Dimensional volume of space that I can access with my body without shifting my weight to change my stance. (Psychological Kinesphere: The space I can – attend to.)'. Many survivors' initial clinical presentation is one of a retracted kinesphere, as the case study describes. This complex relationship to kinespheric space, the space around us, and inner or interoceptive space in a body that can feel like a minefield, makes it difficult to work directly and intensively with space early in treatment.

Time is a dimension from LMA framework that we naturally explore later in life. Time and space orientation, by definition, are absent in states of dissociation, quite common to survivors of extreme interpersonal violence, and in physiological shut down or immobilized states. Our movement in time is related to the sagittal dimension and our ability to interact with the environment, based on our appraisal of the safety, or lack of, in the environment (or space around us). Traumatized individuals by definition perceive the world as unsafe; their nervous systems have shifted into states of chronic fear or terror and they continuously mis-appraise the environment as unsafe even when it practically speaking is safe. Our relationship to time, in this framework for the restorative process, reflects our ability to move towards what we choose, or want, in our own timing, and move away or withdraw from that which we do not wish to engage. This ability is undermined by the fear that is core to the experience of being traumatized. Because the time dimensions are relational, it is often relatively safer for clients to begin in the vertical dimension of the preceding circle although out of sequence developmentally. This promotes mindful re-establishment of boundaries and allows defenses to deconstruct. If clients can mobilize and slowly re-engage in more active play states with less and less fear present, they can regain enough comfort to begin to re-engage with the world. Relationships are fundamental to our humanity, and the perverse abuse of the power differential in relational trauma can make relationship scary. One's sense of self, as experienced through the present moment experience of weight, may need to be the first portal to embodiment restored before one can find the trust (yield) to interocept and rest and relax. Relating outwardly to the world rests on this foundation of space/trust/yield/horizontal, and weight/mobilize/push/vertical.

Rhythmicity is core to polyvagal-informed DMT and CM. The entire approach is based on coherence in internal, or endogenous, and external or exogenous, biorhythms. Sadistic abusers, as described in the preceding section on relational trauma, will intentionally increase suffering for their own vicarious pleasure. This intentional abuse often purposefully resets important biorhythms, such as digestion and elimination, respiration, heart rate, etc. This intentional mis-wiring of these core-to-well-being rhythms literally cause us to 'lose our beat', which has profound effects on our external rhythmicity, i.e. how we move in the world. Rhythm and rhythmicity is worthy of an entire book, and is the focus of a chapter on polyvagal-informed DMT and CM (Gray, 2018). For the purposes of this chapter rhythmic feedback loops are fundamental and core to our internal physiological states and external, fluid movement, actions, and engagement with the world, and are the essence of rhythmicity as a secondary portal. Rhythmicity might be seen as the most integrative of the portals, because when we can align our internal and external realities and rhythms, we can move to our natural beat again.

Conclusion

The arts have been the voice of suffering, celebration, mourning, ritual, and rites of passage, far longer than medicine or psychology. Because traumatic experiences and exposures are a daily global occurrence, people and communities in all countries and cultures benefit from and deserve novel and informed approaches that build on tradition and what has worked historically to heal the wounds of violence and abuse. The embodied and creative nature of DMT and RMP makes trauma-informed applications of this work more accessible for survivors of trauma in a variety of contexts, and may offer a relevance to their restorative process that other approaches do not.

References

American Dance Therapy Association (ADTA). (2016). *FAQs*. Retrieved from https://adta.org/faqs/.
American Dance Therapy Association. Retrieved from https://adta.org/.
Bainbridge Cohen, B. (2012). *Sensing, Feeling and Action: The Experiential Anatomy of Body-Mind Centering*. Toronto: Contact Editions.
Bartenieff, I., and Lewis, D. (1980). *Body Movement; Coping with the Environment*. New York: Gordon and Breach.
Begley, S., (2007). *Train Your Mind, Change Your Brain: How a New Science Reveals Our Extraordinary Potential to Transform Ourselves*. New York: Ballantine Books.
Buk, A. (2009). The mirror neuron system and embodied simulation: Clinical implications for art therapists working with trauma survivors. *The Arts in Psychotherapy, 36*, 61–74. (Original work published 1988)
Chace, M., Sandel, S., and Chaiklin, S. (1993). *Foundations of Dance Movement Therapy: The Life and Works of Marian Chace*. Columbia, MD: American Dance Therapy Association.
Cottingham, J., Porges, S., and Lyon, T. (1988). Effects of soft tissue mobilization on parasympathetic tone in two age groups. *Physical Therapy, 68*, 352–356.
Courtois, C. A., and Ford, J. D. (2013). *Treatment of Complex Trauma: A Sequenced, Relationship-based Approach*. New York: The Guilford Press.
Cozolino (2013). *The Social Neuroscience of Education: Optimizing Attachment and Learning in the Classroom*. New York: Norton.
Cozolino, L. (2014). *Norton Series on Interpersonal Neurobiology: The Neuroscience of Human Relationships: Attachment and the Developing Social Brain* (2nd ed.). New York: Norton Books.
Damasio, A. (2005). *Descartes' Error: Emotion, Reason, and the Human Brain*. London: Penguin Books.
Danieli, Y. (1998). *International Handbook of Multigenerational Legacies of Trauma*. New York: Plenum Press.
Espenak, L. (2005). Psychomotor therapy with a varied population. In F. Levy (Ed.), *Dance/Movement Therapy: A Healing Art*. (Chapter 3). 2nd Revised Edition. Virginia, USA: American Alliance for Health, Physical Education, Recreation and Dance.

Evan, B. (1992). Creative movement becomes dance therapy with normal and neurotics. In F. Levy (Ed.), *Dance/Movement Therapy: A Healing Art.* (Chapter 2). 2nd Revised Edition. Virginia, USA: American Alliance for Health, Physical Education, Recreation and Dance.

Freyd, J. (2008). Retrieved from http://dynamic.uoregon.edu/jjf/defineBT.html.

Gray, A. E. (2015a). The broken body: Somatic perspectives on surviving torture. In S. L. Brooke and C. E. Myers (Eds.), *Therapists Creating a Cultural Tapestry: Using the Creative Therapies across Cultures* (pp. 170–190). Springfield, IL: Charles C. Thomas.

Gray, A. E. (2015b). What language does your body speak: Some thoughts on somatic psychotherapies in international contexts. *Somatic Psychotherapy Today, 5*(4), 30–37.

Gray, A. E. (2015c). Dance/movement therapy with refugee and survivor children: A healing pathway is a creative process. In C. Malchiodi (Ed.), *Creative Interventions with Traumatized Children* (2nd ed., pp. 169–190). New York: Guilford Press.

Gray, A. E. (2018). Roots, Rhythm, Reciprocity: Polyvagal Informed Dance Movement Therapy for Survivors of Trauma. In S. W. Porges and D. Dana (Eds.), *Clinical Applications of the Polyvagal Theory: The Emergence of Polyvagal-Informed Therapies* (pp. 207–226). New York: Norton Books.

Gray, A. E., and Porges, S. (2017). Polyvagal-informed dance movement therapy. In C. Malchiodi and D. Crenshaw (Eds.), *What To Do when Children Clam Up in Psychotherapy: Interventions to Facilitate Communication* (pp. 102–136). New York: Guilford Press.

Grof, S., and Grof, C. (2010). *Holotropic Breathwork: A New Approach to Self-Exploration and Therapy.* New York: Excelsior Editions.

Halifax, R. J. (2014.) Personal communication, 2nd June 2014.

Hanson, R., and Mendius, R. (2009). *Buddha's Brain: The Practical Neuroscience of Happiness, Love and Wisdom.* Oakland, CA: New Harbinger Publications.

Herman, J. L. (1992). Complex PTSD: A syndrome in survivors of prolonged and repeated trauma. *Journal of Traumatic Stress, 5*(3), 377–391. Retrieved May 2017 from http://eds.a.ebscohost.com.emils.lib.colum.edu/eds/pdfviewer/pdfviewer?sid=0b54d06f7a24-46af-a168-bbdd747191a3%40sessionmgr4001and vid=11andhid=4110.

Herman, J. L. (2015). *Trauma and Recovery.* New York: Basic Books.

Hindi, F. S. (2012). How attention to interoception can inform dance/movement therapy. *American Journal of Dance Therapy, 34*(2), 129–140. doi:10.1007/s10465-012-9136-8

Iacoboni, M. (2009). Imitation, empathy and mirror neurons. *Annual Review of Psychology, 60*, 653–670. Retrieved from arjournals.annualreviews.org.

Klimecki, O. M., Leiberg, S., Matthieu, R., and Singer, T. (2014). Differential pattern of functional brain plasticity after compassion and empathy training. *Social Cognitive and Affective Neuroscience Advances, 9*, 873–879.

Konie, R. (2011). *A Brief Overview of LABAN MOVEMENT ANALYSIS.* Retrieved March 2017 from www.movementhasmeaning.com.

Lewis, P. (1986). *Theoretical Approaches in Dance Movement Therapy* (Vol. 1). Dubuque, IA: Kendall/Hunt Publishing Company.

Maslow, A. H. (1943). A theory of human motivation. *Psychological Review, 50*, 370–396.

McGonigal, K. (2013). *The Neurobiology of Willpower: It's not What You'd Expect.* Storrs, CT: National Institute for the Clinical Application of Behavioral Medicine.

Perry, B. D. (2017). *The Moving Child: Supporting Early Development through Movement* [Film]. Vancouver, BC, Canada. Retrieved from www.themovingchild.com.

Porges, S. W. (2008). Personal communication, 2nd October 2008.

Porges, S. W. (2011). *The Polyvagal Theory: Neurophysiological Foundations of Emotions, Attachment, Communication, Self-Regulation.* New York: W.W. Norton.

Psychological First Aid. (2006). *Field Operations Guide* (2nd ed.). Retrieved March 2010 from www.ptsd.va.gov/professional/manuals/psych-first-aid.asp.

Salter, A. (1995). *Transforming Trauma: A Guide to Understanding and Treating Adult Survivors of Child Sexual Abuse.* Thousand Oaks, CA: Sage Publications.

Siegel, D. (2012). *Bringing out the best in kids: Strategies for working with the developing mind. A webinar session.* The National Institute for the Clinical Application of Behavioral Medicine. Retrieved from www.nicabm.com.

Siegel, D. (2013). *The mind lives in two places: Inside your body, embedded in the world. A webinar session.* The National Institute for the Clinical Application of Behavioral Medicine. Retrieved from www.nicabm.com.

Siegel, D. (2014). *Mind: A Journey to the Heart of Being Human.* (Norton Series on Interpersonal Neurobiology). New York: W. W. Norton & Company.

Singer, T. (2014). *Feeling Others' Pain: Transforming Empathy into Compassion.* Retrieved from www.cogneurosociety.org/empathy_pain/.

Singer, T., and Klimecki, O. M. (2013). Empathy and compassion. *Current Biology, 24*(18), R875–R878.

Spinazzola, J., Ford, J., van der Kolk, B., Blaustein, M., Brymer, M., Gardner, L., . . . Smith, S. (2002). *Complex Trauma in the National Child Traumatic Stress Network.* Retrieved May 2017 from www.nctsn.org/sites/default/files/assets/pdfs/Complex_TraumaintheNCTSN.pdf.

St. Just (2000). Personal communication, 13th October 2000.

Tobey, H. (2003). Personal communication, 13th October 2003.

UNHCR. (2014, June 20). Annual Global Trends. *News Stories.*

van der Kolk, B. (2014). *The Body Keeps the Score.* New York: Viking.

Winters, A. (2008). Emotion, embodiment and mirror neurons in dance movement therapy: A connection across disciplines. *American Journal of Dance Therapy, 30,* 84–105.

Yellowhorse-Braveheart, M., Chase, J., Elkins, J. and. Altschul, D. B. (2011) Historical trauma among indigenous peoples of the Americas: Concepts, research, and clinical considerations, *Journal of Psychoactive Drugs, 43*(4), 282–290, DOI: 10.1080/02791072.2011.628913

13

PLAYING THROUGH DANCING STORIES

Sylvie Garnero

Introduction

Phenomenologists consider the inter-corporeal dialogue as the basis of human subjectivity. Dance is a living art and the body is the instrument of the dancer. It is an original way of symbolisation, emphasising the value of bodily senses. Links between body, emotions, and memory are examined considering emotions from a perspective of inter-body phenomena, as well as discussing the place of affects in dance as a performing art.

This chapter presents methods of treatment carried out with Clara, a teenager who had been diagnosed with Borderline Personality Disorder. Dance Movement Therapy (DMT) was introduced in the therapeutic setting. Considering Clara's evolution it was decided to focus on the issue of the historical trauma of the Holocaust and its effects transmitted through the generations as an embodied experience. This chapter seeks to document how the DMT creative process forms a narrative that tells us about the experience, and highlights the importance of forming body narratives, cross-checking our clinical data with questions of aesthetics and anthropology. There is a focus on how transgenerational trauma is understood and how a person is able to work through that in DMT.

Meeting Clara

Clara is a 16-year-old teenager coming by herself to the consultation at a day care psychiatric centre. She complains of various disabling disorders such as anxiety, depression, insomnia, binge eating, and school phobia. She confides that she is in remission of a physical disease and seems to be optimistic, thanks to the doctors. From the outset, she asks me not to meet with her parents. She speaks about her difficulties with family relationships, especially with her mother. Clara belongs to a Jewish family who survived the Holocaust. Through her questions, the family history is paradoxically very present.

Managing this situation is complex and Clara's treatment team have some diagnostic confusion between adolescent problems, which involves generations, and a borderline structure. After a long time, Clara accepts a therapeutic, multifocal work, a therapeutic space for her, and a separate space for her parents. I invite Clara into a conversational space.

Clara is in an intense state of anxiety in her first sessions, noticeable even in her body. The family atmosphere she describes evokes a sense of boundaries. She is intelligent, has capacity for insight yet experiences

161

difficulty bringing together the different aspects of herself. My colleagues propose using analytic relaxation techniques, but Clara is unable to accept this proposition. Therefore, we decide to adjust the therapeutic setting from a solely verbal intervention to DMT sessions, which Clara accepts.

I decide not to question the traumatic family history and take time to listen to Clara's different ways of expression. This flexibility helps us to maintain continuity and enhances our capacity to face the psychic discontinuity that we see in this teenager. In this approach, dance is essential to the session's structure and to the therapeutic process of the individual. This framework holds the most archaic elements of the personality and gives shape to body language, which allows the emergence of thoughts. The sessions with Clara freely combine dance in a therapeutic space and open her to a possible psychic transformation in which she engages. We have been working together for more than 2 years with weekly individual sessions. Clara gradually readjusted psychologically. She felt less depressed and began investing herself in a social life with peers. She went away, far from her family, to engage herself in studies at the university.

Clinical perspectives

In terms of her evolution, the significant improvement of Clara put into question the diagnosis of personality disorders by the medical team. The elements that emerged during the work in DMT introduced a window, which gave a new clinical point of view. These approaches have put forward the concept of trauma that enabled us to make connections between symptomatic manifestations, both physically and psychically. Knowing that the traumatic stories – deportation but also suicides in her mother's family – were related to historical events that she had not experienced herself but had occurred during WWII (World War 2) to the generation of her grandparents. Next arose the question of transgenerational transmission of trauma and its emergence facilitated by DMT.

Regarding the approach of trauma, Janet (1919) and Freud (1920/1977a) centre their theories in the psychological sphere. Janet (1919) was one of the first to have proposed a phase-oriented model in the treatment of trauma, and recent researches validate his clinical work (van der Hart, Brown, and van der Kolk, 1989). Along with this psychodynamic model, Selye (1956) developed a concept of neurophysiological stress that echoed contemporary neuroscience research. It is accepted that trauma affects the psychological organisation as well as physiologically, which leads to transform one theory into another (Georgieff, 2010). Findings on trauma attempt to integrate both and emphasise the value of the infrasemantic level in psychotherapy (Cozolino, 2002; Gedo, 2005; Schore, 2001; Wilkinson, 2010). According to neurosciences, several authors contribute to understanding the relevance of embodiment in trauma treatment (Koch, Caldwell, and Fuchs, 2013; Ogden and Minton, 2000; van der Kolk, 2006).

DMT research on trauma proposed recent overviews from qualitative literature and suggested that DMT specifically creates a trauma healing process (Levine and Land, 2016; Pierce, 2014). Reca (2011) described treatment with 'disappeared persons' in Argentina. Recently, Stanek (2015) stressed the role of body-to-body transmission of trauma down generations.

Returning to Clara with reference to her psychological functioning, a neurotic appearance coexists with a more archaic appearance and allows access to the symbolic function. The transgenerational trauma concerns a teenager and symptoms coinciding with puberty. She faces, in the register of her body, a new image and finds herself blurring the fields of identification. The resurgence of identity and narcissism presents a potential trauma, which, in Freudian terms, is an unbinding process (Freud, 1920/1977a). There is a risk of rupture in the feeling of self-continuity.

When Clara came for the first time without the wig she wore because of her disease, she addressed her concerns about her femininity, evoking the narcissistic injury related to her illness.

The knot between the original conflict and that of the Oedipal conflict was then understood. It can be considered that the process of adolescence was a trigger to the crisis moment she went through.

Adolescence is a time of transmission between generations (Kaës, 1993). For Clara, who descends from a line of deeply wounded women, to access a temporality in which to situate herself was really problematic. Faced with the difficulties of appropriation of her sexual body and her history, Clara had to untie these knots, but also accept this same link as recognition of belonging to her family.

A poetic experience

This section discusses Clara's ability to approach the therapeutic relationship starting with dance movement and how she evolved step by step, along with some elements of understanding which can be derived from a range of authors, crossing the fields of aesthetic and psychology.

Dance is the art of movement, of all movements. It mobilises the body and the psyche together. 'Dancing is an inner adventure . . . the gesture is like a self-thought, the thought becomes material from the feeling of movement' (Piollet, 2014, p. 117). Clara shared an invitation to dance, opening a dancing dialogue. Reflections from the therapist:

> *The first time Clara sat in front of me, she was stable in her base, in contrast with her blocked torso and short breathing. However, she was very present, with large black sad eyes looking at me and also beyond me. I thought about the moon reflections on a lake.*
>
> *Her hands caught my attention. They were elegant hands, making small movements into different directions, as if Clara was trying to find winding paths through the space.*
>
> *But when she spoke to me with carefully chosen words, I felt I wanted to sleep. Her voice was clear but extremely monotonous, as if the words came back to her in a timeless loop that could not reach me.*
>
> *I enlarged her hand gesture. Fortuitously, a play began between us. She looked at me and accentuated the movement of her feet. I felt her heavy. We continued to explore the sensation of the weight, in relation to breathing, which led us to explore new forms of dances.*

The recreational exploration of dance movement constituted a feeling of play between us, in terms of playing (Winnicott, 1971). Clara's hand gestures invited us to find a wingspan to my proposal developed in this dance space, she responded with her feet, giving it rhythm. Space for art meets space for play, 'where experience and creativity interact' (Wigman, 1963/1986, p. 13) and introduces transitionality. She also found security. DMT leads to dynamic situations in which the patient experiences an act directed by his/herself. The absorption in the act creates a bubble of absence as well as a recall to being. It starts with coming–going movement that finds an emergence of the dance. Relaxation leads to a passive position, agonising with regard to the traumatic issue, hence Clara's non-acceptance. The therapist reflects:

> *Then she spoke with a monotone voice, without emotion about the traumatic life of her family during WWII. I felt a sensation of emptiness strangely full; the wish to escape.*

The splits perceived in her evoked a division between body and mind. They represent a vital defence to respect, also an obstacle to psychic integration. Consequently, the focus was on the creative process experience, rather than a direct body-approach, which felt too threatening for Clara.

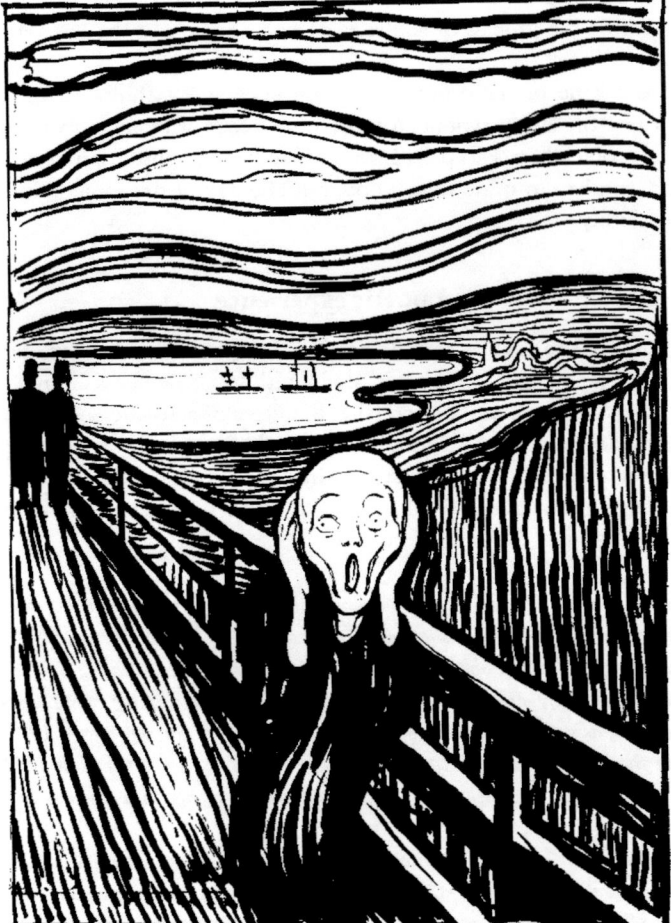

Figure 13.1 E. Münch – the scream.

The discovery of poetic attention occurred to us through a 'seeing/to be seen' in movement (Tortora, 2006, p. 236). Referring to attention is relevant to understanding our aesthetic relation to the world and is particularly rich because the more it mobilises our attention, the more intense the immersion becomes in the experience (Schaeffer, 2015). This special focus jointly on the same cultural object – the dance – played a trigger role in the flow of movement and aided us to tolerate a necessary step of 'formlessness' (Winnicott, 1971, p. 50). Levine (2009) emphasises the importance of this passage in the management of trauma. It makes possible the emergence of a 'creative use of symbolic formations' (Levine, 2009, p. 104).

Moving through the dance, the dance therapist carries inside a deep subjective experience that is presented to the patient. Through 'joint action' and 'joint attention', both patient and dance therapist actively build a reciprocal process supported by kinesthetic empathy (Gallagher and Payne, 2015, p. 73). Clara is caught by surprise to be in motion by a simple improvisational suggestion: exploring first with elements of dance (Laban, 1950/1988) and the fundamentals of movement (Bartenieff, 1980; Hackney, 1998) allows her to enrich her repertoire. Improvisation is an art of the present that enables the unexpected to arise by giving some structures for spontaneity. The therapist reflects:

> *After a long period, Clara reached a higher level of body awareness, and that allowed her to link the way that she expressed her feelings to her body. She was now becoming clearer in the way she distributed her body weight, and her movements showed more strength. She started to play with fall and recovery. Breathing gave life to her dance. In the repetition of movements done thoroughly, a phrasing appeared.*

By discovering the expressive power of her dance, Clara has carefully been listening to how movement is felt throughout the body. Dance, 'as embodied insight' (Hawkins, 1991, p. 17), represented for Clara a step which was better than separation from her internal world.

We sustained the creative transformation process without interpretation of content. The development of the incipient body movements into space brought to consciousness the natural impulses that contained. This allowed rhythmic forms of vitality (Stern, 2010). The strength given to the movement reveals this play between space and time, and Clara's movement intention. By appropriating the play with gravity and the grounding through fall and recovery, she experimented through dancing that it is possible to fall without falling down, and to recover. The therapist reflects:

> *During one session, she suddenly grabbed me. There was now a lot of strength in her fingers and at the same time sweetness to the touch. I stopped moving to wait an impulse emerging from her. We breathed together in the same rhythm, and I felt an energy around us. She stopped dancing. She could not speak. Next session, she began by sitting on a chair, bent over herself, her head heavy and looking far away. I stood a little away from her. Her hands that day found their elegant movement and began to explore her new feeling of strength. Clara repeated the same phrase and a rhythmic structure appeared. A presence emerged from her and I chose to share this special moment as a witness in the silence. I had to contact myself at a point full of nostalgic tenderness. She danced a wild struggle for life.*

The tactile contact allows for reciprocal impregnation (Paxton, 1993/1999). Clara effects emotion in me. The emergence of the 'grasping' – a reflex movement at the dawn of life and often the last before dying – from her hand's gesture was accompanied by intensification of energy. It is in this dynamic attunement, that each body held the experience of the other. Clara engaged herself in a constructed and vital, singular, and shared dance. The therapist reflects:

> *As she stopped dancing, she looked at me with her big black eyes. She was crying, but a light animated her eyes. She sat next to me, quietly catching her breath and then sat opposite me.*
>
> *She began a long story full of emotion. 'People say I look like my grandmother, we have the same eyes' she confided to me, linking her present experience and memory of the past. Upset, Clara began to tell the fate of a line of women. She is the only girl in her generation, she was able to name them by their first names, she evoked similarities, and talked about the survivors . . . her inner dance had meaning for her. A feeling of imprisonment in me.*

Afterwards, I thought of Wigman's ballets: 'Das Totentanz' and the later 'Totenmal', in which a string of women 'form a procession of mourning . . . in the space of oblivion', a body of suffering (Wigman, 1963/1986, p. 89).

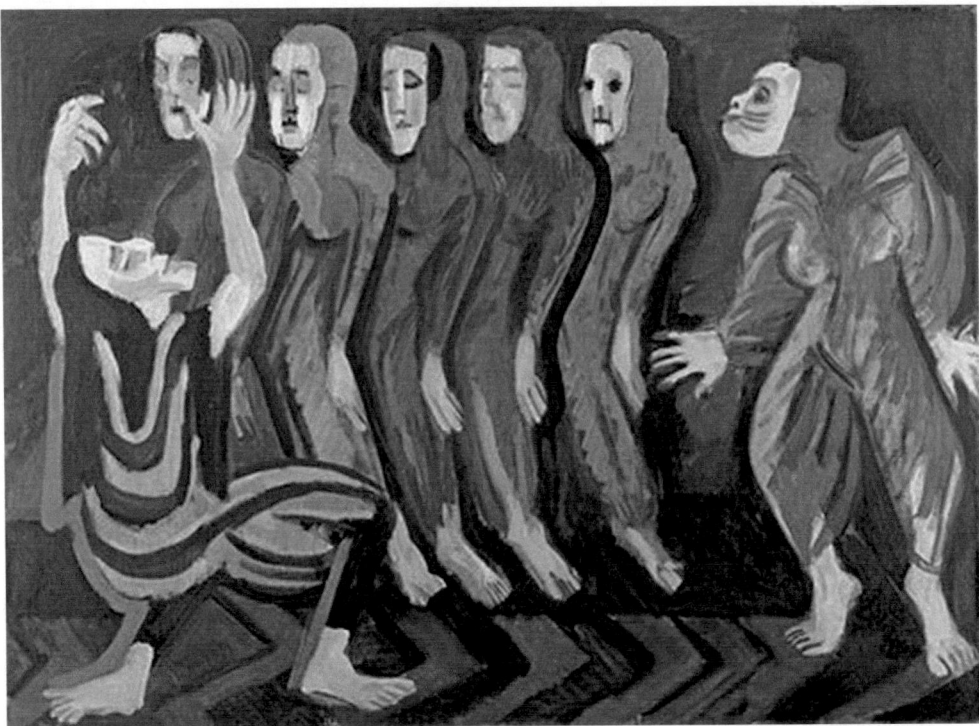

Figure 13.2 E. L. Kirchner, 'Totentanz der Mary Wigman'

The body deeply shows the marks of the injuries continuity down a long line of women. As metaphor of war and death, 'Totentanz' awakened in me the image of kinaesthetic weight of a memorial body (Pandolfi, 1991).

The creative process constituted for Clara an emerging process. An encysted content deep within her movement was released and gave access to a metaphorical movement. 'Movement metaphor is the communication of one's inner state through embodied movement symbolism' (Victoria, 2012, p. 169). The meaning that unfolded in the dance is a key stage of the therapeutic process in DMT (Meekums, 2002). The therapeutic development with Clara belongs to symbolisation logic, included in all artistic process. Roussillon (2012, p. 28) accurately describes the three functions: 'phoric' (to hold), 'semaphoric' (to form) and 'metaphorical' (to symbolise). In this process, the therapist is a 'metaboliser'. The artistic transposition, as the alpha function (Bion, 1962/1984) which transforms unthinkable psychic contents into elements devoid of toxicity, reveals itself essential is dealing with trauma. Moreover, Chouvier (2000) highlights why and how the dance gives specific material to symbolisation. Building on body expression, it involves concrete and visual thinking that 'stands nearer to unconscious process than thinking in words' (Freud, 1923/1977b, p. 189) and opens to a primary symbolisation, as in dreams and play. In this passage, patient and therapist find themselves side by side, which is what Clara very insightfully remarked at the end of her dance.

Dance is a culturally embodied practice in which the body appears saturated with meaning. 'Mass, rhythm, intensity and speed are the appendages of the archaic image of the body' (Dolto, 1981, p. 76). These are the same elements that dancers explore through movement. Dance returns to the time of the constitution of the subject. In the context of transference, dance mobilises the sensory and perceptual substrate of the primal representations (Freud, 1923/1977b). Playing with archaic material, DMT provides access to experiences that haven't been elaborated upon and shapes them into subjective experiences. It allows a dramatisation of archaic registers below the verbal aspect, starting from a kinaesthetic scenario that boosts the metaphorisation faculty. The structuring force of the dance is situated in the 'moving in relation to an image' (Dosamantes-Alperson, 1979, p. 26) that makes possible a working script in which the inner logic of feelings can be narrative. I proposed here to name it 'gesture psychodrama'.

Embodied memories and narratives

Which unconscious contents are then passed from body to body, and how? By being attentive to the way the experience is received in the body, from his/her own body movements, the dance movement therapist can understand what is happening in the patient. In these particular transference dynamics, the therapist engages the body in different ways. In loaning his/her body to dance, the dance movement therapist allows the other to feel, albeit virtually, the dancing. He/she also captures the emergence and possible shaping of dance dialogue. There can only be a witness (Adler, 1987/1999), a reflective mirror of the dance from one to the other and circularity is established that is rooted in inter-corporeality (Merleau-Ponty, 1945).

Neuroscience rediscovered the concept of empathy by demonstrating the existence of neural systems mirrors which are activated in action, or by watching others act (Rizzolatti and Sinigaglia, 2006). Created to reflect the aesthetic experience, this concept refers to a process that can accommodate the world of the others, without confusing yourself and others and highlights DMT practice. It explains the ability of dance therapists to perceive the meaning of gestures and feelings and to mutually resonate with the patients (Gallese, 2009).

Relating to Clara, expanded mirroring and later witnessing created an attunement, both physical and emotional, which allowed Clara's painful world to be shared. The first eye contact with the therapist eventually led to the embodied identification with her grandmother. Kinaesthetic empathy also jointed up emotional reactions derived from the experience of movement.

Fuchs and Koch (2014), offer us an understanding of the 'embodied affectivity'(p. 5). They analyse the reciprocal relationship between movement and emotion for each individual, and especially shed light on what is playing at this level between two people. Regarding Clara, we observed diffraction in the circularity of the process, revealing the traumatic fragmentation. The bottom of continuity is established in a circularity built together, in a shuttle between which emerged from one or the other, to crystallise around the circulation of an image and associated shared feelings. This allowed Clara a conscious integration of fragmented parts of her experience.

Such consideration is particularly relevant for the understanding of the intergenerational trauma transmission, that which is transmitted reflects precisely what is being suffered in the same process of transmission (Kaës, 1993). Psychosomatic practitioners describe the process of embodiment in the case of very young allergic children, as an early form of child over-adjustment. We directly participate in the recognition of others' emotions, by mutual body 'resonance' (Gallese, 2009, p. 523). Such implicit sharing was involved in the early relationships between Clara and her mother, as Clara was caught in the traumatic history of her mother and protected her parent through an early adaptation.

DMT facilitates access to the emotions and the buried memories through body memory (Koch et al., 2013; Reca, 2011; Stanek, 2015). The trauma is indeed memory impairment. It is important to understand how to work with this body memory. Paxton's (1993/1999) reflections on contact improvisation open a path for DMT. He emphasises the existence of 'gaps' in the

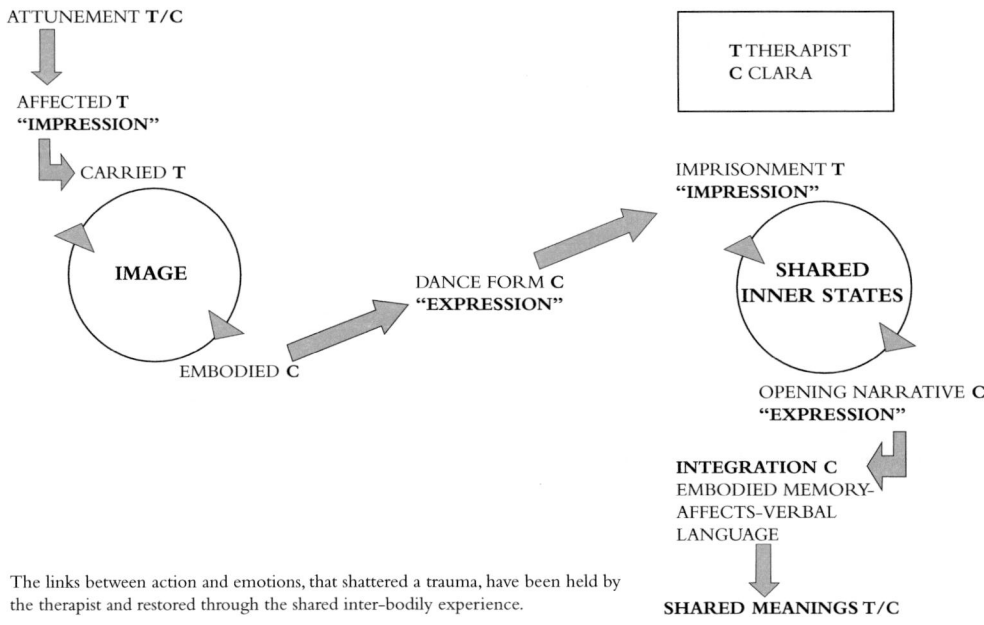

Figure 13.3 The model of the embodied way out of traumatic experience

consciousness of the body in motion, through which operates a body-to-body transmission, without consciously knowing the content. The induction of movements in contact constitutes a phenomenon 'too fast for thought' (Paxton, 1993/1999, p. 108). This process would explain the moments in which there was metaphorical movement inside Clara.

Cognitive psychology distinguishes two kinds of memory (Graf and Schacter, 1985): declarative, which unresolved trauma leaves its mark, and procedural memory, which refers to body memory. Dance, in drawing the body memory, reactivates implicit memory. Dance involves the different forms of body memory (Fuchs, 2000, 2012, as cited in Koch et al., 2013, p. 83), particularly the situational body memory. By structuring space and time, dance creates a contextualisation that supports the working memory. In traumatic memory, images have an important place in connection with intense emotional or sensory states. Kinaesthetic empathy facilitated the emergence of images, which in turn nourished the movement (Dosamantes-Alperson, 1979).

In the example of Clara, I felt a sensation of emptiness strangely full, while experiencing the weight together. This allowed us to follow a thread of associations to the image of memorial body (Pandolfi, 1991). Clara found a grasping gesture, which was the starting point to build her dance. This dramatisation was closely connected to emotional states she expressed through her body. This helped her to become able to relate with emotion the traumatic life of her family. The body memory also gave shape to her experience, opening the way to an imagination that preceded her, and revealed embodied emotional contents of words. This is one key to understanding possible links between the two types of memory, which open on real narrative skills. Moreover, the body remembers through action (Koch et al., 2013).

According to anthropologists, embodiment allows us to understand the body as a source of sensory experience between perceptual and cultural experiences (Csordas, 1990, 1993; Taussig, 1993), but 'often forgets its expressive anatomy' (Surralès, 2004, p. 65). Dance uses body movement in an 'extraordinary' way, far from a functional use (Mauss, 1936/1950). We empha-sise the value of dance as a performing art. Dance explains a world by articulating the body's performance capacity to the affects in a movement's symbolic order. Clara's evolution revealed an important change when she reached the expressiveness of movement. Clara went through a dance state resembling the trance.

It is reminiscent of the ritual action Turner mentions (1982/1986). Something is acted through possession. Ritual represents a mediation to change the world. The ritual staging is read in the symbolic order of the other, which gives it 'symbolic efficiency' (Levi-Strauss, 1958, p. 213). Pandolfi (1991) highlights the value of ritual dance of Tarentism in comparing the pos-session enactment to bodily complaints of women today. However, Clara demonstrated a reverse path. Possession contains in itself an event: as if by revealing a foreign presence in oneself enables a return to oneself. Levine considers that traumatic aftermath takes part of 'identificatory incorpo-ration' that 'can be overcome only by its mimetic embodiment in a performative mode' (Levine,

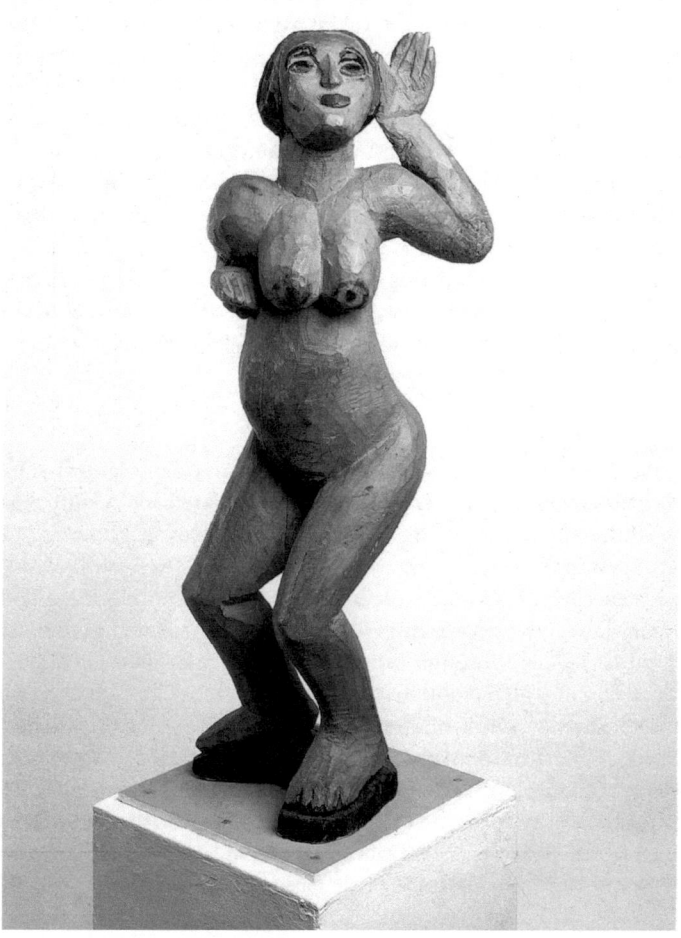

Figure 13.4 E. L. Kirchner, 'Tanzende Frau'

2009, p. 64). Dancing also 're-enacts the past through the body's present performance' (Koch et al., 2013, p. 85). Both aspects are involved in a DMT setting. Dance is an art of representation. The symbolic interpretation of what is given to see makes dancing a symbolic organiser of therapeutic work. Through dancing images, which are mimetic, Clara found a way for addressing trauma.

As in the rites of possession, there is in DMT an unstable point of transition to fiction (Schaeffer, 1999). A work of fiction introduces a narrative element in the mimetic set, because mimesis gives structure to time's experience (Ricoeur, 1983). Medical anthropology has pointed out the importance of forming narratives in the communication of suffering, and has explored its embodied nature (Kleinman, 1988). There are several levels of narrative that do not necessarily take the form of verbal language.

A logical set of dance movements is a choreographic sequence. It shows a level of expressiveness that sequences the dance, which gives meaning in another sense of the articulated language. 'The significance of the gesture . . . the sense and non-sense as sensitive' (Piollet, 2014, p. 117). We saw with Clara how dance gives structure and nuances to what is embedded in her, in an intimate resonance between body and emotions. The body, to deliver its emotions, needs the gap offered by the poetic transposition that introduces a 'distance from ourselves to ourselves' (Schaeffer, 1999, p. 325). Fiction and emotions mean a negotiation constantly replayed in our relationship to the world. We also saw there's a narrative level where the passage of words becomes possible thanks to the staging work that connects the body memory to the declarative memory.

Life is structurally organised into coherent sequences, shattered by the ontological shock of trauma. The continuity of coherent narratives repositions past experiences in a temporality and gives it a meaning. (Crossley, 2000; McDonald, 2013). Clara's narrative skills reintroduced the order of time, where the path of embodied memories revealed the chain between collective history and personal story. Through acting a 'memory of duty', Clara is linked by memory to the members of her family, while differentiating, and she situated herself in the present of her own life story. In our setting, the play between the stage of the body and the subject of narration enabled Clara to become a person and to resume the permanent self-narrative.

Conclusion

DMT is a creative therapeutic approach whose strength is experienced through the body. A dance movement therapist's clinical experience is in the forefront of different scientific findings. In the case illustrated, linking elements from several fields of knowledge highlighted the complexity of Clara's transgenerational traumatic experience, as well as the DMT contributions.

The trauma is experienced above all, especially including the subjective body, and requires attention to both an interactive approach as well as insight, facilitated by kinaesthetic empathy. Witnessing allowed us to share through movement, a speechless horror. DMT opens a poetic and narrative dimension in which emotions take a special place. Through expressiveness we share the reflexive consciousness of arisen emotions. Its performative value emphasises how dance is a rich symbolic vector. The narrative transposition creates space between emotions and disease and enables a modulation of emotions.

With the example of Clara, we found the continuity of the effects of transgenerational trauma between embodied memory and history. Dance movement in a psychotherapeutic context gives access to body memory, before thoughts can articulate the experience in words. The body tells us stories as well as history. Where words often loop back to the real trauma, dance opens an alternative path that allows one to overcome the traumatic experience through artistic transformation process and nourishes the links to language. Attuning to each patient, DMT particularly helps to change through a step-by-step structured process. It represents a highly integrative approach, which finds its relevance in supporting patients with traumatic pathologies.

References

Adler, J. (1999). Who is the witness? A description of authentic movement. In P. Pallaro (Ed.), *Authentic Movement. Essays by Mary Starks Whitehouse, Janet Adler and Joan Chodorow* (pp. 141–159). London: Jessica Kingsley. (Original work published 1987)

Bartenieff, I. (1980). *Body Movement: Coping with the Environment*. New York: Gordon and Breach.

Bion, W. R. (1984). *Learning from Experience*. London: Karnac. (Original work published 1962)

Chouvier, B. (2000). *Matière à symbolisation* [Material for Symbolisation]. Lausanne: Delachaux-Niestlé.

Cozolino, L. (2002). *The Neuroscience of Psychotherapy*. New York: W.W. Norton.

Crossley, M. L. (2000). Narrative psychology, trauma and the study of self-identity. *Theory and Psychology, 10*(4), 527–546.

Csordas, T. (1990). Embodiment as paradigm for anthropology. *Ethos, 18*(1), 5–47.

Csordas, T. (1993). Somatic modes of attention. *Cultural Anthropology, 8*(2), 135–256.

Dolto, F. (1981). *Au jeu du désir* [Desire's Play]. Paris: Seuil.

Dosamantes-Alperson, E. (1979). The intrapsychic and the interpersonal in movement psychotherapy. *American Journal of Dance Therapy, 3*(1), 20–31.

Freud, S. (1977a). Au-delà du principe de plaisir [Beyond the Pleasure Principle]. In *Essais de psychanalyse* [Essays of Psychoanalysis] (pp. 7–81). Paris: Payot. (Original work published 1920)

Freud, S. (1977b). Le moi et le çà [The Ego and the Id]. In *Essais de psychanalyse* [Essays of Psychoanalysis] (pp. 177–234). Paris: Payot. (Original work published 1923)

Fuchs, T., and Koch, S. C. (2014). Embodied affectivity: On moving and being moved. *Frontiers in Psychology, 5*(508), 1–12.

Gallagher, S., and Payne, H. (2015). The role of embodiment and intersubjectivity in clinical reasoning. *Body, Movement and Dance in Psychotherapy, 10*(1), 68–78.

Gallese, V. (2009). Mirror neurons, embodied simulation, and the neutral basis of social identification. *Psychoanalytic Dialogues, 19*(5), 519–536.

Gedo, J. E. (2005). Trauma and its vicissitudes. In J. E. Gedo (Ed.), *Psychoanalysis as Biological Science* (pp. 72–79). Baltimore: Johns Hopkins University Press.

Georgieff, N. (2010). Psychanalyse, neurosciences et subjectivités [Psychoanalysis, neurosciences and inter-subjectivity]. *Neuropsychiatrie de l'enfance et de l'adolescence, 58*, 343–350.

Graf, P., and Schacter, D. L. (1985). Implicit and explicit memory for new associations in normal and amnesic subjects. *Journal of Experimental Psychology, 11*, 501–518.

Hackney, P. (1998). *Making Connections*. New York: Gordon and Breach.

Hawkins, A. M. (1991). *Moving from Within*. Chicago: Cappella Books.

Janet, P. (1919). Les médications psychologiques [Psychological Medications]. Paris: Alcan.

Kaës, R. (1993). *Transmission de la vie psychique entre générations* [Psychic Intergenerational Transmission]. Paris: Dunod.

Kleinman, A. (1988). *The Illness Narratives*. New York: Basic Books.

Koch, S. C., Caldwell, C., and Fuchs, T. (2013). On body memory and embodied therapy. *Body, Movement and Dance in Psychotherapy, 8*(2), 82–94.

Laban, R. (1988). *The Mastery of Movement*. Plymouth: Northcote House. (Original work published 1950)

Levine, B., and Land, H. M. (2016). A meta-synthesis of qualitative findings about dance/movement therapy for individuals with trauma. *Qualitative Health Research, 26*(3), 330–344.

Levine, S. K. (2009). *Trauma, Tragedy, Therapy*. London: Jessica Kingsley.

Levi-Strauss, C. (1958). L'efficacité symbolique [The symbolic effectiveness]. In *Anthropologie Structurale* [Structural Anthropology] (pp. 213–275). Paris: Plon.

McDonald, M. C. (2013). Trauma, embodiment and narrative. *Idealistic Studies, 42*(2/3), 247–263.

Mauss, M. (1950). Les techniques du corps [Body Techniques]. In *Sociologie et anthropologie* [Sociology and Psychology] (pp. 363–386). Paris: PUF. (Original work published 1936)

Meekums, B. (2002). *Dance Movement Therapy*. London: Sage.

Merleau-Ponty, M. (1945). *Phénoménologie de la perception* [Phenomenology of Perception]. Paris: Gallimard.

Ogden, P., and Minton, K. (2000). Sensorimotor psychotherapy: One method for processing traumatic memory. *Traumatology, 6*(3), 149–173.

Pandolfi, M. (1991). *Itinerari delle emozioni* [Routes of Emotions]. Milano: Francoangeli.

Paxton, S. (1999). Esquisses de techniques intérieures [Drafting interior techniques]. In *Contact Improvisation* (pp. 38/39, 103–122). Bruxelles: Nouvelles de danse. (Original work published 1993)

Pierce, L. (2014). The integrative power of dance/movement therapy: Implications for the treatment of dissociation and developmental trauma. *The Arts in Psychotherapy, 41*, 7–17.

Piollet, W. (2014). *Aventure des Barres flexibles* [Flexible Barre Experience]. Paris: Sens and Tonka.

Reca, M. (2011). *Tortura y Trauma* [Torture and Trauma]. Buenos Aires: Biblos.

Ricoeur, P. (1983). *Temps et récit, 1* [Time and Narrative]. Paris: Seuil.

Rizzolatti, G., and Sinigaglia, C. (2006). *Les neurones miroirs* [The Mirror Neuron System]. Paris: Odile Jacob.

Roussillon, R. (2012). Propositions pour une théorie des dispositifs thérapeutiques à médiations [Theoretical frameworks for the therapeutic use of art]. In A. Brun (Ed.), *Les médiations thérapeutiques* [Therapeutic Mediums] (pp. 23–25). Toulouse: Erès.

Schaeffer, J. M. (1999). *Pourquoi la fiction* [Why the Fiction]. Paris: Seuil.

Schaeffer, J. M. (2015). *L'expérience esthétique* [The Aesthetic Experience]. Paris: Gallimard.

Schore, A. (2001). The effects of relational trauma on right brain development, affect regulation, and infant mental health. *Infant Mental Health Journal, 22*, 201–269.

Selye, H. (1956). *The Stress of Life*. New York: McGraw-Hill.

Stanek, D. (2015). Bridging past and present: Embodied intergenerational trauma and the implications for dance/movement therapy. *Body, Movement and Dance in Psychotherapy, 10*(2), 94–105.

Stern, D. N. (2010). *Forms of Vitality. Exploring Dynamic Experience in Psychology and the Arts*. Oxford: Oxford University Press.

Surralès, A. (2004). Des états d'âme aux états de fait. La perception entre le corps et les affects [From the moods to the facts. The perception between body and affects]. In F. Héritier and M. Xanthakou (Eds.), *Corps et affects* [Body and Affects] (pp. 59–75). Paris: Odile Jacob.

Taussig, M. (1993). *Mimesis and Alterity*. London: Routledge.

Tortora, S. (2006). *The Dancing Dialogue*. Baltimore: Paul. H. Brookes.

Turner, V. (1986). *Dal rito al teatro* [From Ritual to Theater]. Bologna: Il Mulino. (Original work published 1982)

van der Hart, O., Brown P., and van der Kolk, B. A. (1989). Le traitement psychologique du stress post-traumatique de Pierre Janet [Psychological treatment for PTSD]. *Annales Médico-Psychologiques, 9*, 976–980.

van der Kolk, B. A. (2006). Clinical implications of neuroscience research in PTSD. *Annals of the New York Academy of Sciences, 1071*, 277–293.

Victoria, H. K. (2012). Creating dances to transform inner states: A choreographic model in dance/movement therapy. *Body, Movement and Dance in Psychotherapy, 7*(3), 167–183.

Wigman, M. (1986). *Le langage de la danse* [The Language of Dance]. Paris: Papiers. (Original work published 1963)

Wilkinson, M. (2010). *Changing Minds in Therapy: Emotion, Attachment, Trauma and Neurobiology*. New York/London: W.W. Norton.

Winnicott, D. W. (1975[1971]). *Jeu et réalité* [Playing and Reality]. Paris: Gallimard.

14

PSYCHOLOGICAL RE-SOURCES IN INTEGRAL DANCE AND DANCE/MOVEMENT THERAPY

Alexander Girshon and Ekaterina Karatygina

Introduction

The concept of personal and psychological resources is common in various areas of social work and psychotherapy. Some studies show that a marked improvement in the realisation of personal resources during psychotherapy can show significant correlations to the improvement of symptoms in clinical setting (Kati, Stumpf, Heuft, Burgmer, and Schneider, 2015). At the same time, the definition of resources varies from therapist to therapist. It seems that there is no clear and distinct picture of what resources actually are, and how and where to look for them. We would like to propose a model of resources, which is based on an integral approach, positive psychology and dance movement therapy practice.

Context

Our model of resources is inspired by the integral approach of the contemporary philosopher Wilber (2000, 2003). The intention of integral approach is to place a wide diversity of theories and thinkers into one single framework. It is portrayed as a 'theory of everything' ('the living Totality of matter, body, mind, soul, and spirit'), trying 'to draw together an already existing number of separate paradigms into an interrelated network of approaches that are mutually enriching' (Wilber, 2003, p. xii).

Within this approach, we can connect the modern understanding of physiology and neuroscience with findings in somatic techniques; a dance movement therapy approach with the theoretical frame of transpersonal psychology, contemporary performance techniques and contact improvisation, mindfulness practices and ecstatic meditation, depending on the requirements, needs and abilities of clients and groups. This approach is used successfully in Russia, Lithuania, Ukraine, Belarus, and Israel in work with children with special needs, in mental health clinics, in private practices, and in creative and personal development training. When practicing dance movement therapy in a training course or in individual therapy, we often turn to the concept of a resource. The basic principle here is: before you tackle a problem, check the availability of resources.

The term 'resources' is primarily associated with economics and geology. This could be because in Soviet Russia children often heard about 'our native resources', as Russia is reliant on its natural resource economy. These associations imply that resources are something deeply hidden, difficult to extract, and exhaustible. Other sources mention that resources are finite, can be easily wasted, and that it is important to manage them well. We are interested in the alluring beauty of the English etymology of this word – 're-source', i.e. 'return to the source', or more precisely, 'recover the source'. This is something fluid and free: resource as a process. These are resources that we can continuously replenish. So what resources can we recover and replenish in dance movement therapy?

Conceptual framework

To understand resources in the context of psychotherapy and personal development, we can turn to Ken Wilber's integral approach which utilises three main perspectives: objective (material, third person resources, it/this), subjective (inner resources of the individual itself, first person resources, I), and intersubjective (resource relationships and communities, second person re-sources, We or I–You resources). In this article, the main focus will be on the first person resources, but we will also address the other two areas. We will start with safety as a prerequisite and key resource for therapy.

Safety as a resource

Safety, which engenders confidence, is one of the key factors in therapy. It is provided by boundaries, contract, and by the therapeutic setting overall. It is important to understand that real safety and a sense of safety may not be one and the same. In situations of trauma and stress our bodies and our unconscious do not perceive the world as a safe place. So how do our bodies and our unconscious react to trauma? We get an answer from the polyvagal perspective developed by Porges (2001). According to the polyvagal theory, the well-documented phylogenetic shift in neural regulation of the autonomic nervous system passes through three global stages, each with an associated behavioural strategy. The first stage is characterised by a primitive unmyelinated visceral vagus that fosters digestion and responds to threat by depressing metabolic activity. Behaviourally, the first stage is associated with immobilisation behaviours. The second stage is characterised by the sympathetic nervous system that is capable of increasing metabolic output and inhibiting the visceral vagus to foster mobilisation behaviours necessary for 'fight or flight'. The third stage, unique to mammals, is characterised by a myelinated vagus that can rapidly regulate cardiac output to foster engagement and disengagement with the environment. The mammalian vagus is neuroanatomically linked to the cranial nerves that regulate social engagement via facial expression and vocalisation (Porges, 1995, 2001).

Thus, it is important to supplement the usual triad of the fight–flight–freeze stress responses with a newer component that Zoe Lodrick called 'friend'. Friend is the earliest defensive strategy available to us ontogenetically and the last one developed phylogenetically (Lodrick, 2007). At birth the human infant's amygdala is operational (Cozolino, 2002), and they utilise their cry in order to bring a caregiver to them. The non-mobile baby has to rely upon calling a protector to its aid, in the same way that the terrified adult screams in the hope that rescue will come. Once mobile the child may move towards another for protection, and with language comes the potential to negotiate, plead, or bribe one's way out of danger. Throughout life when fearful most humans will activate their social engagement system (Porges, 1995).

Thus restoring safe communication in a stressful situation is an evolutionarily more recent, more complex and a more fragile coping strategy. To take the client out of their sense of unsafety, the polyvagal theory advises talking to the person quietly and gently, to lower the timbre of our voice in order to engage the person's listening mechanism. This would provide the client with a calm environment without any loud extraneous sounds and noises.

It is also important to gather physical safety resources such as posture, movement, and position in space that are associated with an experience or memory of a safe environment and to share them with the therapist or group. In this sense, the experience of safety is a renewable and manageable resource.

These techniques have been used when working with people living near the Ukraine military conflict area. Verbal and rational methods could not adequately assist people who expected their homes to turn into a war zone at any moment in coping with their heightened anxiety. But physical exercises and mutual physical support helped reduce anxiety and led to open discussion about their anxieties and their options for action.

First person resources

Much has been written about inner resources. Concepts such as motivation, intuition, discipline, stress resistance, etc., are all included in this category. The multifaceted term 'energy' is often used to refer to the basic level of activity and good mood. We consider three important concepts: power, pleasure, and meaning. These correspond to research in positive psychology. In well-being theory by Seligman (2011) there are five measurable elements:

- Positive emotion
- Accomplishment
- Meaning and purpose
- Engagement
- Relationships

No one element defines well-being, but each contributes to it. Some aspects of these five elements are measured subjectively by self-report, but other aspects are measured objectively. When comparing these models, we see that Positive emotions correlate with Pleasure, Accomplishment – with Power – and Meaning is Meaning. And, in line positive psychology research, we can add to this Engagement. Relationships correspond to second-person resources in our model. Thus, we get a clear and simple checklist of resources that we can test:

Pleasure

We can answer the question: What brings me satisfaction? Are there enough events and things in my life that bring pleasure (but do not cause damage)? How often do I feel comfortable, nice, or cool? How often do I find pleasure in the simple joys of life?

We do not need super-efforts to obtain the basic enjoyment from life (there are, of course, clinical exceptions). Our body is adapted for pleasure, and the internal reward system is constantly running; we just need to not interfere with the natural process and find ways to work with and be in balance with it.

In this context, we would like to share a parable about a Zen master. Students gathered at his deathbed to get the last instructions, many hoped for some wise saying about the Dharma. 'Master, tell us!' – a senior student asked. The old man opened his eyes and said: 'Do you hear squirrels rustling on the roof? How lovely!' And he died.

We can start a workshop by asking participants to perform the most pleasant and comfortable movement. Could you find one right now? It could be stretching, or a deep inhale and a relaxed exhale, a shake, or a jump – any movement that feels natural and brings you pleasure.

Dance movement therapy provides a wide variety of tools to obtain not only 'simple', but also 'complex' enjoyment from life. Those which relate to satisfaction of social, spiritual, or self-affirmation needs for example. So first, the very nature of dance movement therapy gives us the opportunity to develop complex movements that bring special pleasure to mind and body. And then the various sophisticated methods used within the approach, such as improvisation and performance, contact improvisation, authentic movement and etc., provide multi-faceted opportunities for learning how to take pleasure in 'complex' aspects of life. In completion, this unique, compound pleasure can be assimilated in all languages of consciousness and shared with other people. It would be difficult to overestimate these possibilities for modern culture.

When working with 'pleasure', the important issue of 'sufficiency' comes up. How much do I really need to get pleasure from something? What makes my pleasure 'pure', in general, and useful as a resource? How do I choose the ratio of quality and quantity of what brings me pleasure? I (Ekaterina Karatygina) remember how, in an Integral Somatic lesson by Alexander Girshon, while working with the senses we explored 'taste'. After breaking off a piece of dark chocolate and slowly putting it in our mouths, each of us carefully scrutinised our feelings and emotions. Shades of flavour, its shape, the temperature, changing on contact with the tongue, observation of how the chocolate is melting and gradually coated the inside of the mouth, dripping down the throat into the oesophagus, – all of that mattered and unexpectedly brought a lot of joy to me. And it was just one small piece. Active and consciously sustained attention, sharing this unique pleasure with others, as well as the intellectual background of what was happening, were helping me greatly. This made a lot of sense. Pleasure backed by the meaning – which we will address later – is a special pleasure.

Engagement

What do I find interesting? What captivates and fascinates me? Things can be interesting even without any direct practical benefit – but sometimes because of a practical benefit. As children, we have many different hobbies: I (Alexander Girshon) was engaged in aeromodelling, was soldering schemes of some strange devices with friends, attended a photography club and even briefly karate and other activities. But more than anything I loved reading. I read for hours, sometimes skipping school, forgetting homework and everything else. My father had collected a good library at home, so I could always dive into it. I think we all have an experience of a healthy immersion into feelings, into the flow of experience, being swept along on a wave of interest. This can happen in work or in relationships. It happens when I dance, when the movement itself, the music, or my internal and external environment take total control of me and lead me entirely.

When did you last experience this feeling of engagement, of moving with the stream? What helps you get in there and return safely? In dance and movement, it is quite easy for us to get into the flow of engagement. Music, rhythm, working with partners, and a group pattern of motion – all that can bring not only pleasure, but engage us as well. In developmental lessons and therapy sessions, a good question to ask is: In what way, and with what quality of motion would you be most interested in dancing right now? We can also work on developing the sensitivity of different sense organs.

Power

There are two types of questions which are relevant:

- What can I do? What am I capable of? What action or situation can give me a sense of power, control, achievement, and overcoming?
- And how can I 'allow' myself to use my power? How can I use it with a sense of self-esteem? How can I present it to the world and, in particular, to significant people?

Example 1 (Alexander Girshon): My favourite form of dance is a contact improvisation. We share weight within this form, so in the flow of movement supports come naturally, and it can be that my partner is on my back or shoulders, or vice versa. Largely due to the fact that, to me, support in dance is associated with the 'I can' feeling, it has always been easier for me to take my partner's full weight, than for me to let them take all of mine. When I teach students how to take a partner's weight safely and effectively, I see the same 'I can' excitement and pleasure. This feeling is easy to reach if we carefully measure the steps of development and the individual's ability.

Example 2 (Alexander Girshon): One of the most exotic forms of dance I work with, is a dance in the water. We sometimes use this dance during our travel training sessions in warm countries. It is no secret that many people have a fear of diving. Usually this is linked to a bad swimming experience in childhood or trauma. It is not a fear that hinders us in our daily life: people can swim well with it but lowering their face into the water creates an unpleasant experience. And this can be an obstacle for underwater dance training. One of the participants during a training trip to Thailand 2 years ago wanted to overcome this fear. We carefully divided her dives into small steps and actions she could take. We took as many steps as was necessary and worked with as much energy and aspiration as was possible. Two years later, she participated in a somatic water dance laboratory, performing various complicated and disorienting movements under water, in the sea and in a swimming pool. As she said, this experience didn't only give her the freedom to swim and dance underwater, but also taught her to deal with complex and frightening tasks in her life.

Where and when do you have the 'I can' feeling? What actions and abilities is it connected with? Can you organise a number of practices where this experience of yourself can be strengthened until it could be reasonably transferred into other areas of your life?

We believe that 'power' is one of the key resources (along with 'meaning') that we need both to meet our needs and to solve problems, and also to help us survive and cope with dangerous and stressful situations. When we work with 'power' in the context of traumatic experiences, the session may include a 'moving forward', but also an 'escape', not only an 'expression of anger', but also 'managing' it, and not only 'action', but also 'inaction'. It is necessary to make a deliberate choice of the optimal strategy, regardless of how it is 'generally accepted' in the social system, which usually exerts a strong pressure on our understanding of 'power' and 'weakness'.

Meaning

What is important to me? Are there any activities, events, projects, or people in my life that are truly and deeply important to me? Meaning is a special and hard to define category of human experience. There are different perspectives of interpreting meaning. Idealistic – when meaning is a special idea, with its own existence and status, different from 'objective' and 'subjective' (Plato, Frege, 1979). Systemic – when meaning is the role that an action or event plays in the context of the whole. Analytical-pragmatic – when meaning is a utility or utilisation ('Meaning-is-use', Wittgenstein, 2001, p. 14). Existential – when meaning is what a person creates. Empirical – which views meaning as an experience ('felt-sense', Gendlin, 1996, p. 26). The abundance of perspectives may indicate that meaning is one of the keys for understanding human nature.

In a practical, therapeutic context, it is important to consider the concept of 'sensed' or 'experienced' meaning and the connection of the meaning and values embodied in a person's life. I (Alexander Girshon) have one perspective example: my personal value of 'freedom' is embodied in the fact that I am self-employed (no outside control), in my passion for travel (freedom of movement), or in a choice of improvisational dance forms (freedom of motion), etc. I (Ekaterina Karatygina) have another perspective example: my personal binary value of 'synthesis and uniqueness' is embodied in the fact that in my various work fields (art, psychology, and business) I like to combine very different types of art, developmental, or healing techniques and methods, depending on the 'needs and senses of the moment'.

When was the last time you experienced the feeling of a moment's significance? What action, environment, or quality of existence caused that feeling? When we see and feel that the special space of dance and the beauty of emotions experienced in a group, a pair or an individual dance appear, we call it a 'moment of grace'. This feeling is difficult to describe, and impossible to retain, but it is this quality of presence and feeling that gives an inner meaning to what is happening. Yet, this does not preclude the possibility of a practical use.

Resources and shadow

It should be noted that each of the resources if it is not optimally used, can become an anti-resource, a 'black hole', which is able to destroy life. We can say that each resource has a 'shadow'

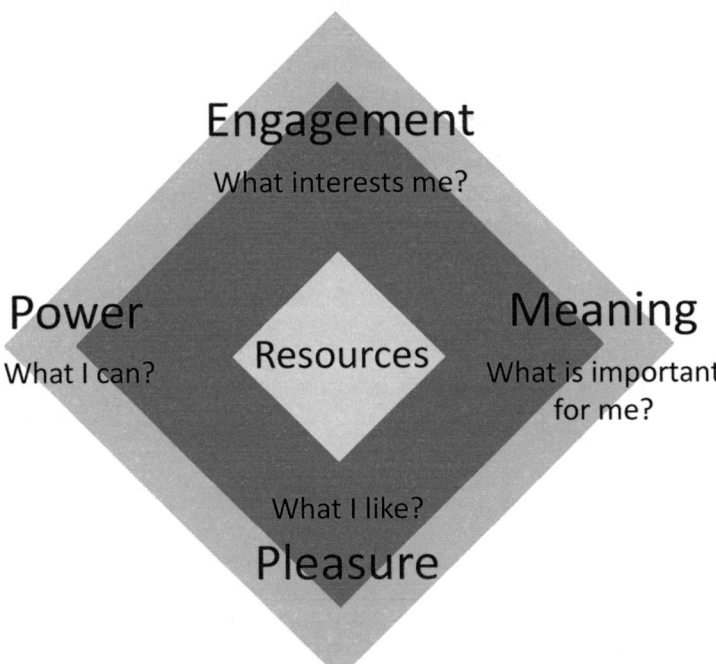

Figure 14.1 Engagement, power, meaning, pleasure

side, which is evident when resources become an independent value, when we lose touch with a larger context of human life. Then pleasure turns into the primitive pursuit of fun, with its simple dopamine spikes, its minimum investment and maximum side effects. Engagement becomes an addiction and power turns out to be a demand for hyper-control or adrenaline injection, while the super importance of meaning turns into fanaticism and an 'idée fixe'. And conversely, 'shadows' can turn into potential resources.

Resource positions

It is important to remember that we should consider not only WHAT the resource is in the context of life, but also HOW and from what position (WHO) I deal with it. Within the resource position we answer the question: Exactly what condition and attitude helps me to move, grow, and cope with difficulties? As a result, we use three such positions in dance movement therapy:

1   Scientific – when there is pleasure and interest in how things work; ability to distinguish between different driving and cultivating forces of internal and external events; it is based on a searching behaviour and assumes an advanced cognitive level.
2   Creative – when there is pleasure and interest in creating completed or instantly disappearing artefacts made of feelings; attention to beauty-in-process; and based on the instinctive game behaviour.
3   Reflexive – the pleasure of detachment, with its interest in life-as-it-is-whatever-it-is and power-in-silence.

And it is clear that there are practices and levels of skills in each of these positions, and there are other heroes (somewhere in other subjective worlds); but ask yourself, which position am I using when considering a situation in my life?

Second person resources

One of the ways of understanding the human psyche is that the subject evolves from the inter-subject or, in the words of Igor Kalinauskas: 'People made of people' (Kalinauskas, 2011, p. 19). In the integral approach we work with self-relationships, other people, the world, and eternity. Self-relationships mean healthy relationships with our own body and feelings, along with a balanced self-esteem and self-acceptance. When working with relationships with other people, we work with the ability to establish and maintain contact, express our own wishes and feelings, and define and protect our borders, etc. Relationships with the world can be seen as relationships with groups, communities, 'socium', or nature.

Relationships with other people can be a non-resource as well as a resource, sometimes they can be destructive and dysfunctional. In the context of psychotherapy and personal development, it is important for us to find re-source relationships and/or ways and strategies of behaving that can support the healthy aspects of relationships. We proceed from the fact that we already have the 'therapist-client' re-source relationships where the clients can learn ways to ask for support, demonstrate the right for their own space and time, and learn ways to really see The Other, without projections and expectations. In the realm of relationships, the dance gives plenty of opportunities to explore loneliness/contact balance, adequate and changing distance, the shift between leading and following, and other aspects of relationships.

Another interesting point – the same relationships can be a resource in one context, and a non-resource and a hindrance in another. Second person resources could be hypothetically divided into:

- People (living or dead) may be a resource due to the feeling of emotional connection with them.
- The nature of the relationship may be a resource in itself – support, acceptance, etc.
- Some aspects of relationship may support, while others may destroy then it is important to monitor the level of creative aspects in these relationships or keep track of balance within the bigger picture.
- There may be forms and methods of resource relationships with which people are not familiar.
- And there may be relationships that require the acquisition of certain resources, before a person can fully support them (for example, in relationships with significant loved ones).

All these forms of resources can be found with the help of dance, real, or symbolic, and with the people in the room, or people from other aspects of our lives that are not present at this moment.

Third person resources

Material resources, such as money, property, and free time do not often feature as major aspects of dance movement therapy, but we can work with them to see how a person handles these resources in their daily life, and what scenarios and patterns are expressed during the dance with them.

Example 1: I (Alexander Girshon) really love my job, I like to hold classes, explore the world of movement, support people in their dance with life. Today I have a sufficient level of work all the time. Meanwhile, 5–6 years ago it became clear that I needed weekends and holidays, so as not to burn out at work. Besides, my full immersion in work could interfere with family relationships. So I started planning special vacations, where I could spend time with my family and children, without doing any great or important projects.

Example 2: Sometimes the topic of money is related to the 'give/take' balance, feelings of unworthiness, or a lack of the right to material reward. Acceptance is not only a psychological concept, it is always an internal action which has momentum. In dealing with this subject, we can study the 'receive-accept-take' spectrum of actions, which is associated with an increase in muscle tone and strengthening the aspect of Agency (author's position). A good exercise for this topic: we share money with full awareness of the action, taking it on inhale and giving it on exhale.

Resources in a time continuum

At the beginning of this chapter, referring to the etymology of the resource, we said that re-source can be seen as a 'return to the source'. In addition, when working with psychological resources, it is also important to consider the ability to 'let go' and 'provide' yourself with new sources. In this approach, we can refer to resources from different time zones: the past (including fields of traumatic experiences), the present (resources revision often occurs here), and the future – in the form of appealing to resources as something to master within a given task (for example, to realise our own values).

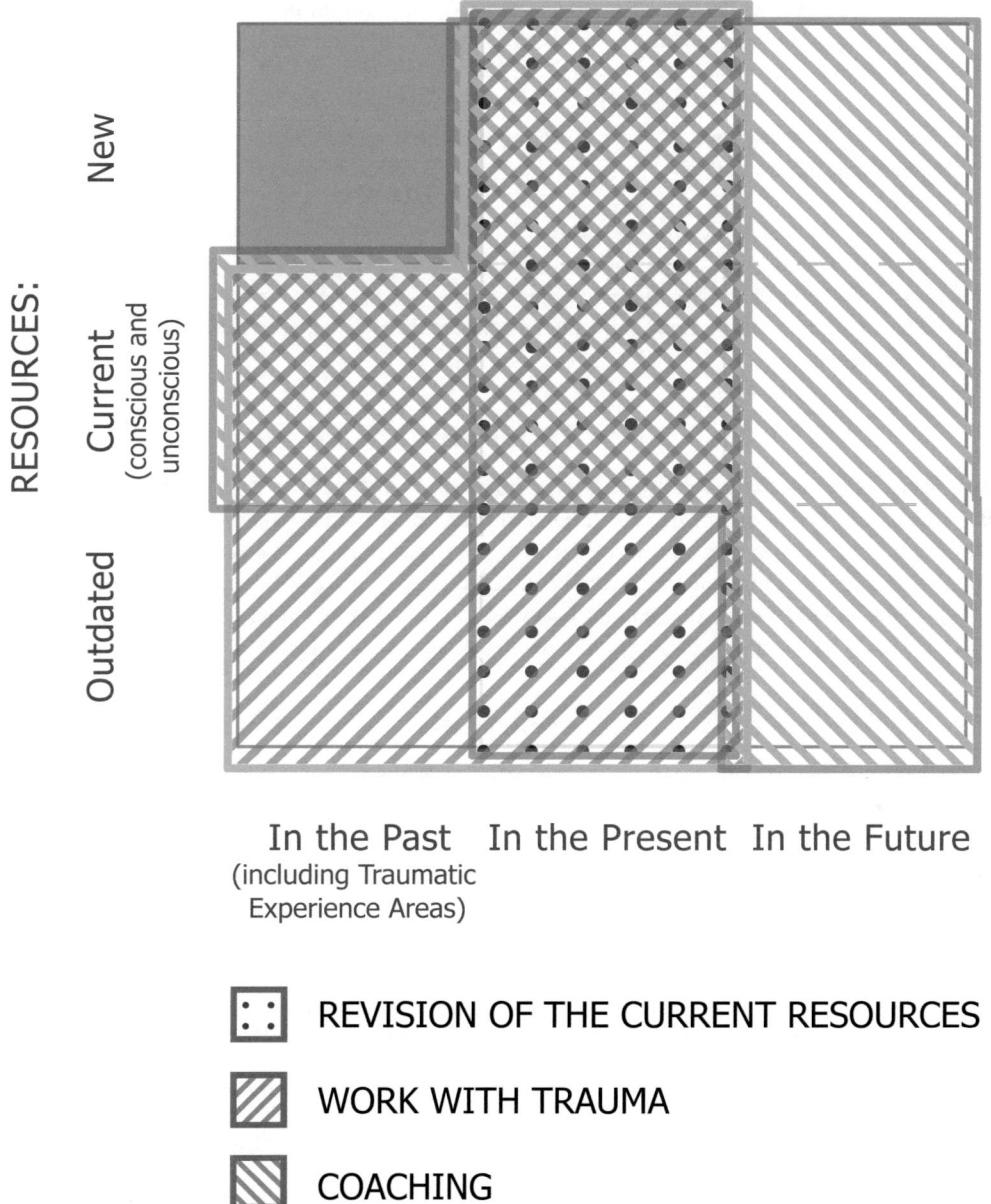

RESOURCES:

New

Current
(conscious and
unconscious)

Outdated

In the Past   In the Present   In the Future
(including Traumatic
Experience Areas)

⠃ REVISION OF THE CURRENT RESOURCES

▨ WORK WITH TRAUMA

▨ COACHING

Figure 14.2   Resources in a time continuum map

On the other hand, we can distinguish three groups of psychological resources:

1   Forgotten or poorly perceived in our everyday life; they return us to our own resource landscape.
2   Re-Sources, unknown before – they were unrealised and not 'fitted', or used; this is a new way of moving.

I try it, and it works out well; I like it and can benefit from it. Sometimes all you have to do is to notice them, sometimes you have to absorb them, or permit yourself to use them – then we will turn to 'shadow' re-sources.

3   Obsolete resources. Here we should revise existing resources: what helped me yesterday, what may interfere today. Next it is important to give them up or, if necessary, replace with something more suitable.

As a result of reviewing these various psychological resource realms, we have created the 'Resources in a Time Continuum Map' (see Figure 14.2). We made this map when we were working simultaneously with different people in three different formats: developing, psychological, and coaching, as we had not had a clear understanding which resources to turn to within a particular format.

Summary

We have tried to list the psychological resources that we work with in dance movement therapy. This helps clients best handle their material resources, understand how they can build resourceful relationships, and how they can find their own internal resources. The main idea, which is the basis of this article is that you and your clients have access to many different resources, some that are available now and some that you need to work on. Or, slightly paraphrasing Erickson (1991), people always have enough resources for those changes that they need.

References

Cozolino, L. (2002). *The Neuroscience of Psychotherapy: Building and Rebuilding the Human Brain*. New York: W.W. Norton.

Erickson, M. (1991). *My Voice Will Go with You: The Teaching Tales of Milton H. Erickson*. New York: W.W. Norton.

Frege, G. (1979). Dialogue with Punjer on Existence. In H. Hermes, F. Kambartel, and F. Kaulbach (Eds.), *Posthumous Writings* (pp. 65–67). Chicago: The University of Chicago Press.

Gendlin, E. T. (1996). *Focusing-Oriented Psychotherapy: A Manual of the Experiential Method*. New York: Guilford Press.

Kalinauskas, I. (2011). *Alone with World*. Moscow: Zikr Shop.

Kati, A., Stumpf, A., Heuft, G., Burgmer, M., and Schneider, G. (2015). Personal resources in inpatient psychotherapy – Relationships and development. *Zeitschrift für Psychosomatische Medizin und Psychotherapie/Journal of Psychosomatic Medicine and Psychotherapy, 61*(2), 139–155.

Lodrick, Z. (2007). Psychological trauma – What every trauma worker should know. *The British Journal of Psychotherapy Integration, 4*(2), 18–28.

Porges, S. (1995). Orienting in a defensive world: Mammalian modifications of our evolutionary heritage. A polyvagal theory. *Psychophysiology, 32*, 301–318.

Porges, S. (2001). The polyvagal theory: Phylogenetic substrates of a social nervous system. *International Journal of Psychophysiology, 42*, 123–146.

Seligman, M. (2011). *Flourish: A Visionary New Understanding of Happiness and Well-being*. New York: Free Press.

Wilber, K. (2000). *Integral Psychology: Consciousness, Spirit, Psychology, Therapy*. Boston: Shambhala Publications.

Wilber, K. (2003). Foreword in Frank Visser's book. In *Ken Wilber: Thought as Passion* (pp. xii–xiii). New York: State University of New York Press.

Wittgenstein, L. (2001). *Tractatus Logico-Philosophicus*. London and New York: Routledge Classics.

15

MOTHER–SON TRANSGENERATIONAL TRANSMISSION OF EATING ISSUES IN A CO-TREATMENT METHOD USING THE WAYS OF SEEING APPROACH

Suzi Tortora and Jennifer Whitley

Introduction

The parent–child case presented in this chapter describes a unique multifaceted co-treatment method called *Ways of Seeing* (WOS) developed by the first author, combining the principles of dance/movement psychotherapy, creative arts therapies, infant mental health, and Laban non-verbal movement analysis (Tortora, 2006, 2016).

The therapists gain a deeper understanding of the underlying psychic and inter-relational dynamics of the dyad through careful attention to both the parent and the child's nonverbal movement styles using Laban Movement Analysis (Bartenieff and Lewis, 1980) in tandem with their verbal statements and dance-play storylines. Infant mental health theory and transgenerational transmission of trauma research and literature provide the theoretical foundations that support this method as outlined in Figure 15.1 below.

Background

In dance/movement psychotherapy (DMT) body-based activities are used to encourage emotional expression and the unfolding of deeper psychic material. Extensive training in nonverbal observation and a deep understanding of the body as an expression of one's felt-experience provide a secure environment to bring awareness to and safely explore one's experiences. This is especially helpful with post-traumatic symptoms, which often create a disassociation between the mind, body, and emotional experiences.

In Ways of Seeing (WOS) the concept of a "body-mind-emotion continuum" (B-M-E continuum), describes the circular synergistic relationship between how a person responds to life events in relationship to each of these aspects of self (Tortora, 2015a, p. 260). It describes how experiences in the body inform how an individual thinks about and develops images and

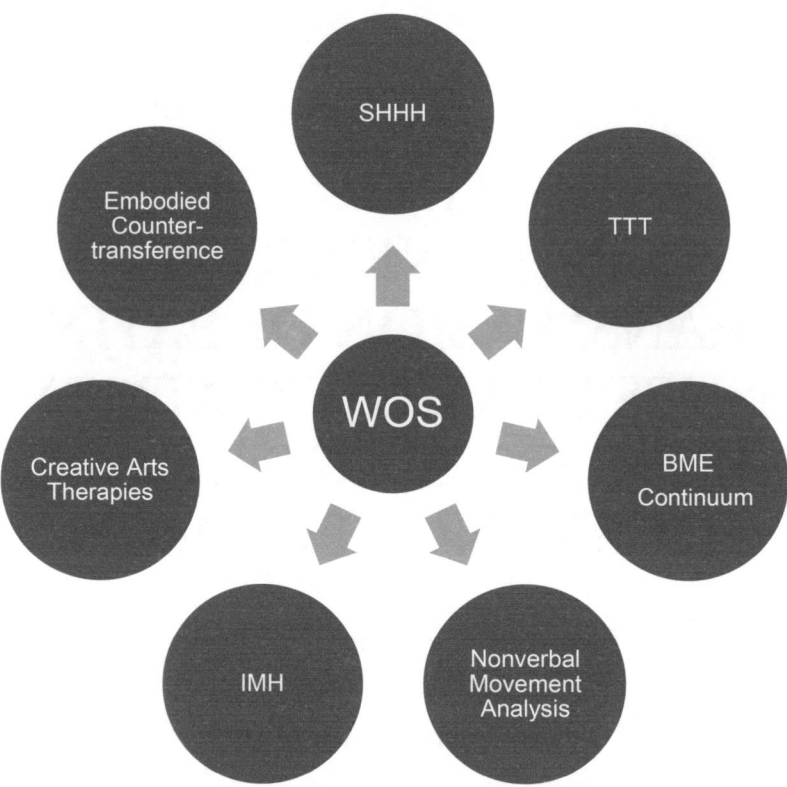

Figure 15.1 Components of Ways of Seeing

SHHH = Seen, Heard, Held, Hugged; TTT = transgenerational transmission of trauma; BME Continuum: Body-Mind-Emotion Continuum; nonverbal movement analysis; IMH = Infant Mental Health; the use of dance/movement psychotherapy and other creative arts therapies for healing; and the role of the therapist's embodied countertransference.

responses to these experiences, and the emotional reactions that evolve from these experiences. The B-M-E continuum grounds the WOS dance/movement psychotherapeutic milieu by creating three levels of entry into one's self. Starting from any of these three components, session activities involve a systematic investigation of body actions, thoughts and feelings through self-initiated creative explorations. This enables the mover to discover his[1] own B-M-E connections within his own timing and control. Though one can start anywhere in this continuum to explore how each element relates to the others, WOS highlights the role of the body for it is the primary way dance/movement therapists enter into the therapeutic relationship.

The felt-experience of the moving body provides an "embodied narrative" (Tortora, 2017) of the mover's life story, which is honoured, explored, and dialogued with through physically active storytelling. Embodiment describes the felt-experiential nature of being in one's body as a way of knowing and perceiving oneself. Embodiment is a central organising aspect of bodily, cognitive and emotional experience. Building upon Sheets-Johnstone's (2011) description, "a fluid dynamic relationship exists between perception and action, emotion and movement" (Tortora, 2017). How one perceives and forms an image and understanding of oneself is greatly influenced by one's bodily, moving experience. In WOS it is through the integration of the body, mind, and emotions that true healing occurs.

Conceptual framework

Transgenerational transmission of trauma references the concept that traumatic themes and symptomatic behaviours can permeate family histories, and can get passed down from one generation to another (Braga, Mello, and Fiks, 2012). Often occurring outside of conscious awareness, it can be evident in early parenting patterns. Scheeringa and Zeanah (2001, p. 799) created the term "relational posttraumatic stress disorder" to describe the co-occurrence of post-traumatic stress behaviours in the adult caregiver and her child. A particular feature of this disorder is that symptoms intensify through the relationship with the caregiver, as symptomatology of one member of the dyad exacerbates the other. This diagnosis includes vicarious traumatic effects, in which the child has not been exposed to the trauma the caregiver experienced. The caregiver's preoccupation with traumatic thoughts impedes her ability to effectively monitor or respond to the child, evidenced in constrictive, overprotective or fear-driven parenting behaviours.

Influenced by this intergenerational process, Pat-Horenczyk et al. (2015, p. 344) created an analogous term "relational emotional regulation," during their research studying the association of maternal posttraumatic stress symptoms and children's emotional dysregulation behaviours. Relational emotional regulation references the process of transmitting emotional regulation capacities and difficulties from parent to child.

Mechanisms of transgenerational transmission in infancy and early childhood

The nature of the parent–infant attachment relationship develops through the co-constructed nonverbal exchange between the parent and infant (Beebe and Lachmann, 2002). It is built upon each dyadic member's self-regulatory abilities, for an individual's skill in regulating internal and external input will influence their ability to attend and engage with their partner. The quality of interactive co-regulation is affected by the presenting behaviours of each member of the dyad. The research findings of Pat-Horenczyk et al. (2015) suggests that maternal capacity to develop adaptive emotional regulatory strategies after stressful and traumatic experiences can act as a protective factor in the child's emotional regulatory skill. Similarly, maternal posttraumatic symptoms can contribute to emotional and behavioural regulatory difficulties in the child. The mother-child relationship and the mother's adaptive coping patterns post the traumatic stress crucially effect the child's adaptation to the trauma and capacity to emotionally regulate and manage behaviours such as anger, fear and sadness. In understanding these findings, it is essential to be careful not to blame parents, for traumatic stress must be analyzed within the context of the dynamic caregiver relationship (Scheeringa and Zeanah, 2001, p. 811). Dyadic treatment is recommended, for the most powerful potential for change is through the caregiver relationship.

Ways of Seeing principle

Dyadic treatment is at the core of the WOS creative arts approach. WOS is founded on the significant role body experience plays within the context of the individual's interactions; the primary caregiver attachment relationship as the essential influential relationship of early childhood. Exploring difficult and unconscious material through a creative arts approach is discussed across the creative arts therapies (McCarthy, 2007; Tortora, 2006). Unique to the WOS approach is the specifically structured collaborative co-treatment of the parent and the child by separate therapists. This collaborative approach provides a safe therapeutic environment for both family members to feel seen, heard, held, and hugged (SHHH) a WOS concept that refers to a basic need for every individual that begins at birth (Tortora, 2015a). Based on Winnicott's statement "When I look I am seen so I exist" (Winnicott, 1971, p. 114) the acronym SHHH extends this concept to highlight the felt-experiential core of all individual's need to be seen.

Embodied multi-arts structure of the WOS session

The specific structure of this multi-arts approach allows the therapist to examine the patient's embodied experience and unconscious from several angles, providing the patient with several layers of containment to express deep and difficult emotions. This model is similar to that of sand tray work described by McCarthy (2007) who discusses the use of the sand tray in his body-centred approach to play therapy as being a highly supportive container for the child's unconscious to emerge. Through play, symbols, and metaphors begin to rise to consciousness.

Symbols are a depiction of the inner psyche, the unconscious, and the metaphor within. They emerge "when the child makes a drawing, tells a story, or makes a scene in the sandbox" (McCarthy, 2007, p. 30). The WOS space represents one very large sand tray box. Symbols emerge and are identified through the use of items in the room during dance-play, embodied improvisational story-telling and art-making. Children speak in the language of play (McCarthy, 2007; Winnicott, 1971) and McCarthy explains, "The child can say through symbols things that are unspeakable in any other form" (p. 31).

In this sacred WOS space, there is a myriad of dolls, stuffed animals, and props to allow the child to not only build his story through characters, but to be the story, completely encompassing his whole body and psyche in the action. The B-M-E continuum is exercised, by providing the patient with the tools to understand what these symbols are saying as specific emotions, thoughts, and body experiences are identified and shared through the movement stories. Bringing awareness to the symbols revealed in stories processes feelings that manifest in the body.

Specific components of the WOS session

Figure 15.2 below illustrates the four components in each session.

Check-in: The body, mind, and emotions are engaged during an initial check-in enabling the therapist to assess the patient's nonverbal communications. The patient discusses what is on her mind related to events of the past week, using emotion picture charts and books, and multi-sensory body awareness activities including the Speed Spiral™ – a chart designed by the first author to identify body feelings (Tortora, 2015b). The B-M-E continuum is physically explored through the Speed Spiral™ by embodying and identifying body sensations, energy levels and tempos while moving up and down four colours representing different movement speeds on the spiral. This essential element of the WOS method, when working with trauma, supports the patient to acquire a somatic sense of control and regulatory capacity in the immediate moment.

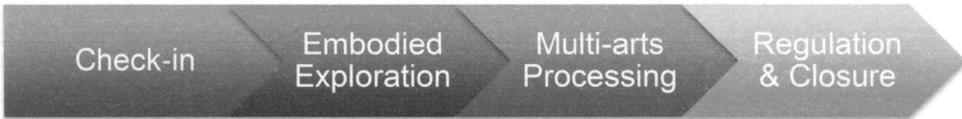

Figure 15.2 Four components of the Ways of Seeing session

Embodied exploration: The information gathered from the check-in is used to create a dance- and movement-based exploration. Music, chosen by the mover, may be used to support the emotional theme. These enacted dance-play stories (Tortora, 2006) must include a beginning, middle, and end and have a conflict. The conflict is essential for it enables the child's psychic struggle to arise. The therapist may be an active participant in the story; silent witness; verbal narrator; or bring unconscious themes that are arising to conscious awareness through verbal interpretation. Working with a sense of collaboration and understanding that only the mover knows his truth, the latter role is very carefully worded. Open-ended questions such as, "What happens next?"; "What should he do?" and "I wonder what will happen?" provide guidance without leading the solution. With all verbal statements the goal is not to change the storyline but rather to glean an understanding of the symbolic meaning that is being expressed.

Often unsolved problems in the child's everyday life can be a great source of challenging behaviours (Crenshaw, 2004). This approach provides the child with skills in problem solving and increases his ability to communicate more clearly. As the child is asked to identify the feelings of the characters, he uses his cognitive abilities to build stories that have a sequence of events and an opportunity to explore new solutions.

Multi-arts processing: Next, the mover is encouraged to first process his embodied story by depicting some aspect of it, through art-making, including drawing, painting or clay/play-dough, providing an additional way to explore and contain the emotional content. Verbal processing of the experience follows. The storyline is written down and includes a title. It is read out loud to see if anything needs to be added and to determine if it is "The End" or "To Be Continued."

Regulation and closure: Body and breath awareness activities are used both throughout the session and at the end. These actions provide emotional and physical regulation any time the patient feels the need to slow down or is overwhelmed. At the end of the session, a specific ordering of these activities creates a closing ritual to provide preparation for the transition, which can be very difficult.

Embodied countertransference

WOS also investigates and makes use of the dance therapist's embodied countertransference (Tortora, 2006, 2016). As contemplative movers dance/movement therapists are deeply sensitive to how movement dynamics create communicative discourse (Tortora, 2017). Embodied countertransference further deepens the core DMT principles of witnessing, mirroring, empathic reflection, and moving with other (Levy, 2005).

The therapist pays particular attention to her embodied presence by attending to the role her own responses play in deeply understanding the patient's journey. The terms witnessing, kinaesthetic seeing, and kinaesthetic empathy are used in WOS to describe the therapist's process. Witnessing (W) refers to immediate thoughts and images; kinaesthetic seeing (KS) refers to body reactions and experiences; and kinaesthetic empathy (KE) refers to emotional reactions (Tortora, 2006). As the layers of complexities surrounding a relationship created by transmission of trauma are opened, staying present with the mover is essential. By processing the mover's actions, story development, and dyadic interactions to analyse personal issues that arise when observing and engaging the patient, the patient's non-verbal communication becomes meaningful, guiding the therapist to make appropriate interventions. Three note keeping forms are used to process the therapist's experience (Tortora, 2006). The Daily Notes Form systematically outlines each element of the session as it unfolds providing an overview of key elements of the session. The Behavioural Descriptions Worksheet provides an in-depth analysis of the meaning of a specific action of the mover. The therapist analyzes her personal responses to a specific action or section of the session with the Interactional Behavioural Log. A salient component of the analysis is to look for movement metaphors defined as, "a specific, personally stylised nonverbal qualitative element, posture, or sequence of movements that frequently recurs within a person's repertoire" (Tortora, 2006, p. 77), and have symbolic meaning.

Co-treatment structure

Sessions occur with both the parent and child in attendance; separate sessions with the child and parent with the same therapist; and two therapists working with each member of the family individually. The separate sessions for mother and child allow them to work through their own processes in relationship to each other. Each patient has complete freedom in a non-judgmental and safe environment to express difficult feelings in ways that may not be tolerated or easy to fully express at home. The parent can engage with feelings about her child that she may not be allowing herself to experience.

The therapists hold regular meetings using three forms to discuss countertransference issues within the context of both current family dynamics and transgenerational themes. The therapists build a deeper understanding of the family and channel reflection and processing back into treatment sessions making connections through the metaphors revealed in stories and artwork.

Two case studies

At age eight, Roberto's presenting symptoms include rigid and restrictive eating; a highly energetic dysregulated movement style; argumentative behaviours, and attention issues. During the initial 2-month assessment phase of treatment the first author sees the family in both dyadic sessions and separate individual sessions.

In Eloisa's first private session she discusses wanting support to know how to provide safe food choices for Roberto. She is very restrictive with his diet due to concern that certain foods can poison him. Further inquiry leads to a lengthy discussion about her confusion and lack of trust in knowing how to feed Roberto that began in infancy. During these early stages of treatment Eloisa discusses her own eating disorder during her adolescence and young adulthood. These behaviours are linked to her extremely difficult relationship with her mother. She has guilt about how her eating disorder history affects her parenting style. She knows her experience of being parented by a very controlling mother deeply impacted her ability to read her infant's basic cues. "My mother did not confirm my feelings. She told me how I was feeling. I could not decide for myself when I was full."

Unknowingly Eloisa is doing this with Roberto evidenced in statements such as "A child can't know when he is full. Roberto can't know if he is cold and needs a coat." She counters this more controlling parenting by having difficulty setting limits, fearing Roberto might feel rejected. This is evident in her lack of clear personal boundaries observed when Roberto aggressively climbs all over her, despite her nonverbal posturing, which clearly communicates discomfort.

The concept of relational emotional regulation is discussed with the possibility that a vicarious traumatic transference has occurred through her fears with food, ultimately symbolising her desire to keeping Roberto safe. The dyadic emotional themes portray a merging between self and other and a need for individuation and self-regulation. Additional stresses due to fluctuating economic insecurity and marital pressures contribute to a chronic crisis level of stress throughout the treatment period. In Eloisa's individual treatment, embodied explorations focus on building her embodied sense of self as a capable woman and mother by uncovering how her own psychic attitudes and early experiences with her mother influence her difficulties with Roberto's food choices. The initial goals of Roberto's treatment are to provide a safe environment for him to express his anger about his mother; bring order to his chaotic, hopeless underlying psychic themes; and provide physical explorations that create somatic organisation and regulation.

Early session: Eloisa

During the check-in with the first author, Eloisa describes, "A foggy feeling in my body that is most intense in my heart and is encased everywhere, even in my hearing." This image is used to initiate her movement exploration:

> *Requesting no music, Eloisa seems to float up to standing, as the tension in her body exudes a sense of weightlessness. Her arms drift midair, subtly pushing away the air surrounding. Her eyes gazing around her without a focus, add to this feeling of density. Slowly Eloisa ends this improvisation by floating back down to the floor. Carefully wrapping her arms around her legs as she folds them into her concave torso, she encloses herself into a small ball, gently almost imperceptibly rocking as she lies on her side.*

The first author notes her embodied countertransference reactions:

> *(W) As Eloisa's arms drift up, the lightness of this action belies an inner tension. As she pushes the air around her, I am struck by an image of moving through something dense that is not letting up (KS). I find myself wanting to take a deeper breath. (W) As I do, I notice that her breath is shallow, barely perceivable in her torso (KE). I feel helpless, unsafe and alone.*

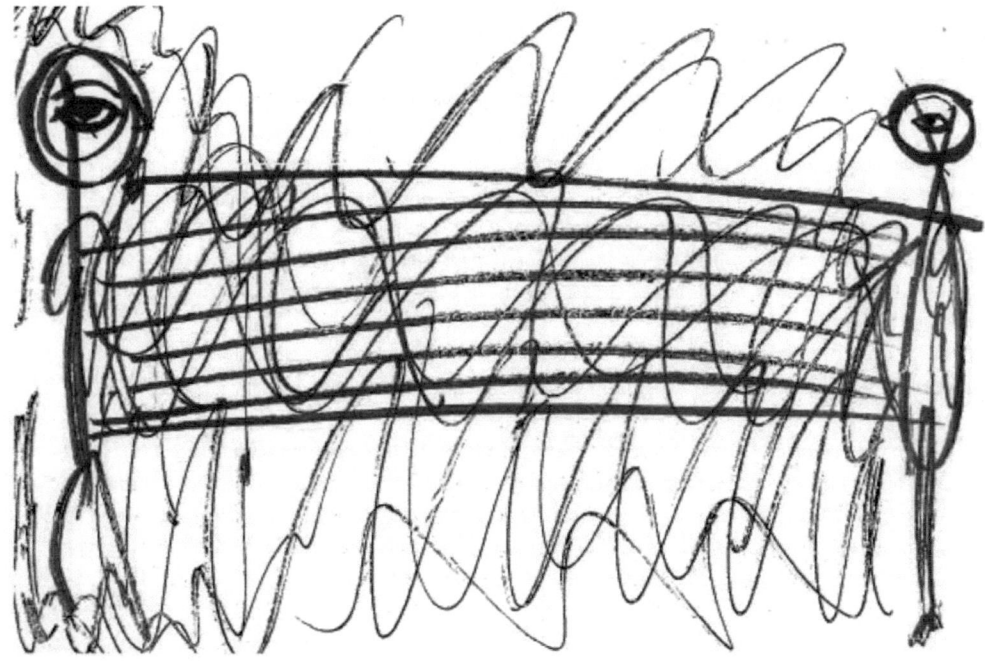

Figure 15.3 Eloisa's drawing: Gap between what I see and what I feel

Figure 15.3 shows her drawing of this experience. During her verbal processing she states, "I experienced a gap, a void between what I see and what I feel. I look into the mirror and do not get a reflection back." She relates this experiential to the lack of resonance she experienced with her mother. Connecting this familiar felt-experience to her early parental relationship is illuminating, creating a Body-Mind-Emotion (B-M-E) continuum of awareness. She longs to be seen and to have her own voice. Eloisa realises that Roberto has the same need, which has manifest through his controlling behaviours around food. She agrees to encourage Roberto to make his own decisions about food choices letting him eat as much of anything he selects, to support him to sense when he is full. Her continuing anxieties about his food consumption are processed in her sessions with the first author.

Early session: Roberto

In Roberto's early sessions his internal sense of bombardment and confusion are visible during the check-in when he creates his own feeling chart using words such as "out of control . . . weird . . . proud . . . frozen . . . deadly . . . happy . . . I feel like I am poison." His play themes are enduringly negative, aggressive, and lack hopefulness. They include very physical interactions with his mother, only restraining his aggression through his use of passive weight. After 2 months the first author refers Roberto to the second author to provide him with an opportunity to safely explore these difficult emotions.

Roberto meets her for the first time in a joint session attended by Eloisa, and both therapists. He walks in with excitement having difficulty containing his moving body. It is clear he wants to jump immediately into his story as if to show his new therapist who he is and what he is feeling emotionally. The first author provides a strong, rhythmic drumbeat for him to move in cadence with as a support for his story as it unfolds:

> *Roberto crouches his body down onto all fours like an animal on the prowl, and begins his "hunt." He uses contra-lateral movement patterns moving all around the room in this animal-like crawling position. At times, he becomes disorganized, falling into a homo-lateral movement pattern. Suddenly, he pounces forward and his body collapses onto the ground, crashing onto his abdomen, appearing to lack core support and core-distal body connections. Lying prone, he uses his limbs to creep forward slowly then quickly returns to all fours continuing his exploration and then pounces up and down again. He repeats this sequence several times, growling throughout as if he is embodying a wild animal on the prowl. The therapist and the boy appear to be in conversation as she synchronizes the drumbeat to his speeds, moving from fast into slow, then medium and into fast again.*

Roberto draws his story, narrating the storyline as follows:

> *"Grrrrr! Aowwww! Scratch! Scratch! Scratch! Hit! Hit! Hit arms flying. HHHHHHHHHH-HHgh! Hind legs up butt up wait! Low growl! Sharp Growl! Lock and veer. Predator and prey lock eyes! Prance, the predator pounces on the prey charge! The predator is growling down on the prey. Aowwwww! The Predator calls for his clan. The clan is coming. The Predator is running to a volcano to call an owl. The End."*

After the dance-play story, Roberto has difficulty regulating his body. He is unable to sit during the discussion. He eventually crawls over to Eloisa and climbs onto her. Eloisa does not establish her own body boundaries during this interaction, sitting very still without moving her limbs, which are planted tightly in her lap. Her rigid, stiff body is held with tension, as Roberto seems to be vigilantly searching for connection.

As the therapists process this session together they have an image of Roberto needing to literally be on top of his mother to feel her presence. As he flails his body around, the therapists hypothesise that he needs a boundary to push against to feel his body. There appears to be no sense of separation between them as their bodies overlap. They are physically connected but this close proximity coupled with the rigid quality of their physical contact creates a sense of discord in their co-regulated relationship.

This initial dance-play story offers a symbolic connection to his need to be the Predator on the prowl looking for Prey, or in Roberto's case, food. The movement metaphor in Roberto's actions shows the high intensity in which he feels this hunger and the feelings associated with this theme. The Predator is not safe, he cannot rest or be calm, there is potential for destruction. The story ends in unresolved action and threat; things did not work out, he stays in crisis and a fearful place.

The second author discusses her embodied countertransference during this first session:

> *(W) As I watch Roberto sitting on top of Eloisa, I think about Roberto, an 8-year-old boy still needing to feel and be in contact with his mother's body. Is he becoming too old to need this much physical contact? (KS) I feel uncomfortable in my own body, becoming tense, as I watch this. My body feels stuck. I have no room to move. (KE) As I witness Eloisa trying to not accommodate Roberto's body on top of hers through non-verbal suggestions, holding her body still and tight seeming to reject his very presence, (KS) I feel restricted in my own body. I begin to wonder if Eloisa is feeling restricted in her own body, in her own life. (KE) As I watch Roberto, trying on his experience in my own body, I feel unseen as if Mom does not experience me. I don't feel accepted, but I so much want to be. (KS) My body feels like its flying. I am trying to find someone or something to anchor me down and ground me. (W) Roberto is not being truly seen, understood, or mirrored. This dancing dialogue between Eloisa and Roberto, asks us, the witnesses in the room "Where is Mom?"*

Mid-treatment: Eloisa

Eloisa progressing, finding her voice through explorations that focus on her embodied experience of being in her body by listening deeply to and moving from somatic sensations and images that arise as she dances. As marital and financial stresses increase, Eloisa struggles to accept monetary and emotional generosity from her friends. Having difficulty taking in and receiving is a familiar dilemma for her. Eloisa explores the action of receiving through a dance improvisation.

> *Eloisa places herself in the center of the room and pauses. Slowly she reaches her right arm out in front of her in a shaping gesture – gently carefully scooping the air creating a circular gestural path back toward herself. Her left arm follows in the same manner. As she extends her arms in this way while stepping her feet firmly in front of her, Eloisa begins to take up more space. She builds her momentum reaching high and low, front, side and behind her creating curving pathways all through the room. She lifts her head high and gazes around as if seeing for the first time.*

During the discussion, she notes that her typical enclosed vertical posture keeps her separate from others. She is able to give to others but cannot receive. She connects this to her experience with anorexia, "I can't take in. I do not feel worthy. I am fearful of being judged." The therapist's words, shared with a warm smile, resonate this back, "Yes, you are not good at taking. You work so hard at giving, but you don't attune to your own needs for you judge yourself." They discuss the importance of placing herself in the centre, signifying that she matters. She states, "I am feeling my internal energy and felt-sense of being in my body as a way to find my authentic self. I can trust my body intelligence." The flowing actions depicted as curving lines outward define her positive attributes. As the symbolism of her embodied exploration is illuminated, Eloisa adds these awarenesses to her drawing: "Seeing clearly and being seen . . . having a voice about what feels authentic to me . . . I can trust these feelings . . . Beauty! Gratitude! Feel worthy. Feel good. Feel un-judged. Out of the courtroom!"

Mid-treatment: Roberto

Roberto's internal chaos manifests in cathartic embodied stories of battles between worlds, in which thunderstorms/tornados destroy everything, as he fights with dragons, giants and meteors. In their joint meeting, the second author discusses the movement metaphors in Roberto's stories. The Giant is disorganised, but strong, perhaps symbolising the parts of Roberto that are hard to accept: his anger and chaotic internal experiences. There is confusion, uncertainty, and stories are left unresolved with little peace or comfort as each session requires a high level of energy and discharge. Life appears to be in constant dysregulation and high arousal. They discuss the chronic stress at home; Eloisa's self-judgment; and parenting fears reflected in confusion about potentially poisoning Roberto through specific foods. They focus on the importance of confirming Roberto's experience of chaos while supporting his independence and resilience.

As chaos continues a therapeutic intervention to refine his regulatory capacity is prompted by an incident at school. Roberto reacts explosively when a friend takes his seat. During the check-in, Roberto uses the feeling chart to identify how he felt during and after the incident. Describing his feeling after the fight, he points to the depressed and frustrated faces. Using the Speed Spiral™, he identifies how he felt on a body/sensorial level pointing to the tip-of-pink, the super-fast speed representing out of control, He states that he started in green (medium) almost orange (fast), then went directly to pink (super-fast) as he became frustrated. Moving up and down all the colours the therapist makes sure Roberto is truly feeling each speed, verbally processing how his body transitions from each speed. Roberto brings the emotional chaos of this school incident into his story:

> *Roberto divides animals into a "weird" and "friend" pile. The "weird" pile includes cute teddy bears and stuffed toys with human-like features. The "friend" pile consists of dragons and typically evil characters, like snakes, spiders, and toys with harsher features. Throwing physio-balls up into the air, and letting them fall, Roberto explains, "This is a huge meteor shower." He throws the "meteors" onto the "weird" animal pile. As he moves from one side of the room the "meteors" bounce around and on him. The therapist, asks, "Who is attacking whom?" He declares, "It is the weird ones vs. the good ones." Asked how he wants to end the session, he states, "With a big meteor storm." They throw the balls around creating a big storm until Roberto lands on the ground in exhaustion as the story ends. He replies, "I think I need to zip-up!" referring to one of the WOS regulatory activities.*

Figure 15.4 is Roberto's drawing of the meteor storm. Relating the characters in his story to the incident at school, he says, "The meteors were about what happened. The fight felt like a meteor shower. It felt good and bad. A meteor shower happened, and the weird animals got crushed by the meteors."

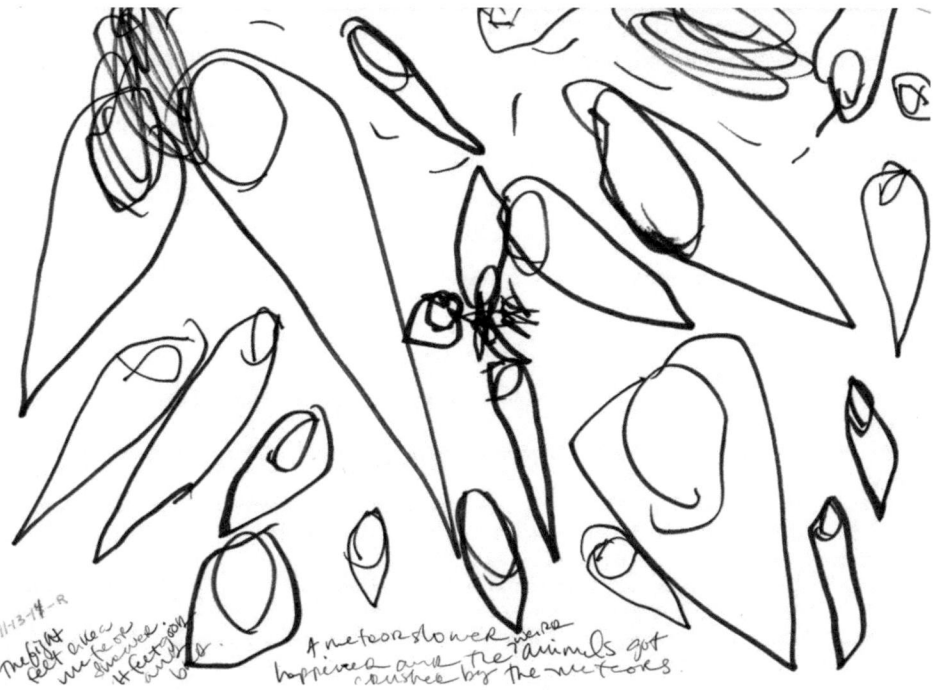

Figure 15.4 Roberto's drawing: Meteor shower

The following week, Roberto comes in with excitement stating that he has a new feeling he wants to share during the check-in. It is the feeling of "out of control, but in control," which becomes a feeling he uses and speaks about for the next year.

This session is a pivotal moment for Roberto in identifying, embodying, and internalising control over the super-fast, tip-of-pink feelings, which are the embodiment of his frustrated, aggressive and fearful emotions. The meteors are a depiction of his internal bombardment, conflict and chaotic dysregulation. Exploring his internal experience Roberto allows himself to feel his anger. As he moves through the story, from a level of dysregulation to slower speeds with more regulation, and states that he needs to "zip-up" at the end of the story, Roberto demonstrates self-regulatory capacity. Through his battles between worlds, Roberto explores good versus evil, independence, and struggles with power to combat not feeling protected.

Conclusion

Safety, a prominent theme vicariously transmitted from Eloisa to Roberto, originates in Eloisa's own parental experiences and manifests in a fearful pre-occupation with feeding her child. As Eloisa becomes more attuned to her own voice, Roberto simultaneously explores his intense feelings. Through his self-identified "out of control, but in control" state, he is embodying a new sense of understanding about himself. Roberto's growing sense of independence parallels his ability to enjoy an expanded range of foods of his choice.

The WOS co-treatment model creates a safe holding environment that supports the needs of each family member within the context of complex transgenerational transmission of family dynamics. Each therapist acts as a witness to all parts of the patient in a multifaceted session.

A transformation occurs, as the patient is able to bring implicit and unconscious material into consciousness awareness through action, art-making, verbal reflections, and verbal processing. By generating an embodied narrative, this structure organises all three components of the B-M-E continuum, creating a felt and experienced knowingness that is an essential component of therapeutic healing.

Note

1 His and her and he and she will be used interchangeably to prevent gender bias.

References

Bartenieff, I., and Lewis, D. (1980). *Body Movement: Coping with the Environment.* New York: Gordon and Breach.

Beebe, B., and Lachmann, T. (2002). *Infant Research and Adult Treatment: Co-Constructing Interaction.* Hillsdale, NJ: Analytic Press.

Braga, L., Mello, M., and Fiks, J. (2012). Transgenerational transmission of trauma and resilience: A qualitative study with Brazilian offspring of Holocaust survivors. *BMC Psychiatry, 12,* 134. Retrieved July 19, 2015, from www.biomedcentral.com/1471-244X/12/134.

Crenshaw, D. A. (2004). *Engaging Resistant Children in Therapy: Projective Drawing and Storytelling Techniques.* Rhinebeck, NY: Rhinebeck Child and Family Center Publications.

Levy, F. (2005). *Dance Movement Therapy: A Healing Art* (Rev. ed.). Reston, VA: American Alliance for Health, Physical Education, Recreating and Dance.

McCarthy, D. (2007). *"If You Turned into a Monster": Transformation Through Play: A Body-Centered Approach to Play Therapy.* Philadelphia, PA: Jessica Kingsley Publishers.

Pat-Horenczyk, R., Cohen, S., Ziv, Y., Achituv, M., Asulin-Peretz, L., and Vlanchard, T. R. (2015). Emotion regulation in mothers and young children faced with trauma. *Infant Mental Health Journal, 36*(3), 337–348.

Scheeringa, M. S., and Zeanah, C. H. (2001). A relational perspective on PTSD in early childhood. *Journal of Traumatic Stress, 14*(4), 799–815.

Sheets-Johnstone, M. (2011). *The Primacy of Movement.* Philadelphia, PA: John Benjamins.

Tortora, S. (2006) *The Dancing Dialogue: Using the Communicative Power of Movement with Young Children.* Baltimore, MD: Paul H. Brookes.

Tortora, S. (2015a). The importance of being seen – Winnicott, Dance Movement Psychotherapy and the embodied experience. In M. Spelman and F. Thomson-Salo (Eds.), *The Winnicott Tradition: Lines of Development – Evolution of Theory and Practice Over the Decades* (pp. 259–272). London: Karnac.

Tortora, S. (2015b). Mindfulness and movement. In C. Willard and A. Saltzman (Eds.), *Teaching Mindfulness Skills to Kids and Teens.* New York: Guilford.

Tortora, S. (2016). Dance movement psychotherapy in early childhood treatment and pediatric oncology. In S. Chaiklin and H. Wengrower (Eds.), *The Art and Science of Dance/Movement Therapy: Life is Dance* (pp. 159–181). New York: Routledge.

Tortora, S. (2017, Spring/Summer). Stories our bodies tell. *The American Psychoanalyst, 51*(2), 16–18, 24–25.

Winnicott, D. W. (1971). *Playing and Reality.* New York: Basic Books.

16

THE BODYMIND APPROACH AND PEOPLE AFFECTED BY MEDICALLY UNEXPLAINED SYMPTOMS/SOMATIC SYMPTOM DISORDER

Helen Payne

Introduction

This chapter outlines a new and novel clinical service in primary care in National Health Service (NHS) England for patients with persistent bodily symptoms [such as fibromyalgia, irritable bowel syndrome (IBS), chronic fatigue, chronic pain, non-cardiac chest pain, dizziness, skin conditions, etc.] for which tests and scans come back negative, termed medically unexplained symptoms (MUS). The service is based on preliminary research (Payne and Stott, 2010) and several pilots (Lin and Payne, 2014; Payne, 2014; Payne and Brooks, 2016, 2017) of delivery with positive outcomes for patients and savings to the NHS. The intervention is termed The Body-Mind Approach™ (TBMA) which employs an animated (Sheets-Johnstone, 2016) methodology emanating from dance movement psychotherapy and the recent neuroscience research (Gallese, 2011; Shore, 2012) integrating body and mind (physical and mental health).

Participants are General Physician (GP) or self-referred to 12 session groups with one-to-one meetings with the group facilitators prior to, and following, the group experience. Phase two engages patients in non-face-to-face contact over 6 months to embed their self-designed action plan based on their new perceptions following the group process. Assessments for anxiety, depression, symptom distress, functioning/activity and well-being are conducted pre, post and at six months' follow up. GP and hospital visits are monitored together with social support, employment and leisure pursuits.

The findings from the delivery of TBMA as a MUS Clinic in primary care thus far have mirrored the original research outcomes including that participants reduce in their scores for symptom distress, anxiety and depression. Furthermore, they increase in activity/functioning and well-being and were able to self-manage their symptoms far better as a result. It can be cautiously concluded that this intervention may offer a useful solution to the vast numbers of patients in primary care with MUS for whom cognitive behaviour therapy (CBT) has been rejected or tried and found unsatisfying.

Medically unexplained symptoms

MUS are a long-term condition and a global problem with very high health utilisation resulting in large costs and wastage. Patients with MUS account for an estimated 15–30 per cent of all primary care consultations (Kirmayer et al., 2004) and GPs report that these can be among the most challenging consultations they provide. Other studies in primary care show 19–50 per cent visits are for MUS (Barsky and Borus, 1995; Preveler, Kilkenny, and Kinmonth, 1997; Reid, Wessely, Crayford, and Hotopf, 2002). MUS account for a more than 20 per cent of all outpatient activity among frequent attenders (Reid et al., 2002), mainly in neurology, gastroenterology, rheumatology, cardiology, gynaecology (Burton, 2003; Hamilton, Campos, and Creed, 1996; Jackson et al., 2006; Kooiman, Bolk, Brand, Trijsburg, and Rooijmans, 2000; Nimnuan, Hotopf, and Wessely, 2001). MUS is the fourth most costly population in primary care and the costliest diagnostic category of out-patients. The cost in 2009 was over £3 billion per year rising to £18 billion if quality of life, benefits and absence from work are included (Bermingham, Cohen, Hague, and Parsonage, 2010).

There is a wide range of symptoms falling into MUS and there are no effective treatments except pain relief medication for some, and, for IBS and chronic fatigue, CBT, found to be no more effective than routine care for generic MUS (Sumathipala et al., 2008). Less than 10 per cent of MUS sufferers receive anti-depressant treatment or accept psychological therapy, leaving the majority to "learn to live with it" (as has so often been said to them) (Fink, Rosendal, and Toft, 2002; Hamilton et al., 1996; Hansen et al., 2001; Mangwana, Burlinson, and Creed, 2009). Some GPs are rather good at working with such patients, but many are not, feel frustrated and at a loss.

Consequently, the author, after noticing this large and varied population without support or hope for change, conducted a four-year research programme to explore whether an embodied group methodology might offer support for this patient population in the NHS. Subsequently, and following market research and cost effectiveness studies, a spin-out clinic from within The University of Hertfordshire was funded called Pathways2Wellbeing. This service is based on biopsychosocial and recovery models designed specifically for people with MUS, some of whom have fearful attachment and/or trauma. It is delivered as a sort of pre-therapy, starting at where the patient is, i.e. with their bodily distress. The patient's relationship with the symptom is worked with by employing practices derived from, and adapted to, this patient group. The initial focus is on creating distance between the symptom and the patient through symbolic and metaphoric practices from the arts, bodymindfulness and dance movement psychotherapy, for which the arts are a vehicle. These practices enable a strong sense of safety and holding for the unconscious, and unknown knowns about the symptom to emerge into consciousness.

It should be noted that in 2013 the DSM 5 was introduced (American Diagnostic and Statistical Manual of Mental Disorders, 2013). DSM 5 replaced somatoform disorders with a new category, Somatic Symptom Disorder (SSD), consisting of a new set of criteria including positive psychological ones. The presence of MUS is no longer a criterion for the diagnosis of an SSD. Among the reasons for this decision were patient and GP dislike of the term MUS, low inter-rater reliability and questionable validity of physicians' judgments as to whether somatic symptoms are medically explained or not (Fink, Rosendal, and Olesen, 2005) as well as the fact that many symptoms change back and forth between being considered medically explained or unexplained (Klaus et al., 2013). Therefore the "A" criteria include the presence of at least one very disabling or distressing physical symptom (explained or unexplained). The "B" criteria include several psychological features such as health anxiety (Barsky and Borus, 1995), disproportionate and persistent thoughts about one's symptoms (Verhaak, Meijer, Visser, and Wolters, 2006), and excessive time and energy devoted to these symptoms or to health concerns (Jackson and Passamonti, 2005). The indicator of severity is no longer based on the number of somatic symptoms, but on the severity of psychological features specified under the "B" criteria. The "C" criteria addresses chronicity i.e. typically a duration of symptoms of at least 6 months.

These new criteria have been criticised. They were described as clinically unhelpful (Mayou, 2014). Furthermore, they seem to cover an extremely heterogeneous group of patients (Rief and Martin, 2014). Research (Khan, Khan, Harezlak, Tu, and Kroenke, 2003) has shown that rarely are doctors incorrect with their diagnosis (0.69 per cent). The members of the DSM somatic symptoms workgroup have stated that the usefulness and reliability of the criteria remains to be determined (Dimsdale et al., 2013). Consequently, the author continues to employ the term medically unexplained symptoms.

The BodyMind Approach™

The clinic being delivered by Pathways2Wellbeing in the primary care section of the health service in England employs a research-informed group work methodology termed The BodyMind Approach™ (TBMA). It offers experiential learning through exercises involving the body bearing the symptom/s in mind. Over time participants make mindful and meaningful connections. The name arose from interviews with patients (co-researchers), in an early research study, who referred to their experience of the group process as enabling them to make significant associations between their bodies and their minds.

John Dewey (Davidson, 2004, p. 198), the philosopher, identified that deeply connected paths of knowing, where body and mind overlap, becoming entwined. Dewey termed this the "Body-Mind" (Dewey, 1998, p. 245); "it is the movement which is primary, and the sensation which is secondary, the movement of body, head and eye muscles determining the quality of what is experienced" (Dewey, 1896, p. 358). Dewey used a hyphen between the two words, joining them together to form the term Body-Mind to represent that the two are not distinct but complementary aspects. The capitalised M in Mind reminds us of the equal importance of the mind with the body and the term capitalises on the inter-relationship between the two. Body is written first in the term, as opposed to the usually written "mind-body" since it is the body which is the focus in this methodology. Through addressing the sensory experience in the lived body, the mind becomes apparent.

For the purposes of this chapter the definition of embodiment is both the recognition that cognitive processes are embedded in the brain and that the origin of these processes are in the sensory-motor experience. Acting and perceiving are therefore not understood as a physical-mental dichotomy, but as interlinked (Fuchs and de Jaegher, 2009). The lived body (i.e. the subjective body) has an impact on the mind. Conseqeuntly a focus on experiencing the sensory body and its action can be employed to help change the minds of patients.

The emphasis in TBMA is on nurturing a re-association with the body (and its symptom/s), engaging with a new perception and thus a different lived body experience. It acknowledges the interaction between the inter-corporeal aspects of the knowing body. It has a focus on the changing and always embodied present moment that allows for the experiential sensation of the symptom to be addressed in unique and novel ways. Because TBMA works directly at the site where much of the distress and damage occurs, the lived body, TBMA trained facilitators are uniquely positioned to address the embodied consequences of persistent unexplainable bodily symptoms on the patients' lived body experience. By helping patients to accept and learn from their symptom they feel empowered and less restricted in ther lives despite the symptom.

TBMA is not a cure but a methodology to help patients to learn to live well with their symptoms. Having said this, some patients do fully recover from their symptoms. TBMA employs metaphors and experiential exercises in response to negative sensory symptoms such as pain or discomfort. There is an exploration of personal values whereby goals and practices are arrived at to improve overall quality of life in an action plan that is drawn up towards the end of the course. TBMA is particularly accessible to the many MUS patients who reject CBT.

Some patients report that they cannot feel their bodies; sensations from the body are only experienced as fatigue or pain, for example (Payne, 2015, 2016). There is a lack of experiential joining of body signals with the sense of being moved by the world around them. Somatic autonomous processing of experiential content such as the quickening of the heartbeat or minimal breathing in the upper chest become isolated into somatic pathways and reported as medical symptoms. Many patients have overwhelming concerns about their somatic well-being but are frequently unable to connect this content to their current or past life situations. TBMA enables patients to explore their symptoms safely, leading to meaning-making and connections with life experience e.g. trauma/attachment issues.

TBMA reduces overall distress, as well as the patient's preoccupation with MUS, by initially teaching coping strategies, for example, progressive muscle relaxation; diaphragmatic breathing; activity regulation; kind attention to, and caring of, the body and somatic and emotional awareness increasing adaptive interpretations of the self and the world. Employing imagery and visualisation can reduce bodily tension providing a different experience of the body. Activity regulation can involve problem solving rather than avoidance or withdrawal as habitual reactions to adversity. Self-monitoring and bodymindfulness help patients increase somatic and emotional awareness. Through employing the arts – for example, mark-making, clay, creative movement and writing – patients learn to change interpretations of the self and the world (e.g. feelings of being overwhelmed, all-or-nothing attributions or catastrophising). In a facilitated group setting they also learn communication skills such as interpersonal processes and assertiveness. Personalised action plans, enacted following the group experience, arise from the new learning and psycho-education. They focus on embedding different behaviours and coping strategies which help to minimise discomfort and increase functioning despite the presence of symptoms.

TBMA facilitators nurture the development of narratives that connect somatic symptoms with psychosocial factors and where possible with past experiences and patients' cultural beliefs. Due to the complexity of medical and psychosocial presentations, it is important to help patients understand how everything fits in. The arts, through symbol and metaphor, can help patients discover new explanatory models (rather than solely the preferred physical) empowering them to embrace self-management through lifestyle changes, leisure pursuits, social activities, emotional regulation, relaxation or stress management, as well as the kindly acceptance of symptoms. Cultivating alternative narratives tailored to patients' specific symptoms and culturally-based beliefs helps alleviate the distress associated with living with the unknown; having no explanation for persistent symptoms.

The TBMA model reassures patients that their symptoms are real; diffusing the emotional charge, and helping patients feel understood and believed. The non-judgmental, accepting group culture assists patients in letting go of the tendency to feel the need to convince others of the legitimacy of their symptoms.

By addressing the subjective body experience, whereby emotion, sensory-motor-body experience, cognition, action, and perception are unified, change in self-experience, emotions and behaviour is possible and resilience is promoted. Emotion and cognition are mirrored in movement and body posture; however, they are also influenced by them (Koch and Fuchs, 2011). We can all feel in our bodies how, by expressing an emotion such as "sadness" in our posture, for example, retreating and sinking, head bowed, hands to upper body, collapsing in the chest, a change in self experience results (perhaps you, dear reader, might try this posture now to see what feelings arise). Furthermore, according to Carney, Cuddy, and Yap (2010) dominant versus submissive postures can even change testosterone levels, saliva secretion and risk-taking behaviour. Emotion and movement/posture are inextricably connected.

Embodied approaches emphasise the meaning of the sensorimotor experience for cognition, affect, and interaction, operating at the centre of emotional processing and self-regulation. Somatic sensations can become a vehicle for an unknown/unconscious or nonconscious attitude, trauma, or affect that has become detached from its motivational context (Sass, 2000). The consequence is that the patient is incapable of making sense of felt emotions as well as adequately expressing or following them; subsequently, somatic symptom/s can emerge as a replacement for this expression. By integrating sensory and emotional awareness through corporeal practices, the range of affect, communicative and expressive behaviours can be expanded, and symptoms explored safely.

TBMA integrates embodied approaches with mindfulness and behaviour change strategies, offering a distinctly flexible and versatile intervention appealing to the whole person, including physical etc. i.e. the cognitive, physical/kinaesthetic, sensory and emotional aspects. Consequently, it can reach a wide range of patients and facilitators. By directing kind attention and mindfulness to the body and its connection to the self, practices in TBMA meet the symptom distress to change the subjective relationship with the symptom/body. The facilitated group setting promotes social attention and the group interactive practices encourage attention towards the bodily mediated emotions of others and their impact on the self.

Typical profile of a patient suffering medically unexplained symptoms

Ms G is a 45-year-old woman, married, and is a mother of two. She formerly worked as a teaching assistant and is now on disability benefits. She initially presented six years previously with abdominal pain located in the right upper quadrant, gradual in onset, very severe in intensity, aching in character and non-radiating. The pain was constant temporally with no remissions. She rated the pain as 10/10 at its worst and 7/10 on average. During the first visit, no aggravating, relieving or precipitating factors were identified. Her abdominal pain was associated with mild headache aggravated by stress. There was no history of appetite or weight loss, dyspepsia or alcohol abuse. Ms G had undergone appendectomy for acute abdominal pain 10 years ago with little long-term relief. In the last 2 years she had referrals to two gastroenterologists; both reported negative findings after extensive investigations.

Ms G was not relieved by these findings and continued to be very distressed during GP visits. She complains of unwavering pain and how overwhelmed she feels with trying to manage her health and care for her family. Although she appears to experience some relief with reassurances that "there is nothing wrong with her physically" and even leaves some visits with a sense of boosted self-efficacy and optimism, she deteriorates during visits to the point of crying uncontrollably. Worrying statements such as, "I can't take this anymore. I don't know how I can go on living like this," result in the GP having to "talk her down from the ledge." It feels like nothing helps her in the long run.

The frequent visits to the GP often end with adjustments to medication or an agreement to discuss the value of continued investigations, imaging and medical procedures. The GP breathes a sigh of relief each time she leaves but doubts the effectiveness of any agreed treatment or investigation.

The GP is concerned about Ms G's mental health and believes there is a connection between her anxiety, frustration and somatic symptoms. Ms G though vacillates on stress as a factor in the exacerbation and maintenance of her abdominal pain. She refuses referrals to psychological services, and since there is no pending psychiatric risk the GP has not insisted. Eventually, after 6 years the GP invites Ms G to consider a Pathways2Wellbeing group course for people suffering persistent physical symptoms for which tests and scans come back negative. She reassures Ms G that others have enjoyed the courses and found them beneficial so asks her "why not give it a try?" She asks lots of questions to which the GP can respond with reassuring answers. At last she agrees to follow through with this referral.

Ms G was given the leaflet about Pathways2Wellbeing, advertising the course, by her doctor. The doctor suggested she might try this clinic in the meantime. She came to her first individual meeting saying that she felt desperate and wanted to try this group as she thought it was something different from what she had been offered so far by the NHS. In the group from the very first session she showed a willingness to engage in whatever she was asked to do, although she found it a little challenging in view of her continuous abdominal pain. She missed two sessions out of 12 (Sessions 3 and 5); in both cases she was in too much pain to be able to attend. However, in each attended session she showed an interest in others. She found it useful talking about her pain and also to listen to others sharing about their difficulty to cope with their painful body, their surrendering attitude, not being listened to properly and not being understood. These were common themes, participants were listened to well and could share their struggles in dealing with pain as they felt understood without judgment.

During the group process Ms G was invited by her facilitator to be kinder to herself, as, in her language there was a derogatory regard towards herself. In session six she announced to the group that she was "a wonderful person." It meant a lot for her to say this to her group without feeling judged. She told the group that she was repeating this to herself and that it was convincing, she started to believe it. There was no self-blaming and no self-denigrating anymore. She told the group that she was starting to see her depression lifting. In the group, during the body movement practices she had the most sensitive perception and was able to capture in another person's movement, something about them. She started trusting herself more and her self-esteem visibly increased.

Week after week she was telling the group how she was much more relaxed, understanding and compassionate about her condition. Her emotional pain seemed to be located in her stomach; her voice was broken as she was talking but the awareness of her tension in her stomach seemed to soften her muscles and she felt better. All this took place in only ten sessions.

At the exit meeting she said that at the beginning of the course she did not know what to expect, was fearful and resistant and felt really down. The group helped her to feel less isolated, she learnt how to make use of the optimal diaphragmatic breathing that she had practiced in the group and this had helped to ease the pain in her abdomen for quite some time. She also learnt that the body movement helps to release her tension and lift her mood.

Individual monitoring

Data was collected the week before the group began, the week after it ended and at 6 months follow-up. The following tools were employed to collect the data at these time points:

Measure yourself medical outcome profile scores (MYMOP2)

The MYMOP (Measure Yourself Medical Outcome Profile)2 is an individualised patient rated outcome questionnaire. It is problem-specific and measures two symptoms chosen by the patient. It also includes general well-being and impact of symptoms on a chosen activity. The greater the score, the more severe the symptoms are.

Primary healthcare depression scale (PHQ 9)

This is a client rated tool for depression. It scores each of the 9 depression DSM-IV criteria as "0" (not at all) to "3" (nearly every day). Depression severity is graded based on the PHQ-9 score 0–4 none; 5–9 mild; 10–14 moderate; 15–19 moderately severe; 20–27 severe.

Generalised anxiety disorder (GAD 7)

This is a client rated measure for assessing generalised anxiety disorder on a 7-item self-rating scale. It scores each item as "0" (not at all) to "3" (nearly every day) for each item. Severity of generalised anxiety is graded based on the GAD 7 score 0–4 none; 5–9 mild; 10–14 moderate; 15–21 severe.

The global assessment of functioning scale (GAF)

This is a clinician rating tool used to measure overall level of psychological, social and occupational client functioning on a scale ranging from 1 to 100. The higher the score, the higher the level of functioning there is. GAF covers the range from positive mental health to severe psychopathology.

Further data is collected via a tailor-made questionnaire

For this patient her perceived social support pre-course was satisfactory; post course it was good. She continued with medication pre and post course.

With reference to psychological insight Question 1 asks "Do you believe the way you think and feel can affect your physical symptoms?". Question 2 asks "Do you believe that your physical symptoms can affect the way you think and feel?". A strong belief in the mind body connection was evident at post course and follow up.

Her individual monitoring is shown in Table 16.1:

Table 16.1 To show comparison of pre to post course outcomes for this patient

Measurement tool	Pre course	Post course
MYMOP2 Wellbeing	4	4
MYMOP2 Activity	5	3
MYMOP2 Overall	5	4.2
MYMOP2 Symptom distress	Pain 5	4
PHQ-9	12	10
GAD7	6	1
GAF	62	70

From the scores it appears that Ms. G has increased her activity from pre- to post course, as well as her general functioning levels. This ties in with her perceived social support being better at post course than at pre-course. This may be as a result of feeling a sense of belonging in the group thus reducing her isolation. Feeling less anxious and depressed might be due to being able to endure or tolerate both, or to their decrease post course when compared to pre course. It is interesting that she has a much stronger belief in the connection between mind and body following the course experience as compared with her belief before the course began. Despite her well-being score remaining the same level pre- to post course there is an indication that the pain has reduced, and overall MYMOP scores reduced slightly.

Conclusion

There is some evidence that TBMA applied as group work in primary care for people affected by medically unexplained symptoms, albeit with small numbers so far, can be an effective way to help people self-care and live well with their symptoms. By gaining an understanding and self-compassion within a supportive group environment it seems this new perspective changes their way of being with their symptoms. There is more to be done to evidence the methodology however an encouraging start has been made.

Acknowledgements

Appreciation goes to the participants, the team at Pathways2Wellbeing and to the University of Hertfordshire for the support they have provided.

References

American Psychiatric Association. (2013). *Diagnostic and Statistical Manual of Mental Disorders*. Washington, DC: American Psychiatric Publishing.

Barsky, A., and Borus, J. (1995). Somatization and medicalization in the era of managed care. *Journal of the American Medical Association, 274*(24), 1931–1934.

Bermingham, S., Cohen, A., Hague, J., and Parsonage, M. (2010). The cost of somatisation among the working-age population in England for 2008–09. *Mental Health in Family Medicine, 7*, 71–84.

Burton, C. (2003). Beyond somatisation: A review of the understanding and treatment of medically unexplained physical symptoms (MUPS). *British Journal of General Practice, 53*(488), 231–239.

Carney, D. R., Cuddy, A. J. C., and Yap, A. J. (2010). Power posing: Brief nonverbal displays affect neuroendocrine levels and risk tolerance. *Psychological Science, 21*, 1363–1368.

Davidson, D. (2004). *Problems of Rationality*. New York: Oxford University Press.

Dewey, J. (1896). The reflex arc concept in psychology. *Psychological Review, 3*, 357–370.

Dewey, J (1998). *Experience and Nature* (pp. 248–298), Chicago, Ill: Dover Publications Ltd.

Dimsdale, J. E., Creed, F., Escobar, J., Sharpe, M., Wulsin, L., Barsky, A., . . . Levenson, J. (2013). Somatic symptom disorder: An important change in DSM. *Psychosomatic Research, 75*(3), 223–228.

Fink, P., Rosendal, M., and Toft, T. (2002). Assessment and treatment of functional disorders in general practice: The extended reattribution and management model – An advanced program for non-psychiatric doctors. *Psychosomatics, 43*(2), 93–131.

Fink, P., Rosendal, M., and Olesen, F. (2005). Classification of somatization and functional somatic symptoms in primary care. *Australia and New Zealand Journal of Psychiatry, 39*(9), 772–781.

Fuchs, T and de Jaegher, H. (2009). Enactive intersubjectivity: Participatory sense-making and mutual incorporation. *Phenomenology and the Cognitive Sciences, 8*, 4, 465–486.

Gallese, V. (2011). Neuroscience and phenomenology. *Phenomenology and Mind, 1*, 33–48.

Hamilton, J., Campos, R., and Creed, F. (1996). Anxiety, depression and management of medically unexplained symptoms in medical clinics. *Journal of the Royal College of Physicians of London, 30*, 18–20.

Hansen, M. S., Fink, P., Frydenberg, M., Oxhoj, M. L., Sondergaard, L., and Munk-Jorgensen, P. (2001). Mental disorders among internal medical inpatients: Prevalence, detection and treatment status. *Psychosomatic Research, 50*(4), 169–204.

Jackson, J. L., and Passamonti, M. (2005). The outcomes among patients presenting in primary care with a physical symptom at 5 years. *General International Medicine, 20*(11), 1032–1037.

Jackson, J., Fiddler, M., Kapor, N., Wells, A., Tomenson, B., and Creed, F. (2006). Number of bodily symptoms predicts outcome more accurately than health anxiety in patients attending neurology, cardiology and gastroenterology clinics. *Psychosomatic Research, 60*(4), 357–363.

Khan, A. A., Khan, A., Harezlak, J., Tu, W., and Kroenke, K. (2003). Somatic symptoms in primary care: Aetiology and outcome. *Psychosomatics, 44*, 471–478.

Kirmayer L. J., Groleau D., Looper K. J., and Dao M. D. (2004). Explaining medically unexplained symptoms. *Can J Psychiatry.* Oct, *49*(10), 663–672.

Koch, S. C., and Fuchs, T. (2011). Embodied arts therapies. *Arts in Psychotherapy, 38*, 276–280.

Kooiman, C. G., Bolk, J. H., Brand, R., Trijsburg, R. W., and Rooijmans, H. G. M. (2000). Is alexithymia a risk factor for unexplained physical symptoms in general medical outpatients? *Psychosomatic Medicine, 62*, 768–778.

Klaus, K., Rief, W., Brähler, E., Martin, A., Glaesmer, H., and Mewes, R. (2013). The distinction between "medically unexplained" and "medically explained" in the context of somatoform disorders. *International Journal of Behavioral Medicine, 20*, 161–171.

Lin, Y., and Payne, H. (2014). The BodyMind Approach™, medically unexplained symptoms and personal construct psychology. *Body, Movement and Dance in Psychotherapy, 9*, 3.

Mangwana, S., Burlinson, S., and Creed, F. (2009). Medically unexplained symptoms presenting at secondary care – A comparison of white Europeans and people of South Asian ethnicity. *Psychiatry in Medicine, 39*(1), 33–44.

Mayou, R. (2014). Is the DSM-5 chapter on somatic symptom disorder any better than DSM-IV somatoform disorder? *British Journal of Psychiatry, 204*(6), 418–419.

Nimnuan, C., Hotopf, M., and Wessely, S. (2001). Medically unexplained symptoms – An epidemiological study in seven specialities. *Psychosomatic Research, 51*(1), 361–367.

Payne, H., and Stott, D. (2010). Change in the moving bodymind: Quantitative results from a pilot study on the BodyMind Approach (BMA) as groupwork for patients with medically unexplained symptoms (MUS). *Counselling and Psychotherapy Research, 10*(4), 295–307.

Payne, H. (2014). The BodyMind approach™: The treatment of people with medically unexplained symptoms. *The Psychotherapist,* Summer (57), 30–32.

Payne, H. (2015). The body speaks its mind: The BodyMind approach™ for patients with medically unexplained symptoms in UK primary care. *Arts in Psychotherapy, 42*, 19–27.

Payne, H. (2016). The BodyMind approach™. *Healthcare, Counselling and Psychotherapy Journal, 16*(4), 14–18. (British Association for Counselling and Psychotherapy).

Payne, H., and Brooks, S. (2016). Clinical outcomes and cost benefits from The BodyMind Approach™ for patients with medically unexplained symptoms in primary healthcare in England: Practice-Based Evidence. *Arts in Psychotherapy, 47*, 55–65.

Preveler, R., Kilkenny, L., and Kinmonth, A. L. (1997). Medically unexplained physical symptoms in primary care: A comparison of self-report screening questionnaires and clinical opinion. *Psychosomatic Research, 42*, 245–252.

Reid, S., Wessely, S., Crayford, T., and Hotopf, M. (2002). Frequent attenders with medically unexplained symptoms: Service use and costs in secondary care. *British Journal of Psychiatry, 180*, 248–253.

Rief, W., and Martin, A. (2014). How to use the new DSM-5 somatic symptom disorder diagnosis in research and practice: A critical evaluation and a proposal for modifications. *Annual Review of Clinical Psychology, 10*, 339–367.

Sass, L. A. (2000). Schizophrenia, self-experience, and so-called "negative symptoms" reflections on hyper-reflexivity. In D. Zahavi (Ed.), *Exploring the Self: Philosophical and Psychopathological Perspectives on Self-Experience* (pp. 149–182). Amsterdam: John Benjamins.

Sheets-Johnstone, M. (2016). *Insides and Outsides. Interdisciplinary Perspectives on Animate Nature.* Exeter, UK: Imprint Academic.

Shore, A. (2012). *Norton Series on Interpersonal Neurobiology: The Science of the Art of Psychotherapy.* New York: W.W. Norton.

Sumathipala, A., Siribaddana, S., Abeysingha, M. R. N., de Silve, P., Dewey, M., Prince, M., and Mann, A. H. (2008). Cognitive-behaviour therapy v. structured care for medically unexplained symptoms: Randomized controlled trail. *The British Journal of Psychiatry, 193*, 51–59.

Verhaak, P. F. M., Meijer, S. A., Visser, A. P., and Wolters, G. (2006). Persistent presentation of medically unexplained symptoms in general practice. *Family Practice, 23*(4), 414–420.

17

THE DISTURBANCE OF THE PSYCHOSOMATIC BALANCE

Haguit Ehrenfreund

Introduction

Dance Movement Psychotherapy (DMP) was institutionalized as a therapeutic discipline in 1966 in the USA. Its particularity is in the focus on body movement as a way of enlarging the emotional repertory, treating the body and the mind simultaneously. Movement patterns give the therapist the possibility of learning the patient's history, and the way he expresses himself in the world (Chaiklin, 1975a; Chaiklin and Wengrower, 2009; Schoop and Mitchell, 1974).

In DMP it is considered that physical behavior reflects emotional states (Fuchs and Koch, 2014; Shahar-Levy, 2004). Changing the patterns of movement can lead to the mobilization of psychic forces. For that reason, the focus is on returning to somatic reality, and awakening the initial source of the psychic experiences. Emotional-movement is employed, also named dance-movement, aiming to harmonize the body and mind relationship when disturbed by mental disorders (Bartenieff and Lewis, 1980; Chace, 1953; Fischman, 2009; Schoop, 1978).

This chapter aims to theorize (meta-theory) the disturbance of the psychosomatic unity as a disorder of the body-mind relation. Medicine uses the term psychosomatic to designate psychic disorders manifesting in the body, when there is no organic cause. In the last years the term 'psychosomatic' was replaced with 'medically unexplained symptoms' and more recently with 'somatic symptom disorder' in DSM-5. However, the conception of that term relies on the inter-relation between psychic processes and somatic processes. The word 'psychosomatic' is engaged in this chapter to remind readers of its psychodynamic orientation. When the concept of imbalance of the psychosomatic identity is used in this chapter, always to be heard as a disturbance of the body-mind relation, the author arises to it as an emotional disorder.

This pathological state means that as long as the correlation (cause and effect) between the body and the thinking process is not invested by an emotion (an affect), the patient cannot form a representation of their own psychosomatic self (Chemouni, 2000; Marty, M'Uzan, and David, 1963; Sami-Ali, 1977; Stora, 1999). In fact, it is through the action of the body, movement and the emotions that this process arises, and that it becomes possible for the patient to recognize the connection between body, emotion and speech. Once this process is accomplished, the patient is capable of naming and feeling, which in the absence of words, was kept out of consciousness (McDougall, 1989). For certain patients the transition via the body and its movement is a necessary step, in order to reach a conscious psychological organization of their life experiences.

We have observed the disturbance of the psychosomatic balance in our practice with different patients, suffering from diverse psychopathologies. In this chapter the pathology will be analyzed relying on psychoanalytical theories of mental pathologies, using Freudian concepts to build a hypothesis of psychosomatic disorder. The discourse of patients suffering from eating disorders will be exposed to enlighten the clinical consequences, because the disturbance of their psycho-somatic identity is particularly clear.

This procedure should enable us to theorize as to the disturbance of psychosomatic balance as a pathology of the body-mind relation, and to conceptualize dance-movement psychotherapy as a psychosomatically informed discipline. The chapter will start by presenting the uniqueness of the DMP discipline and its therapeutic use of movement, to follow with a meta-psychological description of body expression that will serve to ground the concept of psychosomatic identity. The consequences of psychosomatic imbalance will be discussed, illustrated by the discourse of patients suffering from eating disorders. Finally, the author will outline her therapeutic approach and a technique for body-mind awareness: body cartography.

'It is not gymnastics, it is an awareness process' (Bejart, 2001, p. 20). At the beginning of the twentieth century a revolution took place in the art of dance. The emphasis was turned from the technical performance of movement as a form of emotional expression (Bartenieff and Lewis, 1980; Chaiklin and Wengrower, 2009; De Mille, 1963). Dancers participate in the revolution. The message that those artists bring to the world relates to the importance of body expression, to the freedom of emotional expression, and the place of the individual in society. The leading dancers of this period are Isadora Duncan (1878–1927) in the USA; Mary Wigman (1886–1973) in Germany, one of the pioneers of expressive dance; Rudolf Laban (1879–1957) the initiator of the Labanotation system (Laban, 1956, 1960; Laban and Laurence, 1974); Maurice Bejart (1927–2007) in Europe whose writings speak of philosophy through the interpretation of the dancer's place in society (Bejart, 1982, 1994, 1998, 2001); and Martha Graham (1894–1991) in the USA, whose choreographies and teachings remain relevant today (Graham, 1973, 1992). It is in that historical, artistic and social context that dance-movement therapy emerges. The pioneers of DMT in the USA, Marian Chace (1898–1970), Mary Whitehouse (1911–1979), Trudi Schoop (1903–1999), Blanche Evan (1909–1982) and Irmgard Bartenieff (1900–1981), were all accomplished dancers.

The body-mind relation, the role of emotions, the need for expression and the place of dance in society were the impulses for those dancers to use movement as a psychotherapeutic tool (Levy, 1992). Each of them developed their therapeutic approach and working tools, which form the base of dance-movement psychotherapy today. The dancers that followed have developed train-ing programmes in order to teach and systematize this new form of therapy. (Chaiklin, 1975b; Chodorow, 1991; Adler, 2002; Lewis, 1986; Shahar-Levy, 2004). This has led to the publication of clinical cases and exchanges among practitioners that raised new questions. And so, it was left to the third generation, to which this author belongs, to conceptualize the meta-theory. This chapter belongs to that effort of theorizing.

Dance movement: Its therapeutic use

In a dance movement therapy session, speech is not the privileged tool, which does not mean that it is not present. Movement allows the patient's memories to rise from the unconscious and join the present (Adler, 1999; Chodorow, 1999; Whitehouse, 1970, 1999). Dance-movement is a process of free emotional association on the psychosomatic level, in the sense of a body-mind process. The transference occurs on the body-movement level between the patient and the therapist (Gallagher and Payne, 2015; Whitehouse, 1999). At a certain point of the session, in order for the free emotional association to pass from sensual–gesture energy to speech, a process of mental consciousness is needed (Adler, 2002; Chodorow, 1991). This transition structures the physical experience in verbal language and permits the appropriation and elaboration of the contents experienced. When the physical expression is broadened, the gestural expression and the verbal expression integrate and complete each other (Modlingere, 1997).

This psychotherapeutic approach is especially precious when we work with patients suffering from mental or psychosomatic disorders. In these kinds of pathologies, the body becomes the speaker for the psychological apparatus, and sometimes the principle form of expression, communication and learning (Stora, 1999). The physical-gestural language operates as the moderator between body, emotion and thought, allowing the patient to find a body–mind balance (Fischman, 2009; Payne, 2009). This method requires the therapist have knowledge of the body, of movement and of psychopathology. It also requires the capacity to stay tuned to the body–mind relation through movement. Furthermore, it is recommended that the therapist is trained to employ other body disciplines such as yoga, dance styles, relaxation, etc. These conditions restrict the number of persons qualified to practice this discipline. For dancers drawn by the understanding of the psyche and the desire to be a therapist, this method presents unique possibilities.

The body is a physical-emotional-psyche space. Movement actively expresses the needs and drives of the person. Thus, creating a dialogue with the environment. Cognitive science has started to recognize the importance of the interaction brain-body-environment. The principal idea of embodying meaning is that mental process is embodied in physical activity and embedded in the environment (Lakoff and Johnson, 1999; Thompson and Varela, 2001). In DMP we consider that every exchange between two persons implicates an embodied process, through posture, gesture, facial expression or any other physical expression and reaction (Fuchs and Koch, 2014; Gallagher and Payne, 2015). As described by Freud in his early work, every psychic state and every mental process has an affective component and are all accompanied by a physical manifestation and the capacity to modify the somatic process (Freud, 1980).

Our body is a moving body, whose language is structured by physiological rules (nature) and psychological representations. Movement is a repertoire, a language that tells us how the individual apprehends the world, and the way he manages his internal forces (Bartenieff and Lewis, 1980; Dychtwald, 1986). One of the principal advantages of working with the body is the possibility of expanding the repertoire of physical and emotional expression (Chace, 1953; Chaiklin, 1975a). The ability to release muscular tensions while conserving the body forces softens the physical and psychological efforts that life requires (Bartenieff and Lewis, 1980; Shahar-Levy, 2004).

When body and speech is approached through danced-movement, the capacity of the individual to express himself in harmony is exploited: body-emotion-mind (Chodorow, 1991; Ne'eman and Bartal, 1992). This reconciliation meets the patient's need for holistic expression, engaging her/his entire being, and offers her/him a tool for acting by, and in her/himself. The body is then conceived of as not only an extraordinary machine, or a way of communicating with others, but also as a way of enabling the patient to recover his or her psychosomatic balance.

Meta-psychology of movement

Sigmund Freud proposed speech as the method of treatment because of its capacity to provoke psychological modifications (Freud, 1980). The psychoanalytic method concentrates on delivering repressed psychological content to consciousness through speech and the process of free association (Freud, 1920/1981). Helping the patient create the link between her/his memories and her/his present relations and behaviors helps her/him redraw his history and prepares her/him for new life choices which are more conscious and more adaptive (Freud, 1937/1985; Hoffmann, 2008).

DMP proposes movement as a method of treatment because of its capacity to restore balance on the psychosomatic level. It concentrates on investing body action, and the patient's communication with emotion (Chace, 1953; Fischman, 2009; Schoop, 1978). Helping the patient restore her/his psychosomatic identity, considered to be the body-mind balance, gives an emotional color to her/his gestural choices and reinforces her/his self-esteem and body image. The transition from an improvised unconscious movement to conscious movement invested with affect improves her/his kinesthetic sense and her/his capacity for making the link between movement, emotion and thinking.

Body movement is conceived of as an emotional process, therefore it is possible for us to discuss it in terms of a meta-psychology. It is proposed that it is possible to equate Freudian meta-psychology, meaning the dynamic, the topic, and the economics of psychological process (Freud, 1915/2008b), with this conception of movement. Body movement can be discussed on the levels of: gesture, organization, and flow. A meta-psychological presentation of movement would mean describing the flow of movement, to put it differently: the physical patterns, in terms of emotional fluidity and complexity. Discussing movement as a psychological act in that perspective would mean observing body movement as an organized flow system, with non-movement indicating unconscious repressed conflicted content, while fluidity indicates free expression of the emotional self.

Free movement is created by a harmonious coordination of the limbs, in their variety of action, toward a rhythm of contraction and relaxation (Graham, 1992). Such a movement is fluid and peaceful, does not suffer from any obstruction, and is economical in terms of energy. It also allows gathering forces operating with speed and precision when such are needed (Humphrey, 1959/1992). Through such knowledge of the body and its movement, the person acquires a sensation of self and space control. They can recognize the possibilities of change directly or indirectly, feel comfortable with that sensation and use it openly for meeting needs and self-expression. This physical coordination is based on the perception of the body structure, of its weight, of space and time. It enables one to choose the best support points to keep one's balance: a balance that is the key to body management (Graham, 1992). In fact, an imbalanced movement creates muscular tension and discomfort resulting from effort, psychical as well as physical. As a consequence, the capacity to liberate the limbs that do not participate in the action, to be able to choose the best considered movement for the task, avoiding surplus effort and conserving the body forces, softens the psychic effort that physical expression requires. Moreover, it allows for an adjustment of movement to the emotional rhythm of the personality.

An obstruction in movement signifies a blockage in the body action fluidity, or a blockage of emotional expression. This interception is an indication of an unexpressed conflict that prevents movement from accomplishing the act of discharge, followed by relaxation (Schoop and Mitchell, 1974; Shahar-Levy, 2004). Around each obstruction muscular-emotional tension is created that accompanies the contraction of the physical zone. This constant contraction creates pain that the person will try to avoid by repressing the emotion, and by establishing diverted gestural courses that will become movement habits (Shahar-Levy, 2004). The result of this defense mechanism, psychic as well as physical, is the development of what we name a 'dead zone'. This part of the body, which is not integrated into the gestural vocabulary of the person, is a landmark on the map of the body. The uncomfortable or painful sensation felt by the patient, when one of these obstructions is evoked during a DMP session, reconnects the emotion to the body, awakens the memory, and offers the patient the possibility of perceiving his needs and emotions through movement and speech (Fischman, 2009).

The psychosomatic identity

When Freud (1915/2008b) presented his hypothesis of the unconscious, modern psychotherapy was born, and a treatment method for some mental disorders became possible. Freud postulated that psychic processes are all unconscious. The representations, the affects and the drives of the psyche are only partially known by the individual. In order for a representation to become the object of consciousness, it needs to be invested by the word that represents it. Hence, a conscious knowledge is formed in the mind, to put it differently: a thinking process is constituted. The link between the conscious representation invested by words and unconscious memories is activated during psychoanalytical therapy by the discourse of the patient (Freud, 1915/2008b).

In dance movement psychotherapy, we use the term subjective link (Chodorow, 1999) after to refer to the perception of our own body formed by the sensation of movement. Subjective link is formed and is used to form the identity of the patient affected by pathology.

Freud enlightened us as to the development of identity, beginning with the perception of the difference between external and internal via muscular activity (Freud, 1915/2008b). When this separation (external and internal body) is not affected by pathological reasons, the difference between physiological stimulations and drive stimulations does not exist. The consequence of that interrupted process is the disturbance of the patient's identity on the psychosomatic level (Marty, M'Uzan, and David, 1963; Sami-Ali, 1987). In those cases, introducing movement in the therapeutic process enables this separation, and begins to construct the psychosomatic unity. In order for the process of separation and unification to take place, the subjective link between the body and the psychic process (the mind) has to be perceived, so it can become an object of consciousness. The perception of 'my body' needs to be attached to a representation and a sensation for it to become an identity. Because dance-movement psychotherapy uses body movement and the emotions this process awakens, it is the most direct method to restore psychosomatic balance and treat psychosomatic identity disorder.

The hypothesis of the unconscious developed by Freud brings an additional element to the understanding of the psychosomatic imbalance. The destiny of affect after repression can take one of three courses: being repressed without leaving any trace, manifesting as another emotion, or transforming into anxiety (Freud, 1915/2008a; Marty, M'Uzan, and David, 1963; McDougall, 1989). The body movement awakens the unconscious content and gives it the drive strength to become conscious.

Through the use of movement the representation is reinvested with an emotion and the somatic force due to the movement impulse. The body action allows the affect (the emotion) to develop, while the subjective link between the body movement and the revealed emotion brings the memory back to the surface. When the source of the experience was not verbalized, because of the pathology or because the event happened in an early stage, the transition through the body becomes necessary in order to be transformed into words.

The disorder of the psychosomatic balance

The key function of the psychic apparatus, using its specific mechanisms, is to keep the individual at the lowest level of tension. Pleasure, through this psychic logic, is the satisfaction resulting from the reduction of inner tension. Displeasure corresponds to the increase of the level of tension, which usually indicates the possibility of danger (Freud, 1920/1981). In certain pathological conditions, pleasure is obtained by the sensation of body contraction (high tension) (Chemouni, 2000; Sami-Ali, 1977; Stora, 1999). In this case, this contraction that we can also call pain, connects the person to his body. Keeping the tension high and increasing the contraction becomes the emotional and physical structure of the psychopathology. The scene of psychic conflict is transferred to the body, which becomes the enemy. Examples of this psychic functioning in patients suffering from unexplained headache, back pain, non-cardiac chest pain or severe eating disorders (Chemouni, 2000; Payne, 2009; Stora, 1999). Working with movement, reconnecting the body to an emotional reality, liberating the tension due to the restricted movement, are all part of dance-movement psychotherapy tools. Bringing sensations back to the body allows the patient to restart the psychosomatic balancing. The emotional experience of the body in movement helps patients to restructure their body image, and revives the psychosomatic identity.

Clinical examples: Patients with an eating disorder

In the case of eating disorders (anorexia, bulimia), it can be observed how the psychosomatic identity can cause an emotional split between the body and the mind. Words of the patients, when asked to complete the sentence 'I am a body . . .' at the beginning of a dance-movement psychotherapy session include: 'I am a mute body', 'I am a body without space, a body that doesn't belong', 'I am a body ball (and chain), heavy, captive', 'I am a miserable body, we should split', 'I am a body unfortunately', 'I am not a body', 'I am a tormented spirit', 'I have suffered too much, and it makes the persons close to me suffer', 'Why won't it die, this body?'.

When asked about the body and mind relationship they answer: 'In me it's the mind criticizing the body instead of them supporting each other', 'I would like to be able to make the connection between the cause, the feeling of stress and my eating behavior, but it has been so long, so it is necessary to go back at the beginning, go untie the knots and find the source', 'I am a very sensible person, and I have difficulty holding it all back and feeling, that is why I digress and cut out the emotions', 'The body is intelligent, but in daily life I don't let it talk, I don't let it act', 'Most of the time I feel like the body does not exist' and 'I am a mind without body'.

By working with movement with this population the aim is to reinvest each part of the body with sensation and emotion, in order to reach the psychosomatic balance that was disturbed by the absence of emotional mediators. Through the emotional-movement experience, patients can find again the affective level of speech, and the capacity of expression and sensation of the body. When they are asked at the end of the session to complete the same sentence 'I am a body . . .', the answers are the following: 'I am a calmed body'; 'I am a living body'; 'I am a body that needs sun'; 'I am a wise body'; 'I am a good body'; 'I am a present body'; 'I am an extended body'; 'I am a moving body'.

With such patients in order to reconnect with the psychosomatic self and wake the power of healing, they need to develop a representation of the body-mind relationship and restart the capacity to hear the body messages. Experiencing pleasure in their contracted body, being able to recognize different emotional states, and not fearing the felt body sensations, can transform the perception of the body. Contrary to what is often assumed, working with the body in movement does not bring the patient into an overexcited emotional state, nor does it risk driving them into a psychologically decompensated state. On the contrary, it allows them to reach a calmer state due to the discharge of exaggerated tension, and to the expression of the repressed emotions. The clinical illustration confirms that for certain patients the transition via the body and its movement is necessary in order to find an emotional continuity between body sensations and thoughts processes.

Body cartography

There follows a description of the author's therapeutic approach to the body-mind awareness process. Mapping the body is a procedure aiming to guide the patient into an intermediary state between relaxation and tension. The objective of this process is to eliminate excessive tension, in order to open the channel to a physical sensational-emotional receptiveness, and active expression (meaning emotional movement). The body cartography is an adaptation of warm-up exercise in dance practice, to guide a process of body-mind awareness. This will include: placing the body in space, naming the limbs, bringing movement to each part of the body, thus establishing a body cartography that will later be set in motion.

The term 'body cartography' refers to both a physical and cognitive process. All parts of the body are invested by the sensation of movement and perceived by the knowledge of the body organization. Thus, the body map is laid out, not just as a static image but as a moving body that the patient can use for expression. By helping the patient clarify and enlarge movement, identification with his body and involvement in the expression of feelings can be unified (Chace, 1953). The body becomes a known place that the patient can signify as their own, while movement becomes their personal expression.

For every person, in particular those suffering from diverse pathologies, it is useful that the different parts of the body be named, and for patients, to be reminded how they are structured in order to make them present in their consciousness. This warm-up phase is for an isolated sensitization of the body (only the shoulders, or only the pelvis, etc.), in order to focus attention on areas of tension and contraction. In fact, it is impossible to start moving without first preparing the body.

If the patient wishes, music of their choice can accompany this phase. It is desirable to let the patient lead the body cartography for three reasons: in an instructive approach teaching how to release muscular tension, or encouraging them to take charge, or for the affirmation of the 'self'. In a group session, the 'Chace circle' protocol is followed, adding to it the body cartography. The body mapping process promotes interaction, every participant proposing a movement that will be integrated in a collective choreography, as Marian Chace illustrated (Chaiklin, 1975a; Chaiklin and Wengrower, 2009). Before ending this part of the session, every participant is asked how they feel, and if there is any part of their body that needs additional attention. This sequence is frequently used to work separately on each part of the body, giving specific attention to areas of tension and to the mechanical function of the limbs. This procedure aims to prepare the patient for a fluid physical-emotional expression, where all the parts of the body participate.

During this process, the therapist uses their body as a mirror for the patient, helping them to elaborate their own body perception. Words accompany these moments, naming each limb and guiding the form of movement (circle, undulation, right/left, etc.). As mentioned before, with time some patients guide the process themselves. The use of the body as a mirror for the patient's movement is unique to dance-movement psychotherapy. The initial movement of the patient is employed by the therapist to establish the therapeutic relationship, and to transmit a message of acceptance (Chace, 1953). For her, mirroring is not about imitating the patient's movement, but rather embodying its sense, so that the therapist can accompany the patient.

For the psychoanalyst Jaqcues Lacan (1996), the mirror stage is a crucial moment in the relationship that a person will develop with his body, and with the others that resemble him. The infant identifies with his image reflected in the mirror. In order for that to happen, the mother has to be present and confirm that it is indeed the infant's own reflection. The mirror stage allows the child to establish a relationship with reality, through the capture of his spatial body. This process will mark the mental development of the child, and later it will shape the social bond.

When the therapist's body is used as a mirror for the creation of the body cartography, the physical form from space (the gestalt) needs to be outlined, in order to establish a conscious balanced center. When the body map is posed and centered, movement can occur in space, the impulse arriving from the body toward the outside world.

The perception of the body is structured through what the patient sees and imitates in the therapist, but also by the internal sensation that her/his own movement creates. After the body cartography has been posed and the limbs invested with a feeling, the patient can express her/his movement in space and deliver her/his emotional experiences.

Conclusion

Dance movement psychotherapy is practiced in diverse settings, and if there are differences in its conceptualization, which can modify the style or the techniques, the basic theories of movement stay the same. In order to understand the physical expression of the patient, the therapist needs a real knowledge of the body and movement and she must be familiar with the art of expressive and improvisational dance. Movement patterns, the fluidity of expression, the range of movement, are all of essential importance to the psychotherapeutic use of dance movement (Gallagher and Payne, 2015).

The basics of dance are employed in order to understand the patient's movement, in order to join them, to enable transference, and to propose new movements. As Sharon Chaiklin insisted, the simple fact of being able to move does not constitute the ability to use movement as a therapeutic tool (Chaiklin, 1975b).

The author has presented and proposed a tool, body cartography, which it is hoped will add to the reservoir of therapeutic techniques used to awaken body-mind awareness. Grounding the emotions in the body sets the healing forces in motion.

The particularity of dance movement psychotherapy is the approach centered on the integration of psychic contents with psychosomatic manifestations; we can also call it the psychotherapeutic awareness of the body-mind relation.

This chapter has attempted to theorize the imbalance of this relation, and the effect that it can have on the patient's mental health. This psychosomatic imbalance, which can be defined as the shortage of emotional mediators between the body and the mind, can be the pathology itself, or it can accompany another psychopathology. In both situations the psychosomatic identity is essential for the apprehension and the treatment of the patient. One of the objectives of the dance-movement psychotherapists is to help the patient recover and develop the flow of information between the body and the psychic level. This process will support the healing forces, helping the patient to improve his emotional awareness and his message to the environment (Bartenieff and Lewis, 1980).

It is time to define dance movement therapy practice more precisely as a psychosomatic psychotherapy, based on the understanding of the body-mind relation, and the place of emotions in the balance of this unity. This will allow us to further develop the practice and theory of our unique discipline, and to find our place in the discussion concerning psychopathologies, what causes them and what can heal them.

References

Adler J. (1999). Integrity of body and Psyche: Notes on work in process. In P. Pallero (Ed.), *Authentic movement* (pp. 121–131). London: Jessica Kingsley publisher.

Adler, J. (2002). *Offering from the Conscious Body: The Discipline of Authentic Movement.* Rochester: Inner Tradition.

Adler J., Whitehouse, M. S. & Chodorow, J. (1999). *Authentic Movement*. London: Ed. P. Pallaro.

Bartenieff, I., and Lewis, D. (1980). *Body Movement: Coping with the Environment*. New York: Gordon and Breach Science.

Bejart, M. (1982). *Memoires, tome 1: Un instant dans la vie d'autrui* [Memories vol. 1: An instant in the life of another]. Paris: Flammarion.

Bejart, M. (1994). *Le ballet des mots* [The ballet of words]. Paris: Les belles lettres.

Bejart, M. (1998). *Memoires, tome 2: La vie de qui?* [Memories vol. 2: The life of who?]. Paris: Flammarion.

Bejart, M. (2001). *Letters to a Young Dancer*. Paris: Acte Sud.

Chace, M. (1953). Dance as adjunctive therapy with hospitalized patients. *Bulletin of the Menninger Clinic, 17*(6), 219–225.

Chaiklin, H. (1975a). *Marian Chace: Her Papers*. Columbia, MD: American Dance Therapy Association.

Chaiklin. S. (1975b). Dance therapy. In *The American Handbook of Psychiatry* (Vol. 5, 2nd ed., pp. 701–720). New York: Basic Books.

Chaiklin, S., and Schmais, C. (1979). The Chace approach to dance therapy. In P. Lewis (Ed.), *Theoretical Approaches in Dance Therapy*. Dubuque, IA: Kendall/Hunt.

Chaiklin, S., and Wengrower, H. (Eds.). (2009). *The Art and Science of Dance/Movement Therapy*. New York/London: Routledge.

Chemouni, J. (2000). *Psychosomatique de l'enfant et de l'adulte* [Psychosomatic of the child and the adult]. Paris: Editions In Press.

Chodorow, J. (1991). *Dance Therapy and Depth Psychology: The Moving Imagination*. New York/London: Routledge.

Chodorow, J. (1999). To move and be moved. In P. Pallaro (Ed.), *Authentic Movement: Essays by Mary Starkes Whitehouse, Janet Adler and Joan Chodorow* (pp. 267–278). London: Jessica Kingsley.

De Mille, A. (1963). *The Book of Dance*. New York: Golden Press.

Dychtwald K. (1986). *Bodymind*. New York: Pantheon Books.

Fischman, D. (2009). Therapeutic relationships and kinesthetic empathy. In S. Chaiklin and H. Wengrower (Eds.), *The Art and Science of Dance/Movement Therapy* (pp. 33–52). New York/London: Routledge.

Freud, S. (1980). Psychic treatment (soul treatment). In *Results, ideas, problems*. Paris: PUF, 1984.

Freud, S. (1981). *Essais de psychanalyse* [Essays in psychoanalysis]. Paris: Payot. (Original work published 1920)

Freud, S. (1985). *L'analyse avec et sans fin. Résultats, idées, problèmes 2* [Analysis with and without end. Results, ideas, problems 2]. Paris: PUF. (Original work published 1937)

Freud, S. (2008a). Repression. In P. Rieff (Ed.), *General Psychological Theory: Papers on Metapsychology*. New York/London/Toronto/Sydney: Touchstone. (Original work published 1915).

Freud, S. (2008b). The unconscious. In P. Rieff (Ed.), *General Psychological Theory: Papers on Metapsychology*. New York/London/Toronto/Sydney: Touchstone. (Original work published 1915)

Fuchs, T., and Koch, S. (2014). Embodied affectivity: On moving and being moved. *Frontiers in Psychology, 5*, 508.

Gallagher, S., and Payne, H. (2015). The role of embodiment and intersubjectivity in clinical reasoning. *Body, Movement and Dance in Psychotherapy, 10*(1), 68–78.

Graham, M. (1973). *The Notebooks of Martha Graham*. Boston: Houghton Mifflin Harcourt.

Graham, M. (1992). *Blood Memory*. Paris: Babel. (Original work published 1991)

Hoffmann, C. (2008). *Introduction à Freud: le refoulement de la vérité* [Introduction to Freud: the repression of the truth]. Paris: Hachette.

Humphrey, D. (1992). *The Art of Making Dances*. Paris: Babel. (Original work published 1959)

Laban, R. (1956). *Principles of Dance and Movement Notation*. London: MacDonald and Evans.

Laban, R. (1960). *The Mastery of Movement* (L. Ullman, Ed., 2nd ed.). London: MacDonald and Evans.

Laban, R., and Laurence, F. C. (1974). *Effort: Economy in Body Movement*. London: MacDonald and Evans.

Lacan, J. (1996). *Écrits* [Works]. Paris: Seuil.

Lakoff, G., and Johnson, M. (1999). *Philosophy in the Flesh. The Embodied Mind and Its Challenge to Western Thoughts*. New York: Basic Books.

Levy, F. J. (1992). *Dance Movement Therapy: A Healing Art*. Reston, VA: National Dance Association of AAHPERD.

Lewis, P. (1986). *Theoretical Approaches in Dance-Movement Therapy*. Dubuque, IA: Kendall/Hunt Publishing Co.

McDougall, J. (1989). *Theaters of the Body*. Paris: Gallimard.

Marty, S., M'Uzan, M., and David, C. (1963). *The Psychosomatic Investigation*. Paris: PUF.

Modlingere, M. (1997). *In Another Languish*. Tel-Aviv: Hapoalim.

Ne'eman, N. & Bartal, L. (1992). *The Metaphoric Body: Guide to Expressive Therapy Through Images and Archetypes*. London: Jessica Kingsley Publishers.

Payne, H. (2009). Pilot study to evaluate a dance movement psychotherapy (The BodyMind Approach) with patients with medically unexplained symptoms: Participant and facilitator perceptions and a summary discussion. *Body, Movement and Dance in Psychotherapy, 5*(2), 77–94.

Sami-Ali, M. (1977). *Corps réel, corps imaginaire* [Real body, imaginary body]. Paris: Gallimard.

Sami-Ali, M. (1987). *Penser le somatique* [Thinking the somatic]. Paris: Dunod.

Schoop, T. (1978). *Motion and Emotion. American Journal of Dance Therapy, 22*(2), 91–101 (republished 2000).

Schoop, T. & Mitchell, P. (1974). *Won't you Join the Dance?*. US: Mayfield Pub. Co.

Shahar-Levy, Y. (2004). *The Visible Body Reveals the Secrets of the Mind: A Body-Movement-Mind Paradigm (BMMP) for Analysis and Interpretation of Emotive Movement*. Jerusalem: Author's Hebrew Edition.

Stora, J. B. (1999). *Quand le corps prend la relève; stress, traumatisme et maladies somatiques* [When the body takes the lead; stress, traumatism and somatic diseases]. Paris: Odile Jacob.

Thompson, E., and Varela, F. J. (2001). Radical embodiment: Neural dynamics and consciousness. *Trends in Cognitive Science, 5*, 418–425.

Whitehouse, M. S. (1970). Reflections on metamorphosis. *Impulse* (Suppl.), 62–64.

Whitehouse, M. S. (1999). The transference and dance therapy. In P. Pallaro (Ed.), *Authentic Movement: Essays by Mary Starks Whitehouse, Janet Adler and Joan Chodorow* (pp. 63–72). London: Jessica Kingsley.

18

MODULATING VERBAL AND NON-VERBAL LANGUAGES IN DANCE MOVEMENT THERAPY

Moving conversations with neurotic adults in private practice

Teresa Bas, Diana Fischman, and Rosa Mª Rodríguez

Introduction

What are the particularities of Dance Movement Therapy (DMT) when working with adults who cope with neurotic difficulties and have a strong enough ego structure to ask for help and reflect on their situation? How is it similar to and different from other psychodynamic or body approaches? What becomes meaningful to a dance movement therapist? What are some of our tools and intervention modes? This chapter is an invitation to reflect upon these topics, under the scope of a relational, enactive and embodied approach in DMT (Koch and Fischman, 2011). DMT is a form of psychotherapy that aims to integrate implicit and explicit communication, making conscious some of the unconscious, linking verbal and non-verbal languages (Fischman, Rodríguez, and Bas, 2016).

Psychotherapeutic processes with normal neurotic adults[1] capable of reflecting on themselves are seen here as evolving dancing dialogues between patient and psychotherapist, in which many levels of human interaction, communication and understanding are being played out. From the clinical intervention perspective, such a variety of levels includes: movement exploration and words, primary processes of experience and secondary processes of reflection, psychodynamic concepts and the use of movement analysis systems; also, evoking images or metaphors and embodying them through dance and body awareness techniques. All of which mainly pursues body–mind integration.

Neurotic adult patients

If we focus on the patient, it becomes necessary to define what we mean by normal neurotic adults with a strong enough ego. Winnicott (1975) showed us the path towards embodied inter-subjectivity with what he termed the *psychesoma*. The psyche indwelling in the soma describes the successful outcome of the process of personalisation that occurs as a result of the mother's handling of her infant during the holding phase, where dependence is absolute. The psyche is the imaginative elaboration of somatic parts, feelings and functions, related to inner reality and Self. If the child does not receive good enough handling during their early development, they may never feel as one within their body, and a mind/body split occurs. Winnicott spoke extensively about the mind to describe an intellectual functioning, which he related to dissociation, considering that the mind becomes a kind of entity the individual feels as not being part of their sense of Self. Winnicott and DMTs have described some patients as persons living in their heads or their mind, being disconnected from the *psychesoma*; in other words, disconnected from the felt sense of body experience (Fischman, 2009). Following Winnicott, we postulate that neurosis is related to post Oedipus level, but there is much more in the patient related to pre-Oedipus developmental pre-verbal stages that might remain un-integrated in neurotic adults.

Later on, and following Winnicott's path (1975), Stern (1985) presented a new construct to understand human development: the *sense of Self* and its domain of relatedness. He described four levels of them, all of which go on developing throughout life: the emergent, the core, the intersubjective and the verbal. These concepts are very significant for DMT because they provide further theoretical bases for our pioneers' work, which was already addressing the first three pre-verbal senses of Self, completely rooted in the body. That is, the senses of Self by which somebody experiences themselves as an emergent organism which connects information coming from different modes of sensing, owns a cohesive body from which impulses and actions arise, becomes agent of their own actions and is, at the same time, affected by the interaction with the environment. Gradually, considering the intersubjectivity by which one creates and shares meaning, attention and intention, comes the capacity to put words and narratives to experiences while one gets to a verbal domain of relatedness.

Many neurotic sufferings we see in our clinical experience are related to the narcissistic stage, in Freudian terms (Freud, 1914), and to somewhat impaired pre-verbal senses of Self, in Stern's (1985) terms: over-adaptation, living in the head, lack of boundaries, lack of a sense of being agent of one's actions, body-mind splits and not feeling one's body. So, we can say that normal neurotic patients who come to DMT have developed a 'good enough' sense of themselves to relate verbally and reflectively to themselves and others but are still struggling with a certain lack of completeness in their pre-verbal senses of Self. DMT directly addresses the emergent and core senses of Self (Hartley, 2004), as well as the intersubjective, and focuses on this kind of unsolved body needs related with embodied self-awareness. So, DMT offers new opportunities for the development of pre-verbal domains of relatedness more rooted in the body.

Conceptual background

DMT: A relational enactive embodied psychotherapy

The epistemological view adopted here comes from contemporary relational, enactive, embodied perspectives (Lakoff and Johnson, 2003; Lyons-Ruth, 1999; Maturana, 1984; Varela, Thompson, and Rosch, 1991) which DMTs have reunited and intertwined in order to integrate basic DMT assumptions within a wider scientific frame (Koch and Fischman, 2011).

Relational perspectives in psychotherapy gather ideas from Stack Sullivan (2001), for example, who is recognised as one of the first relational psychotherapists and influenced Marian Chace (Chaiklin, 1975), an early pioneer in DMT in the USA. He postulated that we get anxiety, and also heal, within relationships (Barton, 1996). Later, Stern (1985), showed us how the infant's sense of Self first and foremost develops within the relationship with his/her parents who treat him/her from birth like a complete social being with feelings and sensitivity. Lyons-Ruth (1999) states that the psychoanalytical encounter is mutually co-constructed between two active participants, so that the focus is on the point of contact between them. So, with this perspective on DMT, we are mainly interested in how the person developed their ways of moving within the context of their significant relationships and how they express themselves in relation to us, the dance therapist.

Under an *enactive* approach, human beings are considered living systems that actively participate in a creative co-construction of the worlds they live in, where action, perception, emotion and cognition come together (Varela et al., 1991). The term *enaction* synthesises the effectiveness of dance/movement therapy, as it works on the repertoire of the patient's movement patterns, bringing them to a conscious level, and offers an unprecedented opportunity to expand this range through new intersubjective experiences (Koch and Fuchs, 2011). In this sense, we could say that verbal and non-verbal conversations in DMT processes evolve around *enactments*, which are opportunities to reach new meaning for interpersonal experiences that the patient lived in the past.

From the current perspectives of embodiment, we now have more evidence of the psychological significance of body memory or the embodied grounds of metaphor (Koch, Fuchs, Summa, and Müller, 2012). Neuroscience studies support how much the body is a key aspect in the development of our ways of being and relating to others (Damasio, 2000). The discovery of mirror neurons, which shows that the same neural processes are activated when an expressive act is executed and perceived (Gallese, 2009; Gallese and Goldman, 1998; Rizzolatti, Fogassi, and Gallese, 2001), constitutes a step further in the neuroscientific understanding of empathy. Dance movement therapy is by definition an embodied form of psychotherapy that has, from its early developments, worked with body memory and metaphor and intuitively understood how human experience is rooted in the body.

Verbal and non-verbal phenomena involved in change in DMT

From its origins, dance movement therapy was concerned with body action and symbolism, the subtleties of non-verbal communication, bodily movement patterns and kinesthetic empathy to connect with patients' feelings and sufferings. Through verbal and non-verbal processes DMT was always trying to reach some of the unconscious hidden in the body and bring it closer to consciousness (Lewis, 1986). Moreover, in The Boston Change Process Study Group (2010) terms, DMT was also working with the implicit[2] phenomena in the relationship (Stern, 2004; Stern et al., 1998); that is, with making explicit some of what is non-conscious (but not repressed in the sense of the unconscious). This refers to proceedings or relational patterns not said with words but which can be read through paralinguistic aspects in body expression (tone, intensity, volume, etc.).

All unconscious and implicit phenomena happen at a non-verbal level of communication and are, for the most part, imbued in the body and its movement patterns which come into play in the DMT relationship. Movement analysis systems used in DMT, particularly Laban Movement Analysis (LMA) (Laban, 1960), and in more detail the Kestenberg Movement Profile (KMP) (Kestenberg-Amighi, Loman, Lewis, and Sossin, 1999), show us how movement patterns and preferences speak about a person's needs and their relation to themselves, their emotions, others and the environment. So, DMT processes interweave conscious/unconscious and explicit/implicit phenomena within movement and verbal interactions between patient and psychotherapist.

Relational psychoanalysis has also underlined the concept of *implicit relational knowing* (Stern et al., 1998), which concerns all the non-conscious implicit realm of what is enacted in a given relationship and not expressed explicitly. The implicit or *enactive domain* only becomes manifest in doing, says Lyons-Ruth (1999). Moreover, enactive knowing does not necessarily need translation into symbolised reflective knowing, and paradoxically, putting words to embodied experience might not always become an important therapeutic tool. As we know, DMT can be a very powerful tool for meaningful conversations to take place at the non-verbal non-explicit domain. Also, dance movement therapists are concerned with *implicit relational knowing*, for example, when supervising to understand somatic transferences and explore them in movement and when mirroring or attuning through their voice and movement with the patient's affects; in short, when they study and use movement analysis tools and body awareness techniques to approach the non-verbal aspects of the patients' issues.

Nowadays, psychotherapists know how the change process in psychotherapy is very much rooted within the implicit level of communication between patient and therapist (Burke, Danquash, and Berry, 2015; The Boston Change Process Study Group, 2010). Change is not only based on interpretations and narrativisation of life stories at an explicit and conscious level. It also happens in implicit phenomena such as non-specific vivid relational encounters related to spontaneous interchange between patient and therapists and in *present moments of meeting* between them (Stern, 2004). In his book 'The Present Moment in Psychotherapy and Everyday Life', (ibid.) Stern states that the lived experience can be observed in present moments, among which are the moments of meeting. The latter are meaningful experiences that can be framed, described and analyzed during 7-second interactions in which much meaningful intersubjective dialogue happens. What is interesting in DMT is that the lived experience is expanded beyond verbal interactions along movement explorations or creative dance interactions, so present moments can be experienced during both parts of conversations with patients.

Thus, we can say that DMT incorporates basic relational psychoanalysis assumptions and at the same time has an important difference and contribution. DMT uses movement exploration, mindfulness, dance, and movement techniques that mirror-match isomorphically that which the patient brings in words and, vice versa, gives words and narrates the emergent experience of movement sensing. In this way, DMTs allow patients to become aware of the lived body experience while they give words to the unnamed, by moving, playing, art-making, dancing, chatting and reflecting patient and therapist expand transitionality (Winnicott, 1975) and free association. The unconscious is accessed through action and imagination, through conversations and through doing (Maturana, 1984).

Modulating verbal and non-verbal languages: Clinical interventions

Dance movement therapy processes with normal neurotic adults develop into verbal and non-verbal conversations where body action and the lived experience are central for psychotherapeutic change. Manifestly, these patients might come for anxiety, depression, somatic symptoms, body pain or eating disorders, among others. Emotionally, it is frequent to see them feeling very ashamed of themselves, hating parts of them or feeling guilty in different ways. Regarding the body, they feel disconnected from it, or they would like to express more with it and gain self-awareness. They might also experience it as a constant source of pain and tension. They do not understand what is happening to them and they would like to feel more relaxed and find pleasure. Through DMT, they learn how to pay attention to body language and regain trust in the body felt experience. Depending on the emergent manifestations during the sessions, the dance movement therapist decides what to underline, mirror or propose for exploration.

Clinical processes in DMT can take many roads as each case and relationship is unique, however, when working with individuals capable of expressing themselves in movement and reflecting on their sufferings, some particularities can be seen as repeated DMT interventions. These are discussed and illustrated below.

Bringing change by going with the patient and exploring opposites

As Freud (1920) stated, psychotherapists should not have a direct goal to produce change in the patients by removing their symptoms as do surgeons. Patients have very good historical reasons to hold onto their symptoms and difficulties. He told us much about resistance and how symptoms satisfy some unconscious desire, or they come as a negotiation result between two opposite needs in conflict. So, psychotherapists learned that it is in a relational process through time that the Self unfolds, and symptoms melt. In DMT we conduct this process by attuning to the patients' experience and by adding very small quantities of change that they can accept. Moment by moment, in some way, we become similar to the patient and we also introduce some difference that allows an escape from the fusion by differentiation.

Moreover, DMT considers that our personal history has brought us to develop movement patterns which give us a certain sense of ourselves and of how we see the world, as well as a tendency to react automatically towards stressful situations. Some somatic techniques also work with a similar view but considering only body tension patterns. For example, the Duggan French Approach (DFA) (Hansmann, 1997) focuses on the core tension pattern. DFA holds an interesting idea that is parallel to that of DMT: the pattern cannot be modified by trying to push or pull from it or massaging the muscles in a manner to force their relaxation. The transformation is considered to happen by going with the pattern and physically holding the posture it provokes. In this way, the pattern of tension can gradually let go while being held and the novelty of letting go becomes recognised as own, not as something external and strange. From there, it is argued that the person will find new ways of responding when interacting with the world and will expand their range and flexibility of movement. This physical holding that DFA uses also reminds us of the holding that Winnicott (1975) articulated around taking care of baby body-needs. In DMT, this translates into a psychophysical relational holding that allows patients to listen to a certain aspect of themselves; feel less guilty, scared or ashamed of it; and maybe find new meaning in it.

Notice we are describing change in quantitative terms. Having repeated micro doses of change in every DMT session turns into a qualitative change that can be recognised through the therapeutic process. Amplifying a movement relational repertoire between the two participants, in addition to enlarging the patient's resources to interact in life, becomes a kind of equivalent to widening the possibility of free association through imagination and creativity. That is why we state that facilitating free association as in the Freudian perspective, developing play and transitionality, as in a Winnicottian approach, and fluidity, considered as an optimal experience of wholeness (Csikszentmihalyi, 1990), are goals to achieve in DMT. In other words, DMT pursues reuniting Self-domains, integrating body–mind while coupling with the environment.

Ruth

Ruth is an intelligent, well-educated woman who feels very lost professionally and always 'stressed inside', unable to relax and enjoy. For a few years now, she can't seem to stay long enough in any job she is offered. In her transference, she shows little patience with my questions and always enters the room in a hurry, breathing heavily and talking very quickly. She seems to have so much contained in her chest and in her mind. Soon in the process she shows me how she is trapped in an accelerated, strong, abrupt and contained kind of inner rhythm that suffocates her. She does not know how to stop it. She actually longs for the possibility to relax or let go but is very afraid of falling into a depressive state. In movement terms, she translates those feelings by punching rapidly with her fist and forearm against the space in front of her, as if her fist was a hammer, while she shouts 'boom, boom, boom'. In the first sessions, I invite Ruth to first try to engage in different ways with this strong and hectic movement and find different nuances to it, while I accompany her in movement.

Then, through my questions while she moves, she explores the sensations and meanings of that movement: how does this movement make you feel? What do your arms seem to be doing with it? What do other parts of your body want to do with it? Also, by mirroring and engaging in affect attunement with my voice (playing for her a strong and sort of 'techno' rhythm she seems to enjoy), she gradually plays with other parts of the body and other accents. Eventually she seems to find interest in moving from what she experiences is the other extreme of such a movement. In this case, finding pleasure in playing lightly with her fingers in the air. That movement brings her back to being a child in her room, when for a while her mother would not be yelling at her or trying to diminish her by saying she would never accomplish anything good in her life.

So, as the therapeutic relationship builds up and a general theme emerges, the dance movement therapist may propose a movement exploration that 'goes along' with the distressful aspects the person would like to 'get rid of' (i.e. the tendency to live in a hectic rhythm, or to function under tension). Together, they see what these aspects are saying about her unconscious, what relational and emotional information they contain, what function they play for her survival so far. In Ruth's case, the hectic rhythm of constant accomplishment is a survival mode to prove her mother wrong. The patient liberates herself from an inner tension and at the same time feels confirmed in the right to feel what she feels, not having to deny it, suppress it or 'be a good girl'.

A few sessions later, Ruth is able to explore opposites, such as 'accelerating-decelerating' and 'strong-light', and soon finds herself just pausing for a while close to the floor. There she cries as she experiences the possibility to let go. Gradually throughout the process, she starts expanding the awareness of her particular needs and movement preferences, especially around the theme of rhythm. The therapeutic process seems to help her as she takes the decision to take some time for herself to think about her career.

Exploring certain opposites through body movement qualities is considered during DMT sessions in order to recognise pattern preferences, avoidance, difficulties or rejections. It is an opportunity to go from a binary world of opposites, elections and exclusions to a wider variety of possibilities and creativity, understanding complexity and multiplicity of options.

Accessing non-verbal senses of self

As suggested in the theoretical frame we present, we can say that when adults look for DMT as their psychotherapy, they are implicitly looking for an opportunity to feel, to be able to play more freely, to connect more fully with their body spontaneity. That is, to regain direct access to that realm of the non-verbal senses of Self with which we lose touch as we enter the verbal domain of relatedness, as Stern (1985) explains so well. Indeed, the emergent, core and intersubjective domains of relatedness remain beyond verbal language. DMT offers plenty of opportunities to expand the lived experience and access these non-verbal domains as well as to integrate them with the verbal domain. It does so by inviting patients to explore through movement improvisations and body awareness exercises coming from the work developed by our pioneers (Bartenieff and Lewis, 1980; Lewis, 1986) and a vast variety of dance techniques and somatic approaches. The particularities of authentic movement (Adler, 2002; Chodorow, 1991), where the therapist witnesses and resonates with a mover who is in contact with their inner impulses while moving with eyes closed, and some exercises that Body–Mind Centering™ (Bainbridge-Cohen, 2003) offers for experiential anatomy, are two strong tools for the emergence of present moments in the lived experience.

Maria

Maria was moving for a while with her eyes closed to an African percussion song and was exploring the sensation of a 'plug in the chest', as she would often feel. She would feel trapped in that tension in the chest and struggle to let go. She was trying to breathe deeper, swinging her arms in different directions. I noticed my own breathing was rather small while observing her and wished she would bend her knees since I felt their stiffness was separating the experience of the upper and lower parts of the body. I then just said 'I wonder if your legs have anything more to say right now and if they know they can count on the ground beneath them'. At that moment, to my surprise, Maria suddenly dropped her arms, took a deep breath and let her knees bend. Her lips drew a soft smile, as did mine. She loosened up all her lower joints and liberated a lot of the air imprisoned in her chest, engaging in a bouncing joyful movement with the music. In my resonance, I could feel some air and energy that nourished a sense of vitality in my muscles. I could connect to the great pleasure she was finding in her bouncing and a clear presence in the vertical dimension. She later would express how that movement gave a clear sense of being supported by her two legs, as if she was fully discovering them. It made her clearly feel 'This is me; here I am' for the first time. As a witness in Authentic Movement would do, I acknowledged her experience by echoing her words as I described how I saw her moving and how I heard her saying how it felt. This moment became meaningful along the process since she continued exploring in different ways with her legs and connected more meanings to her capacity to use them. Over time she could feel more and more who she was in the vertical plane, she learned to say 'no' to others while she would connect to the floor under her feet and take steps towards her autonomy as a young adult.

In Stern's (2004) terms, a form of *present moment of meeting* happened between Maria and the dance movement therapist. More than that, Maria experienced what we could call a 'dancing dialogue within herself'. A real present moment of integration and wholeness, through which some new implicit meaning arose in her core sense of Self; the sense where one feels a cohesive body and a sense of being the author of one's own actions (Stern, 1985).

Sensing and making sense

As shown in the illustrative cases, dance movement therapists are also concerned with a person's particular way of sensing and perceiving themselves, others and the world. How movement is sensed and how it is linked with the meanings of movement is central to our view (Koch and Fischman, 2011). Freud (1920) stated that curing neurosis was related to linking the affect with the idea that part of the Self is repressed or suppressed or takes the symptom's path (Fischman, 2009). When working with patients who can reflect on themselves, on what is implicit in the therapeutic relationship, and who have a strong enough psychological structure to become aware of unconscious aspects that arise in their bodies, the complexities of sensing and making sense can unfold.

In order to develop these senses and meanings, we ask ourselves questions like: how do they feel through their bodies? What is their own way of regulating their emotions in relation to the situations? How is it to move close to the floor or towards verticality? What does the dance of 'me always fighting against the world versus me letting go' bring to their awareness and how does that relate to their personal history? So, indeed, as they move, we are there observing, mirroring, attuning, containing their experience while asking some questions. The role of questions while the person is in movement is of crucial importance. It gives space for the person to continue moving while shifting their attention to certain parts of their body, their breathing, or the emotions, sensations and images they connect to. The balance in asking questions but not disturbing the person's movement process is delicate. So, the dance movement therapist must adapt and be sensitive in each case. Sharon Chaklin and Claire Schmais (Lewis, 1986) explain well how Marian Chace (Chaiklin, 1975) would sense how much she could approach her patients physically or verbally, or when she had to stop enhancing interaction.

Intertwining the implicit and explicit, the conscious and unconscious

DMT sessions and processes with these high functioning patients often evolve from some bodily felt image or sensation explicitly expressed by the patient, or some behaviour seen by the therapist as an emerging relational pattern in the patient's transference, then exploring them through movement and dances. Subsequently, verbal reflections on the experiences take place. This process connects movement-sensing and sense-making by integrating feelings, emotions, memories and reflections, bringing a new awareness to the person. Going back to movement exploration to further explore the bodily felt nuances becomes possible. That is, we are offering a safe context to continuous embodied experience, which in turn brings new layers of verbal narrative that help the person better cope with their difficulties. One last example helps us illustrate how the verbal and non-verbal realms of implicit/explicit and conscious/unconscious can be modulated in DMT.

Clara

Clara comes to DMT wanting to improve some insecurities and better understand her tendency to be closed in when she actually enjoys the company of friends. In her transference, she makes things feel easy for me, always smiling and saying how things go well, yet her movement patterns unconsciously tell me about some discomfort. She looks muscled and strong, but her chest narrows sideways (reminding me of a sense that she cannot trust her environment, according to KMP) and displays only light movements. As we get to know each other, I understand she is implicitly following a rule in the family where tensions are not spoken about. Gradually, these tensions appear in the sessions.

One particular session she talks about having trouble sleeping and feeling an agitation in her head and chest, as if she 'had seen a hundred movies in 10 minutes'. With the purpose of exploring the images and sensations mentioned, I invite her to warm up and see if she finds a movement for that sensation. She shakes her hands around her head, shaking also the head while keeping it down. I invite her to follow and exaggerate the movement. I can see fear in her facial expression; her chest bends downwards while her lower body shows a low tone. In my bodily countertransference, I can feel a lot of vulnerability and the lack of a strong floor under my legs. When asked what her hands and head seem to be doing and if there is any feeling or association coming up, she mentions a certain fear in her chest, the desire to hide and become small in an eggshell, and says her hands are trying hopelessly to get rid of the images in her head. She also realises her legs feel disconnected from the rest of the body at that moment.

Keeping in mind the hypothesis she will benefit from exploring the images mentioned but also that her agitation might be stronger if her body cannot 'count' on the floor, I invite her to awake the rest of the body in whatever way she wants. She then starts massaging her legs, shaking them as well as the torso, taking in somewhat deeper breaths and doing spirals in her spine by using the floor with her hands and legs. I describe and attune through my voice with some of her 'push' and 'drifting-like' movements. After a while she mentions a sense of relief in touching the floor, feeling her legs stronger.

Going back to moving her previous images and feelings (while asking myself 'what role does her need to hide in an eggshell play in her experience?'), I invite her to embody and move that image of becoming small. She brings her head down and curves the spine, closing her limbs inwards in shape of an eggshell. An image of being the smallest in a set of 'matryoshkas'[3] and a feeling of protection comes up. What could you be protecting yourself from?' I ask.

Rising her torso suddenly and with a clear voice she says to me straight 'From all the shouting, fighting and pain in my family'. Her eyes are wide open and her chest breathes more openly than any moment before in the session. She also connects with an interpretation I suggest around the 'matryoshkas', where she might be containing some feelings related to the history of the women in her family. She recalls a traumatic event in her mother's past that she heard about once and that she had never mentioned to me before. She seems to have found new meaning in her image and her necessity to be closed in. Gradually over the following sessions, she explores further with the opposites of closing in and reaching out and makes conscious great fears she experienced witnessing scenes of violence during childhood. New dialogues open up in her family as she also starts asking more open questions about the past to her parents.

Conclusion

Within the integrative spirit of DMT, by its very nature, the authors have proposed some answers to the 'hows' and 'whys' of the work with neurotic adults in private individual settings. The work of a dance movement therapist includes taking into account the explicit and implicit knowing within the client-therapist relationship, conscious and unconscious processes, movement analysis tools such as LMA or KMP, and body awareness ideas shared with somatic approaches such as Body-Mind Centering™. Such moved conversations, back and forth from words to images, to embodied experience, to reflections on the experience, enrich the narratives, the movement patterns and the relational procedures of these women's lives and bring new knowledge about themselves. Also, novelty and creativity to their forms of existence.

Non-verbal communication is always central to DMT. However, when working with adults who can reflect on their situations and seek help through movement, the accent of the work can be more specifically placed in the modulation between verbal and non-verbal language, in the integration of the implicit and the explicit levels of communication. In this way, as conceived by Lakoff and Johnson (2003), metaphors and metaphorical thinking become the means by which words were created when emerging from the body felt experience. We are co-constructing meaning in a non-verbal relationship that achieves verbal symbolism, while at the same time, reversibility allows imagining body-felt experience by analyzing the latent meaning imbued in the narrative. In some ways, we are mirror-matching body and mind experiences integrating them into one.

Trudy Shoop (cited in Lewis, 1986) wisely envisioned that if psychoanalysts and dance movement therapists worked together, it would probably be more difficult for patients to maintain their mental illness. In the current developments of dance movement therapy, integrating *embodiment*, *enactment* with relational psychoanalysis theories, we believe such an encounter is taking place within the limits of DMT itself. In other words, such an approach to psychotherapy might be a very deep form of transformation for neurotic adults and can righteously be called Dance Movement Psychotherapy.

Notes

1 To distinguish this population from adults suffering from psychotic symptoms.
2 The concept of 'implicit' is first referred to in psychology regarding implicit (procedural) memory and explicit memory. The authors wish to be careful with the use of the term, since the Boston Change Process Study Group have been the ones to develop it in detail.
3 Russian dolls contained one in the other.

References

Adler, J. (2002). *Offering from the Conscious Body: The Discipline of Authentic Movement*. Vermont: Inner Traditions.

Bainbridge-Cohen, B. (2003). *Sensing, Feeling and Action, The Experiential Anatomy of Body-Mind Centering®*. Northampton: Contact Editions.

Bartenieff, I., and Lewis, D. (1980). *Body Movement. Coping with the Environment*. New York: Gordon and Breach.

Barton III, E. F. (1996). *Harry Stack Sullivan. Interpersonal Theory and Psychotherapy*. New York: Routledge.

Boston Change Process Study Group, The. (2010). *Change in Psychotherapy: A Unifying Paradigm*. New York: W.W. Norton.

Burke, E., Danquash, A., and Berry, K. (2015). A qualitative exploration of the use of attachment theory in adult psychological therapy. *Clinical Psychology and Psychotherapy, 23*, 142–154.

Chaiklin, H. (1975). *Marian Chace: Her Papers*. Columbia, MD: American Dance Therapy Association.

Chodorow, J. (1991). *Dance Therapy and Depth Psychology. The Moving Imagination*. London: Routledge.

Csikszentmihalyi, M. (1990). *Flow: The Psychology of Optimal Experience.* New York: Harper and Row.

Damasio, A. (2000). *The Feeling of What Happens: Body and Emotion in the Making of Consciousness.* Orlando: Harvest Books.

Fischman, D. (2009). Therapeutic relationship and kinaesthetic empathy. In *Life is Dance. The Art and Science of Dance Movement Therapy.* New York: Routledge.

Fischman, D., Rodríguez, R.-M., and Bas, T. (2016, September). *Conversations: Embodying Language through Symbolism and Temporal Qualities.* Booklet of the II EADMT Conference in Milan.

Freud, S. (1914). On narcissism. *The Standard Edition of the Complete Psychological Works of Sigmund Freud, Volume XIV (1914–1916): On the History of the Psycho-Analytic Movement, Papers on Metapsychology and Other Works* (pp. 67–102).

Freud, S. (1920). *A General Introduction to Psychoanalysis* (pp. 388–402). New York: Horace Liveright.

Gallese, V. (2009). Mirror neurons, embodied simulation, and the neural basis of social identification. *Psychoanalytic Dialogues, 19*, 519–536.

Gallese, V., and Goldman, A. (1998). Mirror neurons and the simulation theory of mind-reading. *Trends in Cognitive Science, 2*, 493–501.

Hansmann, B. (1997). *Con los pies en el suelo. Forma del cuerpo y visiis del mundo* [With our feet on the ground. Body shape and vision of the world]. Barcelona: Icaria Editorial.

Hartley, L. (2004). *Somatic Psychology. Body, Mind and Meaning.* London and Philadelphia: Whurr Publishers.

Kestenberg-Amighi, J., Loman, S., Lewis, P., and Sossin, M. (1999). *The Meaning of Movement. Developmental and Clinical Perspectives of the Kestenberg Movement Profile.* New York/Oxford: Brunner-Routledge.

Koch, S., and Fischman, D. (2011). Embodied, enactive dance/movement therapy. *American Journal of Dance Movement Therapy, 33*, 57–72.

Koch, S., Fuchs, T., Summa, M., and Müller, C. (Eds.) (2012). *Body Memory, Metaphor and Movement.* Amsterdam: John Benjamins Publishing Company.

Laban, R. (1960). *The Mastery of Movement.* London: MacDonald and Evans.

Lakoff, G., and Johnson, M. (2003). *Metaphors We Live By.* Chicago: University of Chicago.

Lewis, P. (1986). *Theoretical Approaches in Dance-Movement Therapy* (Vol. I). Dubuque, IA: Kendall/Hunt Publishing Company.

Lyons-Ruth, K. (1999). The two-person unconscious. Intersubjetive dialogue, enactive relational representation and the emergence of new forms of relational organization. *Psychoanalytic Inquiry: A Topical Journal for Mental Health Professionals, 19*(4), 576–617.

Maturana, H. (1984). *The Tree of Knowledge.* Santiago de Chile: Ed. Universitaria.

Rizzolatti, G., Fogassi, L., and Gallese, V. (2001). Neurophysiological mechanisms underlying the understanding and imitation of action. *Nature Reviews Neuroscience, 2*, 661–670.

Stack Sullivan, H. (2001). *The Interpersonal Theory of Psychiatry. International Behavioural and Social Sciences, Classics from the Tavistock Press.* London: Routledge.

Stern, D. (1985). *The Interpersonal World of the Infant: A View from Psychoanalysis and Development.* New York: Basic Books.

Stern, D. (2004). *The Present Moment in Psychotherapy and Everyday Life.* London: W.W. Norton.

Stern, D. N., Sander, L. W., Nahum, J. P., Harrison, A. M., Lyons-Ruth, K., Morgan, A. C., . . . Tronick, E. Z. (1998). Non-interpretive mechanisms in psychoanalytic therapy: The "Something more" than interpretation (The Boston Change Process Study Group, Report N°1). *International Journal of Psycho-Analysis, 79*, 903–921.

Varela, F., Thompson, E., and Rosch, E. (1991). *The Embodied Mind: Cognitive Science and Human Experience.* Cambridge, MA: MIT Press.

Winnicott, D. W. (1975). *Collected Papers: Through Paediatrics to Psycho-Analysis.* New York: Basic Books.

19

THE IMPORTANCE OF SUBTLE MOVEMENT AND STILLNESS IN JAPANESE DANCE MOVEMENT THERAPY

A comparison with the Japanese traditional performing art of 'Noh'

Miyuki Kaji

Introduction

Dance/movement therapy (DMT) is a psychotherapy that utilises the power of embodiment and symbolisation through dance and movement. In DMT, clients express their thoughts and feelings through their body and in turn, their experiences are sensed by their body. In this sense, DMT is a therapy made possible by the process of embodiment. In this chapter, the author will use the term 'Embodiment' to mean the expression of feelings and images via bodily position and movement. DMT was developed in Western countries in the 1940s. It was introduced in Japan in the 1980s and has been practiced mainly at locations like psychiatric hospitals, geriatric homes and day care centres. On the one hand, Western theories and techniques, such as the Chacian method, have contributed to the development of Japanese DMT. On the other, Japanese DMT incorporates culturally appropriate techniques that reflect Japanese-specific styles of expression, physical skills and concept of the body (Onuma, 2015). The specifics of Japanese culture include the following aspects.

There is a Japanese saying 'Not speaking is a flower' (it is sometimes better not to say anything). In Japan, it is considered to be polite not to verbalise everything we think or feel and instead to keep thoughts in one's mind. Due to this tendency, Japanese clients tend to show little emotion in psychotherapy. However, this small-scale emotional expression does not mean they feel little emotion. In clinical settings, there are many occasions on which clinicians are surprised by deep feelings that clients express by modest verbalisation.

There are also Japanese-specific physical training techniques and a concept of the body that reflects a Japanese lifestyle. The traditional Japanese way of living is based on its farming culture. Traditionally, Japanese wear kimonos that can restrict one's movement; they sit on the floor in Seiza style (folding one's legs underneath one's thighs, while resting the buttocks on the heels). This culturally specific movement pattern arose from the aforementioned lifestyle. One of the culturally specific movement patterns is that of internally rotating the limbs toward the centre of the body. Due to this movement pattern, Japanese have less muscle mass and the position of their pelvis is lower compared to that of Westerners. Also, the difference between most Japanese body builds and those of Westerners could encourage different movement styles in Japanese and Western culture (Yasuda, 2014; Yatabe, 2007).

Religious beliefs such as Buddhism including Zen tradition and Shintoism also affect Japanese ways of thinking. Zen and traditional Japanese arts such as the tea ceremony and flower arrangement teach us 'Shin shin ichi nyo' (body and mind are inseparable) (Yuasa, 1990). During Zen training and training to master Japanese traditional arts, confined movement can become meaningful. It is believed that repeating the same work or movement can allow a trainee to achieve psychological maturity. In DMT, repeating fixed choreography sometimes allows clients to develop psychological themes when clients' deep feelings and characteristics are expressed by small movements. To establish a body-oriented therapy like DMT in Japan, it is important not only to learn from Western style DMT but also to incorporate a culturally specific healing process derived from the Japanese lifestyle and concept of the body. 'Noh' is a traditional Japanese performing art, which reflects Japanese physical skills and body concepts. In this chapter, the possibilities for integrating Japanese culture into DMT will be discussed by comparing the healing power of Noh and DMT.

The Japanese concept of the body and mind reflected in Noh

Noh is one of the traditional performing arts that represents Japanese culture. Kanami and his son Zeami contributed sophisticated folk entertainment based on Chinese songs and dances to Noh in the late fourteenth century. Noh became an integrated musical drama consisting of 'Mai' (dancing), 'Utai' (singing a song) and 'Hayashi' (playing music).

Noh is performed with a mask. A direct translation of Noh into English would be 'dance'. However, this does not fully convey the meaning of Mai. A characteristic of Mai is restricted movement. Dancers do not intentionally and actively move their body but wait for internal energy to arise and move them (Yatabe, 2007). It is important not to wilfully move the body although dancers physically can move it. The posture required to dance Mai is unique compared to some Western dance. For some of the Western style dances, such as classical ballet and social dance, dancers balance themselves by pulling their body upwards. For Mai, dancers balance themselves by pulling the centre of gravity of their body downwards by concentrating their energy in the 'Tanden' (the abdomen below the navel), standing with bent knees and putting both feet together. It is considered to be necessary to direct one's centre of gravity downwards in order to integrate body and mind. While dancers widen their chest by pulling up their upper body towards the sky, their shins incline towards the earth. When moving on the stage, dancers shuffle their feet without lifting them. The only body part that is slightly lifted while walking is the toes. This walking technique is called 'Suri Ashi' (shuffling feet). By lowering one's centre of gravity, dancers are enabled to create power through pushing back from inside to outside of their body. This shift of energy from the inside of the body to the outside of the body is Mai, and the way dancers walk in Noh (Yatabe, 2007). Dancers maintain the posture with a lowered centre of gravity and place their body passively on stage. Waiting for internal energy to build up creates tension in the atmosphere. As a consequence of built-up internal energy and tension in the atmosphere, dancers are pushed to dance Mai.

This passive attitude is also notable during the practice of techniques to master Noh. Per the creator of Noh, Zeami, training in Noh should start from learning 'Kata'. Kata (form) is a traditional inherited movement pattern that became simplified and stylised over time. Mai consists of the combination and repetition of Kata patterns.

By constraining their body into Kata and repeating Kata, dancers train the sensitivity of their body, heighten their internal senses and master 'Kokoro' (mind/feeling). Defining Kokoro as the core of the 'self', the beginner's 'Karada' (body) that cannot move as one intends can be considered as creating an 'other' that needs to be controlled by Kokoro. However, repeated training of Kata allows one's body to move naturally without consciously thinking about it. In this embodied stage, it is difficult to decide whether Kokoro or Karada is the core of the self. Because of this embodiment process, Zeami teaches us to train Karada first, and then wait for Kokoro development through the training of Karada. This attitude towards body-mind training is similar to Zen training based on 'Shin shin ichi nyo' (body and mind are inseparable) (Yasuda, 2014; Yuasa, 1990; Zeami, 1400/2013, 1400/1976).

Healing in 'Mugen Noh'

'Mugen Noh' is a Noh style in which 'Shite' (the main character) acts as a local person in the first half of the performance and then becomes a ghost in the second half. On stage, there is another person, 'Waki', who is a monk, acting alongside the Shite. At the beginning of a performance, Waki introduces the setting of the story to clarify the structure of the play. Waki, who is a traveling monk, visits a village and accidentally meets a local person portrayed by Shite. Shite shares folklore about an unfortunate past event that happened in the village. However, Shite starts acting like the main character of the folklore while he is talking, and it is difficult to differentiate the local person in the present and the main character from the folklore. The local person disappears and the monk falls into a deep sleep. The Shite who was the local person appears as a ghost from the past in the last half of the performance. It is difficult to work out if it is a dream or reality. The ghost dances and talks to the monk about his longstanding, unsolved agony. In the end, the monk sends the ghost to Nirvana. The process of the monk releasing the ghost from its haunted past and providing catharsis resembles a healing process. During the first half of the performance, Waki intervenes to let Shite recall his memories. In the last half, Waki stands still with some tension to maintain the structure and to provide a stage for Shite to express his past conflicts in the dream world.

Like Mugen Noh, there is a mixture of reality and one's internal world in a therapy session. It is common that a client expresses their unconscious feelings by talking about his/her dreams, drawing a picture, creating a scene in a sandbox or dancing. This expression of unconscious material often helps therapeutic progress (Bosnak, 2011; Giegerich, Kawai, and Tanaka, 2013).

The relationship of Shite and Waki is sometimes considered to resemble the relationship of a client and a therapist (Morioka and Fujinawa, 1978; Yasuda, 2011). A therapist who provides a structure in which a client feels safe to express him/her self, intervenes with a client to help him/her express his/her story and observes and supports a client to face to his/her psychological themes appears similar to the role of Waki in Noh. DMT is particularly similar to Noh in that a client symbolically expresses his/her internal story through his/her body. Due to this similarity, it is possible to consider that the physical level of relationship between a client and a therapist in DMT is akin to the physicality of Shite and Waki in Mugen Noh.

Case study

Yoko (pseudonym) is a medium built, intelligent and elegant woman in her late 50s. Her husband did not work but indulged himself in doing whatever he wanted. Yoko worked hard to support her family. The couple had a daughter. Her husband's physical and verbal domestic violence started 2 years prior to the initial therapy session. Around the same time, she encountered social issues in a hobby group in which she had participated for a long time. These issues wore her out. Yoko lapsed into major depression and was hospitalised in a psychiatric hospital for a half a year. She voluntarily participated in a DMT group every week while she was hospitalised. However, when the group became more expressive and emotional and depressive themes came up in the last half of a session, Yoko always left the group. She dropped out from attending counselling. She said she felt 'heavy hearted by being forced to talk about my miserable experiences' in counselling. She was divorced while she was hospitalised. After she was discharged, she lived with her daughter. Upon her discharge, her doctor recommended that she participate in a bi-weekly individual DMT session to obtain psychological support and to better understand herself to prevent a relapse. A session consisted of 10 minutes of verbal reporting of her life, 25 minutes of improvisational dance and 15 minutes of drawing and verbal reflection of the session. The sessions continued for 6 years. The total number of DMT sessions was 128.

In this case, Yoko had been repeating a simple dance movement like a Noh's Kata. This Noh training-like repetition appeared to help her integrate her internal energy. She then introduced her dreams into the DMT session to heal herself. Using this case, I would like to discuss the concept of body and mind unique to Japanese DMT.

In the first sessions, Yoko chose mid-tempo instrumental music for her DMT session after discussing her music choice with the therapist. She voluntary moved with the music of her choice. Yoko walked alone, moving her arms up and down like a bird flying. Even when the therapist walked along with her, she did not react to this and continued her flying movement. The movement of her arms was linear, her torso was rigid, her body looked like a stick and her steps were weak. The use of space was limited. She maintained the same level and moved back and forth in the same spot in the room. Her repeating flying movement looked empty and simple like a young child's dance. The therapist had the impression that there was strong resistance to expressing her feelings, coupled with ambivalent feelings about relying on others. The therapist tried to carefully inter-vene without being invasive. When Yoko was dancing, the therapist observed Yoko's dance empathetically to understand her feelings expressed in her movement. The therapist also mirrored Yoko's movement to provide feedback for Yoko to clarify her expression. The therapist avoided asking about Yoko's past until Yoko started voluntary talking about it. Yoko's life was stabilised by obsessively ritualising her daily routine like choice of food and steps of doing housework. Yoko's former husband sometimes visited her. Although she felt anxious and uncomfortable in his presence, she could not decline his visit and was hospitable to him.

After several months of sessions, she added a stronger pressing-down movement with her hands while she performed her flying movement. The therapist mirrored her movement and exaggerated it. Yoko added extra strength in her hands after noticing the therapist mirrored her movement. She developed this movement into creating a wall around her, and then pushed it back. After performing the movement that looked like clarifying a boundary between the self and other, Yoko drew a picture of an angular castle. She said, 'Life with my ex-husband was like being imprisoned in a castle without a gate or a window. I became ill because of this confinement'. A week after this session, she started to move her arms slightly more softly and more three-dimensionally. She twisted her upper body and explained, she was 'taking off cloaks one by one and letting fresh air in'.

About 1 year later, Yoko's feelings of not wanting her ex-husband to visit her became stronger. Also, she was exhausted from dedicating too much energy to her relationships with her daughter and friends. She complained about insomnia and exhaustion. In DMT sessions, she moved more freely and her movement became more expressive. She added a movement that looked like shaking something off to her flying move-ment. This movement developed into a punch. The therapist verbalised this movement as an expression of anger. Yoko admitted that she was expressing her anger. Around this time, Yoko frequently remembered her deceased mother. She started talking about her mother in DMT sessions. Her mother had been exhausted by single-handedly taking care of her large family and died when Yoko was in her 20s.

About 2 years after Yoko started DMT, Yoko and the therapist held hands like a mother and a young child and moved their arms like a wing. While Yoko walked next to the therapist, her body touched the therapist as would a child leaning on his/her mother. While walking next to the therapist, Yoko rhythmically opened and closed her mouth and held her arms in a position as if she was holding a baby. After this session, Yoko dreamt about her deceased mother. Although her mother died young, her mother in her dream was an old woman. Yoko helped her mother, whose knees were bent, to stand up by putting her arms around her mother's body. Yoko said, 'Wow, you worked so hard that your knees got bent'. In the next session, Yoko walked with bent knees. The therapist put her arms around Yoko, helped her to slowly stand up and lower her body down, and said, 'I am so sorry that you need to work so hard' like Yoko did to her mother in her dream. Yoko started crying. Yoko said, 'I have not cried for a long time. I cannot recall when the last time I cried was'. She reported that she dreamed about yelling at her ex-husband's relatives. She started recognising her feelings and expressing them.

After dancing about her dream, Yoko began sleeping well. She resumed cooking her favourite soup and jam. She expressed the desire to separate completely from her ex-husband. She started to dance with her feet grounded on the floor and pulling her centre of gravity low. Her flying movement became rhythmical and strong with flexible chest and shoulder movement. The space she used expanded. A new movement pattern, extending her arms up to the ceiling, collecting sunshine on her palms and taking care of herself, appeared. For closure, Yoko put her hands and the therapist's hands on her chest as one might while in prayer.

In the fifth year, Yoko's life stabilised and she was enjoying her hobbies. She was active and moving on to a new life, for example by declining her ex-husband's visits and getting rid of her old possessions. In DMT sessions, Yoko showed negative feelings towards the therapist as if the therapist was her violent and controlling ex-husband. She came to the hospital without an appointment and accused the therapist of missing the session. She complained, 'DMT is tiring' and moved passive-aggressively. The therapist supported Yoko's expression and attuned to Yoko's movement. She also felt empathy with Yoko's anger and powerlessness. Yoko cried and said, 'I always put up with things, even when I was exhausted. This was the cause of my illness. It was good that I could complain about my situation to you'. After this incident, Yoko stopped pushing to devote herself so much to others.

The number of movements that looked like nurturing, and charging her energy, increased. Her movements expressed lightness, quiet strength, freedom and sadness mixed together. By then, Yoko used her entire body to perform her flying movement. Her flying movement was also slowed down. For the ending of each session, she often freely walked in the space alone or held the therapist's hand and walked together with her. Then Yoko stopped and put her hands on the therapist's hands to feel closeness and subtle sadness. After a while, Yoko released the tension in her body. Yoko said she could not believe how much richer her movement repertoire had become. She continued to move in a similar manner for a while, then the DMT was terminated. Around this time, she had recovered so much, that she needed almost no medication. In the last session, Yoko said, 'I am continuing dancing in my own way'.

Discussion

Interpretation of the case from the Mugen Noh viewpoint

Yoko had difficulty in recognising and expressing her feelings. DMT appeared to be a good modality for her, because it did not require her to verbalise her feelings but instead allowed her to express them freely in a nonverbal way. Projecting her feelings onto her movement might have made her feel safe enough, so that her defence mechanisms and resistance to therapy were lowered. Yoko confined herself into the rigid and repetitive flying movement but the limitation in movement also provided her with structure and safety. The therapist carefully intervened with Yoko's process without being disruptively invasive. The therapist encouraged her to express herself physically. Sometimes the therapist observed Yoko without moving and set up a stage for her to safely and freely expresses her feelings. The therapist accompanying Yoko's journey to understand herself physically resembles how Waki supports Shite. When Yoko and the therapist established rapport and trust, her movement repertoire was expanded.

Once Yoko started to symbolise her experience into her movement, she reported on the dream about her deceased mother who had sacrificed herself to take care of the family. Dancing this dream was a turning point in this case. While dancing about her dream, she was Yoko and her deceased mother at the same time, like Shite is a local person and person in a folklore at the same time. Yoko also recognised repressed emotions through dancing the dream of her mother, like Shite dances in his dream-like states talking about his unfortunate past. Yoko realised that she also sacrificed herself like her mother to take care of her family. Yoko embodied her long-standing anger and sadness by dancing her dream. This experience allowed her to cry and to heal. Yoko deepened her understanding of herself and developed a rich variety of self-expression by embodying her difficulties and feelings.

After recognising her anger and sadness, Yoko slowly changed her life by prioritising her own needs. Yoko complained to the therapist out of transference. When the therapist encouraged Yoko to express her anger and accepted Yoko as she was, Yoko cried with joy that she was able to complain to others. She reflected upon her life of being overly devoted to others at her own expense and obtaining key knowledge and insight about herself. The relationship of a therapist and a client consists of respect for the client's expressions and the mutual search for their meaning mirrors the relationship of Waki and Shite in Noh. Yoko acquired new insights and behavioural patterns through DMT sessions by embodying her internal experiences. Her determination to continuing dancing after the DMT was terminated is evidence that the embodiment of internal experience helped her heal.

Looking at the case from the Noh's concept of body

Yoko repeated the flying movement from the first session to the last. Obsession with the same movement can be viewed as a resistance to a treatment, because it limits the development of expression and strengthens defence mechanisms resisting processing of emotional material. In this case Yoko's initial flying movement was simple and non-characteristic. However, Yoko concentrated on performing the same flying movement. The therapist did not think that the repetition of the movement was meaningless, so she did not try to encourage Yoko to change her movement. Instead, the therapist supported the repetitious movement. The flying movement changed its quality as the sessions progressed. The quality of the flying movement had changed from rigid and flat movement to strong and dimensional movement, and further to a light and flexible movement. This change in the movement quality represented changes in Yoko's internal world. The flying movement did not simply represent flying but it was a channel to express her internal world at the time. As previously mentioned, traditional Japanese arts and Zen training include repetition of a particular type of simple movement or activities to achieve physical and psychological growth. When body and mind become one and inseparable, a trainee can naturally embody his/her feelings. It could also be true for DMT to use a simple repetitious movement to foster the growth of body and mind if clients are willing to concentrate on the repetitive movement.

As therapy progressed, Yoko's ungrounded and weak feet became grounded and strong. Also, her centre of gravity settled in her lower body. Locating the centre of gravity in the lower body, maintaining bent knees and remaining strongly grounded to the earth even when walking or jumping is a unique characteristic of Asian dances, including Noh and Japanese dance. Maintaining one's centre of gravity in the lower part of one's body can limit movement of the lower limbs and whole body movement. On the other hand, this lower centre of gravity provides strength and stability. Yoko's body slowly changed to utilise a silent strength to push against gravity and the space around her like a Noh master. Towards termination, Yoko stood still and concentrated on sensing the environment around her. She enjoyed sensing movement arising in her body. What she was doing looked like choosing to stand still and contain her movement internally, instead of stopping her movement. After standing still for a while, Yoko relaxed her body and made relieving vocal sounds. This gave the therapist the impression, that Yoko enjoyed standing still and containing her movement internally. This incident could be evidence that mindfulness and internally embodying what she was sensing were meaningful to Yoko. Restrained movement in Mai (dance) of Noh is also meaningful. In the Noh's theory, it is considered that choosing to contain one's movement within one's body, instead of moving to express oneself, can provide a different experience and an alternative way to express oneself.

Conclusion

Self-expression and non-verbal communication through dance/movement are considered to be important elements of treatment in many DMT techniques. To achieve dance/movement with this healing power, Western techniques often require expressive and possibly dynamic movement. For example, the theory and technique of Marian Chace, one of the founders of DMT, introduced clarifying expressional movement and then developed the movement further. At the same time, there is a Chacian technique, empathic reflection, that may focus on a client's subtle movement. In empathic reflection, a therapist mirrors a client's posture and movement. It is important that a therapist not only pick up a client's overt movement but also looks for underlying subtle movement (Chaiklin and Schmais, 1993). In clinical experiences with Japanese clients, the author has the impression that interventions involving the therapist clarifying and/or developing a client's movement makes the quality of the movement change and can stop the client's internal development process. This tendency is particularly true when a client has a strong defence mechanism against recognising and expressing his/her feelings and when clients utilise subtle movement to connect with his/her feelings. The author thinks that a technique like empathic reflection, particularly focusing on underlying subtle movement, is important when working with Japanese clients. In a clinical setting, what a talkative client says sometimes sounds empty. Fluent and dynamic physical movement with wide variations can be empty like the words of a talkative person and the movement might not represent a client's internal world. As Yoko's case depicted, choosing to limit movement or concentrating on a simple repetitive movement can foster an experience of connection to one's deep internal world.

For Japanese clients, not only are dynamic movement and clear self-expression meaningful in DMT, but also stillness and silence. The characteristic posture of holding one's abdomen as a centre of gravity as in Noh generates subtle movements including stillness. Those subtle movements, stillness and simple and repetitive movement patterns are also meaningful in DMT for Japanese clients. Non-dynamic movement, a repetitive movement pattern and mindfulness of own body and internal movement could also be meaningful for non-Japanese clients. For future DMT training, therapists themselves need to experience not only dynamic and active movement but also subtle movement and stillness, as in Noh training, where one senses internal movement and waits for it to mature. When a therapist experiences the embodiment of his/her mind through subtle movement, he/she would be better able to observe and support their clients' own subtle movements and even stillness.

References

Bosnak, R. (2011). *Embodiment: Creative, Imagination in Medicine, Art and Travel* (Nihon Embodied Dreamwork Kyokai, Trans.). Osaka, Japan: Sogensya. (Original work published 2007)

Chaiklin, S., and Schmais, C. (1993). The Chace approach to dance therapy. In S. Sandel, S. Chaiklin, and A. Lohn (Eds.), *Foundations of Dance/Movement Therapy: The Life and Work of Marian Chace*. Columbia, MD: The Marian Chace Fund of the American Dance Therapy Association.

Giegerich, W., Kawai, T., and Tanaka, Y. (2013). *Giegerich yume seminar* [Giegerich dream seminar]. Osaka, Japan: Sogensya.

Morioka, M., and Fujinawa, M. (1978). Chiryosya = Waki ron jo [Theory of clinician = Waki: Prologue]. *Nihon Geijyutsu Ryoho Gakkai Shi, 9*, 145–146.

Onuma, Y. (2015). Dansu serapi no genzai – sono 1: Nihon no dansu serapi no genzai [Current states of dance therapy 1: Current states of Japanese dance therapy]. *Nihon Geijyutsu Ryoho Gakkai Shi, 46*(1–2), 43–51.

Yasuda, N. (2011). *Ikai wo tabi suru Noh: Waki to iu sonzai* [Noh traveling in otherworldly: Existence of Waki]. Tokyo, Japan: Chikuma Shobo.

Yasuda, N. (2014). *Awai no chikara* [The power of Awai]. Tokyo, Japan: Mishima sha.

Yatabe, H. (2007). *Utsukushii nihon no karada* [Beautiful Japanese body]. Tokyo, Japan: Chikuma Shinsyo.

Yuasa, Y. (1990). *Shintai ron* [BODY: Toward Eastern Mind-Body Theory]. Tokyo, Japan: Kodansya.

Zeami. (1976). *Zeami geijyutsu ron syu* [Arts theory by Zeami] (T. Tanaka, Tran.). Tokyo, Japan: Shincho Sha. (Original work published 1400)

Zeami. (2013). *Shin yaku Fushikaden* [Fushikaden: New translation] (K. Kanze, Tran.). Tokyo, Japan: PHP Institute. (Original work published 1400)

20

EMBODIMENT OF SPACE IN RELATION TO THE SELF AND OTHERS IN PSYCHOTHERAPY

Boundlessness, emptiness, fullness, and betweenness

Rainbow Ho

Introduction

'Space is a hidden feature of movement and movement is a visible aspect of space' according to Laban (1966, p. 4). Space is a physical concept that usually refers to the three-dimensional geometric occupancy on Earth or in the Universe in which an object or a person can fill. Although space is usually physical, it can also refer to psychological space (mind and affect) in the context of psychotherapy, spiritual space in Eastern philosophy, and social relations in all cultures. The symbolic expansion of space can also be extended to personal boundaries and limitations, which can further relate to a person's flexibility, freedom and integrity.

In dance/movement therapy, the physical spaces inside and outside the body are usually the entry points for dealing with issues related to the person and the person's relationships with others and the world based on the premise of the interconnectedness of the mind and body. Inner space relates to a person's internal mind and status in dance and movement therapy, and awareness of it can remind an individual of her emotions and feelings, thus facilitating the growth of acceptance.

In a psychotherapeutic context, the awareness of space outside the body and its relationship to the self, with the consideration of culture, reveals patterns of personal boundaries and social relationships. An individual can develop his or her own identity and healthy relationships with others if appropriate space among people can be maintained. Because embodiment and body work in psychotherapy are closely related to culture (Dosamantes, 1992; Pallaro, 1997; Pruzinsky and Cash, 2002; Schilder, 1950/1935), the concept of space, due to its relationship to the body self, others, and the social environment, cannot be separated from the context of culture.

Eastern and Western concepts of space and the body

In both the East and the West, the space inside and outside the body refers to the distance and relationship between the self and others or the external world. In Eastern cultures, people may value the space that includes both the self and others based on their interdependent nature (the self in others); however, in Western culture, people may pay more attention to the distance between the self and others due to their more independent nature (Markus and Kitayama, 1991). Although the degree of exposure and exchanges may vary among different cultures, some prominent differences in the perception and interpretation of space remain between the East and the West.

Space and relationships between of the body, the self and others

The Chinese language, which is metaphoric and expressive, has specific words related to space to indicate relationship issues between oneself and others. The words that refer to the space in the heart or the chest are particularly used for describing a person's character and virtues, as well as the way a person thinks and acts toward the other. For example, in Chinese *xin xiong guang kuo* (心胸廣闊), literally meaning a 'spacious' heart and chest, refers to a generous and broad-mind. People even describe a heart as like a spacious ocean in which one can row a boat. *Xin xiong xia zhai* (心胸狹窄) literally meaning 'a narrowed heart and chest', refers to a person who is narrow minded and calculating and has little tolerance. *Da kai xin fei* (打開心扉) literally meaning 'opening the window of the heart', refers to the openness or honesty of a person. Similarly, Western psychology, in particular psychoanalysis, also uses the concept of space to describe personal characteristics. However, it is related more to the person himself/herself rather than the relationship with the others. Bloom (2006) writes:

> An overextension of one's sense of space lends itself to omnipotence; a shrinking of one's space may imply feelings of persecution or claustrophobia, or worse perhaps, the lack of interest in 'being in space' at all, which could be described as complacency or mindlessness.
>
> *(p. 78)*

Apart from personal characteristics, the space inside the body in general is more related to a person's spiritual side in Eastern philosophy. Mindfulness meditation, which is an Eastern spiritual practice, can enhance the awareness of one's inner space and enhance the ability to embrace and endure the ups and downs of the journey of life (Pollatos, Kirsch, and Schandry, 2005).

Boundlessness: Space between the self and the others

Space usually refers to specific geometric occupancy. However, there is a special concept of space in Eastern philosophy: boundlessness (*wu ya* 無涯). It is a Buddhist concept and is not material and thus neither chemical nor physical. The body, or more accurately, the 'egoless nature of the body', is defined as 'a space enclosed by bones and sinews, flesh and skin' (Nikaya, 1995, p. 278). Since space in Buddhism is 'an imperceptible entity as it cannot be perceived by the senses except by the mind' (Madurai, 2007, n.p.); experiencing the space inside or outside the body is thus about 'entering into infinite conscious' (Madurai, 2007, n.p.).

This boundlessness concept of space forms the concepts of the 'self' and 'big self' (*da wo* 大我) in Chinese and some other Eastern cultures in which the 'big self' (the bigger, boundless space) is perceived as an extension of the self (the I'ness, the space enclosed by skin and bones) into the eternal space without limitation (Madurai, 2007). A typical example, which demonstrates this relationship between the self (inside the body) and the big self (outside the body), is Traditional Chinese Medicine (TCM), in which the system inside the body resembles the environment and the Universe (the space outside). Both systems contain the same five elements – wood, fire, earth, metal and water (*Wu Xing* 五行), which are governed by the *Yin and Yang* (陰陽) and with '*qi*' (氣) as the energy source.

The concept of boundlessness also shapes the acceptance and comfort of connecting and being with others in Eastern collective cultures, which creates the sense of harmony in interpersonal relationships. In the psychotherapeutic context, however, putting too much emphasis on the other without taking care of the self; or becoming too involved in another's life, become some of the issues arising from this boundlessness concept in space.

In Western culture, on the other hand, space has two clear definitions: one refers to the cosmos or the universe, and the other to the cylindrical or spherical occupancy of a body or an object. On earth, space is material and physical and has a clear boundary. In this regard, the physical body is clearly separated from the external environment, whereas the concept of self, which mostly refers to the conscious or mental presentation of the body, is not connected directly or merged with the outside world. The relationship between the self and others thus becomes independent and there are clear boundaries for the self and also the others.

Emptiness, fullness, and betweenness: Space between the self and the world

'Empty space does not exist' (Laban, 1966, p. 3). While the concept of space in relation to the body and the external world differs between the East and the West, the two cultures also have different emphases when talking about space itself and how it is occupied. From the Western perspective, when an object is placed in a space, the space is partially or fully filled; otherwise, it is empty. Emptiness versus fullness thus becomes the focus. Western interior design to some extent reflects this emphasis, as a Western house is usually filled with furniture and cushions. Since the space between objects is viewed as empty from Western perspective, two objects or persons that stay in two different geometrical spaces are independent and do not affect each other.

On the other hand, from the Eastern perspective, the emphasis is more on the space or emptiness between objects rather than on the 'occupancy'. The Chinese word space (*kong jian* 空間) is composed of two words: the former means 'emptiness' (*kong* 空) and the latter means the 'space between' (*jian*間). Emphasis and attention are always given to the space that is not occupied. In fact, in the Eastern concept, unoccupied space is not really empty; it is viewed as a field (*chang*場) which is fully filled with energy or '*qi*' (氣), although it is invisible. Therefore, all objects are connected, and the space between them is just as important as the space being occupied. The interior design of a Japanese house or garden, which may have a lot of empty space, is one of the exemplars of this concept. In this regard, any two objects or persons are never independent and always affect each other through chi or energy connection.

The emphasis on the 'betweenness' in Eastern culture affects how Easterners perceive relationships. This idea, originally suggested by the Japanese philosopher Watsuji Tesuro (1889–1960), was further elaborated by his student Yasuo Yuasa: 'This betweenness consists of the various human relationships of our life-world. To put it simply, it is the network which provides humanity with a social meaning, for example, one's being an inhabitant of this or that town or a member of a certain business firm. To live as a person means in this instance, to exist in such betweenness' (Yuasa, 1987, p. 37). Individuals connect with others regardless of distance, space, and even time.

Interestingly, the size of space between two persons is perceived as an important measure in social relationships in modern Western culture and psychology. Hall (1968) is the anthropologist who has established the concept of proxemics, which is the study of a person's use of space in relationships. In this context, the individual can use distancing from his/her body to regulate contact and social relationships with others (Low, 2003). In Hall's work, personal space can vary from the smallest intimate space to the largest public spaces dependent on culture and situations (Hall, 1973) and can be measured in physical units. Therefore, space between bodies carries important meaning in social relationships in both the Western and Eastern cultures.

Embodiment of space in psychotherapy

'We reveal space whether we intend to or not, But if we choose to intentionally invest in space, we are rewarded richly' (Hackney, 2002, p. 242). The concepts of boundlessness, emptiness, fullness, and betweenness play an important role in psychotherapy, particularly when personal space, boundaries, relationships and connections with others are the key concerns. In body-oriented psychotherapy, the embodiment of the concept of inner space and personal space (kinesphere) facilitates the creation of a peaceful and private space for self-soothing and development. It also forms the base from which an individual can develop a sense of security and beyond which freedom, exploration, and risks can be taken so that the individual can expand and extend his or her contact with the outward social space and external world (Ho, 2015). As Winnicott described, 'spontaneity only makes sense in a controlled setting. Content is of no meaning without form' (Winnicott, 1965/1984, p. 213). Space may help create a form or an invisible container in which the individual can develop a sense of security and even allow for spontaneity. Nevertheless, when working with space and the body, special attention should be placed on cultural appropriateness and acceptance.

Freeing space inside and outside: Emptiness versus fullness in creating personal and inner space

Awareness of personal space inside and outside the body relate closely to the psychological status and sense of self of the individual. This relationship has not only been addressed by many pioneers and scholars in the field of dance/movement therapy and somatic movement therapy, but also confirmed by recent evidence in neuroscience (Gallese and Sinigaglia, 2011). The kinesphere, or personal space, is always the first space concept related to the body to be explored in embodiment (Taylor and Dragonosky, 1979). However, not every individual has the concept of space around the self, for instance, cultures that focus on interdependence do not necessarily value personal space. In this case, the use of images of an empty circle such as a bubble around the body or putting a string on the floor to form a circle can usually help in grasping the concept of personal space. By exploring the near and far extent of space around the body, the individual can gain a sense of self from which autonomy can be regained within the personal space which is not fully occupied by something.

Case study: Anne

When Anne (aged 55 years) was invited to imagine there was a bubble around her body and she could do whatever she wanted to do, she closed her eyes and stretched her limbs widely. Later on, she moved her hands slowly, doing a tai-chi-like movement. After a while, she lifted her leg trying to flip and kick, and did a little jump and hop. She smiled and moved faster and faster like a little child playing in the bubble playground. After the movement, Anne shared that she felt like she had been returning back to her very young childhood in which she could move and play freely. She continued to talk excitingly but with a little sadness on her face that she did not move like that for so long and she almost forgot how to move and play around. She always had some things to do and with someone else in her life. Her time and space had been completely filled up without any space to breathe and move. But she now could really feel free to move without obstacles.

Traditional Chinese culture in the Confucian tradition emphasises discipline and rules, as well as interdependence; playfulness and spontaneity are not particularly encouraged as an individual grows more mature. A mature person should also be aware of the others' needs and take care of the others. The image of returning to childhood within the individual's control brings about freedom and authenticity. The joyful experience of regaining some free space to do whatever he or she wants to do revitalises the body as well as the life.

Also, from both the Western psychosomatic and Eastern Traditional Chinese Medicine (TCM) perspectives, emotion is one of the important causes of illness, including mental illness such as depression and physical illness such as cancer. According to TCM theories, intense negative emotions that are not well ventilated may cause stagnation of the blood and energy (chi), blocking the flow and circulation of all of the systems in the body (Ng et al., 2006). In this situation, passive methods such as acupuncture and massage can help, but exercise and movement are more effective because they are more active. Movement can definitely be a starting point to help mobilise energy, resulting in better physical and mental health. Therefore, traditional forms of Chinese mind-body exercise such as tai chi and qi qong all serve this function, and there is evidence for their health benefits (Chan et al., 2012; Ho et al., 2013; Wang et al., 2013). Anne's experience of joy and ease from moving in a less occupied personal space brought her to the place where she rediscovered her body-self as well as psychological self (authenticity and autonomy).

Inner space for self-soothing

Although movement can greatly help to ventilate tangled emotion when there is a lack of felt space within the body, obstruction and stagnation can also be created. Freeing some empty space inside is then important in order to give the individual room for self-soothing and further self-exploration.

Case study continued: Anne

Anne closed her eyes and started to follow my verbal guidance of imagining 'putting' the personal space into the body, in particular, to the region of her chest. She breathed deeply in and out and gradually moved her hands following her breath spontaneously. Finally, she placed her hands over her chest and smiled, and sat down onto the floor. A few minutes later, Anne, with tears in her eyes, shared that it was the first time she felt she could have a space inside her body in which she could really breathe freely. In her life so far, she had been spending all her time taking care of others, first, her original family, and then her own family after she got married. She never ever thought about spending time on her own for herself. This was the first time that she felt she could also have a quiet and private space herself and no longer needed to have anyone else there.

Although Anne passed away 1 month after that session, her contented and smiling face is still in my mind even though it has been 12 years since our work together. As Chinese people, we treasure staying in the same space with others because we value interpersonal harmony and relationships, and also because of the cultural concept of boundlessness. However, we may also become too enmeshed with others and lose ourselves. The concept of space and the embodiment of personal space inside the body can bring about a concrete feeling and experience. In fact, the concept of personal space, inside and outside the body, also exists in Eastern philosophy. Contemplative practices such as mindfulness meditation, in which the participant is reminded to observe instead of intervening in the thoughts and images that emerge during the practice, offer an opportunity for the participant to become aware of the free space that she can have.

From personal space to social space: Boundlessness and independence

Eastern culture emphasises interdependence, which corresponds to the concept of boundlessness, fullness and betweenness as explained before. Individuals in a specific community, i.e. family, community, and society, are all 'under the same roof', and thus in the same space. However, this can sometimes create a sense of self-extension, which means that the individual becomes too involved or wanting to control others who are in the same space. This issue is often seen in the relationship between an adolescent and his or her parents, in particular the mother. Because the child originally is part of the mother's body during pregnancy; and the mother must care for the child closely before he or she can survive independently; mother and child inhabit the same space before the child can survive independently. However, when the child enters adolescence, during the search for identity and recognition, he or she will struggle to leave the mother's space – the circle of control.

Case study: May and Jane

May (35 years) and her daughter Jane (14 years old) always argued because of small things like what time Jane came home at night, or whether Jane had taken a shower, etc. Jane became very irritable and emotional and May became impatient and frustrated. They seldom talked to each other and whenever they started a dialogue, they would end up in a big quarrel. In one session, I asked May and Jane to make their own circle on the floor (using string) with a size in which they felt comfortable. Interestingly, the circle Jane made was much bigger than that made by May, although Jane's body was smaller than her mother's. May was very surprised by that. I then asked them to take the string circles closer until the two circles touched each other. I asked May to extend her arms towards Jane. Since Jane's circle was big, May could not reach Jane and after a while, tears came down from her eyes. She cried and sat down on the floor and said, 'I just know now, she likes to keep such a distance from me . . . she is not a small child anymore . . . she always wanted to be around me before . . .'. I asked Jane what she would like to say to her mother. Jane said, using a small voice, 'I am not a child anymore mom, I know you care about me, but I also want you to leave me alone sometimes . . . I want to have my own space . . .' May nodded her head. She finally became aware of the needs of her child.

May and Jane experienced what can be termed the process of individualisation (Jung, 1921) and separation. With the concrete experience in the body, they could easily articulate the concept of physical space and psychological space without any verbal or theoretical explanation. Perhaps the parents' letting-go may not be as difficult in Western culture as in Eastern culture, as children may grow up to be more independent. However, similar situations can also arise between a couple, siblings, or any family and community.

Space and loneliness: The concept of betweenness as the link

Although independence must be emphasised when relationships are too enmeshed, creating distance may sometimes induce a feeling of loneliness, in particular, in Chinese or Eastern cultures. In this case, the invisible connection, the betweenness of space in Eastern culture, can be taken as a perspective for resolving the situation.

Case study: Chris

Chris (50 years old) felt very sad and depressed whenever she thought of her mother who died when she was young. She used to live with her divorced mother; but 1 day, her mother suddenly disappeared. She later learnt from her grandma that her mother had taken her own life. For many years, Chris felt very lonely and had a repeated dream in which her mother came back to take care of her. She could not remember very well how her mother looked except that she had long hair. In one session, when Chris mentioned her dream again, she cried and fell into depression. I kept silent and made two circles on the floor using scarves. I put a black scarf in one circle, and around the place where Chris sat, I made another circle. I then asked Chris to touch my two hands in a pushing position. Since I knew that Chris practiced tai chi regularly, we moved our hands slowly as if doing tai chi's push-hands exercise. I asked Chris to move away from my hands when she felt the qi (energy) between our hands. Once she started leaving my hands, I walked away from her and gradually went to the circle with the black scarf. While I was doing that, I kept checking with Chris if she could feel the qi between our hands. Finally, we were in two circles. When I asked Chris whether she still felt that we were connected, with the qi, her tears came out. She was so clever that she knew immediately what the two circles, the black scarf and our qi meant to her. She went to my circle, holding the black scarf, and cried loudly. After a while, she felt released and understood what we had done.

A few weeks later, in another session, Chris told me that she still dreamed of her mother, although not as often as before. However, she no longer felt lonely and sad when she thought of her mother because she felt that they were connected in some invisible way. In this way, a continuous bond was created to connect two people, regardless of time and space – the fullness (with qi) in betweenness.

From where to where: Which space to start?

The understanding of the self helps the understanding of others. However, there is no fixed sequence that should be followed when exploring different spaces in the therapeutic context, such as from inner to personal and to general space. It depends on the readiness of the individual. For those who may not have much of a concept of inner space or personal space, but boundlessness in Eastern culture, moving in a general space may be an appropriate way to start.

Case study: Kitty

Kitty was a middle-aged woman, 45 years of age, with late stage lung cancer. She was slim and about five feet tall. She joined a six-session dance movement therapy group. In one session, we focused on the theme of space. For an easy start, I asked the group to move in the general space in the room. Kitty showed her excitement when she tried to move across the floor. She moved to every corner of the room and explored the upper and lower space by stretching up and lying down.

Moving in general space can be taken as moving in everyday life. The major difference is that in the therapeutic context, the movement should be in a more mindful state. The individual should be ready to accept all possibilities and have the curiosity to learn from the unknown and re-learn from the known.

Conclusion

The relationships between space and body movement have long been emphasised and utilised in body-oriented psychotherapy, in particular, in dance/movement therapy. Some of the concepts of space explained in this paper echo with the fundamental principles established by pioneers in field of dance/movement therapy. Penny Lewis has explained the work of Marian Chace (Chaiklin, 1975) from the perspective of psychoanalytic theory, in which the process of dance therapy resembles the stages of symbiosis, separation and individualisation during development (Lewis, 1993). Through rhythmic group activity and body action, participants first moving in synchronistic group movement (symbiosis stage) can establish the self (individual body) and finally find out the optimal distance and relationship between the self and the others (kinesphere, personal space) as well as the world (the group, the social and general space) (Lewis, 1993). The continuous struggle and development during this process can be reflected as the process of finding the embodied senses of fullness, emptiness, boundlessness and betweenness. Mary Starks Whitehouse also mentioned her unique model of working with people using authentic movement as the process of individualisation. The concepts of the 'Self' (the big self) and 'self' she acknowledged in Jungian psychology resonate with the Eastern concept of boundlessness (Self) as well as the Western concept of fullness (the person's self). She described that the individual, through working on the 'self', can unfold the wholeness (big self) that is already there (Whitehouse, 1986). Joan Chodorow, when discussing the transcendent function of dance therapy, also cited Trudi Schoop's concept of *Ur'* (Schoop, 2000) which refers to the unlimited space (Chodorow, 1999) – the boundlessness. Many other dance/movement therapists have been using concepts of space to guide their practice. The concepts of fullness, emptiness, boundlessness and betweenness in fact appear in some stages during the process of growth and development of an individual, as well as his/her relationships to the others and the world, which are all the cardinal goals in dance/movement therapy.

Lastly, while the concepts of space can be applied in different cases and situations, we should pay special attention to the cultural context. Eastern culture emphasises interpersonal harmony and values boundlessness and selflessness, which may result in loss of the self and difficulty in separation and independence. In contrast, Western culture encourages the development of an individual self and suitable social distance, which may create a sense of loneliness and isolation. However, this is not completely true for every case. As we are human, we all need a balanced development of personal space and social engagement. The application of these concepts thus should be fluid and dynamic. Nevertheless, no matter what perspective we have, the embodiment of the concepts of space makes the understanding more concrete and direct; and a better understanding and development of these concepts helps establish healthier relationships with the self and others.

Acknowledgement

I would like to express my sincere gratitude to all the individuals who gave me permissions and consents to be included in the case studies of this chapter.

References

Bloom, K. (2006). *The Embodied Self: Movement and Psychoanalysis.* London: Karnac (Books) Ltd.

Chaiklin, H. (Ed.) (1975). *Marian Chace: Her Papers.* Columbia, MD: American Dance Therapy Association.

Chan, C. L. W., Wang, C. W., Ho, R. T. H., Ho, A. H. Y., Ziea, E. T. C., Wong, V. C. W., and Ng, S. M. (2012). A systematic review of the effectiveness of qigong exercise in cardiac rehabilitation. *The American Journal of Chinese Medicine, 40*(2), 255–267.

Chodorow, J. (1999). Dance therapy and the transcendent function. In P. Pallaro (Ed.), *Authentic Movement: Essays by Mary Starks Whitehouse, Janet Adler and Joan Chodorow* (pp. 236–252). London/Philadelphia: Jessica Kingsley Publishers.

Dosamantes, I. (1992). Body-image: Repository for cultural idealizations and denigrations of the self. *The Arts in Psychotherapy, 19*(4), 257–267.

Gallese, V., and Sinigaglia, C. (2011). How the body in action shapes the self. *Journal of Consciousness Studies, 18*(7–8), 117–143.

Hackney, P. (2002). *Making Connections: Total Body Integration through Bartenieff Fundamentals.* New York, NY: Routledge.

Hall, E. T. (1968). Proxemics. *Current Anthropology, 9*(2), 83–95.

Hall, E. T. (1973). Mental health research and out-of-awareness cultural systems. In. L. Nader and T. W. Maretzki (Eds.), *Cultural Illness and Health* (pp. 97–103). Washington, DC: American Anthropological Association.

Ho, R. T. H. (2015). A place and space to survive: A dance/movement therapy program for childhood sexual abuse survivors. *The Arts in Psychotherapy, 46*, 9–16.

Ho, R. T. H., Wang, C. W., Ng, S. M., Ho, A. H. Y., Ziea, E. T. C., Wong, V. C. W., and Chan, C. L. W. (2013). The effect of Tai Chi exercise on immunity and infections: A systematic review of controlled trials. *Journal of Alternative and Complementary Medicine, 19*(5), 389–396.

Jung, C. (1921). *Psychological Types* (H. G. Baynes, Trans.). New York: Routledge.

Laban, R. (1966). *The Language of Movement: A Guidebook to Choreutics* (annotated and edited by Lisa Ullman). London: MacDonald and Evans.

Lewis, P. (1993). The use of Chase techniques in the depth dance therapy process of recovery, healing and spiritual consciousness. In S. L. Sandal, S. Chaiklin, and A. Lohn (Eds.), *Foundations of Dance/Movement Therapy: The Life and Work of Marian Chace* (pp. 154–168). Columbia, MD: Marian Chace Memorial Fund of the American Dance Therapy Association.

Low, S. M. (2003). Embodied spaces: Anthropological theories of body, space and culture. *Space and Culture, 6*(1), 9–18.

Madurai, B. B. (2007, September 19). The Buddhist analysis of space. *Lanka Daily News.* Retrieved from http://archives.dailynews.lk/2007/09/19/fea05.asp

Markus, H. R., and Kitayama, S. (1991). Culture and the self – Implications for cognition, emotion, and motivation. *Psychological Review, 98*(2), 224–253.

Ng, S. M., Chan, C. L. W., Ho, D. Y. F., Wong, Y. Y., & Ho, R. T. H. (2006). Stagnation as a distinct clinical syndrome: Comparing "Yu" (stagnation) in traditional Chinese medicine with depression. *British Journal of Social Work, 36*(3): 467–484.

Nikaya, M. (1995). *Mahahatthipadopama Sutta:* The greater discourse on the smile of the elephant's footprint (28:26). In B. Nanamoli, and B. Bodhi (Trans.), *The Middle Length Discourses of the Buddha: A New Translation of the Majjhima Nikaya* (pp. 278–287). Boston, MA: Wisdom Publications.

Pallaro, P. (1997). Culture, self and body-self: Dance/movement therapy with Asian Americans. *Arts in Psychotherapy, 24*(3), 227–241.

Pollatos, O., Kirsch, W., and Schandry, R. (2005). On the relationship between interoceptive awareness, emotional experience, and brain processes. *Cognitive Brain Research, 25*, 948–962.

Pruzinsky, T., and Cash, T. F. (2002). Understanding body images: Historical and contemporary perspectives. In T. Cash and T. Pruzinsky (Eds.), *Body Image: A Handbook of Theory, Research, and Clinical Practice* (pp. 3–12). New York, NY: Guilford Press.

Schilder, P. (1950). *The Image and Appearance of the Human Body.* New York, NY: International University Press. (Original work published 1935)

Schoop, T. (2000). Motion and emotion. *American Journal of Dance Therapy, 22*(2), 91–101.

Taylor, A., and Dragonosky, J. (1979). Using personal space in developing a working alliance in dance movement therapy. *American Journal of Dance Therapy, 3*, 51–61.

Wang, C. W., Chan, C. L. W., Ho, R. T. H., Tsang, H. W. H., Chan, C. H. Y., and Ng, S. M. (2013). The effect of qigong on depressive and anxiety symptoms: A systematic review and meta-analysis of randomized controlled trails. *Evidence-Based Complementary and Alternative Medicine, 716094*, 13.

Whitehouse, M. S. (1986). C.G. Jung and dance therapy: Two major principles. In P. Lewis (Ed.), *Theoretical Approaches in Dance-Movement Therapy* (Vol. 1, pp. 61–85). Dubuque, IA: Kendall/Hunt Publishing Company.

Winnicott, D. W. (1984). Do progressive schools give too much freedom to the child? In C. Winnicott, R. Shepherd, and M. Davis (Eds.). *Deprivation and Delinquency* (pp. 209–219). London/New York: Tavistock. (Original work published 1965)

Yuasa, Y. (1987). *The Body: Toward an Eastern Mind-Body Theory* (T. P. Kasulis, Ed., and N. Shigenori and T. P. Kasulis, Trans.). Albany, NY: State University Press of New York.

21

FROM THE ALPS TO THE PYRAMIDS

Swiss and Egyptian perspectives on dance movement therapy

Iris Bräuninger and Radwa Said Abdelazim Elfeqi

Introduction

Swiss and Egyptian perspectives on DMT are influenced by different cultural traditions and differences in education and recognition of the profession and by different health services. Both countries have a long tradition of giving shelter to new and old forms of dance related therapies. From 1913–1918, Rudolf von Laban founded his 'School for Art' on Monte Verità in Ascona, Switzerland, which attracted famous dancers such as Mary Wigman and Isadora Duncan, among others.[1] Laban and Duncan have been described as important influencers on the development of DMT (Levy, 1988). Back in 1992, Howaida El Guindy and Claire Schmais examined one of the oldest dances in Egypt, the Sudan and Ethiopia, the Zar, and discussed the healing aspects of this ritual dance applied in Egypt, the Sudan and Ethiopia, as a way to make it accessible to DMT (El Guindy and Schmais, 1992).

The following two sections of this chapter present perspectives coloured by the two authors' personal reflections on their formations as dance movement therapists in Switzerland and Egypt respectively. The first section by Iris Bräuninger furthermore presents a short overview of DMT education in Switzerland, followed by definitions of how Swiss DMT colleagues explain embodiment, how they apply DMT, and how they visualize the profession in Switzerland. Finally, the first author's personal perception on current and potential challenges in the field with regard to practice and research is described. The second section by Radwa Said Abdelazim Elfeqi offers personal reflections on the formation of a dance movement therapist in Egypt including local research conducted in the field of dance movement therapy highlighting some of the challenges confronted to move forward and develop the profession.

Switzerland: Personal reflections on the formation of a dance movement therapist in Switzerland

Having completed my Masters in DMT at the Laban Centre for Movement and Dance and at City University, London, UK in the early 1990s, and after working several years as a DMT pioneer in the field in Germany, I decided to develop my career and therefore conducted a multi-centred randomised control trial on DMT for my PhD project in order to improve both my personal and professional situation. In the meantime, I was offered a full-time contract at the DMT/Physio/Music Therapy Department at the University Hospital of Psychiatry in Zürich, Switzerland as deputy head of a well-trained team of ten experts in those disciplines. During that time, I was invited to present at the XIII World Congress of Psychiatry's first symposium on the Creative Arts Therapies in Psychiatry in Cairo 2005 (Bräuninger, 2005), which Dr. Radwa Elfeqi had organised. I learned that in some psychiatric hospitals in Cairo, the arts therapies, including DMT, were perceived as an important additional treatment complementing the expensive psychopharmacological treatment in mental health care. I perceived this as a spirit of optimism with new possibilities for incorporating embodied visions and including integrative perspectives.

The following presents different perspectives on DMT in Switzerland with an emphasis on DMT education and recognition, definition of embodiment, application of DMT, and possible future perspectives of and challenges for the profession.

Dance movement therapy education and training

Several private institutions offer coherent part-time or full-time DMT training over 3–5 years (minimum of 125 hours) which include for example DMT skills (such as DMT interventions, interpersonal relationships, therapeutic leading skills), DMT theories and history, movement observation, DMT specific knowledge, individual- and group-specific leading skills, clinical practice hours and a thesis. After completing full training, therapists can be accredited as full members with the Swiss Association for Movement, Dance and Body Therapies (the Schweizerischer Berufsverband für Bewegungs-, Tanz- und Körpertherapien (btk)).[2] From 2018 on, Certificates of Advanced Study Degrees (CAS[3]) have been offered, for example, for 'Needs-based Arts Therapies Treatment Models' by a Swiss University of Applied Health Sciences, which also includes DMT modules. This might be the beginning of the expansion in Swiss DMT education from training courses towards academic training.

On a side note, it is worth mentioning that in the German speaking part of Switzerland, nearly all dance movement therapist's work in health services as well as in private practice is with adults exclusively. Movement-based therapy in schools, special schools, and kindergartens is offered by psychomotor therapists, who complete a BA training (three years full-time, four to five years part-time, respectively).

Dance movement therapy professional recognition

After working for 2 years, dance movement therapists in Switzerland (if they are recognized as full members of the btk), can take the higher professional exam in order to become Federal State Registered as an Arts Therapist with specialisation in DMT[4] or as a Complementary Therapist.[5] This Federal State Registration is relevant, if clients have a supplementary health insurance, because they can get reimbursement for their DMT fees, provided that the dance movement therapist in private practice holds one of the Federal State Registrations. In public health services, DMT is mainly applied in the mental health sector and in neurological rehabilitation. Only a few dance movement therapists work in oncology or somatic medicine (these therapists are mainly located in the Swiss Romandie part). In general, DMT in Switzerland seems to have a good stance and to be well established in mental health services and as a state-recognized profession.

Definitions of embodiment, application of dance movement therapy, and a vision of the profession

A common feature in embodiment approaches, as described by Tschacher, Munt, and Storch (2014), is the unity of body and mind where the body and the physical permanently interact with the psyche and are inextricably linked. The authors believe that dance and movement-based interventions can activate some of the efficacy factors and therapeutic mechanisms, that make psychotherapy successful. This has been used in the Zurich Resource Model (ZRM) (Storch and Krause, 2007), a psychological self-management training, not specific to a particular disorder, which can serve as an integrative model between psychotherapy and body-oriented methods such as DMT (Tschacher et al., 2014). Samaritter and Payne (2013) suggested that '(. . .) shared movement intervention could offer a new perspective for psychotherapeutic intervention in disorders with a disturbed self, like autism, and need researching' (p. 143). Tantia (2013) defines embodiment as '(. . .) the enlivened expressive response to awareness of one's present-moment experience' and '(. . .) the cornerstone of dance movement therapy' (p. 98). Results of the randomized controlled trial with schizophrenic patients by Martin, Koch, Hirjak, and Fuchs (2016) strengthen these assumptions of the body and mind unity as their results revealed that negative symptoms in schizophrenia can be reduced by embodied therapies such as DMT or Body Psychotherapy (BP).

To deliver a true Swiss perspective on embodiment and a vision of DMT for the future, I approached seven accomplished Swiss dance movement therapists, whom I know, via e-mail with the following request:

1   '(. . .) Please give a short definition of embodiment;
2   Please shortly describe your application of DMT (where, when, with whom, since when, how etc. do you use DMT?);
3   What is your vision of the profession DMT in 10 years' time?'

They were informed that by answering they would agree that (excerpts of) their answers could be quoted for this chapter. Three of them answered.

Definitions of embodiment

Two colleagues, Bärbel Preusker (BP) and Françoise Broillet (FB), explained embodiment emphasizing bodily aspects. 'The fine perception of body-sensation and the differentiated reflection on feelings, which want to be expressed by these body-sensations' (BP).

'Embodiment is bound to the developing awareness of what is experienced in the body. It can be triggered by a sensation, an image, it can be stimulated from outside or inside the body. To be embodied means that I am directly connected to my experience via my body, whatever the source is. When I am embodied, I live the world, the others all the way down to my own skin and flesh. To remain consciously connected to one's own body experience is a specific human ability' (FB). Furthermore, a connecting line between Authentic Movement and Embodiment was drawn: 'For me the term of "Embodiment" is very connected to the practice of the discipline of authentic movement developed by Janet Adler' (FB).

Another colleague, Annlies Stoffel (AS), stressed the body and mind connection:

'Embodiment in the narrow sense means giving body, form, shape to something. In the larger sense, as it is used in contemporary philosophy and psychology, the term *embodiment* expresses the *interdependency* between the physical, psychological, and spiritual aspects of a human being' (AS).

Thus, the perceptions of these colleagues seem to be in accordance with leading Swiss theorists such as Tschacher et al. (2014), as the emphasizes lies on the body and mind connection. Additionally, the macro cosmos seems to become reflected in the micro cosmos through one's own body.

The application of dance movement therapy in Switzerland: Three individual perspectives

One colleague located in the Northeast part of Switzerland (BP), with many years of DMT experience in psychiatric settings and work in private practice, expressed the following to the questions:

'I work in a psychiatric clinic, where DMT is provided in all hospital wards. I offer DMT on the ward for addiction treatment and the ward for acute treatment. I have been practicing on these wards for 12 years. The treatment has different goals. The ward for acute treatment is the beginning of a psychotherapeutic treatment. Thus, it has the task of creating a sentiment of acceptance of all the psychological and physical differences and dimensions by the patients. To accomplish these goals, I use the method of Chace-Circle. Furthermore, I use a lot of different materials in order to reintroduce the patients to their motion. The different materials offer something to hold on to and also an exercise at the same time. The work on the ward for addiction pursues higher objectives. It is about experiencing the proper physical boundaries and first attempts to reach relaxation using the body. Overall, it is important for the patients not only to reflect, but also to get actively involved. In a group called "emotion-group", it is all about experiencing and discovering links between emotions, feelings, and body-sensations, such as feelings of rage, grief, shame, guilt, love, and joy. The patients find out in which ways these feelings can be identified and expressed on the body level. On this ward, I also offer deep-relaxation and breathwork. In my private practice, the patients are looking for support in situations of crisis and radical change. A method I typically use here is to recreate the targeted situation of stress to observe the reaction of the body. This is then followed up by an analysis of possible changes to be made and solutions to be found in order to treat the problem' (BP).

Another therapist (FB) is located in the French speaking part of Switzerland with an extensive background in DMT: 'In my private practice in Auvernier by Neuchâtel, since 1992, I welcome adults experiencing various psychological difficulties or life challenges, as well as those wishing to develop new channels of knowing through movement and dance. With body wisdom at the core of my study, I integrate the discipline of Authentic Movement in my dance movement therapy work, as a gateway to discover personal and transpersonal issues. I offer ongoing group meetings, workshops, group and solo retreats and preparation training for a variety of health care workers and people called by presence, awareness and truth' (FB).

The individual perspectives of these two colleagues on how they apply DMT, namely with patients with psychiatric and psychosomatic disorders, seem to be the most widespread use in Switzerland.[6] All three therapists furthermore work in private practice, also common in Switzerland.

The vision of our profession over the next 10 years in Switzerland

All three colleagues responded to the question as to how their vision of our profession would be over the forthcoming 10 years in Switzerland. Their answers cover educational and research aspects, aspects linked to embodiment and personal benefits for clients.

'I perceive that the importance of DMT is growing in advanced training courses and conferences on psychological health. Also, I find that research on DMT and its results are more strongly received by treating physicians. Therefore, I think that in 10 years a psychotherapeutic treatment will always include the body, in whichever way. I am convinced that costs for the healthcare system can be immensely reduced instead of increased by using DMT. I believe that in 10 years' time also clinic managers will have this opinion' (BP).

'In 10 years, when the concept of embodiment will be recognized as a natural given fact in wider circles of society, the taking into account of the body-mind-soul-interdependency will be seen as THE essential, indispensable element in therapy. Therefore, and because of the growing acceptance of DMT since its official national recognition in Switzerland (2011), the profession of DMT and its underlying principles will be better understood, supported, researched and more widely practiced. (This is my optimistic vision)' (AS).

'I am hoping for more visibility and recognition of the profession within health care institutions! With the people I have the privilege to accompany, I notice an increased interest in developing a connection to what "the body says" and I see this as a possible development of the profession' (FB).

These colleagues thus share an optimistic view, assuming that the meaning of the body will be more deeply understood in health care in general, in medicine and in psychology and that the impact of DMT will be consolidated or even expanded.

Final notes

Current and potential challenges in the field of DMT in Switzerland include the following:

- Switzerland, as many other Western countries, faces increasing costs in health services accompanied by cut-backs in treatment and services which could challenge the stance of DMT.
- Another challenge is the need for conducting more intervention studies with randomised controlled trials that evaluate the efficacy of DMT with questions such as: Does DMT foster health-related behaviours and/or reduce symptoms in clients? The challenge here is that many therapists a) are not trained in depth in research methods, b) might not have an explicit task in their employment to conduct research, or c) often do not have the access and means to apply for research grants. To address these challenges the CAS courses from 2018 on are one step. The creation of a MS/MA or a PhD program and the funding of DMT research grants could be further steps to foster DMT research.
- For the future, it would be desirable if therapists not only enter into applied fields but also enter academia and research thereby contributing to the scientific underpinnings of DMT.

Egypt: Personal reflections on the formation of a dance movement therapist in Egypt

Raised up in a scientific medical environment having a paediatric haematologist mother and a psychosomatic psychiatrist father had a great influence on my approach to Creative Arts Therapies and particularly Dance Movement Therapy. My father used to deliberately send my siblings and me to a number of artistic (inquiry) plays and tasks since the age of four years old, prompting us to discover our drawing skills, music playing, and vocalization while he was playing Oud, Flute, and other instruments that he had mastered. Yet, he did not like the idea of me becoming a ballerina, since the fine lady needs to take off her clothes to dance, which he did not appreciate coming from a conservative culture (Capello, 2014).

Nevertheless, I pursued my dream since I was eight years old by joining the Creative Dance Centre led by Dance Inji El Solh and trained there till the age of 14 years, when I joined the Faculty of Medicine at Cairo University and studied medicine at an early age. The urge to dance never stopped calling and in 1997, I received the call of the Carlos Saura movie 'Tango' which started my journey in ballroom and Latin street dance after my early jazz and creative dance. In 2002, I officially joined the Contemporary Dance School at Cairo Opera House and fulfilled my dream of studying ballet, Martha Graham and other contemporary dance approaches. I graduated in 2005 to immediately join the Creativity Centre Workshop (2005–2010) at the Opera House, where I studied drama, scenography, improvisation, script writing and performance.

I was practically living a dual life, a medical student, who turned into a Psychiatry resident in the morning, and a dancer/performer, who taught dance classes in the evening at Arthur Murrey School and spent her dance education in several venues in Cairo (Capello, 2014).

My journey in dance movement therapy started in 1999–2000 at Arthur Murrey School when I observed that my 60-year-old American student who was stuttering and stumbling in his footsteps at the beginning of his first few lessons turned into another person after six months of pursuing his classes and was able to master different rhythms. He had lost a few pounds making him look better and his posture was more erect, and his self-confidence and self-esteem lit the dance floor as he took those steps with other dancers of his class. Next morning, I was searching for something called dance therapy! I found the American Dance Therapy Association on Google and the US was quite far off my radar and I also had no connection there. I was desperate for resources as my mind was set on researching the topic for my master's degree. In 2001, my father shared the brochure of the Royal College of Psychiatrists Meeting taking place in London and here it was a Mind Odyssey comprising a series of workshops on all five modalities of creative arts therapies including music therapy, art therapy, drama therapy, dance movement therapy led by psychiatrist Robin Ellis and poetry therapy was taking place concomitant to the meeting (Ellis, 2001).

Being a doctor, introducing the idea of using dance therapy at the psychiatry department of Cairo University Hospital was often a reason to be made fun of during this time. The fact that Robin Ellis was a psychiatrist herself and conducted her research on four psychotic male patients was a very important argument to employ for the seriousness of DMT as a valid reference to all those other medically oriented psychiatrists.

Dance movement therapy at Cairo University Hospital

After participating in Robin Ellis' workshop (Ellis, 2001), I started tailoring the first pilot methodology for my research with children and adolescents suffering from emotional and behavioural disorders, a sample comprised of seven participants (7–12 years old), testing body image, with the 'strengths and difficulties questionnaire' as the outcome measurement tool (Goodman, 1997, 'self and parent version'). The children were engaged, and the modality seemed to be working, but I had only studied dance at this point and attended only one workshop on four psychotic individuals. To my scientific upbringing and my psychotherapy training at the psychiatry department, this was not enough to assume the identity of a dance movement therapist, although I felt it in my heart and mind that this must be it. I needed to question and supervise my work with an experienced eye.

I tried to contact Goldsmith College, UK but received no answer via phone or email. I risked my very limited financial resources and travelled back to London to find out that they were closed at the moment and offered no links to their professors. I went desperately looking for a dance movement therapist in the yellow pages till I reached Dr. Jill Bunce, head of Dance Movement Therapy programme at Derby University, UK, who received me with unequal generosity after hearing my story and my journey. Dr. Bunce invited me to her house and offered me free supervision on my recorded footage of the pilot and any further assistance that I needed for that research. She approved the methodology and the session module and told me: 'Go ahead'. That was it.

I went back to Cairo, collected a sample of 40 participant (8–14 years old), with the inclusion criteria of being drug naïve or having had a last administered medication dose at least six months prior to engaging in the trial. The sample was collected for the purpose of conducting the first randomised controlled trial using dance movement therapy as a monotherapy to treat Emotional and Behavioural Disorder with or without nocturnal enuresis primary or secondary, according to ICD 10 research criteria (World Health Organisation, 2001).

The methodology comprised 12 sessions over six consecutive weeks, each session lasting 90 minutes. The module included warming up, self-massage and centring techniques, attunement, dyadic play, using props (balls, walls, etc.), dramatic themes, improvisational lapses, therapeutic use of touch, and ended with de-rolling and verbal feedback. The 11th session included the mothers for dyadic techniques and was unexpectedly 100 per cent attended, despite bad weather on that winter's day and the fact that some of those mothers could barely afford the transportation fees. That indicated the appraisal of the mothers to their children's response to treatment prior to post intervention re-assessment with psychometric tools.

The impact of DMT as a monotherapy was quite impressive in comparison to use of tricyclic antidepressants and anti-psychotics with the addressed population. Forty per cent of the participants in the intervention group showed full remission of all symptoms of the manifested disorders on clinical and psychometric assessment, while 20 per cent showed substantial amelioration of all symptoms and 20 per cent showed amelioration followed by relapse after six months follow up and 20 per cent remained refractory to treatment. Waiting list participants showed no amelioration in any of their manifested symptoms.

This study was accomplished in 2006, and presented at several national and international medical conferences and at the 2013 American Dance Therapy Association international panel (Capello, 2014) and most recently published (Fenner, Abdelazim, Bräuninger, Strehlow, and Seifert, 2017). Findings were also shared at associated training workshops on creative arts therapies modalities with a focus on dance movement, at national and international conferences and at venues including Drexel University, Philadelphia, USA (in 2007 in the context of a class on neuroanatomy of dance movement therapy alongside a medical dance movement therapy workshop with Dr. Sherry Goodhill), Buenos Aires (in 2011 in a workshop on the psycho–neuro–immunological impact of dance movement therapy at the WCP (2005–2017)) and in Egypt (in 2005 with Dr. Iris Bräuninger who organized the first Creative Arts Therapies Symposium in Egypt demonstrating evidence-based practice and current research findings).

The challenge to spread the word and prove that dance movement therapy is effective: The Pyramids call for the Alps

The role to advocate for Creative Arts Therapies started young with different misconceptions related to the field and to the word 'dance'! It was quite fascinating what this word could provoke in people before any invitation for them to move. The resistance to endorse 'dance' with research evidence in Egypt has not ended to this day. The first author, Iris Bräuninger, kindly responded to my invitation to join the first symposium on the topic to demonstrate evidence-based material next to the Egyptian randomised trial but this did not seem to be enough to shake the preconceived notions associated with what dance means in my culture. Sufism is a shared Egyptian heritage with other cultures depicting wholly spiritual dance, pharaonic writings on their everlasting temples depicted dancing rituals for healing and communicating with Gods along with acrobatic moves and poses for entertainment and enlightenment of the soul. However, such heritage was unfortunately adulterated by misconceptions related to associating dance with inappropriate behaviours or condescending manners related to misconceptions about belly dance in particular and its sexualised notions in the contemporary mind. Also, the prevailing ideas related to sexualisation of the female body and the need to cover it as a misinterpretation of the Q'ran verses enhanced such distorted conceptions about the body, body image, the female body, and the self in the body, comprising different components of embodiment of the self in being, feeling and existing.

Going through this journey took me to human sexuality and addressing sexuality, the body, movement and dance within a couple and to leading an interactive workshop for psychiatrists from all over the world along the program of the Human Sexuality Section in the World Psychiatric Association WPA Congress. I also joined a creative arts therapies advocacy symposium with Iris Bräuninger and a consortium of established colleagues from Germany, Australia, and the UK, to start a promising new collaboration for further much needed advocacy.

Last but not least, I presented at a television program for two months twice a week called 12+18 addressing psychosomatic disorders, human sexuality, and comprising a segment called 'oxygen' addressing the impact of arts in health, with a focus on the role of dance and movement in particular in 2016. Additionally, writings in the newspapers and assisting in other television programs have addressed the role of dance movement therapy and creative arts therapies in healing and in prevention of disease.

Dance movement therapy education and prospects in the next ten years

Unfortunately, no dance movement therapy training program is available in Egypt yet. However, there are potent contemporary dance schools and dance advocacy moves at the Cairo Opera House that could offer a potential basis for future dance movement therapists, if given the necessary education and formation required to engage with illness and modulate therapies for different symptoms, disorders and populations with supervision. Howaida El Guindy took her training in the US as a dance movement therapist but does not offer any training; she used to treat patients at Behman Hospital, Cairo. I offer workshops in local conferences whenever possible and supervise students who have now also started offering workshops (2007–present).

Also, initiating an aura and raising the demand of dance movement therapy using media channels received positive attention from audiences. It gave space to a number of individuals who employ dance/movement and call it therapy without the 'know-how' and with a lack of experience and supervision of, and in, the modality. Interestingly, some of the psychiatrists who fought the modality, when I first introduced DMT in Egypt, are currently seeking learning with those who claim the practice for business purposes. Not only this, but also hosting dance therapists from nearby countries in an attempt to learn the modality.

From my experience in the field (2001–present), it would be fundamental to collaborate between different departments of contemporary dance and ballet institutes, high institutes of theatre and performance, applied arts universities and different departments of psychiatry at faculties of medicine in Cairo and other governorates of Egypt to come up with a proper foundational training in the field that would be culturally oriented and inclusive of the Egyptian wealth of healing dance and heritage, including Sufism and belly dance.

Definitions of embodiment and application of dance movement therapy

Cairo University Hospital Psychiatry department trains residents in using the integrative approach to the assessment of patients and for managing their suffering. This means psychotherapy training and supervision is fundamental to becoming a psychiatrist in this department beside the use of pharmacotherapy, electro-convulsive therapy and hospitalisation whenever required. Milieu and sports rehabilitation therapy is part of the culture raised in the department by Professor Yehia T. Rakhawy for over fifty years now and fostered by other successive professors such as Shaheen, Omar and others (Rakhawy, 2001). Professor Said Abdelazim former head of the department (2000–2002) founded the first psychosomatic unit in 1990 at the time that Professor Rakhawy was teaching embodiment and its role in assessment and healing.

On my learning journey, I witnessed embodiment at play with every patient starting from the eloquent antisocial addiction in disguise to the mute catatonic psychosis in fear of fragmentation. When I retrieve those experiences and contemplate embodiment the following aspects come to mind:

1) Embodiment entails living with every cell of one's existence, body and soul, whether in movement or in stillness, alone or in the company of/witnessing 'an' other; with every cell restoring a mind of a whole, a feel and a memory; in the here and now.

2) Embodiment entails synchronizing of one's cognition, emotion and memory to one's body, so that the body becomes the implicit and explicit mirror of one's status, body and soul, in the here and now.

3) Embodiment entails a process of exploration and discovery of one's authentic 'state of being' in terms of psyche, emotion, memory and cognition, acknowledged and embraced by one's body, in the here and now.

4) Embodiment entails a sense of awareness for one's own existence in body and mind, transcending from the consciousness of the mind to the consciousness of the body in/and soul/psyche, in the here and now.

Conclusion

While DMT in Switzerland is in the consolidation stage, it is clearly in the foundation stage in Egypt. With no other DMT generation beforehand in Egypt, the professionalization of the field still means pioneering both DMT as professional practice as well as developing a DMT professional training programme. In Switzerland, dance movement therapists can achieve, but are not required to have, federal state recognition. DMT courses in Switzerland offer high quality training courses, however academic training also needs to be established as an additional path.

Notes

1 www.monteverita.org/de/82/chronik.aspx.
2 btk-Schweizerischer Berufsverband für Bewegungs-, Tanz- und Körpertherapien www.bvbtk.ch/
3 A Certificate of Advanced Studies (CAS) requires a university degree and professional experience. A certificate course lasts one to two semesters and comprises between 10 and 15 ECTS ★ credits. CAS courses can be combined in meaningful contexts to a more comprehensive degree (DAS or MAS) at any university. (www.hkb.bfh.ch/de/weiterbildung/weiterbildungsangebot/ translated by the author)
4 www.artecura.ch/kunsttherapeut_in.php
5 www.oda-kt.ch/methodenanerkennung/
6 www.bvbtk.ch/fileadmin/btkAdressenlisten/FormTherapListe.doc

References

Bräuninger, I. (2005, October). *Efficacy of dance movement therapy in improving quality of life and reducing stress. A randomized control trial (RCT)*. Symposium Creative Arts Therapies in Psychiatry: Dance/movement therapy, Music therapy, Art therapy, Poetry therapy, XIII World Congress of Psychiatry, Cairo, Egypt.

Capello, P. (2014). "Why I Became a Dance Therapist": The 2013 ADTA International Panel. *American Journal of Dance Therapy, 36*(1), 28–39.

El Guindy, H., and Schmais, S. (1992). The Zar: An ancient dance of healing. *American Journal of Dance Therapy, 16*, 107–120.

Ellis, R. (2001). Movement metaphor as mediator: A model for the dance/movement therapy process. *The Arts in Psychotherapy, 28*, 181–190.

Fenner, P., Abdelazim, R., Bräuninger, I., Strehlow, G., and Seifert, K. (2017). Provision of arts therapies for people with severe mental illness. *Current Opinion (Review), 30*(4), 306–311.

Goodman, R. (1997). The Strengths and Difficulties Questionnaire: A research note. *Journal of Child Psychology and Psychiatry, 38*, 581–586.

Levy, F. J. (1988). The evolution of modern dance therapy. *Journal of Physical Education, Recreation and Dance, 59*(5), 34–41.

Martin, L. A., Koch, S. C., Hirjak, D., and Fuchs, T. (2016). Overcoming disembodiment: The effect of movement therapy on negative symptoms in schizophrenia – A multicenter randomized controlled trial. *Frontiers in Psychology, 7*, 483.

Rakhawy, T. Y. (2001). Images in psychiatry: An Arab perspective. In A. Okasha and M. Maj (Eds.), *Psychotherapy in Egypt. An overview* (pp. 225–246). World Psychiatric Association Publication, Scientific Book House.

Samaritter, R., and Payne, H. (2013). Kinaesthetic intersubjectivity: A dance informed contribution to self-other relatedness and shared experience in non-verbal psychotherapy with an example from autism. *The Arts in Psychotherapy, 40*(1), 143–150.

Storch, M., and Krause, F. (2007). *Selbstmanagement – ressourcenorientiert. Grundlagen und Manual für die Arbeit mit dem Zürcher Ressourcen Modell ZRM* [Self-management – resource-oriented. Principles and manual for working with the Zurich Resource Model ZRM] *(4. Aufl.)*. Bern: Huber.

Tantia, J. F. (2013). Mindfulness and dance/movement therapy for treating trauma. In L. Rapaport (Ed.), *Mindfulness and the Arts Therapies: Theory and practice* (pp. 95–106). London: Jessica Kingsley.

Tschacher, W., Munt, M., and Storch, M. (2014). Die integration von tanz, bewegung und psychotherapie durch den embodimentansatz [The integration of dance, movement and psychotherapy through the embodiment approach]. *Körper-Tanz-Bewegung, 2,* 54–63.

World Health Organisation. (2001). *International Classification of Diseases ICD-10. Classification of Mental and Behavioural Disorders with Glossary and Diagnostic Criteria for Research (ICD 10): DCR-10. Behavioural and emotional disorders with onset usually occurring in childhood and adolescence (F90-F98)*. Churchill Livingstone.

SECTION III

Theory and practice in body psychotherapy

Introduction

Section III presents sixteen chapters that provide perspectives on psychotherapy from a body psychotherapy approach. In body psychotherapy (also called somatic psychotherapy in the US), attention to embodied experience brings unconscious information to the forefront of a client's awareness. Embodied awareness can also facilitate an interpersonal dynamic with the therapist so that the client can build a greater sense of what they need, which increases self-compassion while finding the source of their suffering so that change may take place. The sections span a rich range of perspectives, from the basic fundamentals of tried and true systems of body psychotherapy to current issues for body psychotherapists. Contemporary perspectives on somatic countertransference, clients' embodied sense of safety, benefits and implications for the use of touch in treatment, awareness of micromovements, emotional regulation and a model for learning sensitivity toward clients' embodied oppression are among the offerings.

Section III begins with Chapter 22, by UK body psychotherapist **Gill Westland** who explores the repair of early stressful and traumatic interactions (insecure attachments) with adult clients. Awareness practices and theory drawn from Buddhist psychology support this. Being aware is being present, registering sensory experiences and being aware of shifting levels of consciousness as they manifest in the body. This is being embodied and is the foundation of embodied relating. This chapter will first discuss the theoretical foundations of this form of body psychotherapy and then illustrate how the application of this theory will offer not only the possibility of healing psychological problems presented by clients, but also the possibility of expanding therapist and client/patient consciousness.

In Chapter 23 **Ursula Bartholomew** and **Ingrid Herholz**, both from Germany, contribute an interesting overview of Functional Relaxation (FR) in psychosomatic medicine. FR is a method developed by Marianne Fuchs well known in German psychosomatic treatment, with increasing evidence-based research. It assumes the unity of moving and sensing and builds upon the Gestaltkreis by physician and philosopher Victor von Weizsäcker in the 1940s.

Next, **Halko Weiss** and **Maci Daye** in Chapter 24 speak to the ways in which a 'bottom up' approach (attention to embodied experience to inform cognition) is not only unique to body psychotherapy, but pertinent to the ways in which true meaning of the self can be revealed. They describe the ways in which reflection, a common process in psychoanalysis is primarily 'top-down' or thought through rather than experienced. Furthermore, they argue eloquently the ways in which mindfulness in addition to a 'bottom up' process in which observation of embodied experience and meaning-making that comes from experience can be more effective in contacting a client's self-compassion.

A UK body psychotherapist **Nick Totton**, in Chapter 25, describes Embodied-Relational Therapy (ERT), which contains a unique blend of Reichian and process-based approaches to psychotherapy, drawing on philosophy and cognitive science. This chapter outlines its history and general principles and approach. It summarises a view of embodied relating as the ground of all psychotherapy, offers a reframing of the body psychotherapy concept of character and illustrates ERT's style of working through a fictional case vignette.

From Switzerland **David Boadella**'s novel quadratic system of body psychotherapy creates Biosynthesis with 'Four Forms of Knowledge' in Chapter 26. The chapter looks in detail at different kinds of bridges of connection within a person and between people, and how it can be applied to body psychotherapy clinical practice.

Chapter 27 presents 'The relational turn in body psychotherapy', by UK based body psycho-therapist **Michael Soth**, in which he explores the different relational stances which body psy-chotherapists can be found to be taking in relation to the client's embodied character, manifesting in the here and now between client and therapist. By rooting the BodyMind process of the therapeutic relationship in a non-dualistic enactive, embodied, embedded and extended account of mind in the context of intersubjectivity in the therapeutic encounter, we can recognise the limitations of the therapist taking a variety of fixed stances (or a combination thereof). We can identify the following therapeutic stances as common denominators in the diverse subcultures of the body psychotherapeutic field: the therapist can position themselves.

Pertaining to the experience of the client, in Chapter 28 by German body psychotherapist **Ulf Geuter**, describes his system of emotional regulation in body psychotherapy that addresses the usefulness for enhancing clients' awareness, regulating pleasantness or unpleasantness and activation-deactivation and transforming discrete emotions such as anger, fear, or joy while assigning different body psychotherapeutic strategies for working with these factors.

Chapter 29 is by **Michel Heller** and **Gillat Burckhardt-Bartov**, both from France, who offer a clinical case describing the often complex and multi-faceted ways in which body psycho-therapy can become a source of healing for a physical condition that has psychological under-pinnings. They describe the ways in which vaginismus is treated through a series of sessions that help a client to discover insight that changes her experience of herself and the way she lives in the world.

The two subsequent chapters by **Tom Warnecke**, from the UK (Chapter 30) and **Asaf Rolef Ben-Shahar** (Chapter 31) focus on the therapist's body as a source of uncovering interpersonal knowledge in a body psychotherapy session. Warnecke describes how the therapist's body can act as a physical utility for both therapist's and client's emotional/biological processing by attend-ing to the therapist's embodied awareness in treatment and describes the value of the therapist's embodied awareness in sessions. Whereas in the contribution from Israel, **Rolef Ben-Shahar's** self-study discusses a case in which he reveals awareness of his own body while treating a client that challenged his sense of vulnerability as a therapist with human emotions.

Furthermore, Chapter 32 by **Rae Johnson** from the US, follows a similar theme of the ther-apist engaging with their body. They write about the importance of embodiment as a means of acknowledging oppression psychotherapy and in society. They articulate the crucial role of the body in navigating experiences of social difference and mediating chronic trauma of oppression. This chapter offers a clear description of how oppression is experienced as a bodily felt sense and illuminates the mostly unconscious behaviours that perpetuate inequitable social relations. Embodied psychotherapy practitioners might bring themselves into an experience of fuller contact with social power, privilege and difference on reading this chapter.

From the US **Christine Caldwell**'s (Chapter 33) innovatory contribution on micro-movements give a fresh perspective on the ways in which a therapist's sensitivity to a client's micromovements can be used in treatment. The 'Mobility Gradient' illustrates the process from immobility to spontaneity with six sub-steps along the way. Caldwell's description is accessible to both somatic and traditional talk psychotherapy practices.

Helma Mair, from Ireland, in Chapter 34, shares an original study which explored the experience of clients' feelings of safety in a psychotherapeutic context, and how their awareness of body sensations can determine the client's experience of safety and danger in the treatment setting. She articulates two main factors: language and embodied aspects of connection/disconnection with the therapist as ways to enhance a client's sense of safety.

Michael Chanagris, from the USA in Chapter 35, offers an argument for the use of touch in the psychotherapeutic session, and discusses from a developmental perspective the role of touch in developing embodiment, where it belongs in a somatic psychotherapy setting, and how it might be codified as part of assessment, intervention and treatment planning. He articulates five types of touch for somatic psychotherapists; attention and intention, attunement and mirroring, and emotional dialogue.

In Chapter 36, **Maurizio Stuppigia**, from Italy, discusses a case of how complex post-traumatic stress disorder (cPTSD) affects body perception and body image, and illustrates a client's experience in treatment who had become 'dis-embodied' following early childhood sexual traumatic experience.

Finally, **Margit Komeda-Lutz** from Switzerland in Chapter 37 develops an important bridge between bioenergetic analysis and neurobiological research mobilised through two clinical cases in which the body psychotherapy process gives a voice to implicit knowledge through body memory.

22

RELATING THROUGH THE BODY

Self, other and the wider world

Gill Westland

Introduction

In individual, depth, developmental psychotherapy the repair of early distressful relationships runs alongside profound moments of interconnection as universal states of consciousness are entered. Repair involves the re-patterning (re-organisation) of early traumatic and stressful relationships (early insecure attachments). These early relationships, where bonding has been problematic, form basic signature patterns of relating and ways of organisation. They are encoded in implicit memory and are out of our awareness. However, patterns of relating are revealed, for example, in breathing movements, which are specific to individuals (Andersen, 2007). These patterns are malleable and 'Deep re-organization occurs through the *deepening and expansion of relational capacity* in the client (and the therapist)' (Carroll, 2005, p. 90, author italics). Through embodied contact in the therapeutic relationship, both client and therapist may cultivate under-developed parts of themselves and jettison unhelpful ways of relating. Changes happen in the present moment with re-organisations of the biological systems of the body and are reflected in new signature postures, movements and breathing. Changes are also revealed in novel speech patterns, ways of thinking and expressing emotions. Changes occur in *non*-conscious, implicit parts of the individuals and are activated by present time physical, sensory and atmospheric experiences, in which the client-psychotherapist dyad join together in moments of meeting.

The non-conscious is to be differentiated from the unconscious. The non-conscious has never been explicitly known and forms implicit memory, which is non-verbal (Rustin, 2013). 'Implicit knowing is nonconscious' (Stern, 2004, p. 116). It manifests in tangible, physical ways. In contrast the unconscious was explicit and became repressed. Changes in people come about through shifts in non-conscious ways of being without any explicit knowledge of how the changes came about. From this viewpoint, change is possible without insight (cognitive understanding), analytical thinking, and verbalisations (Lyons-Ruth, 1998; Marks-Tarlow, 2012; Schore, 2011; von Peter, 2013). This does not exclude the possibility of change through insight, which is more widely discussed in the psychotherapy literature, but the inclusion of non-conscious ways of changing widens the scope of the discussion on how healing comes about.

Buddhist psychology and philosophy contribute to an understanding of how changes occur and underpin the perspective of this chapter. Awareness and mindfulness practices taken from

Buddhist psychology and introduced into psychotherapy provide the vehicles within which to explore experiences. Exploration may have a selective focus on the self, the other, or the wider world, and open different states of being. Central to the change process is *bringing awareness to the dynamics of therapeutic relating*. It is through deep listening and bringing awareness to different dimensions of relating that profound transformation occurs.

Theory
Embodiment and lack of embodiment

When I trained as a body psychotherapist in the late 1970s it was common to hear 'he's in his head, he's not in his body', but theoretical discussions about precisely what this meant were limited. Significantly, the descriptions could be observed by the trained eye and had clinical relevance. The assumption was that many problems could be attributed to, and were character-ised by, a lack of body awareness and 'splits' between parts of the body that felt alive and parts that felt dead, numb, or non-existent. An explanation about a particular experience was less important than having, for example, the *experience* of numbness. Following Reich (1945/1970, 1942/1983) body psychotherapy, along with other psychotherapies such as dance movement psychotherapy took non-dualism for granted (Payne, Warnecke, Karkou, and Westland, 2016). This perspective also saw life and energy synonymously (Reich, 1945/1970, 1942/1983), a viewpoint more consistent with Eastern philosophies than Western ones. Being in the body (being embodied) was a working assumption rooted in empirical work with clients. With it came views about human beings and whether they were merely existing or living vibrant, full lives. Current literature is exploring embodiment or the lack of it more systematically with clinical populations (for example, Fuchs and Schlimme, 2009; Martin, Koch, Hirjak, and Fuchs, 2016).

Being aware of the stream of arising subjective experiences in the body is being embodied. Knowledge of this process is cultivated by focussed awareness. It involves tracking thoughts, feelings and sensations with reference to how they are simultaneously experienced bodily. Any thought has an accompanying collection of physical sensations and emotions; emotions have an accompanying collection of muscle and postural changes, including changes in breathing rhythms. Being embodied is having the capacity for thinking, feeling and sensing at the same time. Through developmental arrests, and 'insults to form' (Keleman, 1985), including trauma, past and present, these functions become split from each other. Being embodied is a fluctuating process representing shifts in our level of consciousness (Clover Southwell, personal communica-tion, 2014). Being in touch with the 'felt-sense' (Gendlin, 1981, 1996), 'somatic body awareness' (Fogel, 2009), and 'somatic markers' (Damasio, 1994) provides information for decision-making, links thinking with the feeling of something and is vital in relationships for effective commu-nication. Furthermore, body awareness is important when a person is talking and attempting to express feelings authentically. Reich writes:

> It is clear that language, in the process of word formation, depends on the perception of inner movements and organ sensations, and that words which describe emotional states render, in an *immediate way*, the corresponding expressive movements of living matter.
>
> *(Reich, 1945/1970, p. 361, original italics)*

When Reich writes here about the 'movements of living matter', he is describing being in contact with the movements of life. Movement distinguishes the living from the dead. Following from this *living in a body* and inhabiting oneself (rather than having a body) means connecting with the movement of life itself. And so, to the extent that we are embodied, we are truly alive.

Imagine a man 'in his head', let's call him Mark. He thinks, he talks, but he lacks awareness of his body. Sensitive observation of him shows that from the occipital region at the back of the head and from his neck down his body barely moves. He lacks vitality. He speaks in a monotonous tone without the contours of emotions being expressed in his voice. If Mark is asked about himself, he explains himself, but not an immediate experience of what it feels like to be him. Mark's thinking is well developed, but he struggles to couple his thinking to his sensations and feelings. Nevertheless, he knows that he is lonely, anxious, somewhat depressed, and that he finds it difficult to relate to other human beings intimately and so prefers solitary pursuits. Mark has developed sensitive-analytic defences (Kurtz, 1990), also known as schizoid character structure/strategy (Lowen, 1958/1971; Reich, 1945/1970), which roughly correlates with Ainsworth's insecure-avoidant attachment style (Ainsworth, Blehar, Waters, and Wall, 1978). These diagnostic models are useful for recognising and thinking about clients and how they relate in a general way. They do not describe immutable states and obviously, clients are more than their defence system. Mark's style of relating protected him from experiencing inhospitable relationships early in his life, but also hinders the development of different aspects of himself, such as feeling and sensing. More importantly it obscures his fundamental sense of connection with life.

Awareness as healing

It is easy to think that Mark's difficulties can be resolved simply by somehow lessening the grip of his protective ways of relating. A different approach, however, is for him to become aware of how he is engaging with feelings, thoughts, and sensations from moment to moment, when by himself, with others, and when engaged in all sorts of activities – eating, walking, sitting, exercising and so on. Awareness is non-verbal and is the physical felt-sense of something, not a description of it in words, although sounds, movements, art, poetry, and imagery can bring some sort of approximation to it. Within psychotherapy awareness has long been known to be transformative (Bugental, 1978; Maslow, 1973; Ogden, Minton, and Pain, 2006; Siegel, 2010).

Although the term awareness is often used interchangeably with mindfulness, 'mindfulness directs us to the details of our experience, [while] awareness refers to the larger context, the space within which experience arises' (Wegela, 2009, p. 58) and 'mindfulness is paying precise attention in the present moment to whatever object we have chosen to observe' (Wegela, 2014, p. 17). Both awareness and mindfulness are important for living life more fully. Meditation teacher Gunaratana writes:

> Awareness allows us to see whether our actions spring from beneficial or harmful impulses . . . When we are mindful of the deep roots from which our thoughts, words and deeds grow, we have the opportunity to cultivate those that are beneficial and weed out those that are harmful.
>
> *(Gunaratana, 2012, p. 2)*

Whilst Western science and philosophy have struggled with mind-body dualism, this is not the case in Eastern philosophy where the perspective is 'of mind/body oneness' and experiential practices taking precedence over theory (Watson, 2002, p. 187). These are 'the foundation for methods of self-cultivation which affect, train, and transform the mind through the body' (Watson, 2002, p. 187). This view sits easily within embodied psychotherapies. Not only does Buddhist philosophy give ways of thinking about human existence, but mindfulness and awareness practices provide tools for the clinician to cultivate disciplined attention to the details of relating. Embodied psychotherapies often draw on phenomenology (Merleau-Ponty, 1962) for their philosophical underpinnings (for example, Gallagher and Payne, 2015; Koch and Fischman, 2011; Payne et al., 2016). This can be valuable as phenomenology attempts to bridge the perceived dualities between mind/body, and man/world, but nevertheless, phenomenological investigation remains mostly an intellectual activity. Cognitive scientist, Varela, and his colleagues observe that current scientific investigation has 'no direct, hands-on, pragmatic approach to experience with which to complement science' and suggest meditation practice gives the possibility for 'skilful and disciplined examination of experience' (Varela, Thompson, and Rosch, 1993, p. xviii). They suggest a combination of mindfulness and awareness meditation practices to structure research experiences. These practices also have a role in psychotherapy and are familiar to body psychotherapies explicitly (Kurtz, 1990; Ogden et al., 2006; Weiss, 2009; Weiss, Johanson, and Monda, 2015; Westland, 2015) or implicitly (Boadella, 1987; Boyesen, 1980; Rosenberg, Rand, and Asay, 1985). In this sense psychotherapy may be seen as experiential research.

Latent potential

Returning to Mark, his therapeutic journey involves him gaining awareness of his ways of relating and qualities of being, rather than selecting some experiences over others and having set goals. Rather than trying to change him, the therapeutic stance is one of accepting him (and oneself) as he is. Mark's psychotherapy might end once he becomes consistently less anxious and no longer depressed, but it might not, since body psychotherapy aspires to more than symptom or problem reduction. A central theme in body psychotherapy is the blossoming of latent potential (Boening, Southwell, and Westland, 2012). Southwell writes:

> from conception onwards each individual has a unique and dynamic potential. This drives his physical growing into his particular human shape: it also drives his passage towards mental, personal, and spiritual fulfilment. We work in alliance with this dynamic inner pressure . . . The dynamic of our client's potential is the motor of the therapy. Our therapeutic relationship is its containing membrane. *We hold the vision of our client's unrealised potential. For us, this is more significant than his pathology.*
> *(Southwell, 2010, p. 11, author italics)*

And Boadella adds:

> The goal of therapy is to restore the person to a state of healthy pulsation in which the basic life activities are rhythmic, give pleasure, and work for enhanced contact with oneself and others.
> *(1988, p. 163)*

Boyesen (1982) describes a person living from the 'primary personality' as in contact with life. This is nourishing and gives meaning to life. This contact with life is visible in people in their actions and general demeanour. She writes:

> The Primary Personality has a natural joy in life, a basic security, stability and honesty . . . There is pleasure in work and in relaxation, a gentle euphoria and a mild

intoxication in the pleasure of living . . . He or she is in touch with the instinctual self, the primitive and animalistic urges, yet this is integrated also with the transcendent . . .

(Boyesen, 1982, pp. 5–8)

In Mark's case, his psychotherapist notices that he becomes most alive when he speaks of his passion for bird-watching; his eyes light up and his face shines. At those times she underscores this by asking him more and engaging in lively discussion about the plumage and habits of the birds that Mark had seen. The invitation to say more validates Mark's pleasure and vitality and offers the possibility of him connecting with his experience in these moments.

Movement towards health

The tendency of all life, including human life, is movement towards health. Life is self-directing, and healing is a self-organising, non-linear process (Capra, 1996; Maturana and Varela, 1987; Wilber, 1995). Many of those seeking psychotherapy will have experienced early traumatic events and relationships. Nevertheless, whether severely traumatised or not, there is always 'an organic impulse to heal, which can be experienced phenomenologically and that moves towards increased complexity and wholeness' (Johanson, 2014, p. 68).

Southwell tells us, 'The dynamic updrift is the key to change in biodynamic therapy [body psychotherapy]' (Southwell, 1988, p. 196). Fosha describes 'transformance', which sounds like Southwell's 'dynamic potential' (Southwell, 1988). Transformance is, '. . . the overarching motivation for transformation that pulses within us . . . Innate dispositional tendencies toward growth, learning, healing, and self-righting are wired deep within our brains and press towards expression when circumstances are right' (Fosha, 2009, p. 174).

The force of 'unrealised potential' is also described as primary impulse(s) or primary communications (Westland, 2015). If early relationships or the atmosphere of the family home is threatening, the primary impulse becomes overlaid and obscured by the 'secondary personality' (Southwell, 1988, p. 182). The acquired secondary personality is developed by the child to protect him or herself from unbearable feelings. This is secondary patterning or secondary communications (Boadella, 1987; Westland, 2015). The lack of movement in Mark's body is an example of secondary patterning, his eyes lighting up, when talking about a bird's primary impulse.

In spite of Mark's secondary patterning, he already possesses everything for his independent well-being. The psychotherapeutic task is to foster conditions in which he, and clients generally, reconnect with life or 'inherent health'. Inherent health is synonymous with 'wisdom', 'core state', 'essential self', 'source', and 'essence' (Boadella, 1988; Boyesen 1976; Kurtz, 1990; Maurer, 1993; Pierrakos, 1987; Rosenberg et al., 1985; Sills, 2009; Southwell, 1988). Wegela, uses the term 'Brilliant Sanity' and also informs us that the therapeutic task is 'to help our clients connect, or reconnect, with their own worthiness, their brilliant sanity' (Wegela, 2014, p. 5).

Theory into practice

Psychotherapy and relating through the body

Psychotherapists must live from a place of embodied connection with life to help clients to connect with Brilliant Sanity. Being relatively embodied and relating through the body are fundamental. However, having a moving, flexible body such as that cultivated through dance or gymnastics does not equate with relating through the body. Embodied relating requires being grounded and centred in the body and using the physicality of the body as a reference point for staying in contact with reality. As the therapeutic relationship develops and different states of consciousness emerge, the task is to maintain an awareness of whatever is being experienced through referencing the bodily experience of it. Being aware involves slowing down the stream of experiences to capture subtlety and nuance. Maurer adds, 'Slowness serves to help one concentrate, to increase one's capacity to spiritually concentrate and to become fully attentive, preliminary to meeting one's wholeness, one's own essence' (1993, p. 88). This invites wholeness in both client and psychotherapist and has implications for the training of psychotherapists and ongoing professional development.

Training

The main way that psychotherapists learn embodied relating is through *experiential* training, including participating in one to one psychotherapy of the same modality that they will be practising. It should be experiential and process oriented. The training of humanistic psychotherapies, which include body psychotherapies and creative arts psychotherapies, has long privileged this sort of experiential learning. Experiential learning becomes embedded in the psychotherapist and is often not known explicitly, but emerges from the psychotherapist spontaneously, when the need arises. It cannot be acquired thorough textbooks and interactive technology. In experiential training something is tried out in an activity, such as a role play, a movement, a posture or different way of breathing and afterwards reflected on. Reflection means further experiencing and recasting of the first experience in the present, as what was experienced is spoken about. This deepens the experience and with it the learning. Meaning emerges through the experience rather than through analytical thought. So the term reflection here is not the same as mentalising as used psychoanalytically (for example, Fonagy, Gergely, Jurist, and Target, 2002). Experiential learning as a student psychotherapist approximates the way learning occurs in embodied psychotherapies. This style of training and clinical work is also described as 'bottom up' (Ogden et al., 2006). That is, it focusses on sensations and emotions and the physicality of these before the 'top down' processes of thinking and analysis.

Intuitive, spontaneous and creative interactions are also the stuff of this sort of training. Analyst Lomas writes . . . 'a good training is one which allows and encourages students to trust, as far as possible, their own intuitive capacity, and to build on their own style of being with people rather than suppressing it and replacing it with a formula for behaviour imposed from without' (Lomas, 1994, p. 136).

Marks-Tarlow explains, 'In psychotherapy, we continually shuttle back and forth between the intuitive mode of the right hemisphere and the deliberative mode of the left one . . . it is the intuitive right side that integrates the whole' (2012, pp. 17–18). Intuitions and spontaneous interactions can be seen as undisciplined and reckless and so 'Intuitions have to be *grounded in and experienced, through the body*; otherwise they really can be wild and unhelpful' (Westland, 2015, original italics).

Ongoing experiences

When training is finished, continuing to relate through the body requires practice within and outside the consulting room. Maurer (1993) suggests psychotherapists help themselves to slow down by engaging in 'relaxation exercises' and 'Eastern fighting techniques' such as Aikido and Tai Chi. Additionally engagement with activities which nurture an ongoing relationship with body experience are essential. These could include dance, walking, meditation, and yoga. These practices help to keep essential therapeutic skills honed, but also help to prevent burn out.

Practice

Awareness in clinical practice

Increasingly there is recognition that every therapeutic relationship is unique, with both client and psychotherapist bringing their personal histories, life experiences and predilections to it. Soth and Young observe:

> There is not just *one* kind of therapeutic relating, but a pluralistic diversity of different – and sometimes contradictory – ways of relating that all seem to 'work' at different times, in different situations, and with different therapists and clients, and *all* these therefore need to be acknowledged as valid, at least in principle.
>
> *(Soth and Young, 2015, p. xvii)*

Being to being

Relating through the body (embodied relating) requires a relatively more right brain way of relating, described by Schore (2012) as a right brain to right brain interactive approach. Schore elaborates:

> At the most fundamental level, the work of psychotherapy is not defined by what the therapist explicitly, objectively *does* for the patient, or *says* to the patient. Rather the key mechanism is how to implicitly and subjectively *be* with the patient, especially during affectively stressful moments when the 'going on being' of the patient's implicit self is dis-integrating in real time.
>
> *(Schore, 2011, pp. 94–95)*

Within this style of psychotherapy there is a lot of scope for intuitive responses (Marks-Tarlow, 2012), since the psychotherapist does not have to understand something intellectually and consciously before responding. Schore explains 'Much of the therapist's knowledge that accumulates with clinical experience is implicit, operates at rapid, unconscious levels beneath levels of awareness, and is spontaneously expressed as clinical intuition' (Schore, 2012, p. 7).

Nevertheless, while it is convenient to describe psychotherapy as right brain to right brain relating, as it offers a way of discussing ideas, in practice *being with clients* is more than one brain relating to another brain. Returning to a Buddhist perspective, being with the suffering of ourselves and others reminds us of the 'inherent connectedness of all life' (Sills, 2009, p. 2). Meditation teacher Thich Nhat Hanh uses the term 'Interbeing' to describe this fundamental interconnection. All human beings, all living creatures and the wider environment including forests, rivers, mountains and minerals are interconnected and 'Interbe' (Hanh, 1998). Intersubjectivity is therefore the natural condition (Fulton, 2014). Sills (2009) describes two axes of relating. The first is 'Source – being – self'. In moments of stillness, in the present moment, universal connectedness (Source) can be entered. The second axis is 'being – to – being' and is interpersonal. Being-to-being relating is relating from beneath any defensive secondary patterning, that either client or therapist carry, and which may evoke reactive responses in either or both. The two axes co-exist and can melt into a profound sense of the interconnection of everything.

Objects of awareness in psychotherapy

Awareness is always connected with something. Within psychotherapy attention can focus on different 'objects', as client and psychotherapist follow their co-arising curiosities. Objects of attention can be breath, body sensations, movements, sounds, smells, feelings, sights, touch, energy, atmospheres, others – loved ones, friends, acquaintances, difficult people, enemies, people in the wider world – nature, and inanimate objects. Any of these can be the portal for personal explorations and expanded states of awareness.

Being with the self

Gunaratana (2012) reminds us that the body and breathing are ever present and can be the starting place for self-awareness. By becoming more self-aware, the psychotherapist becomes more present to him or herself and creates a receptive field for Mark to enter. When Mark arrives, he will sense this welcome without necessarily registering it in his thinking. For Mark, the difference between thinking emotions and physically sensing them and gaining a different sense of self can be cultivated by asking questions about his experience. For example, 'Let's take a pause here, notice what you are sensing in your shoulders and chest. How would it be to move your shoulders a bit? How it that now?' These sorts of questions are commonplace in body psychotherapies and are termed by Ogden (2009) as directed mindfulness.

For clients more traumatised than Mark, reflections on self-experience are often problematic. Those with a diagnosis of Borderline Personality Disorder (BPD), for example, have deficits in mindfulness and these are predictive in BPD pathology. Mindfulness, therefore, has a role in the treatment of BPD (Wupperman, Neumann, Whitman, and Axelrod, 2009). For some traumatised clients an internal focus on themselves whether on the body or a body part or their breathing is too exposing or threatening. These clients, as it were, live at some distance from themselves. An alternative inquiry is with objects in the room. 'As you place your hand on the wall, notice if the wall feels cool, warm from the sunshine or cold'. A short-rein, matter of fact style of discussion is apt (Westland, 2015). This keeps a tight hold on the pace of relating, without silences, and keeps to an everyday level of consciousness, which reduces potential emotional overwhelm.

Being with the other

We are always connected with others, although we may not be aware of it. From a neuroscience perspective mirror neurons (Gallese, Fadiga, Fogassi, and Rizzolatti, 1996) let us resonate with others. They enables us to capture what is happening with clients beneath the spoken word. '*Somatic resonance is the direct experience of the client's feelings, bodily sensations, and thinking. It is more than empathy*' (Westland, 2015, p. original italics). For the psychotherapist the task is to track changes in their physical, subjective internal state and read them *both* as information about themselves, but also the client. Shifting the focus of attention to the actual client sitting in front of the psychotherapist gives further visual information.

So again, taking Mark, as an example, if the therapist senses tightness in her shoulders, she might look at him and see the tension and lack of mobility in his shoulders. When Mark is asked about his experience of his shoulders he might respond 'tense'. He might then be invited to explore further with questions such as, 'What is the shape and texture of "tense"? What happens to the tension if you move a little?' The psychotherapist might then notice her own changing experience of her shoulders.

Often clients will come to learn how to have contact with an internal focus on themselves and be able to sustain it as they are more focussed interpersonally. Clients tend to focus more on the other and loose connection with themselves or vice versa. Traumatised clients, for example, often have highly developed antennae for mood shifts in the other, but underdeveloped body awareness. Those more narcissistically inclined tend to focus on themselves, but do not connect with the other. As a way of addressing the focus on self – other dynamics a pertinent question at the right time is, 'As I say that how do you experience that?' This is quite a challenging question and probably not suitable for Mark until he becomes less fearful about such a direct focus.

Being with the wider world

Focussing attention on the wider world and taking a panoramic viewpoint involves relating to, and having awareness of, objects – the wall, the floor, the picture on the wall. It also includes the atmosphere in the room and relationships with others not present in the room – loved ones, friends, difficult people, and so on. Again whatever the focus, the question is to reflect on what arises. All of these reflections can give different senses of self.

Expanded states of awareness

Whilst it is helpful to become aware of all sorts of aspects of ourselves and our surroundings, Fulton reminds us that the relationship to experience is not raw experience itself (Fulton, 2014). However, from focussing on any one of these objects of attention, it is possible to slip into expanded awareness of the core state. Wegela writes:

> When we are willing to be present, we tap into direct experience: that is experience that is not filtered through our thoughts, expectations, hopes and fears. Instead, we see, hear, taste, touch phenomena, and recognize thoughts and images in the mind without adding judgments or preferences. Things are just what they are. Putting nowness and direct experience together means being awake in the present moment.
>
> *(Wegela, 2009, p. 26)*

Conclusion

Through embodied relating and bringing attention to different experiences gives clients and psychotherapists alike the means to live life more fully. Awareness and meditation practices are not so much about reducing symptoms such as anxiety, although that may happen, but open the way for surrendering into the core state. This is characterised by compassion, loving-kindness, joy and equanimity.

References

Ainsworth, M. D. S., Blehar, M. C., Waters, E., and Wall, S. (1978). *Patterns of Attachment. A Psychological Study of the Strange Situation*. Hillsdale, NJ: Lawrence Erlbaum.

Andersen, T. (2007). Human participating: Human "Being" is the step for human "Becoming" in the next step. In H. Anderson and G. Diane (Eds.), *Collaborative Therapy. Relationships and Conversations that make a Difference* (pp. 81–107). New York: Routledge.

Boadella, D. (1987). *Lifestreams. An Introduction to Biosynthesis*. London: Routledge and Kegan Paul.

Boadella, D. (1988). Biosynthesis. In J. Rowan and W. Dryden (Eds.), *Innovative Therapy in Britain*. Milton Keynes: Open University Press.

Boening, M., Southwell, C., and Westland, G. (2012). *UK Body Psychotherapy Competencies*. Retrieved from www.eabp.org/forum-body-psychotherapy-competencies.php

Boyesen, G. (1976). The primary personality and its relationship to the streamings. In D. Boadella (Ed.), *In the Wake of Reich* (pp. 81–98). London: Coventure.

Boyesen, G. (1980). *Biodynamic Psychology. The Collected Papers* (Vols. 1 and 2). London: Biodynamic Psychology Publications. (Originally published as a series of articles in *Energy and Character, The Journal of Biosynthesis.*)

Boyesen, G. (1982). The primary personality. *Journal of Biodynamic Psychology* (1982) *20*, 3: 3–8.

Bugental, J. F. T. (1978). *Psychotherapy and Process. The Fundamentals of an Existential-Humanistic Approach.* London: Addison-Wesley.

Capra, F. (1996). *The Web of Life: A New Understanding of Living Systems.* New York: Anchor Books.

Carroll, R. (2005). Rhythm, reorientation, reversal: Deep reorganization of the self in psychotherapy. In J. Ryan (Ed.), *How Does Psychotherapy Work?* (pp. 85–112). London: Karnac.

Damasio, A. (1994). *Descartes' Error, Emotion, Reason and the Human Brain.* London: Picador.

Fogel, A. (2009). *The Psychophysiology of Self-Awareness. Rediscovering the Lost Art of Body Sense.* New York: W.W. Norton.

Fonagy, P., Gergely, G., Jurist, E. L., and Target, M. (2002). *Affect Regulation, Mentalization, and the Development of the Self.* New York: Other Press.

Fosha, D. (2009). Emotion and recognition at work: Energy, vitality, pleasure, truth, desire, and the emergent phenomenology of transformational experience. In: D. Fosha, D. J. Siegel, M. F. Solomon, (Eds.), *The Healing Power of Emotion. Affective Neuroscience, Development and Clinical Practice* (pp. 172–203). New York: W.W. Norton.

Fuchs, T., and Schlimme, J. E. (2009). Embodiment and psychopathology: A phenomenological perspective. *Current Opinion in Psychiatry, 22,* 570–575.

Fulton, P. R. (2014). Contributions and challenges to clinical practice from Buddhist psychology. *Clin Soc Work J* (2014) 42: 208–217.

Gallagher, S., and Payne, P. (2015). The role of embodiment and intersubjectivity in clinical reasoning. *Body, Movement and Dance in Psychotherapy, 10*(1), 51–68.

Gallese, V., Fadiga, L., Fogassi, L., and Rizzolatti, G. (1996). Action recognition in the premotor cortex. *Brain, 119,* 593–609.

Gendlin, E. (1981). *Focusing* (2nd ed.). London: Bantam.

Gendlin, E. (1996). *Focusing-Oriented Psychotherapy: A Manual of the Experiential Method.* London: Guilford Press.

Gunaratana, B. (2012). *The Four Foundations of Mindfulness in Plain English.* Boston: Wisdom.

Hanh, T. N. (1998). *The Heart of the Buddha's Teaching. Transforming Suffering into Peace, Joy and Liberation.* London: Rider.

Johanson, G. J. (2014). Somatic psychotherapy and the ambiguous face of research. *International Body Psychotherapy Journal, 13*(2), 61–85.

Keleman, S. (1985). *Emotional Anatomy.* Berkeley, CA: Center Press.

Koch, S. C., and Fischman, D. (2011). Embodied enactive dance/movement therapy. *American Journal of Dance Therapy, 33,* 57–72.

Kurtz, R. (1990). *Body-Centered Psychotherapy: The Hakomi Method.* Menocino, CA: Life Rhythm.

Lomas, P. (1994). *Cultivating Intuition, an Introduction to Psychotherapy.* London: Penguin.

Lowen, A. (1971). *The Language of the Body.* New York: Collier Books. (Original work published 1958)

Lyons-Ruth, K. (1998). Implicit relational knowing: Its role in development and psychoanalytic treatment. *Infant Mental Health Journal, 19,* 282–289.

Marks-Tarlow, T. (2012). *Clinical Intuition in Psychotherapy. The Neurobiology of Embodied Response.* New York: W.W. Norton.

Martin, L. A. L., Koch, S. C., Hirjak, D., and Fuchs, T. (2016). Overcoming disembodiment: The effect of movement therapy on negative symptoms in schizophrenia – A multicenter randomized controlled trial. *Frontiers in Psychology, 7,* 483.

Maslow, A. H. (1973). *The Farther Reaches of Human Nature.* Harmonsworth: Penguin.

Maturana, H. R., and Varela, F. J. (1991). *The Tree of Knowledge.* Boston, MA: Shambhala.

Maurer, Y. (1993). *Body-Centered Psychotherapy: A Multi-Dimensional, Multi-Communicative, Process-Oriented Approach.* Zurich: IKP-Verlag.

Merleau-Ponty, M. (1962). *Phenomenology of Perception* (C. Smith, Trans.). London: Routledge and Kegan Paul.

Ogden, P. (2009). Emotion, mindfulness, and movement: Expanding the regulatory boundaries of the window of tolerance. In D. Fosha, D. J. Siegel, and M. F. Solomon (Eds.), *The Healing Power of Emotion. Affective Neuroscience, Development and Clinical Practice* (pp. 204–231). New York: W.W. Norton.

Ogden, P., Minton, K., and Pain, C. (2006). *Trauma and the Body: A Sensorimotor Approach to Psychotherapy.* London: W.W. Norton.

Payne, H., Warnecke, T., Karkou, V., and Westland, G. (2016). A comparative analysis of body psychotherapy and dance movement psychotherapy from a European perspective. *Body, Movement and Dance in Psychotherapy, 11*(2–3), 144–166.

Pierrakos, J. (1987). *Core Energetics: Developing the Capacity to Love and Heal.* Mendocino, CA: Life Rhythm.

Reich, W. (1970). *Character Analysis.* New York: Farrer, Straus and Giroux. (Original work published 1945)

Reich, W. (1983). *The Function of the Orgasm.* London: Souvenir Press. (Original work published 1942)

Rosenberg, J. L., Rand, M. L., and Asay, D. (1985). *Body, Self and Soul Sustaining Integration.* Atlanta, GA: Humanics Limited.

Rustin, J. (2013). *Infant Research and Neuroscience at Work in Psychotherapy, Expanding the Clinical Repertoire.* London: W.W. Norton.

Schore, A. N. (2011). The right brain implicit self lies at the core of psychoanalytic psychotherapy. *Psychoanalytic Dialogues, 21*, 75–100.

Schore, A. N. (2012). *The Science of the Art of Psychotherapy.* London: W.W. Norton.

Siegel, D. (2010). *The Mindful Therapist. A Clinician's Guide to Mindsight and Neural Integration.* New York: W.W. Norton.

Sills, F. (2009). *Being and Becoming. Psychodynamics, Buddhism, and the Origins of Selfhood.* Berkeley, CA: North Atlantic Books.

Soth, M., and Young, C. (2015). Introduction to the American – English edition. In G. Marlock and H. Weiss with C. Young, and M. Soth (Eds.), *The Handbook of Body Psychotherapy and Somatic Psychology.* Berkeley, CA: North Atlantic Books.

Southwell, C. (1988). The Gerda Boyesen Method: Biodynamic therapy. In: J. Rowan, and W. Dryden, (Eds.), *Innovative Therapy in Britain* (pp. 178–201). Milton Keynes: Open University Press.

Southwell, C. (2010). Levels of consciousness and of contact in biodynamic psychotherapy. *The Psychotherapist, 47*, 10–11.

Stern, D. (2004). *The Present Moment in Psychotherapy and Everyday Life.* New York: W.W. Norton.

Varela, F. J., Thompson, E., and Rosch, E. (1993). *The Embodied Mind: Cognitive Science and Human Experience.* Cambridge, MA: The MIT Press.

von Peter, S. (2013). Exploring embodied perspectives of change within a psychiatric context: Some preliminary remarks from a psychiatrist. *Subjectivity, 6*(2), 212–224.

Watson, G. (2002). *The Resonance of Emptiness, a Buddhist Inspiration for a Contemporary Psychotherapy.* London: Routledge Curzon.

Wegela, K. K. (2009). *The Courage to be Present, Buddhism, Psychotherapy and the Awakening of Natural Wisdom.* London: Shambhala.

Wegela, K. K. (2014). *Contemplative Psychotherapy Essentials. Enriching Your Practice with Buddhist Psychology.* New York: W.W. Norton.

Weiss, H. (2009). The use of mindfulness in psychodynamic and body oriented psychotherapy. *Body, Movement and Dance in Psychotherapy, 4*(1), 5–16.

Weiss, H., Johanson, G., and Monda, L. (2015). *Hakomi Mindfulness-Centered Somatic Psychotherapy. A Comprehensive Guide to Theory and Practice.* New York: W.W. Norton.

Westland, G. (2015). *Verbal and Non-Verbal Communication in Psychotherapy.* New York: W.W. Norton.

Wilber, K. (1995). *Sex, Ecology and Spirituality.* London: Shambhala.

Wupperman, P., Neumann, C. S., Whitman, J. B., and Axelrod, S. R. (2009). The role of mindfulness in borderline personality disorder. *Journal of Nervous Mental Disorders, 197*(10), 766–771.

23

FUNCTIONAL RELAXATION IN PSYCHOSOMATIC MEDICINE

Ursula Bartholomew and Ingrid Herholz

Introduction

Functional Relaxation (FR) is a psychodynamic body psychotherapy method, founded by the German gymnastics teacher Marianne Fuchs (1908–2010) at the University Hospital of Heidelberg in the years after the Second World War. FR aims at rebalancing the organism by releasing muscular tension through soft movements of joints during expiration. During relaxation, patients experience areas of the body intensively through the 'proprioceptive' sense to promote perception of their own body processes. Bodily sensations allow access to unconscious memories, body images and emotions, particularly those associated with very early experiences. This 'inner dialogue' is accompanied by a verbal dialogue with the therapist, and body resonance in the context of countertransference. A constant flow of body awareness enhances the therapeutic process leading to organisation of complex psychological functions such as symbolisation and building of representation.

The intention is to improve self-regulation and to achieve somato-psychological equilibrium, to promote empathy via self-acceptance and to enable patients to have a more relaxed approach to themselves and others. FR has proved to be especially effective for treatment of functional disorders like somatoform and pain disorders as well as anxiety and trauma related symptoms (Arnim et al., 2006; Lahmann et al., 2007, 2008, 2009). The saluto-genetic effect is applied in preventive medicine, e.g. as a manualized approach to stress prevention (Lahmann et al., 2017).

According to Fuchs FR is a 'pragmatic psychotherapy', 'because it acts from the here and now and orients itself at the reality of the living body, by means of which the patient perceives, acts, experiences and suffers (Fuchs, 2013, p. 17). At that time a bodily approach to influencing psychological functions was pioneering. It implied a concept of the body as base of and home to psychological functions and thus represented an early 'intuitive' understanding of 'embodiment'. Fuchs always preferred the older German term 'Leib' for 'body' (instead of 'Körper'), standing thereby in the philosophical tradition of the ambiguity of the body. In contrast to other languages there exist two different German words for body: while 'Körper' means the 'objectively' measurable body ('the body I have'), the older word 'Leib', nowadays rarely used in everyday German language, but still common in metaphors, defines the 'subjective' entity of the body ('the body I am').

Historical background

FR was born when Marianne Fuchs intuitively started to work with her 1-year-old son who suffered from spastic bronchitis. By touching his rib cage and breathing together with him coaxing him to say 'pooh' while exhaling, she was able to stop his respiratory distress. She had found a non-verbal way of communication via access to vegetative functions. According to Fuchs the therapeutic effect was 'a correction of disturbed body functions through alteration of rhythm' (Fuchs, 2013, p. 14).

Fuchs was trained in 'Leibpädagogik', which was influenced by the Life Reform Movement (a political heterogeneous social movement in the late 19th and early 20th century in Germany that propagated a back-to-nature lifestyle, including alternative medicine). She studied at the 'Günther Schule' for Gymnastics, Music and Dance in Munich (founded 1924 by Dorothee Günther and Carl Orff). The pioneers of a new body-orientated approach, represented by Fuchs' teacher Thekla Malmberg, tried to combine physiological function and 'free' physical expression with musical elements and verbal symbolisation. Primarily they did not pursue therapeutic application, but there were crucial elements, which Fuchs adopted for her future clinical work: 'Body development with the principles of inner involvement, release of authentic impulses and above all "the simple and naturalness of moving" (Fuchs, 2013, p. 13). From the Schlaffhorst-Andersen School (Atemschule; breath therapy) she adopted the concept of 'finding one's own natural rhythm' (Fuchs, 2013, p. 13).

During her studies, a major influence came from depth psychology. Creativity was regarded as something emerging from the 'deep dimension', and the unconscious was regarded as an important part of any 'proper' concept of movement. As a psychodynamic method FR believes somatic perception to be the deepest layer of the unconscious.

At the Psychiatric University Hospital of Marburg, Fuchs became acquainted with psychosomatic medicine. After moving to Heidelberg, Victor von Weizsäcker's anthropological medicine became increasingly influential for the method. Weizsäcker's intention was to reintroduce the subject to medicine. He postulated the unity of perception and movement and the equivalence of somatic and psychological phenomena: 'The body represents the soul, the soul the body. Most important, however, in their reciprocation is that they substitute each other' (Weizsäcker, 1985). Both ideas were implemented in FR, leading to the method meaning to influence psychological functions by treating bodily symptoms.

Because of the immediate effect on body symptoms by neurovegetative regulation, FR was regarded as a good supplement to the verbal therapy of neurotic conflicts. With the new method it seemed to be possible to 'access to the vegetative unconscious' (Fuchs, 2013, p. 15) by influencing the rhythm of breathing. Since that time FR has become a significant therapeutic method in psychosomatic medicine in Germany.

Although non-verbal resonance and touch have played an important role from the beginning, language was always an essential part of the process. In FR the individual body perception is verbalised in terms such as 'tight-wide', 'hard-soft', corresponding to phenomenological categories such as space, boundaries, movement, direction, etc. Furthermore, FR offers a wide range of pictorial terms and metaphors to make somatic experience accessible to conscious analysis. Thure von Uexküll (Uexküll, Fuchs, Müller-Braunschweig, and Johnen, 1997), another important representative of academic psychosomatic medicine and Fuchs' life-long scientific companion, characterised the method as 'perception of the unnoticed in one's body' (Johnen, 2010, p. 62).

In the 1990s, Marianne Fuchs and Thure von Uexküll founded a study group called 'subjective anatomy'. It was an interdisciplinary discourse between psychosomatic doctors, body-psychotherapists, psychoanalysts and philosophers and brought forth a book with the same title (Uexküll et al., 1997). The intention was to provide a plausible scientific foundation for body psychotherapy in general, using the accumulated practical experience with FR as an example. The results from baby labs such as Daniel Stern's work were integrated into this approach (Stern, 1985).

After the first publication (Fuchs, 1949) clinical research developed leading to a broad variety of indications with an emphasis on psychosomatic disorders. Case studies showed improvement of symptoms for numerous disorders such as migraine, hypertension, obstipation, anorexia and depression (Herholz, Johnen, and Schweitzer, 2009). Clinical studies proved the effectiveness of the method for asthma (Loew, Siegfried, Martus, Tritt, and Hahn, 1996; Loew et al., 2001; Lahmann et al., 2009; Lahmann, Henningsen et al., 2010), irritable bowel syndrome (Lahmann, Röhricht et al., 2010), somatoform heart disorder (Lahmann et al., 2008) and dental anxiety (Lahmann et al., 2008).

Theoretical background

The physiology and psychology of psycho-vegetative effects of FR

According to Marianne Fuchs, the dynamic core of the method is its link to unconscious forces, which as an organising structure are effective in various physiological rhythms and metabolic processes (Fuchs, 2013). They influence mental states and can be best experienced in the rhythm of breathing. In FR the rhythm of breathing is regarded as a psychosomatic interface, because the autonomous breathing rhythm can simultaneously be consciously and deliberately controlled. 'Blockades' are understood as an unconscious expression of psychological tensions and conflicts. They are visible and palpable as disturbances in the rhythm of breath and as muscular tension. FR intends to dissolve these blockades by restoring one's personal rhythm through accentuated expiration during subtle movements.

The intention is to assist the patient to surrender to the natural rhythm of breathing with its repetition of in- and exhalation. To be in harmony with one's personal rhythm means, in terms of FR, to also be in harmony with the outside world. By balancing the rhythm of breath many other vegetative patterns such as blood pressure, skin temperature, peristalsis, salivation and bronchial obstruction are altered (Lahmann et al., 2009; Loew et al., 1996). Modifying vegetative patterns via intentional breathing means having an immediate influence on many psychosomatic symptoms. Applied to everyday life, this has an enormous effect on the personal sense of competence and the understanding of psychosomatic contexts – in other words the cognition of embodiment.

This physiological process of self-perception and self-regulation is facilitated by a specific somato-sensory competence of the body, the proprioceptive system. Similar to the senses for the outside world (exteroception), this sixth sense has its own organs of perception, the propriocep-tors, found in muscles, tendons and joints, allowing the body to organise itself in space and dur-ing movement. It seems that cutaneous receptors also contribute to proprioception. The system consists of conscious and unconscious parts, together both form 'body schema' and 'body image'. By sharpening the individual's sense of perception FR improves self-awareness. In psychological terms it means a reactivation of the 'sensuality of early childhood' (Fuchs, 2013, p. 20).

The main goal of FR is to replace the deliberate control of one's own bodily and psychological functions by allowing self-regulation to equilibrate vegetative states. It can be experienced as a spontaneous unfolding of the self; observed as sighs of relief, the impulse to stretch, yawn etc. In contrast to other methods such as Autogenous Training (Schultz, 2003), both the parasympathetic and sympathetic are simultaneously activated (Lahmann et al., 2013). A hypothetical explanation was provided by clinical research on effects of FR in asthma and other respiratory disorders (Lahmann et al., 2009; Loew et al., 1996).

The translation of body language in FR and the role of body empathy

'Everything that has been said about psychotherapeutic aims can be discovered and delivered through the body' (Fuchs, 2013, p. 20). Understanding, i.e. cognitive processing, mental representation and personal meaning is as important for FR as working with bodily phenomena such as rhythm and body knowledge. In general, an important issue in psychosomatic medicine is the translation of individual somatic phenomena into verbal discourse and subsequent psychological meaning. Freud called it 'the mysterious jump from the psyche to the body' (Freud, 1969b, p. 259).

In FR, the experienced therapist can read via 'body language' (Fuchs, 2013, p. 21) the patient's mental state: his composure, strain, irritability or assurance. In FR, the therapist also uses touch in a responsible way to help the patient feel. Another unique way of understanding in the sense of body empathy is used by the therapist to perceive sensations responding to those evoked in the patient. Fuchs calls it 'feeling/co-sensing with the patient' (Fuchs, 2013, pp. 18–20) ('Mitspüren'. 'Spüren' comprises both perceiving and feeling and is derived from 'Spur' meaning 'track').

The bodily reaction of the FR therapist may have various forms of resonance phenomena e.g. resembling, opposite or supplementary perceptions and feelings. FR uses body empathy as a continuous parallel lane during the therapeutic process. It is again the rhythm of breathing where resonance phenomena find their best expression. Body empathy enables the therapist to understand the patient's problems in a deeper way without necessarily interpreting them. In fact, language is not even capable of representing all complex and pre-verbal experiences. Body empathy facilitates the container for delicate conditions of the patient, a pre-symbolic bodily state of preserving and commemorating early relational experiences and sometimes-traumatic states. In a condition comparable to Freud's 'free-floating attention' (Freud, 1969a, p. 259; Fuchs, 2013, p. 22), states similar to the relationship between mother and child in early infancy can develop. Also, states of clear differentiation between the self and the other can be experienced in FR, for example, through the skin as a border or by retreating into the inner spaces of the body. In FR, it is necessary for the therapist to have had an intensive encounter with the method. FR not only offers the therapist enriched diagnostic information and therapeutic skills, but also an attitude of self-care.

The methodological procedure within the body-therapeutic process

Although the theory of FR was influenced by various complex theories, its practical application is simple and unique. It is easy to use and follows the principle 'less is more'. This means not unnecessarily wasting energy to hold tight and resist. Instead, one lets loose and trusts in one´s own healing powers. The aim is to find a path into a perception of the body, which does not focus only on symptoms but includes healthy areas of the whole organism. This process begins with awareness and switching one's attention from the outside to the inside. Self-perception is guided by verbal offers made by the therapist. Certain areas of the body are focused through slight movements while exhaling. The following dimensions are central:

- The relationship to outer support systems (floor, chair, couch);
- Bony structures representing the inner support system;

- Inner spaces;
- The skin as boundary.

The most important relational system is the breathing rhythm. The patient learns to surrender to relaxed perception and movement. Small movements while exhaling lead to prolongation of this phase and the quality of the movements change. Through small movements in the joints, it is possible to notice differences in pressure, tension and position. The bodily experience of support and boundaries lead to relaxation perceived as a slacker muscle tone. This profound perception enacts a kind of dialogue with one's own self and respectively one's own body. The patient learns to interact with herself/himself on a deeper level. An extended dialogue takes place by precisely describing perception verbally, expressing feelings, images, memories, impulses and desires, which can be connected to one's biography, especially to important experiences. The following so-called rules guide the body-oriented process:

1) All movement and perception take place during exhalation;
2) All movement is repeated two to three times;
3) After that, no more movement, just perception.

According to Fuchs, exhaling should best be accompanied by a soft sound. The process is tailored to the needs of the individual and takes place in different regions of the body. The aim is to release unconscious tension and blockades and find one's own rhythm and a flexible inner balance. By linking the release of muscle tension to the autonomous rhythm of breath and small impulses to move, diverse psycho-vegetative procedures are precipitated. They can be felt directly e.g. sense of weight, temperature felt due to improved circulation, slower heartbeat or salivation. These phenomena of the body can be perceived as calming or activating e.g. felt as an impulse to stretch. In the long run, they lead to changes in body perception and body image as well as positive modification in self-esteem.

Several authors (Johnen, 2010, p. 65) have pointed out that this process creates a 'playroom', as coined by Winnicott, in which creative solutions are found and autonomic progress takes place in the sense of being alone in the company of another (Winnicott, 1958). The individual's body perception connects to the successful attunement to the early dialogue between mother and child.

Within the body psychotherapeutic process, the reference to the outer support system can represent object relations. Perception of bony structures may stand for autonomy. Experiencing one's own skin boundaries enhances the capacity for self-protection and distance regulation. Experiencing inner space leads to trust in autonomous vegetative changes and the absence of evil objects. And last but not least, the sense of 'giving and receiving and sensuous encounters are enhanced' (Arnim et al., 2006, p. 407) Basically, Stern's concept of basal self-perception (core-self) with its sense of coherence, continuity, agency, activity and affectivity is strengthened (Stern, 1985).

Mentalisation requires psychological representations of the self, others and conscious emotional experience. Many of these representations are deficient in psychosomatic and psychologically disturbed patients. However, it is possible for them to mature through new body-based experiences.

Fictional case

Paul, a 48-year old married accountant with three small children, presented himself with somatoform pain in the stomach. He described himself as very ambitious. He had long ago been diagnosed with irritable bowel syndrome, but had noticed that his stomach pain was related to psychological stress. What he described as pain was actually discomfort in the right top corner of his abdomen. The pain started in the morning when he asked himself 'How is my stomach today?'. He generally felt better in the evening and it helped to lie down.

First session: Paul lay down on the couch, on the sheepskin. He could only identify the couch under his hands. He felt 'something soft and warm'. It then became evident that his perception was very differentiated, and he could describe his contact with the couch very precisely. Letting go of his weight with a soft sound led to an immediate reaction in his stomach, the pain 'loosened itself'. His legs opened slightly, he said he felt 'more relaxed'. He was asked by the therapist where he felt it the most. He answered: 'right leg, my stomach'. He explained he had the feeling he had an egg lying horizontally inside his stomach, the broad side of the egg was on the right at the painful spot. Where, at the beginning, was pain, was now reported by him as a 'cotton wool feeling'. Paul was asked whether something moves if he remains still. His intestines gurgled, 'something is moving' he said. The pain moved to the centre and then dissolved. He described it as 'like a string pulled tight, squashed from the inside like an overtight seam'. Associations were that he was always trying to keep everything together to create order in an obsessive-compulsive way. It was suggested he could 'open the string' with a soft sound. It was difficult for him to let his voice flow. He was asked again 'what is moving?'. He said his heart was beating, his head was heavy, he felt the blood in his arms.

For the therapist it was remarkable that he could not feel breathing movements and indeed they were hardly visible. By putting his own hand on his stomach, he said 'it started flowing to his chest'. He inhaled deeply several times but had no perception of what was happening. His comment was 'it feels good to breathe in and out'. At the end of the session he was asked what had been important. Paul's reply was 'the situation in general, being able to lie down and to do nothing'. He felt more relaxed, had hope.

Second session: Paul lay down and wanted to cover himself with a blanket. He had had persistent stomach ache for 2 days, which he described as a 'storm in my stomach'. A possible trigger was that he had been criticised by his boss for micro-managing. Paul felt his lower back muscles and was encouraged to experiment with movements in his lower back. He remarked 'letting go is great', he said he felt a kind of wave through his stomach, and the knot loosened itself. He reported he remembered the first session a lot, even while jogging. He could then 'switch off' for a short moment, change his position if sitting and experienced a feeling of warmth. Although Paul's expiration hardly changed when letting go of his weight, it was now possible for him to feel his chest moving up and down. Breathing in was perceived as positive, as 'getting strength', breathing out however was, he said, 'rigid and hard'. He was asked by the therapist what had been important to which he replied, 'small movements change something'. His whole body felt different he said, and he said he suspected it had something to do with his breathing.

His stomach ache started to reduce from the third session on. After 29 sessions the ache had disappeared. His abdomen was now perceived as a space within which rhythm, expansion and flow occurred. A turning point. At the end Paul, whose conception was an 'accident' and who had suffered from emotional neglect as a child, was able to abandon his previous identification with family rules that focused on achievement and ambition. He reported that he was more relaxed and flexible, had higher respect for himself and genuinely enjoyed life more.

Summary

Healing processes can be fostered with FR by improving self-perception and self-awareness and at the same time modifying vegetative patterns via intentional breathing. The body's ability to self-regulate, precipitated by FR, provides the base for psychological changes and regulatory processes. Enhanced body awareness is used as access to implicit body memories, feelings and individual bodily needs. Symbolisation and building of representation are enabled. FR's approach is genuine embodiment.

References

Arnim, A. v., Müller-Braunschweig, H., and Joraschky, P. (2006). Körperbezogene Psychotherapie-Verfahren bei traumatisierten Menschen [Body related psychotherapy methods for treating the traumatised]. In A. Remmel, O. Kernberg, W. Vollmoeller, and B. Strauß (Eds.), *Handbuch Körper und Persönlichkeit*. Stuttgart: Schattauer.

Freud, S. (1969a). *Schriften zur Behandlungstechnik* [Papers on treatment techniques] (Studienausgabe, 11th ed.). Frankfurt am Main: S. Fischer.

Freud, S. (1969b). *Vorlesungen zur Einführung in die Psychoanalyse* [Introductory lectures on psycho-analysis] (Studienausgabe, 11th ed.). Frankfurt am Main: S. Fischer.

Fuchs, M. (1949). Über Atemtherapie und entspannende Körperarbeit als Unterstützung der Behandlung vegetativer Störungen [About breath therapy and relaxing body-work supporting the treatment of vegative disorders]. *Psyche, 1949*(3), 538–548.

Fuchs, M. (2013). *Funktionelle Entspannung. Theorie und Praxis eines körperbezogenen Psychotherapieverfahrens* [Functional relaxation. Theory and practice of a body related psychotherapy method] (7th ed.). Berlin: Pro Business.

Herholz, I., Johnen, R., and Schweitzer, D. (Eds.). (2009). *Funktionelle Entspannung. Das Praxisbuch* [Functional relaxation. A practice book]. Stuttgart: Schattauer.

Johnen, R. (2010). Funktionelle Entspannung [Functional relaxation]. In H. Müller-Braunschweig and N. Stiller (Eds.), *Körperorientierte Psychotherapie*. Heidelberg: Springer.

Lahmann, C. (2013). Körperpsychotherapie in Forschung und Praxis. Eine Einführung in die Funktionelle Entspannung [Body psychotherapy in research and practice. An introduction to Functional Relaxation]. *Ärztliche Psychotherapie, 3*, 170–174.

Lahmann, C., Gebhardt, M., Henrich, G., Dinkel, A., Pieh, C., and Probst, T. (2017). A randomized controlled trial on functional relaxation as an adjunct to psychoeducation for stress. *Frontiers in Psychology, 8*, 1553.

Lahmann, C., Henningsen, P., Schulz, C., Schuster, T., Sauer, N., Noll-Hussong, M., . . . Loew, T. H. (2010). Effects of functional relaxation and guided imagery on IgE in dust-mite allergic adult asthmatics: A randomized, controlled clinical trial. *Journal of Nervous and Mental Disease, 198*, 125–130.

Lahmann, C., Loew, T., Tritt, K., and Nickel, M. (2008). Efficacy of functional relaxation and patient education in the treatment of somatoform heart disorders: A randomized, controlled, clinical investigation. *Psychosomatics, 45*, 378–385.

Lahmann, C., Nickel, M., Schuster, T., Sauer, N., Ronel, J., Noll-Hussong, M., . . . Loew, T. H. (2009). Functional relaxation and hypnotherapeutic intervention as complementary therapy in asthma: A randomized, controlled clinical trial. *Psychotherapy and Psychosomatics, 78*, 233–239.

Lahmann, C., Röhricht, F., Sauer, N., Noll-Hussong, M., Ronel, J., Henrich, G., . . . Loew, T. H. (2010). Effectiveness of Functional Relaxation as complementary therapy in irritable bowel syndrome: A randomized, controlled clinical trial. *Journal of Alternative and Complementary Medicine, 2010*(16), 47–52.

Lahmann, C., Schoen, R., Henningsen, P., Ronel, J., Muehlbacher, M., Loew, T., . . . Doering, S. (2007). Brief relaxation versus music distraction in the treatment of dental anxiety: A randomized, controlled, clinical trial. *Journal of the American Dental Association, 139*, 137–324.

Loew, T. H., Siegfried, W., Martus, P., Tritt, K., and Hahn, E. G. (1996). 'Functional relaxation' reduces acute airway obstruction in asthmatics as effectively as inhaled terbutaline. *Psychotherapy Psychosomatics, 65*, 124–128.

Loew, T. H., Tritt, K., Siegfried, W., Bohmann, H., Martus, P., and Hahn, E. G. (2001). Efficacy of 'functional relaxation' in comparison to terbutaline and 'placebo relaxation' method in patients with acute asthma. A randomized, prospective, placebo-controlled, crossover experimental investigation. *Psychotherapy Psychosomatics, 70*, 151–157.

Schultz J. H. (2003). *Das autogene Training. Konzentrative Selbstentspannung* [Autogenic Training. Concentrative Self-relaxation, 20th edition]. Stuttgart: Thieme.

Stern, D. N. (1985). *The Interpersonal World of the Infant*. New York: Basic Books.

Uexküll, T. v., Fuchs, M., Müller-Braunschweig, H., and Johnen, R. (1997). *Subjektive Anatomie* [Subjective Anatomy] (2nd ed.). Stuttgart: Schattauer.

Weizsäcker, V. v. (1985). *Der Gestaltkreis: Theorie der Einheit von Wahrnehmungen und Bewegen* [The Gestaltkreis: Theory of the Unity of Perception and Movement]. Berlin: Suhrkamp.

Winnicott, D. W. (1958). The capacity to be alone. *International Journal of Psychoanalysis, 39*(5), 416–420.

24

THE ART OF BOTTOM-UP PROCESSING

Mindfulness, meaning and self-compassion in body psychotherapy

Halko Weiss and Maci Daye

Introduction

The use of reflection has long been a cornerstone of psychoanalytic and psychodynamic therapies, and for good reason (Shedler, 2010). Reflection provides a meta-level view of the client's psychic life and has the power to uncover vital information on the unconscious roots of emotional suffering (Aron, 1998; Falkenström, 2012; Holmes, 2009). Without meaning, human beings are unable to orient to life and mental health is compromised (Siegel, 1999). While the existential importance of meaning-making has been well established (Bateson, 1979; Frankl, 1997; White, 2007), newer research indicates that self-compassion also plays a vital role in well-being (Neff and Dahm, in press), and is related to the way we understand and look at ourselves (Germer and Siegel, 2012). In this chapter, we argue that meaning derived through "bottom-up" processes (Gregory, 1997, p. 191), aided by mindfulness, is more reliable than reflection, and that it also fosters self-compassion.

In psychotherapy, reflection generally consists of "top-down" processes, such as interpreting, making mental connections, explaining, and creating a coherent story in words. Unfortunately, these processes are subject to social desirability and other cognitive biases that prevent clients from looking at themselves honestly and with kindness. Through case studies, we will show how the experiential use of mindfulness in body-psychotherapy can eliminate these biases. Furthermore, when clients observe normally implicit processes in an open and accepting way, meanings emerge spontaneously, as does self-compassion.

Body-psychotherapists have long taken the bottom-up route (Johnson, 2015), which starts with accessing and studying somatic experiences without attaching meanings for long periods of time. Here, we are drawing on the teachings of Hakomi Mindful Somatic Psychotherapy (Weiss, Johanson, and Monda, 2015). In the years since its inception in 1980, Hakomi has incorporated the findings of affective science and interpersonal neurobiology and refined its methodology accordingly.

The perils of self-reflection

Reflecting on experience to construct a coherent story relies on "top-down" processes and pre-existing mental models (Bateson, 1979; Bishop et al., 2004; Ogden, Minton, and Pain, 2006;

Siegel, 2017). These processes are highly automatic and subject to the following errors and distortions (Harrer and Weiss, 2015):

- *Confabulation*: The mind tends to create interpretations, connections between events, reasons, and "facts" that are entirely made-up while believing they are true (Spitzer, 2002, pp. 331–333).
- *Social desirability*: The mind tweaks and twists facts, often without any conscious intent, to fit what is expected from the social environment and to protect a sense of self-worth (Roth, 2001, pp. 370–372, 2003, p. 38).
- *False memory*: The mind tends to unconsciously distort, create, mix, or alter memories. (Loftus, 1994; Schacter, 1995, 1996).
- *"Infantile amnesia"*: The conscious mind cannot recall autobiographical events (episodic memory) that occurred before three or so years of age (Tulving, 1983).

According to Olendzki (2005, p. 264) "Ours is a universe of macro construction, in which the continually arising data of the senses and of miscellaneous internal processing are channeled into structures and organized into schemas that support an entirely synthetic sphere of meaning – a virtual reality." What's more, the conversion of experience into meaning is the result of re-occurring neural activations (Begley, 2007). For this reason, we are apt to see, hear and think the same things over and over, even when our conclusions are faulty (Lewis, Fari, and Lannon, 2001; Wilson, 2004).

In regard to self-compassion, the mind's penchant for critical thinking, as well as comparing and judging, makes it difficult for many people to accept their egodystonic behaviours, traits, impulses, feelings and internal parts of the self (Rogers, 1961; Schwartz, 1995). For this reason, self-reflection may be anathema to self-compassion; which requires, instead, an all-partisan attitude towards the subpersonalities that comprise a person's inner world, along with care for the way those parts have suffered (Neff, 2011).

Mindful observation as an alternative to reflection

Mindfulness has entered the psychotherapeutic stage comparatively recently but has been warmly embraced by practitioners of many modalities (Bishop et al., 2004; Daye, 2015; Johanson, 2006). It is frequently taught within a structured group setting as an adjunct to cognitive behavioural therapy to enhance affect tolerance (as in Dialectical Behavioural Therapy), manage chronic pain (in Mindfulness-Based Stress Reduction), or prevent relapse into depression (Mindfulness-Based Cognitive Therapy). Recent modalities, such as Acceptance and Commitment Therapy (ACT), use mindfulness to promote psychological flexibility, which enables clients to observe unpleasant states of mind without being held back or driven by them (Falkenström, 2012; Hayes, Follette, and Linehan, 2004). As we will demonstrate, mindfulness can also support meaning-making in psychodynamic therapy.

The classical literature describes mindfulness as pure observation (Gunaratna, 1970; Nyanaponika, 1976). More recently, mindfulness has been defined as the regulation of attention to the present moment, combined with an accepting, open and curious attitude (Bishop et al., 2004). With practice, mindfulness develops the capacity to study what is going on intrapsychically, without preferences or judgements, and without the constraining forces of explicit mental processes.

The "Observing Self" (Deikman, 1982, p. 91ff) is less influenced by automatic interpretations, habitual ways of processing information, or character-driven forces than the reflecting self. It is likewise untainted by confabulation, social desirability or false memory syndrome.

The Observing Self *is* limited by infantile amnesia; however, it can detect remnants of early emotional learning by noting reactions and impulses in the present. For example, a person may notice that they have a contracted belly, sweaty palms and the impulse to cross the street whenever a large dog is approaching, without remembering that they were knocked down by a neighbour's boisterous Labrador retriever as a toddler.

Meta-levels of consciousness

Studies indicate that mindfulness promotes a thickening of the pre-frontal medial cortex and other neuroplastic changes in the brain (Begley, 2007; Lazar et al., 2005; Siegel, 2007). With changed equipment, the observing mind can explore presenting issues from an even higher state of consciousness than self-reflection as it hovers above while a person moves between various self-states (Siegel, 1999). This capacity is sometimes described as a saluto-genetic split of consciousness that allows a person to witness an emotional state without being pulled into it. Buddhist texts call this "dis–identification" (Anderssen-Reuster, Meibert, and Meck, 2013; Hoelzel et al., 2011). Teasdale et al. (2002), call it "metacognitive awareness" (p. 275).

Mindfulness therefore affords a second meta-level above the meta-cognitive level of self-reflection. So, from one meta-level to another meta-level (the first), that can reflect on its object of study (Bishop et al., 2004; Flavell, 1979; Kegan, 1982). This allows clients to observe their habits of self-organisation in real time. This second meta-level is also a boon to self-compassion. By cultivating a warm, curious, and accepting attitude towards present moment experience, the Observing Self develops an all-partisan relationship with the often-conflicted internal parts of the self. The internal observer can also dis-identify from the critical thoughts, ruminations and self-judgements that may lead to low self-esteem and depression (Pyszcynski and Greenberg, 1987; Raes, 2010).

Implicit learning

Implicit memory refers to everything a person has learned without conscious processing or encoding (Cozolino, 2006; Wilson, 2004). In other words, learning that never became conscious because it occurred during infancy or was encoded emotionally and somatically later in life. There are many forms of implicit learning: procedural memory involves the development of motor skills such as standing upright. Once mastered, a person does not have to think about which muscles to use to balance on two legs because the body knows how to do this. Another form of implicit learning is relational. Just as children learn the grammar of language by hearing others speak, children learn a grammar for lifelong relating based on early experiences with attachment figures. These experiences sculpt the brain, imprinting the known but not remembered rules of relating in the neural hardware by 12–18 months of age (Cozolino, 2006; Graham, 2008; Schore, Dagniela, and Sieff, 2015).

Interestingly, self-compassion is believed to also grow out of the caregiving system and is correlated with higher levels of oxytocin, a hormone that engenders feelings of connection, safety, comfort, and trust (Carter and Porges, 2013; Neff and Dahm, in press). A critical caregiving system, on the other hand, is believed to trigger the threat response, generating feelings of depression, anxiety, and elevated levels of cortisol (Goetz, Keltner, and Simon-Thomas, 2010). Neff and McGeehee (2010) suggest that children reared in critical, insecurely attached family systems adapt to their environment by becoming self-critical of themselves.

The power of implicit learning applies to all complex adaptive systems, from a national economy to a single human, as they adapt to their environment *automatically* and without conscious processing. This was demonstrated by early experiments with amoebas (Alsup, 1939). Like humans, amoebas will contract if they are exposed to a single electric shock but will expand again after a refractory period. However, they will remain in a contracted state much longer if the shocks are repeated. This indicates that even amoebas learn to "anticipate the future" (Holland, 1995, pp. 31–34) although they do not have a nervous system or a brain.

From the point of view of Body Psychotherapy, the human body also adapts to its environment automatically. It implicitly learns what kind of world is out there, and organises its physiology accordingly (Bentzen, 2015; Grand, 2015). This level of embodiment is of great interest to body psychotherapists, who observe and explore these physical adaptations to identify the early life lessons implicitly encoded in the body (Kurtz, 1990; Lowen, 1958; Reich, 1933/1972). Here we define embodiment as the: 1) physical expression of a person's prior learning and resulting beliefs about life (whether conscious or not); 2) process of gaining a conscious, bodily felt sense of this implicit learning; and 3) on-going experience of having an integrated body-mind.

Accessing the implicit

It is virtually impossible to access implicit memory data through reflection. However, mindful self-study of the body stimulates the neural circuits associated with emotional learning, rapidly and directly (Fogel, 2009; Kurtz, 1990; Marlock and Weiss, 2015; Varela, Thompson, and Rosch, 1991; Weiss, 2009). The non-judgmental and highly sensitive Observing Self can then decipher the learned but not remembered information revealed in a person's posture, gestures, facial expressions, and internal sensations (Kurtz and Prestera, 1977). In so doing, meanings surface spontaneously, without thinking, analyzing or reflecting.

Case example: Linda

Linda's head is leaning forward as she is speaking about how hard her life is and that she has no one to lean on. The therapist suggests doing an experiment in mindfulness. She offers to support her client right now, by cradling Linda's head. Linda consents to the experiment and becomes mindful as she studies the changing experiences in her body. When the support is provided, she is surprised to notice that instead of relaxing into it, her muscles tense automatically. She detects a "steely" quality in her core, from the stomach to her throat.

Encouraged by the psychotherapist to simply stay with the tensing and see what develops, Linda reports that she senses something "grey" about her emotional state. She becomes aware of feelings of isolation that deepen as she lingers with her present experience. Tears well up in Linda's eyes, as it seems to her now that she needed to provide support to herself, even as a child, and that depending on others would have somehow been dangerous.

Although Linda had no explicit memories attached to this experience, by studying her physical and emotional reactions in mindfulness, she came to understand something essential about how she organises around support. Prior to the experiment, Linda had no idea that a part of her would automatically defend against support because, consciously, this is what she longs for. Now she understands that one reason her life is so hard is that an internal part is protecting her from depending on others. In subsequent sessions, Linda explored this unconscious barrier and allowed herself to gradually receive support from others.

Contact with direct experience opens the door to new experiences (Gendlin, 1996; Perls, Hefferline, and Goodman, 1951; Stern, 1985). The Observing Self (as cultivated in mindfulness practice) can see what is true by studying the automatic process of self-organisation (Markose, 2003) that is evoked when a trigger (such as support for the head) is introduced in the session. Kurtz (1990) called this way of evoking experience *accessing*. It is aided by the neutral Observing Self, which can study habits of self-organisation without evaluating them as good or bad.

Pure observation is thus akin to the empirical approach used by natural scientists. For example, the botanist notices the shape, size and colour of the flower, without preferences for how the flower *should* be. By studying the flower in this open, non-judging way, the scientist becomes a more precise and differentiated observer. Clients can, likewise, train themselves to become astute and non-judgemental observers of their present experience, noticing details in their body-mind that hold meanings that were previously outside of awareness.

Meaning-making through bottom-up processing

Mindful somatic psychotherapy diverges greatly from ordinary conversation, at least for significant parts of a session. To access formative experiences encoded in implicit memory requires an experiential approach (Ecker, Ticic, and Hulley, 2012; Greenberg et al., 1998) that privileges the body (Damasio, 1999). A mindful somatic approach involves gathering raw data from subcortical levels, including sensory inputs, before the higher levels of the brain intercept them. Otherwise, the data will be interpreted in accord with pre-existing templates and mental models which, as indicated earlier, are subject to various errors and distortions.

Neuropsychologists call this "bottom-up" processing (Siegel, 2017, p. 127). Psychotherapists can support bottom-up processing by encouraging their clients to sense, listen, look and feel into themselves before coming up with a story or explanation (Ogden et al., 2006; van der Kolk, 2015). Clinicians can also slow themselves down and allow meanings to unfold from within the client, rather than offering interpretations or reflections on their client's behaviour.

A somatic approach can evoke the core organisers of experience through direct observation rather than by exploring them intellectually (Sparks, 2015). For example, a therapist working with a client who has difficulties with intimacy might design an experiment to study how the client's contracted chest and shoulders contribute to a life stance of withdrawal. The therapist could, for instance, suggest that the client slowly and mindfully experiment with opening and closing their posture while monitoring their feelings and sensations. In effect, the therapist is avoiding reflecting upon memories around intimacy, and choosing to explore how the body is managing the issue automatically.

Case example: Brian

Brian came to therapy to address his "explosive intensity," which would overtake him, especially at work. More than once his supervisor told Brian that he needed to get a hold of himself or he would not last long in his position. Brian didn't understand why he would "lose it" so easily, but he very much wanted to keep his job.

After being oriented to mindful self-study, Brian was ready to explore the internal processes related to his anger. Brian reported that he became angry whenever his proposals were resisted by his colleagues. The therapist asked Brian to identify a statement that might trigger his anger, a statement that would capture the essential feel of the resistance from his colleagues. The statement he chose was, "No, we're not going to do that."

The therapist guided Brian into a mindful state and said: "What happens inside when you hear someone say the words, 'No, we're not going to do that?'". After a short pause, Brian noticed tension throughout his body, particularly in his arms. He had an impulse to jump up and "do something." The therapist encouraged Brian to stay with the tension and study this impulse. After a minute or so in silent self-study, Brian noticed something in his stomach. It feels "tight, dark, and very intense," he reported. Once more, the therapist invited Brian to simply observe his experience with curiosity. After about 30 seconds or so, the therapist asked, "Is there an emotion that goes with the sensation in your stomach?". Brian felt into himself and then said, "It is fear . . . a huge fear."

The therapist assumes that the body has learned something from its environment and is "anticipating the future" (Holland, 1995). Rather than making interpretations she invites Brian to study his fear. Step-by-step Brian goes more deeply into it, activating the neural circuitry connected to his early learning.

An image of Brian's father begins to appear. Brian experiences himself as very small, "almost like a 7-year old." His therapist encourages Brian to stay with the image and the feeling of being a child. It becomes clear to the boy that he is both awed by and fearful of his father. Brian also senses how inferior he feels around his father, particularly when he becomes impatient with Brian. After exploring this for a while, the therapist asks: "What does this boy seem to be learning from this? What kinds of ideas is he getting about himself when his father gets so short with him?". Brian hesitates, struggling to hold back tears, and then says, "I'm not worth anything at all." He reports that the pressure in his stomach is pulling him downward, "like I might collapse into a deep, dark pit of pain."

As Brian says this, the therapist detects a change in Brian's face: his jaw is tightening and hardening a bit. She names her observation.

Brian reports that he is starting to get angry and that he once again feels the tension in his arms and the impulse to do something. The therapist asks if Brian still feels the deep, dark pit of pain in his belly. Brian investigates this and with a slight smile says, "No, I don't. The anger is helping me feel bigger and stronger. It's like it's making sure I don't collapse."

Brian and his therapist were now able to see what lay behind Brian's fury: his angry outbursts rested on feelings of worthlessness and the fear of collapsing into utter despair. Coming up with good ideas was one way the adult Brian had been unconsciously trying to compensate for the implicitly encoded belief that "I don't matter." When his colleagues resisted his ideas, Brian touched back into this worthless state, from which sprung an angry part that helped him feel stronger. Over the next few months, Brian developed a compassionate relationship with the young boy inside as well as the angry protector part of him. He also integrated numerous experiences from subsequent therapy sessions that contradicted and eventually modified this belief. As Brian healed the pain of feeling unworthy, his angry outbursts diminished significantly.

In body-centred psychotherapy, meaning arises by sensing into an activation in the present moment. It is a direct encounter with arising embodied phenomena, unfiltered by mental concepts. Mindful somatic psychotherapy therefore involves: 1) guiding the client into a mindful state; 2) directing attention to what is arising or using experiments to access implicit learning; and 3) supporting meaning-making through observation and direct experience, rather than through reflection.

When clients like Brian see that their adaptive strategies were born of necessity, rather than weakness or some character flaw, feelings of self-compassion often replace feelings of worthlessness and shame. Therapists can also point out that the ways a client learned to protect themself from re-injury were adaptive and resourceful. Self-understanding, accompanied by feelings of self-care, is the next step, which also fosters a reintegration of "exiled" parts (Schwartz, 1995, p. 47) and communication between inner child parts and the compassionate self.

Case example: Bella

Bella, a retired school teacher from Austria, decided to sample body-centred psychotherapy at the recommendation of her physician. Bella reported that despite years of physical therapy, she still had excruciating pain in her neck and shoulders. Bella judged herself for being too "weak," and wondered if she was using her pain as an "excuse" to avoid the stress of daily life.

In her second session, Bella mindfully directed attention to the pain in this area. She noticed a squeezing and pinching at the place where her shoulders met her neck. She also reported some fear in her belly and a sense of confusion. Her therapist encouraged Bella to feel into this activation and notice any images or memories connected to this state.

In so doing, Bella slowly entered a regressed child state. The therapist checked to make sure Bella's Observing Self was still present before proceeding. Bella nodded. Returning to the experience of the child, Bella reported that she sees herself standing at the edge of a cornfield. She is anxiously staring at the distant horizon. Only then does a memory surface: the young Bella is waiting for her father to return from the war. A part of Bella is now activated in a way she had long forgotten. She feels very tense and her shoulders ache very badly. Her young part tells the therapist that she does not know whether her father is coming back or not.

The therapist then asks the child if it would be okay to leave her for a minute to talk to the grown-up Bella. The girl agrees, so the therapist turns to the mindful adult, and asks: "Did your father ever come back?". The adult answers: "No, he did not." The therapist thanks the mindful adult and returns to the "child" who is still waiting at the edge of the cornfield. The therapist says: "I have very bad news for you, little girl . . . your father has died in the war. He is not coming back." Bella breaks down and weeps for a long time while her therapist holds her.

A mindful state allowed Bella to access deep layers of her unconscious and receive a vital experience (in this case the truth) that was missing throughout her life – at least by the levels of her neural circuitry that were holding her distress. Mindfulness can access early learning and regressive states fairly easily, while the compassionate and somewhat detached observer safeguards against 'malign regression' (Geissler, 2015, p. 572). This enables clients to stay curious and calm on a second meta-level while they actively engage in understanding themselves. In this safe and exploratory context, the organisers of experience can be accessed and eventually transformed.

Bella reported that she now understands that her body aches were linking her to an experience long in need of healing. She appreciates the effort her inner child has made to connect with her. As mentioned above, when clients understand themselves, they often feel compassion for the ways they have suffered and the heroic ways they have tried to manage this suffering. They can also take the next steps towards greater levels of freedom. At last, little Bella was able to grieve her father's death in an integrated way. Working with the body in mindfulness thus offers an emancipatory path from the pain of the original wound and the self-judgement that often comes with it.

This process can also be understood as the mindful activation of a prior problematic state, or part, that is "frozen in time" (Schwartz, 1995, p. 105), followed by the therapist's introduction of a corrective experience (Pesso, 1973). This facilitates the neurological process of memory reconsolidation, which occurs after an old memory is activated and paired with a corrective experience in the present (Duvarci and Nader, 2004; Ecker et al., 2012; Hanson, 2013; Nadel, 1994).

Transformation of the implicit in a state of mindfulness

The change that clients seek through therapy, which may be to heal pain, find self-acceptance, and experience themselves and others differently, is born of experience rather than reflection. This is because the core organisers that convert experience into meaning and feeling reside at the biological substrate of the unconscious, or sub-cortical, brain. These structures are highly stable. They can only be modified by integrating corrective experiences that mismatch prior emotional learning, and only when the relevant levels of this substrate are activated (Ecker, 2012, Grawe, 2004).

Experiential, body-based psychotherapies can safely promote activation by employing mindfulness. Once meanings arise into consciousness, such as, "My needs don't matter" or "I'll be hurt if I open up," therapists can offer experiences to the contrary during the session. When these experiences are integrated, existing elements of self-organisation are deautomatized (Deikman, 1982, 2014). This increased freedom from habitual adaptive strategies allows clients to experience life in a fuller way.

Conclusion

Talk therapy, with its emphasis on elaborative cognitive processes, including self-reflection, risks generating meanings that rely on highly automatic and biographically-biased mental activity. Mindful self-observation of somatic processes, on the other hand, opens a comparatively easy and direct path to implicit memory. The latter uses bottom-up processing to access implicitly encoded limiting beliefs to transform them. By suspending meaning-making, the bottom-up approach makes space for novelty, which may involve unearthing significant memories, or bringing into consciousness the impact of early (pre-conscious) experiences on one's structures of self-organisation. When combined with mindfulness, a bottom-up approach also deepens self-compassion for the creative and resourceful adaptations the younger self made to survive within its early environment.

References

Alsup, F. W. (1939). Relation between the response of amoeba proteus to alternating electric current and sudden illumination. *Physiological Zoology, 12*(1), 85–95.

Anderssen-Reuster, U., Meibert, P., and Meck, S. (2013). *Psychotherapie und buddhistisches Geistestraining. Methoden einer achtsamen Bewusstseinskultur* [Psychotherapy and Buddist training of the mind. Methods of a mindful culture of consciousness]. Stuttgart: Schattauer.

Aron, L. (1998). The clinical body and the reflexive mind. In L. Aron and F. S. Anderson (Eds.), *Relational Perspectives on the Body*. Hillsdale, NJ: The Analytic Press.

Bateson, G. (1979). *Mind and Nature: A Necessary Unity*. New York: E. P. Dutton.

Begley, S. (2007). *Train Your Mind, Change Your Brain: How a New Science Reveals our Extraordinary Potential to Transform Ourselves*. New York: Ballantine.

Bentzen, M. (2015). Shapes of experience. In G. Marlock and H. Weiss (with C. Young and M. Soth), *Handbook of Body Psychotherapy and Somatic Psychology*. Berkeley: North Atlantic Books.

Bishop, S. R., Lau, M., Shapiro, S., Carlson, L., Anderson, N. D., Carmody, J., . . . Devins, G. (2004). Mindfulness: A proposed operational definition. *Clinical Psychology: Science and Practice, 11*, 230–241.

Carter, S., and Porges, S. W. (2013). The biochemistry of love: An oxytocin hypothesis. *European Molecular Biology Organisation Report, 14*(1), 12–16.

Cozolino, L. (2006). *The Neuroscience of Human Relationships: Attachment and the Developing Social Brain*. New York: Norton.

Damasio, A. R. (1999). *The Feeling of What Happens*. New York: Harcourt Brace.

Daye, M. (March 2015). The experimental attitude: Curiosity in action. In H. Weiss, G. Johanson and L. Monda (Eds.), *Hakomi Mindfulness-Centered Somatic Psychotherapy*, W.W. Norton & Company, Inc, New York: Norton.

Deikman, A. (1982). *The Observing Self*. Boston: Beacon.

Deikman, A. (2014). De-automatization and the mystic experience. In *Meditations on a Blue Vase*. Napa: Fearless Books.

Duvarci, S., and Nader, K. (2004). Characterization of fear memory reconsolidation. *Journal of Neuroscience, 24*, 9269–9275.

Ecker, B., Ticic, R. and Hulley, L. (2012). *Unlocking the Emotional Brain: Eliminating Symptoms at Their Roots Using Memory Reconsolidation*. London: Routledge.

Falkenström, F. (2012). *The capacity for self-observation in psychotherapy* (Doctoral dissertation). Department of Behavioural Sciences and Learning, Linköping University, Linköping, Sweden.

Flavell, J. H. (1979). Metacognition and cognitive monitoring: A new area of cognitive-developmental inquiry. *American Psychologist, 34*(10), 906–911.

Fogel, A. (2009). *The Psychophysiology of Self-Awareness. Rediscovering the Lost Art of Body Sense*. New York: Norton.

Frankl, V. (1997). *Die Sinnfrage in der Psychotherapie* [The question of meaning in psychotherapy]. München: Piper.

Geissler, P. (2015). Regression in body psychotherapy. In G. Marlock and H. Weiss (with C. Young and M. Soth), *Handbook of Body Psychotherapy and Somatic Psychology*. Berkeley: North Atlantic Books.

Gendlin, E. T. (1996). *Focusing-Oriented Psychotherapy*. New York: The Guilford Press.

Germer, C. K., and Siegel, R. D., (2012). *Wisdom and Compassion in Psychotherapy. Deepening Mindfulness in Clinical Practice*. New York: Guilford.

Goetz, J. L., Keltner, D., and Simon-Thomas, E. (2010). Compassion: An evolutionary analysis and empirical review. *Psychological Bulletin, 136*, 351–374.

Graham, L. (2008). *The neuroscience of attachment; blog: Resources for recovering resilience*. Retrieved from http://lindagraham-mft.net/resources/published-articles/the-neuroscience-of-attachment.

Grand, I. J. (2015). Body, culture, and body psychotherapy. In G. Marlock and H. Weiss (with C. Young and M. Soth), *Handbook of Body Psychotherapy and Somatic Psychology*. Berkeley: North Atlantic Books.

Grawe, K. (2004). *Neuropsychotherapie*. Göttingen: Hogrefe.

Greenberg, L. S., Watson, J. C., and Lietaer, G. O. (1998). *Handbook of Experiential Psychotherapy*. New York: The Guilford Press.

Gregory, R. L. (1997). Visual illusions classified. *Trends in Cognitive Sciences, 1*(5), 190–194.

Gunaratna, V. F. (1970). *The Satipatthana Sutra and its Application to Modern Life*. Kandy, Sri Lanka: Buddhist Publication Society.

Hanson, R. (2013). *Rewiring Happiness*. New York: Harmony.

Harrer, M. E., and Weiss, H. (2015). *Wirkfaktoren der Achtsamkeit und wie sie die Psychotherapie verändern und bereichern* [Effective factors of mindfulness and how they change and enrich psychotherapy]. Stuttgart: Schattauer.

Hayes, S. C., Follette, V. M., and Linehan, M. M. (2004). *Mindfulness and Acceptance: Expanding the Cognitive-Behavioral Tradition*. New York: Guilford Press.

Hoelzel, B. K., Lazar, S. W., Gard, T., Schuman-Olivier, Z., Vago, D. R., and Ott, U. (2011). How does mindfulness meditation work? Proposing mechanisms of action from a conceptual and neural perspective. *Perspectives on Psychological Science, 6*(6), 537–559.

Holland, J. H. (1995). *Hidden Order: How Adaptation Builds Complexity*. Cambridge, MA: Perseus Books.

Holmes, J. (2009). *Exploring in Security. Towards an Attachment-Informed Psychoanalytic Psychotherapy*. London: Routledge.

Johanson, G. (2006). A survey of the use of mindfulness in psychotherapy. *The Annals of the American Psychotherapy Association, 9*(2), 15–24.

Johnson, D. H. (2015). The primacy of experiential practices in body psychotherapy. In G. Marlock and H. Weiss (with C. Young and M. Soth) (Eds.), *Handbook of Body Psychotherapy and Somatic Psychology*. Berkeley: North Atlantic Books.

Kegan, R. (1982). *The Evolving Self: Problem and Process in Human Development*. Cambridge, MA: Harvard University Press.

Kurtz, R. (1990). *Body-Centered Psychotherapy*. Mendocino: LifeRhythm.

Kurtz, R., and Prestera, H. (1977). *The Body Reveals: Illustrated Guide to the Psychology of the Body*. New York: Joanna Cotler Books.

Lazar, S. W., Kerr, C. E., Wasserman, R. H., Gray, J. R., Greve, D. N., Treadway, M. T, . . . Fischl, B. (2005). Meditation experience is associated with increased cortical thickness. *Neuroreport, 16*(17), 1893–1897.

Lewis, T., Fari, A., and Lannon, R. (2001). *A General Theory of Love*. New York: Vintage.

Loftus, E. (1994). *The Myth of Repressed Memory*. New York: St. Martin's Press.

Lowen, A. (1958). *The Language of the Body*. New York: Macmillan.

Markose, S. M. (2003). Novelty and surprises in complex adaptive system (CAS) dynamics: A computational theory of actor innovation. *Physica A, 344*, 41–49.

Marlock, G., and Weiss, H. (with C. Young and M. Soth) (Eds), (2015). *Handbook of Body Psychotherapy and Somatic Psychology*. Berkeley: North Atlantic Books.

Nadel, L. (1994). Multiple memory systems: What and why. In D. T. Schacter and E. Tulving (Eds.), *Memory Systems* (pp. 39–63). Cambridge, MA: MIT Press.

Neff, K. D. (2011). *Self-Compassion: The Proven Power of Being Kind to Yourself*. New York City: William Morrow.

Neff, K. D., and Dahm, K. (in press). Self-compassion: What it is, what it does and how it relates to mindfulness. In M. Robinson, B. Meier, and B. Ostafin (Eds.), *Mindfulness and Self-Regulation*. New York: Springer.

Neff, K. D., and McGeehee, P. (2010). Self-compassion and psychological resilience among adolescents and young adults. *Self and Identity, 9*, 225–240.

Nyanaponika. (1976). *The Power of Mindfulness*. Kandy, Sri Lanka: The Buddhist Publication Society.

Ogden, P., Minton, K., and Pain, C. (2006). *Trauma and the Body: A Sensorimotor Approach to Psychotherapy*. New York: Norton.

Olendzki (2005). The roots of mindfulness. In C. Germer, R. D. Siegel, and P. R. Fulton (2005). *Mindfulness and Psychotherapy*. New York: The Guilford Press.

Perls, F. S., Hefferline, R. F., and Goodman, T. (1951). *Gestalt Therapy, Excitement and Growth in Human Personality*. New York: Dell Publishing.

Pesso, A. (1973). *Experience in Action. Psychomotor Psychology*. New York: New York University Press.

Pyszcynski, T., and Greenberg, J. (1987). Self-regulatory preservation and the depressive self-focusing style: A self-awareness theory of reactive depression. *Psychological Bulletin, 102*, 122–138.

Raes, F. (2010). Rumination and worry as mediators of the relationship between self-compassion and depression and anxiety. *Personality and Individual Differences, 48*, 757–761.

Reich, W. (1972). *Character Analysis* (3rd ed.). New York: Farrar, Straus and Giroux. (Original work published 1933)

Rogers, C. R. (1961). *On Becoming a Person: A Psychotherapist's View of Psychotherapy*. Boston: Houghton Mifflin.

Roth, G. (2001). *Fühlen, Denken, Handeln* [Feeling, Thinking, Acting]. Frankfurt a. M.: Suhrkamp.

Roth, G. (2003). Wie das gehirn die seele macht [How the brain creates the soul]. In G. Schiepek, *Neurobiologie der Psychotherapie* [The Neurobiology of Psychotherapy]. Stuttgart: Schattauer.

Schacter, D. L. (1995). *Memory Distortion*. Cambridge, MA: Harvard University Press.

Schacter, D. L. (1996). *Searching for Memory: The Brain, the Mind, and the Past*. New York: Basic Books.

Schore, A. N., Dagniela, F., and Sieff, D. F. (2015). On the same wavelength: How our emotional brain is shaped by human relationships. In D. Sieff (Ed.), *Understanding and Healing Emotional Trauma: Conversations with Pioneering Clinicians and Researchers*. Oxford: Routledge.

Schwartz, R. (1995). *Internal Family Systems Therapy*. New York: Guilford Press.

Shedler, J. (2010). The efficacy of psychodynamic psychotherapy. *American Psychologist, 65*(2), 98–109.

Siegel, D. J. (1999). *The Developing Mind: How Relationships and the Brain Interact to Shape Who We Are*. New York: Guilford Press.

Siegel, D. J. (2007). *The Mindful Brain*. New York: Norton.

Siegel, D. J. (2017). *Mind: A Journey to the Heart of Being Human*. New York: Norton.

Sparks, T. F. (2015). Observing the organisation of experience. In H. Weiss, G. Johanson, and L. Monda (Eds.), *Hakomi: Mindfulness Centered Somatic Psychotherapy. A Comprehensive Guide to Theory and Practice*. New York: Norton.

Spitzer, M. (2002). *Lernen* [Learning]. Heidelberg: Spektrum.

Stern, D. N. (1985). *The Interpersonal World of the Infant: A View from Psychoanalysis and Developmental Psychology*. London: Karnac Books.

Teasdale, J. D., Pope, M., Moore, R. G., Hayhurst, H., Williams, S., and Segal, Z. V. (2002). Metacognitive awareness and prevention of relapse in depression: Empirical evidence. *Journal of Consulting and Clinical Psychology, 70*(2), 275–287.

Tulving, E. (1983). *Elements of Episodic Memory*. Oxford: Oxford University Press.

van der Kolk, B. A. (2015). *The Body Keeps the Score: Brain, Mind, and Body in the Healing of Trauma*. New York: Penguin Books.

Varela, F. J., Thompson, E., and Rosch, E. (1991). *The Embodied Mind*. Cambridge, MA: MIT Press.

Weiss, H. (2009). The use of mindfulness in psychodynamic and body oriented psychotherapy. *International Journal for Body, Movement and Dance in Psychotherapy, 4*, 5–16.

Weiss, H., Johanson, G., and Monda, L. (Eds.). (2015). *Hakomi: Mindfulness Centered Somatic Psychotherapy. A Comprehensive Guide to Theory and Practice*. New York: Norton.

White, M. (2007). *Maps of Narrative Practice*. New York: Norton.

Wilson, T. (2004). *Strangers to Ourselves: Discovering the Adaptive Unconscious*. Cambridge, MA: Harvard University Press.

25

EMBODIED-RELATIONAL THERAPY

Nick Totton

Introduction

Embodied-Relational Therapy (ERT) has formally existed since 1997, emerging from the training previously developed by Em Edmondson and myself under the title 'Selfheal'. 'Embodied-Relational Therapy' seemed an odd and clunky expression at the time, but has turned out to be rather prescient – there is now a great deal of talk and writing about embodied and relational aproaches, both within and beyond psychotherapy (e.g. Clemmens, 2012; Küpers, 2005; Overton, 2008; Sharpe and Strong, 2015; Sletvold, 2014; Todres, 2008; Wright and Brajtman, 2011).

In 1997, I started a UK training programme in ERT: originally one year, and developing into a two-year modular programme with a third optional year. A group of trainers emerged, who from 2018 will be running the programme without me. The training is postgraduate, for people already qualified in counselling, psychotherapy or therapeutic bodywork; it occasionally accepts someone not already qualified but with exceptional qualities and/or experience, on the understanding that this training alone will not lead to accreditation as psychotherapist or counsellor.

ERT evolved out of previous forms of body psychotherapy, and has continued to develop. I want to focus here on our most recent insights, many of them discussed in my book *Embodied Relating: The Ground of Psychotherapy* (Totton, 2015; see also Totton, 2014; Totton and Priestman, 2012). This recent work is a radical return to the basic nature of embodiment and its link with relationship, allowing a deeper understanding of their inseparability, and the fundamental role of embodied relating for *all* forms of psychotherapy.

ERT has firm roots in Reichian therapy. Both Em and I trained in Post-Reichian therapy with William (Bill) West, and Reich's groundbreaking work remains very important to me (Reich, 1973[1942]; Totton and Edmondson, 2009; West, 1994). We integrated Bill's approach, based on hands-on work with breath and muscular tension, with psychodynamic relational concepts, and Process Oriented Psychotherapy's profound trust in following what is happening in the moment (Mindell, 1985). We also drew from the Hakomi Method (Kurtz, 1985), in which Em was a certified trainer, and from various kinds of energy work.

Reaching an emergent integration of this material was complex, a long conversation between theory, clinical experience, and the experience of leading a training: there is nothing like teaching an idea for testing its validity and coherence to the limit! ERT, I think, *is* now a valid and coherent approach to body psychotherapy, hopefully of long-term value. It is not solely my intellectual property, but belongs also to Em Edmondson, who co-parented it; to my co-trainers, Allison Priestman, Jayne Johnson, Stephen Tame, and Kamalamani; and to everyone who, by training in the approach, contributed to its development.[1]

Summarising Embodied-Relational Therapy

ERT is a self-contained form of psychotherapy (that is, not needing to work in combination with any other method), addressing both verbally-focused and bodily-focused aspects, together with imagery, energetics, political and spiritual dimensions, and whatever else emerges in the therapeutic process. It rejects the current trend to specialism, a separate training for working with every variety of client and issue; instead ERT offers a single, transmodal approach applicable to a wide range of different situations and methods.

ERT is phenomenological: rather than starting out from what *should* be happening, it tries to observe what actually *is* happening, believing that this is also what *needs to* happen – that in any situation the movement toward growth and resolution is already present and seeking expression, although often out of awareness or even defined as part of the problem. ERT supports flexible, open-minded attention to all the many channels of experience in which potential change may be trying to manifest.

Hence ERT does not privilege particular channels – for example, embodiment, or relationship. Everyone is ambivalent about change and growth, we want it and don't want it; its manifestations tend to hover at the edges of awareness, so fixation on specific aspects of experience risks missing what is most important. Empirically, though, we find that the meeting point between embodiment and relationship is very often where the impulse for change will appear, so an emphasis on skilful attention to this meeting point is worthwhile – so long as we do not then miss significant material popping up unexpectedly elsewhere in the field.

Four phases of therapy

The core of ERT practice is a sequence of four therapeutic phases, presenting on every scale from micro to macro: Contact, Information Gathering, Amplifying, and Integrating. The four phases are something between a convenient heuristic device and an objective reality: certainly a lot of what happens can readily be fitted into this framework, providing a useful anchor when the process gets confusing. When we look deeply, each depends on all the others, and each contains all the others nested fractally within.

Contact can be described as a mutual sense of each other's presence and impact. It is central to relational work, and probably even to work not defined as relational; however, the therapist's capacity to enter into and explore contact is often simply assumed. Yet contact issues can block therapy completely, and need resolution before other factors can usefully be explored. ERT sees all contact as ultimately *embodied*, inseparable from a sense of one's own embodied existence in the world.

Information Gathering refers to all the ways we get news about the space we share with the other person: what they say and do, and how they look – but also how we ourselves feel, both emotionally and physically; what thoughts, memories, and fantasies come to mind for either of us, perhaps apparently randomly; and what external events enter our awareness – sounds in the street, changes of light, birds flying past the window. So information gathering includes, but is far from limited to, the actual questions we may ask a client; and our choice of questions is as informative about the situation as the client's answers. There is far more information than we can possibly use; and undue emphasis on any one channel limits our news-gathering, especially since the most important things often happen around the edges. We seek to maintain Freud's 'free-floating attention' (Langan, 1997), letting it follow whatever attracts it, trusting this to be fruitful even if we have no idea right now what it signifies.

Amplifying is a term for all the many ways in which we can support and encourage what is happening to happen *more* – louder, fuller, deeper, clearer. Different modalities have discovered a huge range of effective techniques for doing this; many of them involve bringing in more channels – for example, if the client describes a sensation we might ask them to make a sound which corresponds, or to come up with visual image, or remember a dream. But the most fundamental way of amplifying is simply to bring attention to what is happening, and let it start to unfold.

Integration comes after the activity of amplifying settles down: making sense, making connections, developing a shared narrative, language that links the new material with our existing understanding of key issues. It will always involve a *relational* integration: the client–therapist relationship needs to change shape to incorporate the new material. As 'incorporate' implies, this will also be an *embodied* integration: the two participants' embodiment and their embodied connection will need to alter, often imperceptibly but sometimes strikingly.

Embodied relating

Embodied relating is no more *central* to therapy than verbal or other kinds of work. In ERT, though, we treat it as the *ground* of psychotherapy, the foundation on which other modes of experience and action are grown (Totton, 2015). Phenomena like transference, countertransference and projection, phantasy, and emotional responses in general are founded in embodied, relational interactions happening mainly outside conscious awareness, and activating existing schemas, developed in early interactions, which we call *engrams* (see below).

ERT sees 'embodiment' as having a double meaning. On the one hand, it refers to the *state*, shared by all living human beings, of being a self-aware organism: corporeality. On the other hand, it refers to the meta-level *process* of realising and experiencing that we are this self-aware organism, and that despite appearances there is not really any separate psychological realm divorced from the body, and equally no separate bodily realm divorced from the psyche.

Embodiment is always embedded in a relational context which, at the same time, it *creates*. This context is wider than one-to-one relationships and both forms and is formed by the wider contexts of family, culture, and society (Totton, 2015, Ch 5). Some of our social embodiment is conscious, some preconscious, and some unconscious – repressed because it embodies conflicts between social requirements and individual desires, or between different social forces. As Reich (1973[1942]) showed, preconscious and unconscious aspects are effectively embodied in patterns of muscular tension, which are simultaneously patterns of psychological character: thus, the social world and its power relations directly enter the therapy room, instantiated in the embodiment of both client and therapist.

Recent work on embodied cognition shows the vital role of implicit or procedural knowledge in human learning. For every repeated activity, from riding a bicycle to forming a relationship, we rely on preconscious or unconscious patterns of activation and behaviour developed when first learning the activity (Thelen and Smith, 1994), which move from foreground to background as we absorb them into our subliminal ways of being in the world. Some of the deepest implicit, embodied patterns we hold seem to be those around relating (Boston Change Process Study

Group, 2008). We enter the world as bodies, primed to seek contact with other bodies, eager and expectant to form intense relationships. Throughout our lives we can experience the deepest wounding and the deepest healing in relationship, and from these experiences we learn implicit lessons about how to relate – largely unavailable to consciousness, just as we do not consciously know how to ride a bicycle.

Applying these ideas to the concept of transference, it emerges as not only a psychological but also a *bodily* process, shaped through implicit procedural memories of childhood relationships, learned complexes of emotional and physical response outside and in part repressed from consciousness. Our child body learns ways of positioning self in relation to other which become an automatic part of our adult repertoire: these are what ERT refers to as *engrams*. Each of us has several different embodied engrams of relating available, deployed in response to different stimuli, organising our bodymind behaviour and activating accompanying habitual thoughts and attitudes.

As a very simple example, we implicitly 'look up to' certain people and 'look down on' others, depending on a large set of personal/cultural criteria. In our culture and many others these relational attitudes are anchored in *posture* – a shortening and bending of our body to 'look up', a lengthening and straightening to 'look down', accompanied by differences in how we hold our head and neck, and in the eye contact we make. Which pattern we use will involuntarily affect the other person as a probably preconscious *experience* of being looked up to or looked down on, stimulating a physical/relational response, which either colludes with or challenges the attitude we are expressing – either says 'Yes, you should look down on/up to me' or 'No, you shouldn't'. All these patterns reflect our personal history, and the history of those who impacted us in our early relationships: they are a re-presentation of the past, when we responded to what other people's patterns told us about ourselves: a sort of possession of our bodymind by early ghosts.

Although we can conceptually separate transference (A on B) and countertransference (B on A), we are actually dealing with an *intersubjective field*, which simultaneously conditions both how A experiences B, and how B experiences A (cf. Merleau-Ponty's (1968) concept of intercorporeality). ERT is not primarily interested in identifying the mechanism – more likely, multiple mechanisms – behind this mutual influence; subliminal cues of posture and expression, mirror neurones, pheromones, and much more are no doubt involved, but what matters most is the direct experience of embodied mutuality. If we focus too much on mechanics, we risk missing the full implications of intersubjectivity.

It is now widely accepted that transference and countertransference are sometimes experienced in an embodied way (e.g. Athanasiadou and Halewood, 2011; Egan and Carr, 2008; Field, 1989). This is actually back to front: what we are dealing with is an *embodied interaction that is then usually experienced and conceptualised on the level of transference*. The logic of the case for treating transference and countertransference as fundamentally embodied also implies their mutual dependence (Totton, 2015, Ch 3). Transference and countertransference create and shape each other: they are two sides of one phenomenon, cross-transference.

Trauma and character

Our embodied subjectivity combines traumatic and nurturing elements, often in the same engram, and inherited through generations as well as new-minted (Totton, 2015, Ch 10). Both trauma and nurture are what we *take in* from the world into which we are born. They are the stuff out of which we are made, out of which we make our selves. But unless the self we construct is an open system, open in both inward and outward directions to the world and to others (since we find the world and others within as well as outside ourselves), it is both illusory and deathly. In the play of therapy, it is sometimes possible to expose and explore our deathly defences against openness without destructive effect; but only when the therapist is prepared to join in the serious game.

ERT draws strongly on Reich's (1972[1945]) unfashionable but seminal work on character, as a way to make sense of the different styles of self, which people construct from their traumatic and nurturing early experiences. We treat character not as inherently pathological, but simply as a natural and potentially creative aspect of being human. However, the more trauma and the less nurture, crudely stated, which someone has experienced, the more rigid and limiting their character structure will tend to be, with an impoverished repertoire of relational engrams reflecting their impoverished history. An understanding of character is an enormously helpful basis for grasping a particular person's central concerns and relational style, and for facilitating contact (Totton, 2015, Ch 7; Totton and Jacobs, 2001, Ch 3).

Metaskills

Although they do not directly show up in our clinical work, it is important briefly to mention ERT's 'metaskills' (Mindell, 2016), which are its widest context and its orienting framework: Awareness, Trust, Contactfulness, Spontaneity, Spaciousness, Relaxation, and Wild Mind (ERT, 2012). 'Wild Mind' refers to the inherent intelligence that emerges from identifying with the body as an aspect or part of the whole ecosystem (Totton, 2011). The seven metaskills overlap with one another; they can be thought of as holographic, with each one reflected and contained within the others – for example, contactfulness, spontaneity, relaxation, and spaciousness all depend on and also support trust, but none of them are possible without awareness; and Wild Mind in a sense describes the combined effect of all the other six.

Janice

I will try to illustrate ERT's approach through an imaginary client, Janice. Although the events I describe have not actually happened, they are closely parallel to real interactions with several clients.

Janice is having her first session with me, after a previous initial meeting. Her only previous experience of therapy was a brief course of counselling at university. She is in her late forties, a teacher, childless, and married to a man; she has identified this relationship as what brings her to therapy. Like many of my clients, she has not come seeking body psychotherapy, but when I mentioned this as a possibility she expressed mild interest. Our contact feels cool but friendly; she seems open to exploring what therapy means and what it has to offer.

We are about twenty minutes into the session; Janice has been talking for a while about her relationship with her husband, and I am starting to experience bodily sensations that seem connected to this, although it is not obvious how. My hands and feet are increasingly, unusually cold; and my awareness is being drawn in a non-specific way to my belly. While Janice continues to describe her relationship, quietly and slightly monotonously, I give some of my attention to amplifying this information from my own body.

The more attention I give, the stronger the sensations get: my hands and feet feel like ice, I start to experience chills running up and down my spine, and my guts begin to churn. I feel myself starting to break into a sweat. These seem to be symptoms of fear; but where are they coming from, and what do they mean?

From ERT's perspective, this is not actually the important question right now. The sensations are there; they are part of the relational field, they have caught my attention, and therefore they are significant and relevant to the process Janice and I are engaged in; all the more so because they are at the edge of the field – I have no reason to think that Janice is feeling fear, or indeed that she is aware of her body in any particular way. The fearful sensations are happening outside her awareness – they have become mine to hold and work with.

By giving them attention, I have already started amplifying my sensations; but how can I bring them into the shared space? There are several alternatives. I could tell Janice what I am experiencing, and see what she makes of it; this is often the best option, with the advantages of directness, simplicity, and democracy – sharing my perceptions, rather than keeping them close to my chest. However, Janice and I don't know each other very well yet; our contact is friendly, but also cool, and since Janice has little experience of therapy I am unsure how she could use such sharing at this point.

Another option would be to ask at a suitable moment what she is feeling in her own body. For example, if she talks about an emotion or thought, I could respond 'Are you aware of any reaction in your body when you talk about that?' – letting my own reaction guide me toward the channel of bodily sensation, and inviting Janice to explore that channel. However, I know that she has no experience of body-focused work, and nothing has yet suggested that she is used to finding information in her sensations.

So I decide to wait, and to listen to what Janice is saying in the context of my own experience of physical fear – which is strong but manageable. And almost immediately after I have made that decision, Janice says – very calmly and unemotionally – 'I was gutted when my husband said he had been thinking about a trial separation'.

This word 'gutted' has a powerful effect on me: it seems to slide into place and link several elements of the field. Janet is naming something that she is not expressing, and that relates directly to my own churning guts and sense of impending doom. It seems as though I have been allotted the physical experience while Janice holds the thoughts and words – a common division of labour in therapy. However I am also very struck that a few minutes previously Janice described her husband as a 'cold fish'.

'Cold fish' clearly relates to the bodily chilliness that I am experiencing – and also to the coolness that is perhaps the strongest feature in my experience of Janice so far. But I also now have in mind an image of fish being gutted. And while Janice described herself as gutted, I also make a spontaneous link with the monotony and persistence of her description of the relationship with her husband – the word 'remorseless' had come to mind. Suddenly I am thinking of her as a worker in a fish factory, with the monotonous yet ruthless job of gutting fish one after another all day long – and dissociating from her emotions in order to tolerate the situation.

I have arrived at a powerful image that feels very relevant; but it is not yet clear quite how it applies – who is doing what to whom. It seems as though all three of us, Janice, her husband, and myself, are caught up in this image of the fish gutting line: Janice is being gutted by her husband, and I am being gutted – slowly and remorselessly – by Janice. One can make a reasonable guess that the husband also feels gutted by Janice; but does Janice feel that there is a danger of being gutted by me – of being made to spill her guts, to lose emotional control? People are suffering from each other's coolness, but also perhaps fearing their own and each other's violence and aggression. Predictably, my own role in all this is least clear to me – which of my own engrams have been stimulated? I need to understand more before I intervene actively. At the same time, though, I am aware how strongly I censored myself from activity – asking Janice about her body sensations, or sharing my own – and I wonder whether I have also taken on some of the self-control and emotional coolness that I experience in her.

Having reached this point, I suddenly realise that there is another important perspective. Sitting in the therapy room seeking to make contact with a new client is enormously frightening; but like most therapists, I have grown used to suppressing my anxiety, dissociating from it. To some extent I have turned the process into a routine, like the fish-gutting conveyor belt (and I wonder distantly whether Janice might feel similarly about teaching). It seems that Janice's fear has activated my own and allowed me to become conscious of it. And as soon as I re-own the fear as mine, but also hers, my body symptoms fade, my hands and feet warm up and my guts settle. I am ready for the infinitely complex task of easing us both into deeper contact.

Analysis

Hopefully readers will be able to trace the four phases described previously – Contact, Information-gathering, Amplifying, and Integration – as they weave their way in and out of the session. From one point of view, all the work of information-gathering and amplifying is in the service of an integration, which brings my attention to the contact deficit in our relationship, and offers me clues about how to address it, and about my own part in it. The vignette illustrates how the four phases can operate on a micro-scale, as a portion of a single session; but they can also be identified on a much larger scale, for example in an entire therapeutic relationship.

What does this fictional vignette tell us about ERT's way of working? There are three points I want to emphasise. Firstly, that I started attending to my body sensations simply because they entered my awareness; I did not initially have, or need, any theory for why this was happening or what it might mean. It could have been any of a wide range of phenomena that called attention to themselves, and it seems reasonable to think that any of them would have led me to a similar place. ERT encourages practitioners to become used to noticing as many aspects of what is happening as possible, rather than just a familiar few (often mainly verbal). If I was not in the habit of tracking my embodied experience, it would have taken a lot longer for me to notice what was going on.

Secondly, once I did notice my sensations I approached them with as few preconceptions as possible. In particular, I didn't distance myself from them by assuming that they were information *only about the client*; nor did I keep them out of the field by assuming they were *only about me*. I explored them by playing with them, turning them round to see every facet, allowing them to move through whatever channels of experience appeared – in this case, embodied, verbal, visual, fantasy, and relational. Only gradually did I let a conceptual framework develop for understanding what was going on.

And thirdly, I took responsibility for my own relationship with the material. Nothing from the therapeutic field will express itself in my bodymind unless there is something already there that resonates with it. I needed to identify the cold fish/fish-gutter in *myself* in order to make therapeutic use of the material, and to see why Janice might feel frightened and therefore distant in the here and now. This is both an ethical and a technical requirement: as so often in therapy, the two cannot really be distinguished.

Conclusion

ERT is *integrative* in a sense rather different from the usual one. Rather than integrating TA and Gestalt, for example, or humanistic and psychodynamic models (although in some ways it does do this), it approaches the whole business of therapy from a different angle, which shines new light on what we doing and why we are doing it. It also integrates body-centred and verbal approaches in a much deeper way than is often the case, not bolting the one onto the other, but looking for the fundamental connections between them.

This chapter only allows a brief outline of how Embodied-Relational Therapy works. If ERT has a goal, it is to move toward living more of the time from the seven metaskills which I outlined above. We aim to continually work from and offer these metaskills to our clients, and the times when we find ourselves unable to do so offer useful information about what's happening in the relationship. We are modelling for our clients and for ourselves what it means to be more open, more relaxed, more trusting, more free – because only by doing so can we do our job. So, being a therapist does us good. Being the best therapist we can be is a journey of becoming more ourselves: relaxing into and trusting who we are.

Note

1 I would like to dedicate this chapter to the memory of Pete Kulak, who was involved with ERT for many years, and who died on 1 September 2016.

References

Athanasiadou, C. and Halewood, A. (2011). A grounded theory exploration of therapists' experiences of somatic phenomena in the countertransference. *European Journal of Psychotherapy & Counselling, 13(3),* 247–262.

Boston Change Process Study Group (2008). Forms of relational meaning: Issues in the relations between the implicit and reflective-verbal domains. *Psychoanalytic Dialogues, 18,* 125–148.

Clemmens, M. C. (2012). The interactive field: Gestalt therapy as an embodied relational dialogue. In T. B. Levine (Ed.), *Gestalt Therapy: Advances in theory and practice* (39–48). London: Routledge.

Egan, J. and Carr, A. (2008). Body-centred countertransference in female trauma therapists. *Irish Association of Counselling and Psychotherapy Quarterly Journal, 8,* 24–27.

ERT (2012). Embodied-Relational Therapy metaskills. http://homepages.3-c.coop/erthworks/ERT%20 Metaskills.pdf. (Accessed July 24, 2017.)

Field, N. (1989). Listening with the body: An exploration in the countertransference. *British Journal of Psychotherapy, 5(40),* 512–522.

Küpers, W. (2005). Phenomenology of embodied implicit and narrative knowing. *Journal of Knowledge Management, 9(6),* 114–133.

Kurtz, R. (1985). *Hakomi Therapy.* Boulder, CO: Hakomi Institute.

Langan, R. (1997). On free-floating attention. *Psychoanalytic Dialogues, 7(6),* 819–839.

Merleau-Ponty, M. (1968). *The Visible and the Invisible.* C. Lefort (Ed.). Evanston, IL: Northwestern University Press.

Mindell, A. (1985). *River's Way: The process science of the dreambody.* London: Routledge & Kegan Paul.

Mindell, A. (2016). *Meta-skills: The spiritual art of psychotherapy.* CreateSpace.

Overton, W. F. (2008). Embodiment from a relational perspective. In W. F. Overton, U. Muller and J. L. Newman (Eds.), *Developmental Perspectives on Embodiment and Consciousness* (1–18). New York: Lawrence Erlbaum.

Reich, W. (1972[1945]). *Character Analysis.* New York: Farrar, Straus & Giroux.

Reich. W. (1973[1942]). *The Function of the Orgasm.* New York: Farrar, Straus & Giroux.

Sharpe, H. and Strong, T. (2015). *Embodied Relating and Transformation: Tales from equine-facilitated counseling.* Rotterdam, The Netherlands: Sense Publishers.

Sletvold, J. (2014). *The Embodied Analyst: From Freud and Reich to relationality.* London: Routledge.

Thelen, E. and Smith, L. B. (1994). *A Dynamic Systems Approach to the Development of Cognition and Action.* Cambridge, MA: MIT Press.

Todres, L. (2008). Being with that: the relevance of embodied understanding for practice. *Qualitative Health Research, 18(11),* 1566–1573.

Totton, N. (2011). *Wild Therapy: Undomesticating our inner and outer worlds.* Ross-on-Wye, UK: PCCS Books.

Totton, N. (2014). Embodied relating: The ground of psychotherapy. *International Body Psychotherapy Journal, 13(2),* 88–103.

Totton, N. (2015). *Embodied Relating: The ground of psychotherapy.* London: Karnac.

Totton, N. and Edmondson, E. (2009). *Reichian Growth Work: Melting the blocks to life and love* (2nd ed.). Ross-on-Wye, UK: PCCS Books.

Totton, N. and Jacobs, M. (2001). *Character and Personality Types.* Maidenhead, UK: Open University Press.

Totton, N. and Priestman, A. (2012). Embodiment and relationship: Two halves of one whole. In C. Young (Ed.), *About Relational Body Psychotherapy* (35–68). Stow, UK: Body Psychotherapy Publications.

West, W. (1994). Post Reichian therapy. In D. Jones (Ed.), *Innovative Therapy, A Handbook* (131–146). Maidenhead, UK: Open University Press.

Wright, D. and Brajtman, S. (2011). Relational and embodied knowing: Nursing ethics within the interprofessional team. *Nursing Ethics, 18(1),* 20–30.

26

FOUR FORMS OF KNOWLEDGE IN BIOSYNTHESIS THERAPY

David Boadella

Introduction

In Biosynthesis, we integrate the understanding of ourselves, the other and the world, in terms of four forms of knowledge. These forms of knowledge are part of the human heritage, through philosophy, science, and the human arts (Pieringer and Fazekas, 1996).

First, a few words about knowledge and science. Science comes from the root to know: science means basically knowledge. Related to this is the word conscience, which means inner knowledge. Knowledge itself is closely related to words meaning to handle, to touch, to explore the world. The words of our language are built on a basis of gestures we develop in infancy. Words for speech originate from words related to pointing with the fingers. Daniel Stern has shown us that we have four distinct kinds of self, and only the fourth of these is a linguistic self, a self that speaks. The other three are earlier and are pre-verbal.

This raises the difficulty of trying to communicate about Biosynthesis, a therapy that works with the non-verbal, or pre-verbal, as well as the verbal. Our therapeutic work is constantly involved in the translation from verbal language, to non-verbal language, and back again. This process of communication is either top-down, from words to body, or bottom-up, from body to words. Neurotic conflicts split this integration, so the therapeutic work is trying to re-build the bridges between what we feel and what we say, what we mean and how we express it, what we want and how we move towards it. Each one of the four forms of knowledge described below has been developed in Biosynthesis therapy.

Intra-personal knowledge: "I feel, therefore I am"

Science has not been able yet to understand consciousness, which has resisted attempts to reduce it to functions of the brain. The "what it feels like" of our experience, (the so-called *qualia*) presents the so-called "hard problem" of consciousness studies. It seems that consciousness must be a fundamental property of nature, along with time and space and energy. Certainly, our consciousness is the basis of all our science, and without it no science is possible.

We know, in psychotherapy, that our consciousness sits on top of a vast sea of what has been called the "unconscious." It would be more correct to call this the "sub-conscious." It is what lies under consciousness. This sub-conscious is like a sea underlying the waves of our conscious thinking and feeling. It is the organismic wisdom of the body, evolved over three billion years of life, since the first life forms emerged on earth. It is related to self-regulation, to the repair of cells, to the 50 percent of our energy which goes just to maintain our body and our activities.

If we want to contact it, we need to go inwards, for the first form of knowledge is inner knowledge. Intuition is part of this, listening within. Conscience is part of this "knowing with" our inner sense organs. What Gendlin (1982) has called the "felt sense" is part of this, together with listening to the rhythms of our breathing, sensing the nuances of our muscle tone and following the rhythms of thoughts and feelings and the spaces between them. Dreams are also part of this inner knowledge. Einstein developed his relativity theory after dreaming of riding on a light wave. There are many such examples from the history of science.

In Biosynthesis, this inner knowledge is the foundation of our ability to integrate the other three forms of knowledge. The therapist is focussed not only on the client, but also on his or her own responsiveness: what is termed counter-transference in psychotherapy. In Biosynthesis, we extend this to "somatic resonance," the echo of experience in the cells. This is why self-experience is the centre and ground of psychotherapy training, always returning to the central message of the oracle of Delphi, "know yourself."

One way to know ourselves is to be open to the experience of meditation. Meditation comes from the word "medi," centre, and is related to the ability to centre oneself in awareness; it is a form of self-remembering. In meditation, we get closely in touch with what is going on inside us and with the process of coming into balance. The same root is the basis of the word "medicine," the study of health, the process of supporting well-being.

Our therapeutic work is a kind of meditation on what is happening in the interactions between ourselves and the one who has come to us for help with some kind of problem. Neurotic problems break up the integration between the different levels of ourselves, so that we cannot listen any more to the internal communication. In Biosynthesis we speak of seven different life fields of experience and of expression. We distinguish:

- the somatic level of posture, movement, and muscle tone;
- the energetic level of breathing;
- the level of the primary emotions related to exploration and self-protection;
- the level of heart feelings;
- the level of thoughts and words;
- the level of images and dreams;
- and the spiritual level of fundamental values and deepest aspirations.

In our therapeutic work, we help to reconnect all these seven aspects in the client. We realise that as therapists we are not technicians who can repair human problems with the brilliance of our methods. Rather we are explorers trying to reach behind the problem to find the resource level within the other, as well as within ourselves.

There are resources to be discovered, uncovered, and recovered, at all levels of the life fields. It is no accident that the word "recovery" means to get well, and that the word "remembering" means, literally, to reconnect the members of the body and of the self.

At the resource level, we find our inner wisdom, which is a source of healing. This begins to bring fresh energy to each of the other life fields. We begin literally to move differently, to breathe differently, to experience our affects differently, to have a new connection to the heart, to speak, and think differently, to make contact to regenerative images and to insightful dreams, and to get a deeper and closer connection to our fundamental values.

The healing of therapeutic work is initiated from outside, which is why a person comes to us for help; but the real work proceeds from inside, from the first form of knowledge in each person, from the subconscious resources becoming usable, from the inner healer and the inner teacher.

Inter-personal knowledge: "You are, therefore I feel"

In the bipersonal field of every relationship, we have the paradox that I am sensing you sensing yourself and sensing you while you are sensing me. In Biosynthesis, as in other forms of psychotherapy, this means that the therapeutic relationship is the primary ground for all therapeutic change. If the relationship gets stuck, the therapy gets stuck.

The ancient Greeks, at the time of Pythagoras, studied therapy in terms of concepts such as harmony and empathy. Harmony meant a form of attunement between persons. This primary attunement has been studied between animals (Bowlby, 1969) and between parents and children (Stern, 1991; Schore, 1996). Stern distinguished attunement as taking place between over-stimulation, where the child is bombarded with too many invasive stimuli, and under-stimulation, where the child is deprived of essential emotional nourishment. In the therapeutic relationship, the same processes apply. Therapy is a process of progressive attunement between therapist and client.

This attunement establishes a somatic resonance between the two persons. This resonance was studied by the philosopher Spinoza, who commented: "affects have effects." The client can catch new attitudes and approaches from the therapist, but the therapist can also catch old attitudes and approaches from the client. We can resonate positively or negatively. The negative resonances we feel in response to the client are ways of learning about the kind of problems he had: what does it feel like to be in his skin, from his family, with his problems. By accepting these negative resonances and then helping to transmute them, we give the client a role model of how to cope with trauma, pain, loss, and invasion (Boadella, 2005).

The therapist needs to learn how to handle overwhelming anger, or fear. I call this the process of having one foot in the ditch. If we are too little able to identify with the client's desperation, we are too detached, too far away. If we are over-identified with his problems, we are caught up in them: now the therapist is depressed as well as the client. So the skill of navigating the relational field is to be able both to be in empathic contact, and to remain in good self-contact.

Empathy in Greek means "feeling into." Sympathy, unfortunately, can sometimes become symbiosis in a negative sense, as in the condition known as "co-dependency": therapist and client are bound together helplessly in this suffering. So empathy involves the ability to find the other without losing oneself. It involves both the process of feeling, and being at times, symmetric with the client, so we can humanly mirror back to him in ways where he or she feels seen, heard, and understood. However, we also need, at times, to be asymmetric with the client, so he sees that we are not stuck where he is, and that there is movement and help coming from the outside. In this way, we can become an inviting mirror, a person who offers fresh possibilities, insights, angles of view, and new skills for becoming unstuck. Sometimes we are more active–initiating. Sometimes we are more receptive–responsive.

Fine-tuning these responses is part of our attunement. This dance of interaction between us is an energetic process of communication, rich with information in many channels. Some of the information that passes is conscious and becomes part of explicit learning. Some of the information is subconscious and becomes part of implicit learning. Our body language is the ground for our verbal language; the body of our words grows out of the signals of our body.

In the holding environment of the therapeutic relationship, the client begins to unlearn old habit patterns and character attitudes, and to accept new emotional experiences of relationship, which can build trust instead of mistrust. Since the therapeutic relationship is only a "good enough" relationship, and not an ideal relationship, there will of course be times of what is called "empathic failure," when the therapist was unable to attune, where he misunderstood, overlooked, and failed to listen, or where he offered the wrong interventions. The client can deal with this, provided the therapist is able to admit error, to work, in his supervision, on his own blockages to the client, and to show constant willingness to grow himself, in the contact with the difficulties of the client.

The more disturbed the client is, the more difficult it can be for the therapist to avoid being seen by the client as the difficult therapist. Therapy is a form of verbal and non-verbal dialogue that seeks to take place between the poles of invasion and deprivation. This Biosynthesis model of invasion, deprivation, and dialogue was inspired by the work of Friere (1993), working with communities in South America. We try to open up spaces between these two extremes in the therapeutic relationship, so that real interaction can take place, permitting healing to become possible. This means to gradually widen the tolerance space in the client's awareness, between feeling invaded – the therapist did too much of the wrong things and feeling deprived – the therapist did too little of the right things.

The principle of contact canals in Biosynthesis means that we can seek contact through appropriate speaking, appropriate looking, and appropriate touching. If one of these channels is more difficult than the other, we look for the one that can create more trust and less distrust. In this way, in the dance of interpersonal knowledge, I can contact, in the here and now, the other who is contacting himself while contacting me: a process of mutual reflection, which begins to unwind the spiral of disturbance whose origin lies in there and then.

Impersonal knowledge: "They think, therefore I understand"

The third form of knowledge seeks to find some general patterns of process, some laws of growth and form, which can help us to order the almost infinite variety of human attributes and problems. We seek a frame, which can make sense of our intuitive sensing, and our empathic attunement. How can we reflect cognitively and consciously on these often-implicit forms of experience?

In this way science seeks to be "objective," aiming at certain truths about health and pathology, what is a good intervention and what is a bad one. In our therapeutic work in Biosynthesis, we certainly are looking also for general laws that can guide our work and help us to order our perceptions and our interventions.

One of these fundamental laws, which has guided Biosynthesis since its origins, is the understanding of the tri-partite organisation of the body into three lifestreams (Boadella 1987/2015). The three embryological layers which form 2 weeks after conception provide the ground plan for somatic organisation now. This conceptual tool helps us distinguish and yet connect:

- Feelings (related to the endoderm);
- Actions (related to the mesoderm);
- Perceptions (related to the ectoderm).

Therapeutic work in Biosynthesis seeks to support the client to find better centering in feelings, better grounding in actions, and better facing in relation to communications. Neuroscience has discovered a similar functional simplicity, underlying the immense complexity of the brain (Luria, 1976; Porges, 2011; Yakovlev, 1948).

Trauma research has shown that excessive shock and stress breaks up the interconnectedness of these three systems. Therapy works to reintegrate what has been disassociated, to build bridges, and to dissolve splits.

Nevertheless, in the post-quantum era, we have learned that scientific hypotheses are forever conditional, and can be overturned by new findings. Theories are ways of seeing, and not rigid paradigms. Unfortunately, science can sometimes become a dogma that fixes us into not seeing what we do not want to see and to finding only what we want to find. This is the shadow side of diagnosis if it becomes too reductionist. In order to avoid this, we need to remember that the science of therapy needs to be in balance with the art of therapy.

In Biosynthesis, we work constantly with the concept of polarity: which means that what is good and helpful for one client, at one stage of development, may well be unhelpful and disturbing to another client, or to the same client at a different stage of development. Character theory is also a third person form of knowledge, since it seeks to characterise, to generalise, and to typify. This can easily lead to reducing a person to an outer psychological diagnosis. In our therapeutic work, we seek not to reduce clients to examples of prototypes, but rather to see prototypical tendencies, in various degrees, in others, and ourselves. Under stress, we are pushed into being frozen, or flooded, or we take catastrophic jumps between these two states. Too much stress can over-excite a person into a manic state or lower the life-energy into a depressive state. So, stress can push us from one extreme to the other. These are general processes of human reactivity, which can be studied in research, and even measured physiologically. This has been well studied in catastrophe theory (Thom, 1989), a general scientific theory which can be applied to many phenomena, including weather systems, the stock market, and neurosis. In catastrophe states the system swings wildly between storms and drought, between financial inflation and financial depression, between neurotic panic, and neurotic numbing.

Character theory, in Biosynthesis, seeks to emphasise the resources in a person, which lie beneath and beyond problems. It is therefore also a polar theory, in which we are looking always for ways to come out of the duality of these extreme states, and to recover the natural pulsation between opposite healthy poles of reaction. The therapeutic work seeks to recover the missing middle ground. In states of balance, there is easy movement between the poles of a system, a little more, or a little less: for example, more active, or more restful.

If the therapist understands the general principles of these dynamics, he can help the client to reorganise himself, until the extreme splitting between the dualities is overcome, and a gentler rhythm develops between activation and quiescence. This is then in tune with the organic rhythms of life, and restores a sense of pulsation, which is the basis of health, to the body and to the personality.

For example, we have developed in Biosynthesis the concept of motoric fields (Boadella, 2000). Motoric fields are patterns of movement, which carry with them feelings, relational attitudes, belief systems, and value systems. For example: a baby reaches out towards the mother. There is a gesture, there is an attempt to communicate a need, there is the expectation of a response, and there is an attitude of trust in the other.

On the other hand, there may be the opposite of all these. The motoric fields are shapes of the body, attitudes of mind, and postures of the soul. We understand them as general patterns, which can be studied "objectively" by means of video recordings. But the meaning is not objective, it has to be understood in terms of the total sense of an interaction, so that the objective knowledge once more has to be grounded and validated in terms of subjective, intuitive, and empathic knowledge.

Trans-personal knowledge: "We create: therefore I grow"

The fourth form of knowledge relates to the wisdom of a culture, the shared legacy of art, music, drama, poetry, and myth. In these forms of creativity, the individual is connected to the group so that "I" and "you" are transcended to become "we." This form of knowledge includes the spiritual traditions, which are transpersonal in the sense of uniting each person with a deeper essential source.

Campbell (2003) has shown how many myths can embody the transpersonal aspects of a personal story. Each of us during our life embodies a personal myth, which reflects dimensions of collective stories (Keleman, 2000). We are one and we are many.

One of the earliest myths in the world is the myth of Osiris, Isis, and Horus, from Egypt. We find when we study this myth that there is much to learn about mysteries of life and death, love and hate, vision and deception. There are also deep connections between these three figures. Here is a mythological connection to the theme in Biosynthesis of grounding, centering, and facing. Osiris is related to grounding in the spine and the support system of the body. Isis is related to centering in the belly, the breathing, the lungs, and the sea of emotions. Horus, their child, is related to facing, through the eyes, and the qualities of vision.

In Biosynthesis one of the ways of going beneath the problems is to contact the resources of healing and recovery, through inviting the client into some form of creativity. The foundations of creativity lie in play. Depression is equivalent to the loss of the ability to play.

Play is known to be related to exploration, and to promote new levels of integration in the brain, and in the body. So the heavier the problem, the more important it is to help the client to become exploratory, playful, creative, even if to begin with this is only to a minimal degree. We call this blowing on the flame of resources beneath the ash of the problems.

There are many ways to do this. One way is to encourage the client to write creatively about experiences. A client, who had no sense of the continuity of her past at the start of her therapy, wrote and published a book, at the end of her therapy, called "Room to breathe."

In our interactive work in Biosynthesis, the embodied relationship with the client moves between sitting, standing, lying, moving around the room, and all possibilities between. We are involved not so much in a psychodrama of re-enacting the past, as in a "biodrama" of recreating the present. Catharsis becomes possible in the old Greek sense of a relieving emotional enact-ment. Catharsis here does not mean the discharge of emotion, so much as the cleansing effects of emotional communication.

The dance of interaction between parent and child is similar to the phrases and sequences of a musical melody. Our first language is the music of body gesture, the language of muscle tone, and the tones of sounds existing before speech. When we work with principles of movement and muscle tone, we are helping the client to retune the muscle spindles in different parts of the body. Our therapeutic work in Biosynthesis, grounded in the other three forms of knowledge, is in the end an art, the art of attunement, the dance of relationship, the music of creativity.

So each of the four forms of knowledge offers a taste of a different range of possibilities and qualities, which we need to blend and bring into dialogue with each other. This is the challenge and opportunity, which we face, as therapists, in our day-to-day work on ourselves, with our clients, and in the process of explaining this work to others.

References

Boadella, D. (2000). Shape flow and postures of the soul. *Energy and Character, 30*, 2.

Boadella, D. (2005). Affect, attunement and attachment. *Energy and Character, 34*, 13–23.

Boadella, D. (2015). *Lifestreams: An introduction to Biosynthesis* (Silver ed.). London: Routledge. (Original work published 1987)

Bowlby, J. (1969). *Attachment*. London: Basic Books.

Campbell, J. (2003). *The Hero's Journey*. Novato, CA: New World Library.

Friere, P. (1993). *Pedagogy of the Oppressed*. New York: Continuum.

Gendlin, E. (1982). *Focussing.* New York: Bantam Books.

Keleman, S. (2000). *Myth and the Body.* Berkeley, CA: Centre Press.

Luria, A. (1976). *The Working Brain.* London: Penguin Books.

Pieringer, W., and Fazekas, C. (1996). Die vier primären Erkenntnismethoden als wissenschaftliche Leitlinien für die Selbsterfahrung in der Psychotherapieausbildung [The four primary forms of knowedge as scientific guidelines for self-experience in psychotherapy training]. *Psychotherapie Forum, 4,* 229–338.

Porges, S. (2011). *The Polyvagal Theory.* New York: W. W. Norton.

Schore, A. (1996). *Affect Regulation and the Origin of the Self.* Hillside, NJ: Erlbaum.

Stern, D. (1991). *The Interpersonal World of the Infant.* New York: W. W. Norton.

Thom, R. (1989). *Structural Stability and Morphogenesis.* Reading, MA: Addison-Wesley.

Yakovlev, P. (1948). Motility, behaviour and the brain. *Journal of Nervous and Mental Diseases, 107*(4), 313–334.

27

THE RELATIONAL TURN IN BODY PSYCHOTHERAPY

Michael Soth

Introduction

This chapter presents the author's journey from his struggle with shadow aspects of the body psychotherapy (BP) tradition (Soth, 2005a) toward a re-integration of the split with psychoanalysis and beyond that towards a broad-spectrum embodied-relational integration of therapeutic approaches. A specific key learning in the author's development, located in the mid-1990s, was the 'relational turn'. This constitutes a paradigm shift towards a systemic-holistic phenomenology of the therapeutic relationship in practice and is underpinned by an integration of humanistic and psychoanalytic principles of two-person psychology, beyond the understanding of unconscious dynamics provided by the psychoanalytic conceptualis-ation of transference-countertransference (Soth, 2007). The relational turn is based upon recognition of the paradoxical nature of 'enactment' by which the therapeutic relationship both replicates the client's core developmental woundings and offers the space and crucible for transforming them. This chapter explores the range of therapeutic stances that are cur-rently found amongst body psychotherapists, as these need to be understood flexibly within the dynamic force field of the therapeutic space in order to facilitate the transformative con-tainment of enactment.

Since Reich's expulsion from the International Psychoanalytic Association in 1934, the body-oriented tradition and psychoanalysis have developed along separate trajectories. Within that historically protracted split, significant aspects of the art of psychotherapy have remained isolated from each other, the traditions replicating their special expertise and sensibilities in ther-apeutic subcultures from generation to generation, leaving precious understandings and wisdoms fragmented into segregated communities of practitioners. In spite of our holistic intentions, body psychotherapists have been stuck in habits of therapeutic styles that do not comprehensively meet and manifest the wholeness and fullness of clients, but only those aspects that fit the blueprint of the BP (Body Psychotherapy) tradition. It is only over the last 20 years that body psychotherapists have begun to re-integrate that split between the body-oriented traditions and psychoanalysis. In relation to this point the author wrote:

> . . . by integrating the body/mind sensitivities of the Body Psychotherapy tradition
> and the relational sensibilities of modern psychoanalysis we can arrive at an embodied

notion of countertransference . . . a (re-)integration of their theoretical frameworks may generate an holistic phenomenology of relationship . . . which understands both transference and countertransference as embodied processes manifesting on multiple body/mind levels as well as multiple relational levels.

(Soth, 2005b, p. 40)

On the level of abstract theory a twenty-first-century embodied account of intersubjectivity from the first moments of life has been comprehensively established by infant research, neuroscience and philosophy (Gallagher, 2006; Stern, 1985; Trevarthen, 1993) across the fragmented discipline of psychotherapy. However, on the level of therapeutic practice, a coherent, embodied two-person psychology formulation that does justice to these principles of intersubjectivity and embodied, embedded, enactive, extended cognition (Gallagher, 2006) has not, as yet, been established. What has been developing is a two-person psychology account of psychotherapeutic interaction as 'a meeting of minds' (Aron, 2002, title page). Intersubjectivity (Atwood and Stolorow, 1992) and interpersonal neurobiology (Schore, 2012) are taking steps beyond the traditional Cartesian limitations of the talking therapies, but it is the contention of this author that this has not yet translated into a comprehensive systemic-holistic phenomenology of therapeutic practice, i.e. as an interaction between two body/minds.

In a nutshell, since Reich, body psychotherapists' unrivalled expertise regarding intra-psychic body/mind processes was gained and developed at the expense of an awareness of unconscious inter-personal processes (the special expertise of the psychoanalytic tradition). The 'relational obliviousness' (Soth, 2000, p. 12) of body psychotherapy, a common and valid critique by psychoanalysts, inclines us towards therapeutically 'using the body in habitual ways to minimise, circumvent, and avoid transference pressures and their corresponding countertransference disturbances'.

The paradigm shift inherent in the relational turn described in this chapter makes it conceivable that BP has other options, specifically for the therapist to surrender to their complex involvement with these relational vicissitudes at the 'intimate edge' (Ehrenberg, 1992, title page). Rather than minimizing their counter-transferential sense of conflict, therapists can intensify their sense of conflict by deepening awareness of how their body/mind as therapists is always already involved in intersubjective enactments of wounding dynamics. Being able to fully inhabit the spontaneous relational charge of these enactments depends on the therapist's capacity to apprehend and contain their embodied countertransference (Shaw, 2004; Soth, 2005b) as a meaningful parallel process to the client's internal object relations, and thus to flexibly dwell in a variety of relational positions and integrate them.

Body psychotherapists in the Reichian tradition have available a sophisticated body/mind way of apprehending and working with transference, based upon Reich's functionalism initiating a holistic and biologically-rooted meta-psychology of human relating.[1] However, as a tradition, BP has not extended that understanding into the therapist's side of the therapeutic encounter and applied it to the therapist's body/mind functioning when at work (i.e. into embodied countertransference). Body psychotherapy is largely caught in Freud's classical definition of countertransference as therapists' own character and pathology, which considers it as an interference with optimal contact and thus the therapeutic process (Boadella, 1982; Soth, 2015).

That means that as a tradition BP has not taken on board the 'countertransference revolution' in psychoanalysis (Samuels, 1993), whereby the client's inner world is understood to manifest within the therapist's countertransference process (Heimann, 1950), offering profound and immediate avenues into the client's unconscious experience. This is ironic because the degree of body/mind expertise accumulated in BP down the generations would allow such access in more far-reaching ways than is customary even in modern psychoanalysis. Through vegetative identification (Reich, 1972), somatic resonance, and intricate embodied awareness we can apprehend what other approaches might consider subliminal processes in the therapist's body/mind, including somatic responses triggered by mirror neuron interactions (Rothschild, 2006). Although these body/mind communications inevitably become complicated by the therapist's subjective reactions to them, they nevertheless give access to 'implicit relational knowing' (Lyons-Ruth, 1998, p. 282) and unconscious processes in the therapeutic relationship, including projective identifications which are at the root of 'situational countertransference' (Soth, 2006a).

The accumulated body/mind wisdom of the BP tradition could thus allow extraordinary access to the widely recognised transformative potential of countertransference and enactment. However, that first requires a radical change in body psychotherapy's conventional focus and paradigm, expanding the habitual therapeutic stance to embrace a multiplicity of relational modalities (Clarkson and Wilson, 1994/2003) as a dynamic force field manifesting the relational configurations of the client's character wounding (as well as the therapist's). As a minimum, this requires an integration of Stark's (1999) 'one-person', 'one-and-a-half-person', and 'two-person psychology' stances. Applying Stark's terminology to the BP tradition, I would argue that Reich's original one-person psychology treatment focus was complemented by humanistic two-person psychology principles from the 1970s onward, without acknowledging, let alone integrating the inherent contradiction between the two. As previously argued (Soth, 2008) the medical model has remained a hidden relational modality within BP. As a result, it can be seen that most body psychotherapists are, on balance, operating in a confused one-and-a-half-person psychology mode, combining contradictory stances without differentiating them (which would then make them available for paradoxical integration).

The therapist's relational stance and habitual position

Character analysis explains that the client cannot help but bring their developmental wounding into the 'here and now' of the consulting room (Soth, 2006a) and therefore into therapeutic relationship. But just as the client's character moulds their posture and position in the world and shapes their engagement with others, the same is true for the therapist. Just as the client's ego rationalises unconsciously held attitudes and behaviour patterns, so the therapist's ego rationalises characteristically held fixed therapeutic stances, styles and ways of relating, using therapeutic theory and meta-psychology to justify its *modus operandi* in the therapeutic position.

The underlying reason why body psychotherapists have remained relationally oblivious and, like other approaches, have not thoroughly conceptualised the conflicted body/mind ambiguity of the working alliance, is because BP tends to take that alliance for granted the more it operates within a one–person psychology framework, and assumes that the alliance is a given as long as clients continue to attend sessions. Across the psychotherapy approaches, including body psychotherapy, the working alliance is overestimated, with the client supposedly receptive to the therapist's interventions, aware of their therapeutic intentions and collaborative with the therapist's supposedly benign rationale. This is in spite of the fact that Reich (1972) had a clear grasp that unconscious characteristic issues pervade the client's transferential feelings towards therapy and therapist when he said that, 'unconscious hostile attitudes on the part of the patient formed the basis of the neurosis as a whole. Every interpretation of the unconscious material glanced off from this secret hostility . . . Every patient is deeply sceptical about the treatment. Each merely conceals it differently' (Reich, 1972, p. 119).

Two key assumptions leading to relational obliviousness

The traditional conception of the therapeutic position, whatever stance therapists take, relies on two underlying assumptions:

- the notion that the therapist's stance, responses, and interventions are consciously and deliberately chosen, derived from a therapeutic rationale to aid the process in line with principles of therapeutic theory and technique (this is an unquestioned remnant of late-nineteenth-century one-person psychology assumptions (Soth, 2006a), even amongst therapists who officially eschew a two-person psychology perspective)
- an overestimation of the working alliance between client and therapist (often conceptualised in unhelpful and limiting ways as the cooperation between the client's and the therapist's supposedly healthy parts (Greenson, 1965), traditionally even more reduced to their respective rational intentions and shared understandings manifest in their negotiated explicit contract).

These two assumptions reduce the notion of the working alliance to ego-ego collaboration and guarantee relational obliviousness by minimising the significance of unconscious processes and failing to take into account fundamental psychoanalytic principles: the way in which the client's unconscious constructs the therapeutic space as well as the therapist's experience and behaviour within it.

These assumptions minimise the degree of conflict and wounding which clients bring into therapy (i.e. the extent to which they cannot help but approach therapy *through* their character, its defences and corresponding transferences), implicitly ignoring the degree to which the client's ego cannot and does not accurately perceive and understand the therapist's good intentions and framework. By definition the client's character prevents them from making 'good' use of the therapist and the therapeutic space, and from exploring it openly and fully.

These two assumptions therefore fail to account for the inevitable dynamic by which the client's conflict becomes the therapist's conflict (Soth, 1998a) and precipitates necessary ruptures of the therapeutic relationship which thus end up replicating and re-enacting the client's wounding. Consequently, they deny the inevitable and compelling nature of these enactments (Bromberg, 2001) and the extent to which therapists get drawn into them and contribute to them, in degrees unwittingly and unconsciously.

In simple terms, these assumptions vastly overestimate the degree of conscious collaboration, choice and intention possible in the therapeutic relationship. Furthermore, they underestimate the power of unconscious dynamics and their body/mind manifestations and thus divert awareness away from the entanglements by which therapists find themselves replicating the client's character wounding *through* therapy and *through* their therapeutic stances, ideas, reflections and interventions. All therapeutic theories and techniques, especially those beliefs and assumptions about therapy most cherished by therapists, can become vehicles of enactment.

The relational turn

The recognition of enactment in the mid-1990s constituted a watershed in my own development as a therapist, refined over the following years into the following formulation: 'It is impossible for a therapist to follow a strategy of overcoming or changing a dysfunctional pattern without enacting in the transference the person in relation to whom that pattern originated' (Soth, 2006b, p. 44). A more specific formulation of the relational turn relevant to body psychotherapy and formulated in its language might be: 'It is impossible to pursue a "therapeutic" agenda of breaking through the armour or undercutting the ego's resistance without enacting in the transference the person whom the armour/resistance first developed against' (Soth, 2006b, p. 44).

This recognition divides the author's development into two phases, one before and one after the relational turn, and thus defines the difference between traditional and relational body psychotherapy. Because this principle is relevant in all therapy, regardless of tradition, approach, theory or technique, it can become an integrative foundation for a diverse and pluralistic yet eventually *coherent* field of the psychological therapies, grounded in two-person psychology.

Enactment as the paradoxical linchpin of character transformation

By formulating enactment as a two-person psychology account of what used to be described as transference-countertransference in the psychoanalytic tradition (Soth, 2007), the relational movement has been arriving at the paradoxical heart of a relational theory of therapeutic action and transformation. This depends on the recognition that the healing of the client's wounds *in* and *through* therapy is inseparable from the enactment of the wounding *in* and *through* therapy.

Whilst this paradox has been recognised in many therapeutic approaches, although not always grasped precisely, the necessary consequences for practice remain vague and controversial across the relational movement. There are two main reasons. First, therapists attempt to do justice to the enactment while holding onto their traditional habitual therapeutic positions (not fully recognising that these positions are being deconstructed, destroyed and potentially transcended by the enactment). Secondly, relational therapists as well as BPs are lacking a non-dualistic embodied formulation of enactment that fully embraces its spontaneity and largely non-verbal and subliminal manifestations, and therefore the extent to which it is out of control. The metaphor can be used of a vortex in the sea that can be survived not by struggling and trying to escape, but by therapists surrendering to being sucked down, and thus spat out at the bottom.

A diversity of relational stances in the force field of the therapeutic relationship

An essential condition for surviving transformative enactments is the therapist's flexibility between different relational modalities and stances, recognising all of them as potential externalisations of the client's internal object relations and therefore as parallel processes to the wounding dynamic and character conflicts (Soth, 1998b). Models by Gomez (2004), Stark (1999), and Clarkson and Wilson (1994/2003), who have used different and complementary perspectives to distinguish various relational modalities and kinds of therapeutic relatedness, can be integrated to circumscribe the conflicted force field of the therapeutic space, and the various positions which therapists find themselves taking (Soth, 2003).

The Stances: Authoritative guidance versus mutual exploration

Eight different stances and habitual positions in the field of body psychotherapy can be listed along a spectrum between two poles (see Figure 27.1).

At one end are stances that emphasise the role of the therapist (implying various versions of authority), and at the other end, more in line with humanistic beliefs, the therapist as a person (facilitative, but ultimately another human and an equal). The authority polarity implies some sort of expert position, making guiding, directive interventions or providing treatment as the psychological equivalent of a doctor. The essence of the other polarity, client and therapist meeting

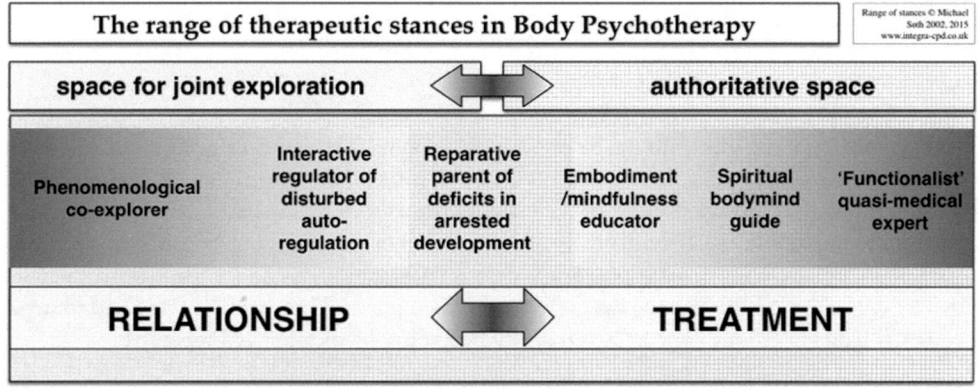

Figure 27.1 The range of therapeutic stances in body psychotherapy

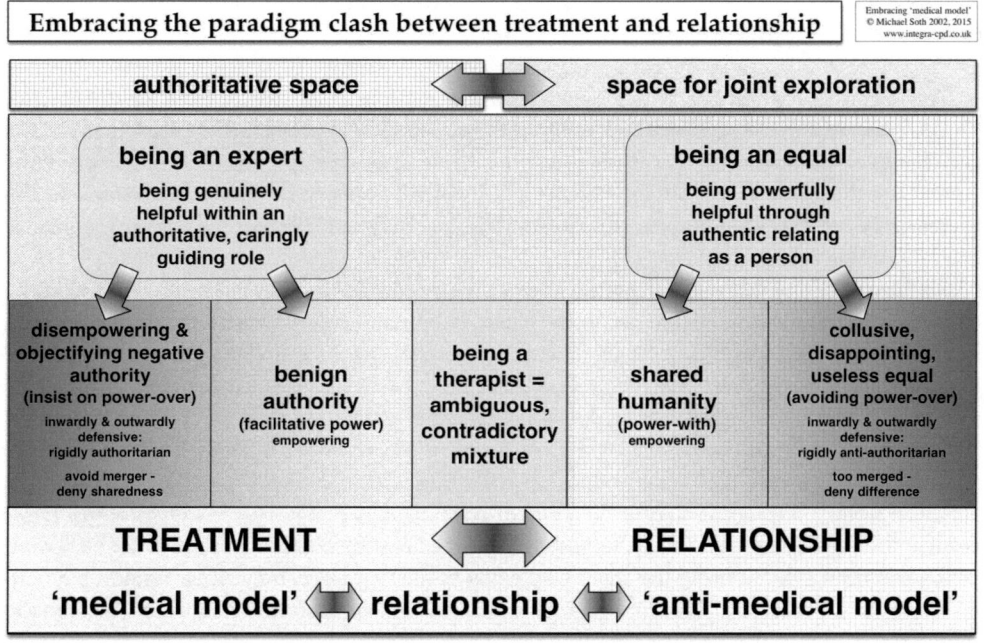

Figure 27.2 Embracing the paradigm clash between treatment and relationship

as equals in a human encounter, implies an invitation into therapy as an experiential space which, in both humanistic and intersubjective contexts, equates essentially to mutual co-exploration. The two ends of the spectrum create different and in significant ways contradictory therapeutic spaces which lend the meeting between client and therapist fundamentally different atmospheres and qualities (see Figure 27.2).

It is a common misconception to equate the authority stance with one-person psychology (with which it was indeed historically associated), and to equate the non-expert human encounter stance only with humanistic approaches, for example, Buber's 'I–Thou' (Buber, 2000). With the increasing cross-fertilisation and integration of the therapeutic field, these are no longer necessary correspondences, as illustrated by two-person conceptions in modern psychoanalysis. The equation authority = one-person psychology = psychoanalysis versus anti-authoritarian equality = two-person psychology = humanistic is no longer helpful, although it has a kernel of historical validity.

Each polarity of the spectrum can be profoundly beneficial, both for the process and for developing a viable working alliance. Equally, both can be unhelpful and counter-therapeutic, either by colluding with defensive features of the client's character or by too categorically confronting and challenging those defences, usually by objectification or pathologising (regarding the tension between colluding versus objectifying, Soth, 1998a). Whichever end of the spectrum a therapist inhabits as a rule, it can be asserted that *any* stance, when pursued in a habitual and fixed strategic manner, is liable to fall into one of two traps by becoming predictable and repetitive:

1   Collusion enactment: too indulgent of client's defences, making it too easy for strategic avoidances to anticipate and manoeuvre around therapist's strategies.
2   Objectification enactment: too rigid in confronting defences, becoming relationally unresponsive from moment to moment, resembling the unattuned wounding characteristics of the client's primary scenario.

Any habitual therapeutic stance, whether unconsciously taken for granted or deliberately chosen and ideologically rationalized, ends up either avoiding or exacerbating the experience of the client's wounding in therapy. Either way, it is liable to unwittingly enact the client's existing patterns, and because the inherent enactment is habitually outside the therapist's awareness, can therefore be seen to have counter-therapeutic effects that limit the transformative potential of the therapeutic space.

To illustrate this, even a benign authority with the best intentions can inadvertently perpetuate patterns of submission and deference in the client, falling into collusion with habits of compliant dependency, when it would be in the client's interest to assert themselves, protest, individuate, and learn to stand on their own two feet. Conversely, the benignly equal therapist may end up failing the client in the opposite way, that is, by insisting on the semblance of adult-adult equality they may end up ignoring the client's regressed aspects (i.e. their dependency needs or primitive hostilities). In this case the therapist ends up colluding with the client's pseudo-maturity, or, in Reichian terms, their façade. Under the guise of creating an exploratory, non-directive space, free from authoritarian impositions, client and therapist can end up colluding to avoid the very roots of the wounding which bring the client to therapy in the first place. Inevitably, this developmental wounding would have occurred in a relational context of profound inequality – a scenario which the therapist may be unconsciously seen to be avoiding.

It should be emphasised that these dangers have little to do with the therapist's conscious therapeutic intentions. Body psychotherapists understand that pre- and non-verbally communicated structures of relationship are more significant than conscious perceptions and deliberations. It would be the actual body/mind relational interactions and positions which client and therapist take vis-à-vis each other in the consulting room which would be exacerbating the client's pattern, outweighing and undoing the effects and efforts of their deliberate collaboration. The helpfulness of any therapeutic stance is not a function of its declared rationale and its associated therapeutic knowledge, skills or techniques, but in how it relates to (i.e. colludes with, challenges or rigidly confronts) the client's pattern and characteristic habits.

Therefore, each of the eight stances to be distinguished here has entirely valid and necessary dimensions, and each has its respective shadow aspects and counter-therapeutic dangers. Each stance can be inhabited as responsive and called for by the client's process on the one hand, and it can be a manifestation of the therapist's dogmatic and habitual investment in that stance (for their own characteristic reasons) on the other. In reality, it is usually a mixture between the two.

The role of power and authority inherent in the various therapeutic stances

The power and authority that the expert insight, knowledge and skill bestows upon a therapist is most clearly visible when the therapist takes a quasi-medical treatment stance, in line with patriarchal stereotypes of masculine authority. The detrimental and iatrogenic effects of unquestioned power implications in the therapeutic position have been challenged and deconstructed by a wide variety of humanistic and existentialist writers. Whatever therapists' attitudes are around power, and regardless whether they own it or disown it, professional authority is explicitly present in all of the first five stances. Only the extreme end of spectrum, the sixth stance (the phenomenological co-explorer) might be considered by some to be free from power differential from the therapist's perspective. But the therapist's philosophical beliefs around power and equality, i.e. whether they subscribe to being an authority or whether they hide, modify or counteract it, are relatively insignificant – what matters is that from the client's unconscious and regressed point of view *all* stances can be experienced as manifestations of a power differential that could either be benign or destructive or both. It is this author's assumption and experience that *any* kind of power differential is likely to evoke at some point in the process an enactment of the original scenario in which human authority was first encountered, and it is *that* scenario which is going to become transferentially projected into the therapy, whatever the therapist's conscious attitude or orientation. The author's conclusion from this is not to avoid power and authority as a therapist, but to be alert to the specific enactments it engenders with each particular client.

The eight different stances and habitual positions in the field of body psychotherapy are described in the following section.

Functionalist quasi-medical expert

At the origin of the BP tradition there was only one stance, that modelled by Reich, which he had absorbed from the dominant culture in psychoanalysis at the time, including Freud himself: it was taken for granted that psychoanalysts deliver psychological treatment pretty much like doctors, grounded in natural science. Where Reich radically departed from his colleagues was in developing a functionalist science (these days it would be called systemic-holistic or integral body/mind meta-psychology, theory and technique), which then framed and shaped the kind of treatment he aimed to provide as a doctor. But there is no sign that Reich ever doubted the quasi-medical construction of his task as delivering objective and objectifying capabilities in the three steps of examination, diagnosis and prescription in administering the appropriate treatment (Cornell, 2015; Soth, 2000).

It was only 30 years later, when the humanistic movement took up the Reichian legacy that the objectifying power implications of the doctor role were questioned and deconstructed. In the anti-authoritarian paradigm shift that followed, the ideas of medical treatment and cure not only lost their highly prized status, but also became inverted as counter-therapeutic fallacies.

However, 'the longing for a cure' cannot be that easily eliminated or legislated against. Whether or not it is realistic or deliverable, the client's longing for an omniscient and omnipotent saviour, who is a transformative object in Bollas' (1987) terms, calls forth in the transference a benign doctor/expert (a kind fairy godfather) or a reparative mother (a kind fairy godmother), who might be able to cure unconscious problems without these ever having to be actually experienced.

In body psychotherapy terms, that cure would essentially involve the dismantling of character-istic defences in order to make vibrant flow of the life-force possible in an integrated body/mind (Soth, 2000). That was the goal pursued by Reich himself, explicitly and systematically, and as a teenager reading Reich and later pursuing Reichian training, that was the fantasy and promise which attracted this author. During the initial years of my practice, I largely saw myself as, and operated as, a body magician able to facilitate profound release on body/mind levels beyond the awareness and control of the client's ego, a therapeutic stance that does appear to invest body psychotherapists with quasi-magical powers. All classical vegetotherapy would be comfortable operating predominantly from this position, and incredibly sophisticated and comprehensive treatment systems can and have been developed based upon modern extensions of Reich's clas-sical stance (Ferri, 2012).

Spiritual body/mind guide

Whilst historically this stance is a fairly recent hybridisation of body psychotherapy with various spiritual practices and complementary therapies, the spiritual body/mind guide falls into the same category as the doctor/expert in terms of the degree of inequality which it involves and evokes in the transference. It can manifest in various forms: as the energy body worker or healer, as an inspirational or instructive guru, an elder or initiator.

Within the BP discipline there is a polarisation between spiritual/mystical/metaphysical and rationalist/scientific branches of the field. Whatever one's belief system within this polarisation, there can be little doubt that both stances (spiritual guide and doctor) evoke, manifest, maintain, and rationalise power differential, and therefore carry the danger of exploitation and damage. On the positive side, both of them take the risk of engaging with, and thus acquiring access to, the more helpless, regressive, merged and dependent aspects of the client, providing an attachment figure to believe in or entrust oneself to. Whether this becomes a healing or re-traumatising experience is not a function of the stance itself but depends upon what transpires in the process between the client and the therapist taking such a stance.

Embodiment/mindfulness educator

In the history of human development, one of the more benign manifestations of power differ-ential is as tutor, mentor or educator. In BP, with its clear analysis of the client's characteristic disembodiment, the educational task is clear: it is to offer experiential practices that will help the client develop the intricate and differentiated self-awareness necessary for establishing embodi-ment, or at least for registering and monitoring their disembodied habits. There is a plethora of possible techniques which can be used to instruct the client, ranging from meditation, relaxation, martial arts, movement, and breathing techniques, to the more psycho-emotional techniques of 'here and now' sensorimotor or Gestalt awareness process.

In recent years the educator stance has gained traction both as psycho-education in somatic trauma therapy as well as in association with the burgeoning field of mindfulness, which in its Buddhist roots always had body awareness as one of its foundations. It then makes sense for the body-oriented therapist to become a mindfulness instructor, providing the principles and prac-tices which extend simple body awareness into a more comprehensive psycho–somatic system. But throughout the body-oriented tradition, mindfulness has effectively been an essential prin-ciple in BP long before it became fashionable (Kurtz, 1990).

However, the concern here is not the validity of the teachings, but the relational configura-tion between client and therapist which the educative stance engenders, and how it counteracts or exacerbates characteristically established patterns in the client's psyche. For some clients the caring guidance of a tutor, attentive to the minutiae of their body/mind process, can become a deeply supportive and healing experience. However, the danger (as with all the authoritative stances) is that the client is so desperate for acceptance that they will deliver the required gestures out of compliance, and the therapist mistakes this for cooperation and therapeutic success, when all that has been achieved is an additional layer of adaptation and contortion. Unless the theoretical recognition of character formation, by definition involving regressed child states, is extended into the transference, the degree to which the client is scanning the therapist for their preferences and agendas may be missed, as unconsciously the client will often do anything to please them. The awareness of the wounded child within character is the foundation for the next stance, the reparative position.

Reparative parent of deficits in arrested development

Whereas Reich and his immediate followers were focused on penetrating and cracking the character armour, it was always understood that within its protective shield lay a soft and fluid living core (i.e. Reich's three layers of core, secondary and façade). Amongst body psychotherapists that understanding manifests in two complementary aspects of the core, the biological and the psychological: in *biological* terms, BP equates the idea of the core with the plasmic motility of the life force, vibrantly and passionately moving through the body; in *emotional and psychological* terms, the core is the human sense of vulnerability, the child dependent on the maturational environment (Winnicott, 1965), whose natural needs and 'rights' (Lowen, 1958) are being denied and frustrated.

The child's spontaneous impulse, arrested by the 'turning against the self' that is implicit in character formation, is understood to be frozen in time, living on unchanged in the depths of the psyche behind walls of repression and defences (as evocatively imagined for the humanistic generation by Pink Floyd's movie 'The Wall'). It was Gerda Boyesen who most explicitly brought a mothering touch to the wounds of character and complemented the traditional harsh, masculine attacks on the armour with the idea instead of melting it by lovingly reaching through the defenses to the hidden child's primary impulse.

This more motherly therapeutic space was explicitly taught by Boyesen (1994) as the midwife approach, waiting with an exquisitely attuned embodied presence for impulses to impinge on the client from within the client. Boyesen's feminine alternative to the typical neo-Reichian bioenergetic stance parallels a similar development in psychoanalysis, with Winnicott shifting the emphasis from the traditional doing of interpretations towards the analyst being a presence capable of providing a relational container. In this way he was paving the way for a significant debate about theories of therapeutic action (Stern, 1994), posing questions such as 'was it the delivering of insight through interpretation, or the provision of a corrective emotional experience which made analysis work?' The equivalent question in body psychotherapy would be: 'is it the confrontation with secondary emotions and their catharsis or the surrender to primary impulses, called the instroke by Davis (2016) and their gratification that leads to healing?'

With the benefit of decades of hindsight, it can be affirmed that this is a moot polarization. From an integrative perspective, clearly both stances are needed. Slightly adapting a point made by Greenberg (1986) it could be said that unless the therapist:

- can provide a new, good experience, the therapy never gets underway (as it might with a therapist who only ever attacks the character armour);

- confronts the defences, the therapy never ends (as it might with a therapist who keeps trying to feed the primary impulses, despite the client being disconnected from them and never really sufficiently receptive).

Both ways of challenging or undercutting the defence are inadequate on their own; both therapeutic stances, the doing and the being, the confronting expert and the reparative parent, are needed. Once the therapeutic necessity for that which Clarkson (1994/2003, p. 12) calls the 'reparative developmentally-needed' stance has been identified, the modern gender stereotypes can be deconstructed beyond the child's needs for mothering to include the need for fathering, too.

Whilst some might argue that the reparative provision of a corrective emotional experience is just a function of ordinary human empathy, and not an explicit therapeutic stance, a differentiated model of the client's arrested development helps the realization we are not simply talking about empathy, but about the highly complex task of re-parenting. Whatever the child was missing due to parental neglect, or whatever protection against inescapable parental invasion developed as necessary, the therapist as the reparative object will want to be precise in meeting the specific deficits implicit in the client's character structure. This might entail the setting of limits and boundaries in some situations just as it might involve nurturing touch in others, depending on the nature of the wounding dynamic and the developmental stage when it occurred (Johnson, 1994). It is not just a spontaneously compassionate authentic attitude that becomes reparative, it requires precise attunement, a perceptive judgement and the therapist taking a deliberate *role* in order for re-parenting to occur.

Interactive regulator of the client's disturbed auto-regulation

Arguably, the therapist as regulator could be classified with the previously described reparative stance, because in developmental trauma this becomes indistinguishable from the re-parenting task. However, with the recent corroboration that BP (especially the somatic trauma therapies) has derived from neuroscience, it makes sense to differentiate it as a separate category. The essence of this stance involves the therapist in monitoring the client's autonomic nervous system and their body/mind oscillations between the trauma symptoms of hyper- and hypo-arousal, attempting to keep the client within their window of tolerance (Ogden, Minton, and Pain, 2006) and thus providing an interactive regulation to compensate for the client's deficient auto-regulation.

Because of a common conflation between the reparative stance and the humanistic principles of dialogical I–Thou relating, the following clarification is necessary: both the regulating and the reparative stance involve the therapist in taking a powerful and authoritative *role*. Within that role, the therapist can be said to be authentically accessing their nurturing empathic self, but this is hardly the same as fully being themselves in the way that authenticity is understood in dialogical, existential terms. Both the regulating and the reparative stance require a power differential for these stances to work. They depend on the therapist taking an asymmetrical rather than reciprocal or equal position, and on deliberately filtering and withholding some of their dialogical responses which would be too wounding or dys-regulating.

Because the reparative and regulating stances are often identified, in a limiting way, with feminine stereotypes (both depend upon intimate attunement and parental love, and thus invite reductions to fantasies of merger and harmony), a crucial point frequently missed is the fact that both depend as a prerequisite on the therapist maintaining a differentiated, objectifying distance. There can be no appropriate repair without prior diagnosis and that means having a separate, un-merged perception that differs from the client's self-perception. Otherwise the reparative efforts, however well-intentioned, become reactive and anxious scatter-gun gestures and intrusions.

Therefore the reparative stance and the expert doctor position (although often construed as mutually exclusive opposites) are in fact completely dependent on each other, and thus inter-linked. In order to arrive at a therapeutic diagnosis the body-oriented therapist needs to draw upon right-brain empathic intuition, as well as the kind of left-brain mental faculties more commonly expected from a doctor. But regardless of the various channels by which a therapist uses their holistic perception to generate data, it is only once they have identified and diagnosed the wounding, from what is necessarily a differentiated stance and implicit power position that they can respond in reparative or regulatory ways.

Phenomenological co-explorer

The humanistic revolution can be seen as liberating the psychological therapies/BP from the dominant grip which the doctor/treatment stance had on the therapeutic profession throughout the first half of the twentieth century, in psychoanalysis, behaviourism and psychology generally. As elaborated elsewhere (Soth, 2006a), the history of psychotherapy over the last century could be described in terms of the successive challenges and deconstructions of the medical model as the taken-for-granted paradigm for all psychotherapy.

Influenced by Buber's (1923) notion of I – Thou meeting, all hierarchical power-over aspects previously presumed to be definitional for the professional role were scrutinised and dismissed, leading to one of the key humanistic principles, that of the client and therapist working towards a meeting as equals. Inspired also by Laing's (1970) anti-psychiatry, the iatrogenic and self-serving implications of maintaining a professional power position were identified and counteracted. Rather than any kind of professional role-bound expertise, the therapist meeting the client authentically in their own existential nakedness and shared humanity was recognised and validated as an essential aspect of what makes the encounter therapeutic.

Over-idealising authenticity and the hidden medical model: Personal reflections

It took me some years of operating as a therapist within the philosophical frame of this anti-authoritarian subculture to realise that I was in danger of throwing out some precious babies with the supposedly dirty, power-over bathwater of inequality. Apart from over-idealising the body *against* the mind, I was also idealising the notion of authentic contact, insisting on it, and imposing it on myself and the client, even when all body/mind evidence in front of me suggested that the client at that moment was not up for dialogical authentic relating [or in Benjamin's (1998) term: 'mutual recognition'].

This would lead to barely veiled exhortations on my part, with me becoming in turn authoritative, educative, pleading in the hope that I might persuade the client to see sense and join me in pursuit of undefended dialogical relating. Sometimes I managed to cajole clients into my value and belief system, but with others my attempts to avoid a power/doctor position and my insistence on intimate mutuality seriously backfired and had disastrous consequences for the working alliance and the process. Trying to get to the root causes of such breakdowns in the alliance, I went through a painful period of questioning many of the cherished assumptions that had first attracted me to the humanistic and Reichian traditions, not least my therapeutic zeal to liberate the client from the prison of their character, only to realise that I was just as fixed in *my* therapeutic identity as the client was in *their* characteristic identity.

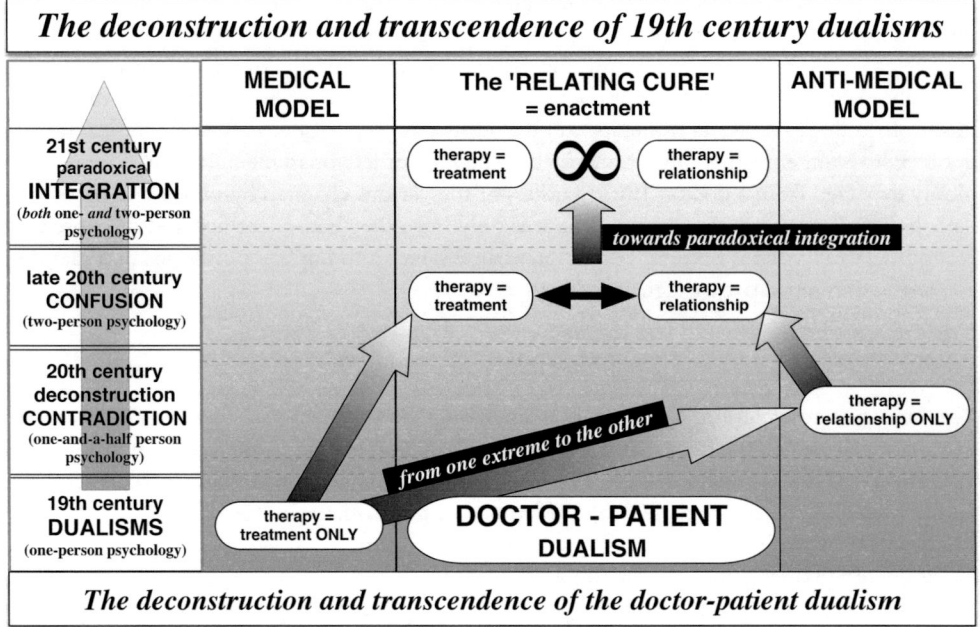

Figure 27.3   The deconstruction and transcendence of nineteenth-century dualisms

I discovered I was consistently giving both the client and myself absurdly confusing double-messages: I was championing the unconditionally accepting atmosphere of a non-hierarchical encounter; and I was passionately invested in an agenda which was inseparable from taking an authority position of 'knowing better'. I came to think of the latter as my hidden and implicit medical model position which was operating within me as a grandiose body magician expert who, true to its Reichian legacy, was trying to 'liberate the animal' and the client's life-force from the prison of their repressive ego. I was constructing my superior therapeutic position as an enemy of the client's ego (Soth, 2006c) while at the same time requiring myself to be authentically equal.

I recognised that both these stances, the humanistic equal and the Reichian doctor, and the polarised conflicts between them, were alive within me, irrespective of the one-sided egalitarian philosophical allegiances of my consciously declared humanistic ego-position. Whereas I had seen only the classical expert stance as authoritarian and oppressive, I now came to understand both as equally matched in their categorical rigidity and dogmatism. This prompted me to formulate them as a clash between the medical and the anti-medical model (see Figure 27.3), initiating my search for a third position that might be able to transcend and include both of these polarities.

Working alliance

The relational turn constitutes a paradigm shift by which therapists, and especially BPs, might no longer focus on the literal validity of each of these six stances and their associated rationales, theories and techniques *only*, but where these can be seen as arising in the force field of the therapeutic relationship as enactments of the client's characteristically internal(ised) matrix of relationships

(Soth, 1998b). The therapeutic relationship can then be conceived of as a two-person body/mind system which oscillates in dynamic tension between the poles of working alliance and enactments in rupture–and–repair cycles (see Figure 27.4).

Working alliance and enactment therefore constitute the last two stances of the eight stances proposed here, corresponding to Clarkson's (1994/2003) working alliance and transference-countertransference modality, respectively. But rather than conceiving of these relational stances as alternate treatment options, with the idea of the therapist choosing between them, all the stances can be considered valid and present *simultaneously* in the dynamic force field of the therapeutic space. The fundamental tension creating that space is between the therapist engaging as an authentic other versus allowing themselves to be constructed as an object by the client's unconscious[2] (Soth, 2014). From a perspective which integrates humanistic and psychoanalytic principles both of these poles can be embraced as equally valid and necessary to the process.

The working alliance then depends on the degree of conflictual enactments currently constellated between client and therapist and obscuring the possibility of mutual recognition. As more

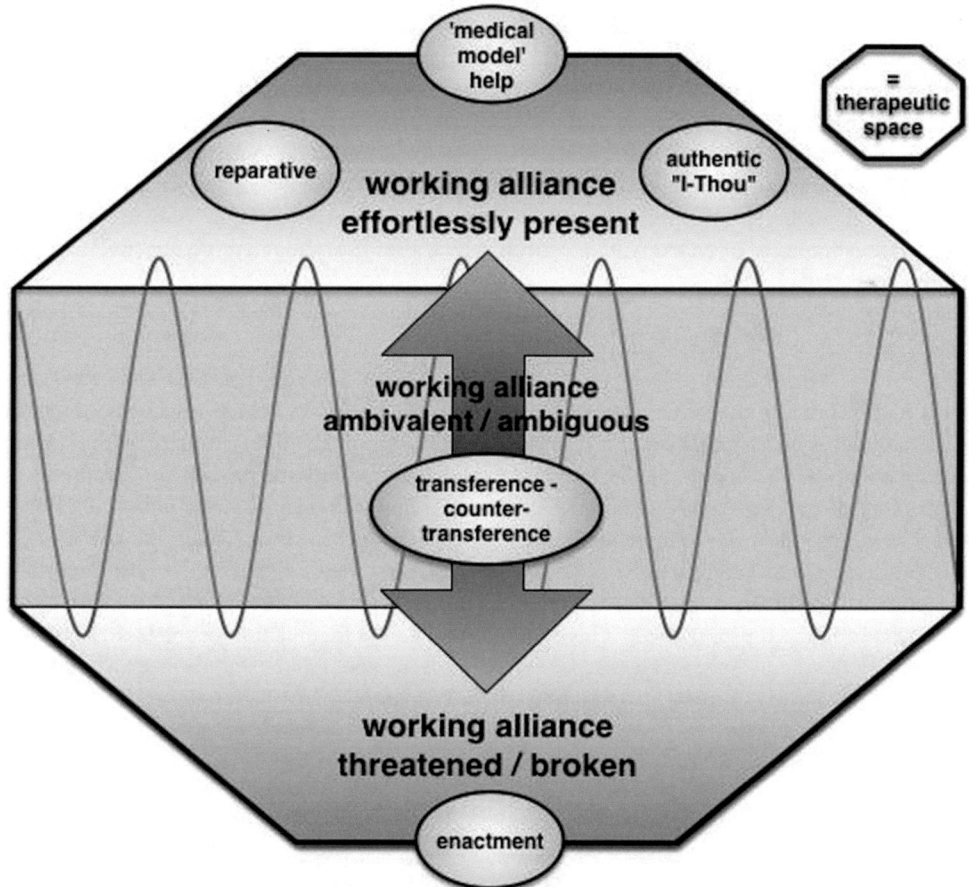

Figure 27.4 The oscillations in contact between working alliance and enactment (rupture and repair)

unconscious material is invited into the space through the safety of the alliance, intensifying enactments disturb the working alliance towards breaking point. If, and when, these enactments can be contained, the therapeutic dyad returns to an even deeper alliance, thus cycling in ever deepening rupture-and-repair cycles which provoke, constellate, repeat and transform successive layers of characteristic structuring throughout the unfolding therapeutic process. As a result, this process resembles the kind of systematic 'un-peeling of the onion' layer by layer of defence Reich (1983) had in mind, except that he was construing it as a one-person psychology treatment process for which he assumed control. An embodied two-person psychology would need to include the therapist's countertransference process as well as their authentic presence, and thus their full human participation in the relationship, acknowledging all their vulnerability and passion, for better or worse.

Enactment

The enactment stance relies on the traditional psychoanalytic notion of 'working through', including Johnson's (1994) organismic response to the wounding object as the third step of character formation. Relational psychoanalysis (Bromberg, 2001; Mitchell and Aron, 1999) has most clearly formulated the validity of the therapist acknowledging and engaging in enactments (Varga, 2005), rather than the analyst doing their utmost to prevent them as purely counter-therapeutic countertransference enactments (Casement, 1985). However, as mentioned in the introduction, the relational movement has not yet developed an *embodied* account of how to survive enactment transformatively (Soth, 2005b, 2013), nor is it using the full range of relational stances outlined in this chapter. BP, if it can recover from relational obliviousness by taking on board the countertransference revolution and then beyond that the notion of enactment, possesses the accumulated body/mind expertise which can take the therapeutic dyad more deeply *into* the spontaneous intensity of enactments, a process which promises deeper, more effective and more lasting characteristic change.

Conclusion

This framework for the different stances or relational modalities which therapists adopt and find themselves enacting provides a foundation to engage in these enactments in ways which do not minimise the charge of the transference-countertransference process and maximise the probability of transformative containment while avoiding strategies of reductionist collusion or dissociative objectification. Apprehending the body/mind processes by which the therapist gets co-constructed into taking diverse relational stances (how they find themselves taking a stance rather than consciously having chosen to adopt it) is an essential feature of surviving enactments and inhabiting them productively. This recognition allows a formulation of the basic conditions required in the therapeutic relational space if BP wants to invite, allow and facilitate the transformation of characteristic patterns including the full range of their unconscious and body/mind manifestations.

Notes

1 'Regression is merely a psychological term describing the actual, present-day effectiveness of certain historical events. Childhood experiences could, however, not be effective 30 years later, had they not actually damaged the process of the coordination of the biosystem. We are dealing with actual, present-day functions of the organism and not with historical events.' (Reich, 1972, p446).

2 The use of the term 'object' resonates with Winnicott's (1965) formulation, and ranges across a whole developmental spectrum and between extremes of love and hate.

References

Aron, L. (2002). *Meeting of Minds – Mutuality in Psychoanalysis*. London: Routledge.

Atwood, G. E., and Stolorow, R. D. (1992). *Contexts of Being: The Intersubjective Foundations of Psychological Life*. London: Routledge.

Benjamin, J. (1998). *Shadow of the Other: Intersubjectivity and Gender in Psychoanalysis*. London: Routledge.

Boadella, D. (1982). Transference, resonance and interference. *Journal of Biodynamic Psychology, 3*, 73–93.

Bollas, C. (1987). *The Shadow of the Object: Psychoanalysis of the Unthought Known*. New York: Columbia University Press.

Boyesen, G. (1994). *Biodynamik des Lebens* [The Biodynamics of Life]. Berlin: Synthesis Verlag.

Bromberg, P. M. (2001). *Standing in the Spaces: Essays on Clinical Process, Trauma and Dissociation*. London: Routledge.

Buber, M. (1923). *Ich und Du* [I and Thou]. Berlin: Reclam.

Buber, M. (2000). *I and Thou*. New York: Simon and Schuster.

Casement, P. (1985). *On Learning from the Patient*. London: Routledge.

Clarkson, P. and Wilson, S. ([1994]/2003). *The Therapeutic Relationship*. Oxford: Wiley-Blackwell. (Original work published 1994)

Cornell, W. F. (2015). *Somatic Experience in Psychoanalysis and Psychotherapy: In the Expressive Language of the Living*. London: Routledge.

Davis, W. (2016). Affective core consciousness and the instroke. *International Journal for Body, Movement and Dance in Psychotherapy, 12*, 21–35. doi:10.1080/17432979.2016.1203356

Ehrenberg, D. (1992). *The Intimate Edge: Extending the Reach of Psychoanalytic Interaction*. New York: W. W. Norton.

Ferri, G. (2012). *Psicopatologia e carattere. L'analisi reichiana. La psicoanalisi nel corpo ed il corpo in psicoanalisi* [Psychopathology and character. Reichian analysis. Psychoanalysis in the body and the body in psychoanalysis]. Rome, Italy: Alpes Italia.

Gallagher, S. (2006). *How the Body Shapes the Mind*. Oxford: Clarendon Press.

Gomez, L. (2004). Humanistic or psychodynamic – What is the difference and do we have to make a choice? *Self and Society, 31*(6), 5–19.

Greenberg, J. (1986). Theoretical models and the analyst's neutrality. *Contemporary Psychoanalysis, 22*, 87–106.

Greenson, R. (1965). The working alliance and the transference neurosis. *The Psychoanalytic Quarterly, 34*, 155–181.

Heiman, P. (1950). On countertransference. *International Journal of Psychoanalysis, 31*, 60–76.

Johnson, S. (1994). *Character Styles*. New York: W. W. Norton.

Kurtz, R. (1990). *Body-Centered Psychotherapy – The Hakomi Method*. Mendocino, CA: LifeRhythm.

Laing, R. D. (1970). *Sanity, Madness and the Family: Families of Schizophrenics*. London: Pelican Books.

Lowen, A. (1958). *The Language of the Body*. London: Collier Macmillan.

Lyons-Ruth, K. (1998). Implicit relational knowing: Its role in development and psychoanalytic treatment. *Infant Mental Health Journal, 19*(3), 282–289.

Mitchell, S. A., and Aron, L. (1999). *Relational Psychoanalysis: The Emergence of a Tradition*. Hillsdale, NJ: Analytic Press.

Ogden, P., Minton, K., and Pain, C. (2006). *Trauma and the Body: A Sensorimotor Approach to Psychotherapy*. New York: W. W. Norton.

Reich, W. (1972). *Character Analysis*. New York: Touchstone. (Original work published 1933/1949)

Reich, W. (1983). *The Function of the Orgasm* (1st UK ed.; US 1942, 1948, 1973). London: Souvenir Press.

Rothschild, B. (2006). *Help for the Helper: The Psychophysiology of Compassion Fatigue and Vicarious Trauma*. New York: W. W. Norton.

Samuels, A. (1993). *The Political Psyche*. London: Routledge.

Schore, A. (2012). *The Science of the Art of Psychotherapy*. New York: W. W. Norton.

Shaw, R. (2004). The embodied psychotherapist: An exploration of the therapists' somatic phenomena within the therapeutic encounter. *Psychotherapy Research, 14*(3), 271–288. doi:10.1093/ptr/kph025

Soth, M. (1998a). *The Client's Conflict becomes the Therapist's Conflict*. Retrieved January 12, 2017, from http://integra-cpd.co.uk/cpd-resource/soth1997_clientsconflict_therapistsconflict_original/.

Soth, M. (1998b). *The Five Parallel Relationships*. Retrieved January 12, 2017, from http://integra-cpd.co.uk/cpd-resource/soth1998_5_parallel_relationships_conflicted_ego/.

Soth, M. (2000). The Integrated Bodymind's View on Body/Mind Integration. *AChP Newsletter*.

Soth, M. (2003). *The Therapist's Relational Stance*. Retrieved January 12, 2017, from http://integra-cpd.co.uk/cpd-resource/soth2003_therapists_relational_stance.

Soth, M. (2005a). Body psychotherapy today – An integral-relational approach. *Therapy Today, 16*(9), 8–12.

Soth, M. (2005b). Embodied countertransference. In N. Totton (Ed.), *New Dimensions in Body Psychotherapy*. Maidenhead: OUP.

Soth, M. (2006a). How 'the Wound' enters the room and the relationship. *Therapy Today, 17*(10), 10–14.

Soth, M. (2006b). What therapeutic hope for a subjective mind in an objectified body? Part 1. *International Journal of Body, Movement and Dance in Psychotherapy, 1*, 43–56.

Soth, M. (2006c). What therapeutic hope for a subjective mind in an objectified body? Part 2. *International Journal of Body, Movement and Dance in Psychotherapy, 2*, 143–154.

Soth, M. (2007). *The Three Relational Revolutions*. Retrieved January 12, 2017, from http://integra-cpd. co.uk/cpd-resource/soth20073_relational_revolutions/.

Soth, M. (2008). From humanistic holism via the 'integrative project' towards integral-relational Body Psychotherapy. In L. Hartley (Ed.), *Contemporary Body Psychotherapy – The Chiron Approach* (pp. 64–88). London: Routledge.

Soth, M. (2013). We are all relational, but are some more relational than others? Completing the paradigm shift towards relationality. *Transactional Analysis Journal, 43*(2), 122–137.

Soth, M. (2014). *The Essential Relational Conflict Inherent in the Therapeutic Position: Object- versus Subject-Relating*. Retrieved January 12, 2017, from http://integra-cpd.co.uk/cpd-resource/soth2014_ therapysessential_conflict_object_vs_subject/.

Soth, M. (2015). Transference, countertransference and supervision in the body psychotherapy tradition. In G. Marlock and H. Weiss (with C. Young and M. Soth) (Eds.), *The Handbook of Body Psychotherapy and Somatic Psychology*. Berkeley, CA: North Atlantic Books.

Stark, M. (1999). *Modes of Therapeutic Action*. New York: Jason Aronson.

Stern, D. N. (1985). *The Interpersonal World of the Infant: A View from Psychoanalysis and Development Psychology*. London: Karnac Books.

Stern, S. (1994). Needed relationships and repeated relationships an integrated relational perspective. *Psychoanalytic Dialogues, 4*(3), 317–346. doi:10.1080/10481889409539020

Trevarthen, C. (1993). The self born in intersubjectivity: The psychology of an infant communicating. In U. Neisser (Ed.), *The Perceived Self: Ecological and Interpersonal Sources of Self-knowledge* (pp. 121–173). New York: Cambridge University Press.

Varga, M. P. (2005). Analysis of transference as transformation of enactment. *Psychoanalytic Review, 92*(5), 659–674.

Winnicott, D. W. (1965). *The Maturational Processes and the Facilitating Environment*. London: The Hogarth Press and the Institute of Psycho-Analysis.

28

EMOTIONAL REGULATION IN BODY PSYCHOTHERAPY

Ulfried Geuter

Introduction

Emotions set the tone of how we experience the world, relate to it and act. They serve to evaluate events, engender and regulate reactions and communicate inner states, intentions and reactions to others (Scherer, 2015). As emotions are adaptive processes they are in constant change and have to be regulated. Emotional regulation is disturbed in all severe mental ill health (Schore, 2003). Nearly all disorders of chapter F of ICD 10 comprise disorders of emotions. Thus, emotion regulation is a component of mental health (Eberhard-Kaechele, 2017).

In psychotherapy, we constantly face dysregulated and maladaptive emotions. Clients repress feelings or inhibit their expression, while others are trapped in an ambivalence to express or to suppress feelings (Greenberg and Bischkopf, 2007). Still others control shame by showing pride, or mask sorrow with anger. Some become inundated by the arousal of anger, sorrow or disgust; others are caught in numbness or torpidity; while yet others react with arousal to dangerous situations or with anxiety to neutral ones (Russell, 2003). Some do not perceive any feelings and/or silence emotions by displacing emotional arousal into bodily tensions or symptoms (alexithymia). Thus, psychotherapy has the complex task of helping clients to regulate emotions. As disorders vary, there is no standard way of doing this (Greenberg and Van Balen, 1998). Moreover, every emotional process is individual and subjective. Therefore, we have to consider models which help us to apply different clinical strategies to different problems.

In this chapter a model of emotional processes which helps to define various body psychotherapeutic lines of emotional regulation is proposed. The model is based on the component process model of emotion (Scherer, 2009a, 2009b), the theory of core affect from Feldman Barrett and Russell (1998, 1999) and the concept of basic emotions (Ekman, 1999). A model from Geuter and Schrauth (2015) is presented below detailing different blockages in an emotional process and to show how these can be treated in body psychotherapy.

Defining emotion

There is a lack of consensus defining emotion (Frijda, 2007). Garvey and Fogel (2008) understand emotions as dynamic patterns of 'relational experiences lived in bodies' (p. 62). Emotions integrate the perception of situations with inner perceptions in order to spark activities to think, to act or to

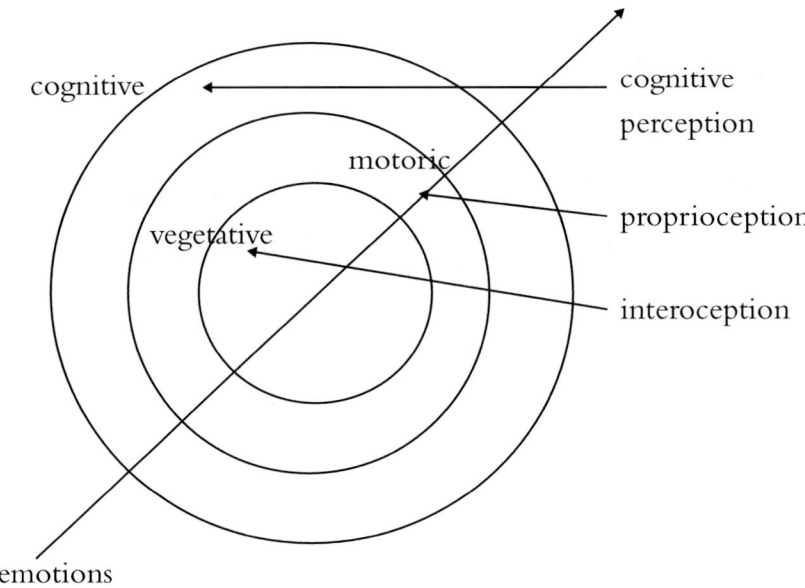

Figure 28.1 Three layers of experience

scale them down (Barlassina and Newen, 2014). They exist in the interaction between a subject and a meaningful situation or object (Frijda, 2009). In this chapter emotions are seen as a person's answers to an internal or external event of subjective importance in the form of reactions such as arousal, torpidity, sorrow, anger or anxiety which interrupt the normal regime of thoughts and actions and engage the person as a whole (Frijda, 2009). Emotional reactions give meaning to situations by signalling how to appraise them and how to 'act appropriately' (Johnson, 2007, p. 61).

Emotions are always bodily felt (Nummenmaa, Gelerean, Hari, and Hietanen, 2014). They become conscious by perceiving our thoughts and fantasies and our signals of visceral and sensomotoric systems (Dalgleish, 2004; Scherer, 2009a). Emotions are also communicated by the body via posture, movement, mimicking or voice. Many can be imparted to others precisely by touch (Hertenstein, Holmes, McCullough, and Keltner, 2009). According to Damasio (1994, 2003) emotions happen on the stage of the body whereas feelings are conscious representations of changes in the state of the organism that are integrated with other information about the meaning of a situation. Emotions sometimes remain subconscious or ineffable. If they are consciously processed and reflected we can give them words and talk about them as feelings.

Following cognitive theories of emotions appraisal is a mental process that elicits bodily reactions. However, if we follow non-dualistic theories bodily reactions themselves are appraisals. In emotions, we do not feel the body as an object, but we feel meaning in relation to something through the body. Within the paradigm of the embodied mind emotions can be seen as a process of embodied appraisal which is experienced on three different layers: first, cognitions, thoughts, imaginations and fantasies; second, proprioceptive perceptions, impulses and motoric actions and third, interoceptive perceptions of vegetative somatic markers (Geuter, 2015, p. 100ff; see Figure 28.1). In an experiential body psychotherapy these levels are not conceptualised as biological layers but as layers of experience (Geuter, 2016). Thus, the first layer is not conceived as mental and the two others as bodily. Whether a thought is emotionally important for us and whether we experience a thought as congruent, we feel bodily. And if we perceive a proprioceptive or interoceptive signal this bodily perception is a mental act. Thus, every experience is both mental and bodily. That is why the concept of mindfulness is one-sided. Awareness for signals on all layers is always mental and bodily and always awareness for something being felt. Therefore, mindfulness is bodyfulness at the same time (Sugamura, Haruki, and Koshikawa, 2006; see also Caldwell, 2014). In body psychotherapy we connect cognitions, perceptions of motoric impulses and inner sensations in exploring and regulating emotions.

Three steps of perception and appraisal in an emotional process

The following model outlined in detail by Geuter (2015, pp. 184–194) concentrates on how emotions arise in an actual situation. In this model we can distinguish three steps in an emotional process (see Figure 28.2) below, followed by an explanation of each step.

In the first step, emotional processes start with an external or internal stimulus or event which is first appraised with respect to its relevance for the subject (Sander, Grandjean, and Scherer, 2005). If a situation is new, different from our expectations, and/or important, attention increases. This appraisal of 'personal relevance' of a situation (Sachse and Langens, 2014) is part of what is sometimes called orientation reaction, which is a pre-condition for emotional perception. A stimulus can also pass the threshold of perception unconsciously and lead to a reaction. To have the experience of an emotion, however, some conscious attention is needed. And it needs a further appraisal as attention itself is not experienced as emotional.

According to the component process model, a second appraisal evaluates the pleasure or displeasure of an event. Pleasant means to be in accordance with our needs and desires, unpleasant

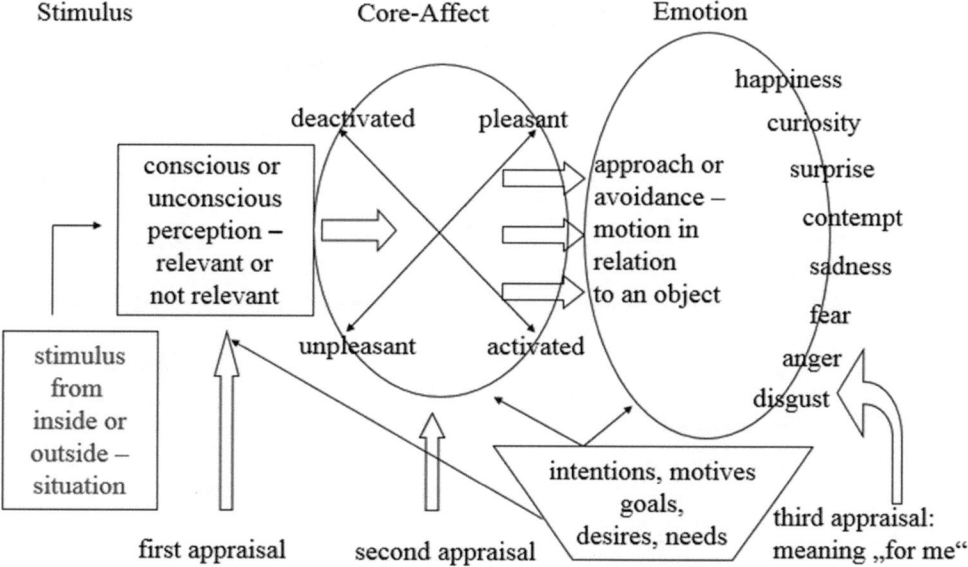

Figure 28.2 The structure of emotional processes
Source: Geuter, 2015, p. 184

the opposite. A theory of Feldman Barrett and Russell (1999) introduces a further dimension. They argue that every emotionally relevant stimulus changes an already existing affective state of the organism, which can be portrayed by two orthogonal dimensions: pleasure–displeasure (or valence) refers to hedonic tone, activation 'to a sense of mobilisation or energy'. This dispositional state of feeling somewhere on the continuum of pleasantness–unpleasantness and activation–deactivation the authors call the core affect (see Figure 28.3). The concept is similar to that which Damasio (2003) designates as background feelings. Zinck and Newen (2008) speak of pre-emotions as unfocussed expressive emotion states. This we also call mood. Feldman Barrett and Russell generally prefer the term 'affective experience', not emotion. The author does not make a clear difference between affect and emotion but uses the term 'affect' more for core affective experiences.

The core affect is 'a continuous assessment of one's current state' (Russell, 2003, p. 149). It is not elicited by stimulus. However, it colours the perception of emotional situations. If a person is in a pleasant–deactivated state of wellbeing events will affect him/her less. If s/he is already tense (activated–unpleasant) s/he will easier tense up. Emotionally relevant situations thus alter the core affective state, for example, they calm us down, tense us up, make us upset or elated. Only by this change in the degree of pleasantness and activation situations are experienced as emotional. If solely the core affect changes without feeling a discrete emotion, a person experiences a shift in mood.

According to pleasure–arousal theory (Reisenzein, 1994) discrete emotions can be characterised by a certain position in the coordinate system of the core affect; for example, being enraged or fearful are both situated in the upper left quadrant. But the same quadrant also contains disgust, disappointment, shame or envy. To explain the different quality of these emotions a further appraisal is necessary.

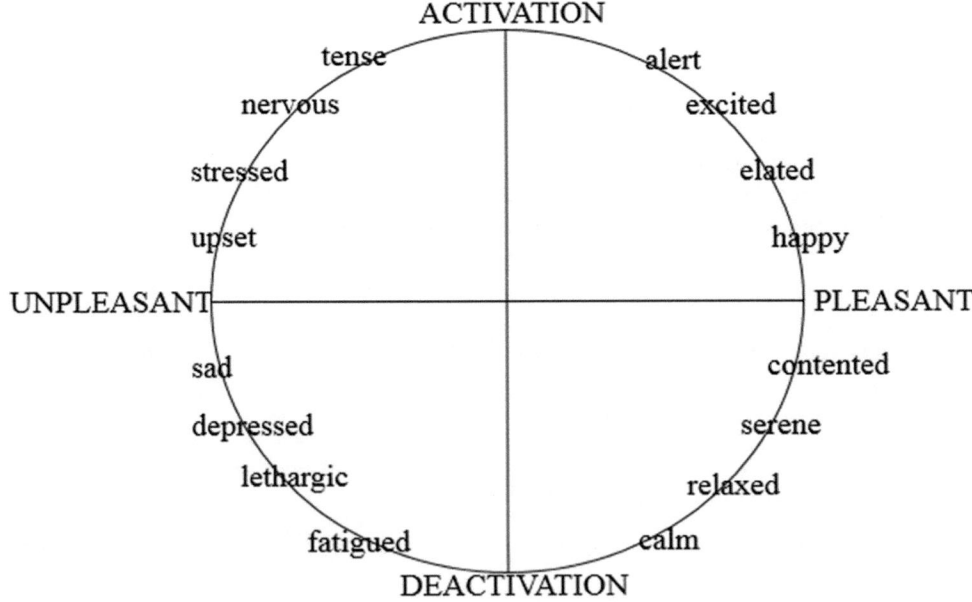

Figure 28.3 The two-dimensional structure of core affect

Source: Feldman Barrett and Russell, 1999

Finally, in a third step of appraisal we experience emotions like fear, rage or disgust. Russell (2003) speaks of 'attributed affects' (p. 194) as here an affective quality is attributed to an event or a person. Following that, a change felt in core affect 'is linked to its perceived cause' (Russell, 2003, p. 149) and filled with a specific meaning. On this level we experience something as making us angry, anxious or sad.

This author prefers speaking of discrete or categorical emotions (Geuter and Schrauth, 2015) because these emotions show discrete qualities in relation to something. For example, happiness is not opposite to sadness on a linear dimension; such bipolarity only applies to the dimension pleasant–unpleasant of the core affect (Feldman Barrett and Russell, 1998). Both happiness and sadness are qualitatively different reaction patterns which have a specific aboutness, stimulate specific action tendencies, and might also be connected with discrete neural patterns of mapping the organismic state (Damasio et al., 2000).

Some discrete emotions interrupt our core affective state. They are mostly situational, time limited and have a cyclical structure of coming and going as well as a brief duration. Ekman (1999) calls them basic emotions and names happiness, anger, fear, disgust, surprise, sadness, contempt and curiosity (see Figure 28.2). They seem to be evolutionary formed affective programs of responding to certain events. With sadness and an attempt at attachment we react to loss and fear, and an attempt to avoid hurt or threat; with disgust when facing something which is detrimental or very unpleasant for the organism; with curiosity to something which seems to be useful, exciting or very pleasant. Needs and desires activate respective motivational seeking systems (Panksepp, 1998) leading us to strive for attachment, solace, safety, avoidance and play.

In his later work, Ekman (1999) added embarrassment, contentment, relief, guilt, pride in achievement or shame to the basic emotions. Other authors regard these emotions as a separate class of so called self-conscious or self-referential emotions (Tangney and Fischer, 1995; Zinck and Newen, 2008). With them an emotional reaction is set in relation to an inner measure of value or to representations of other's thoughts within the process of appraisal. While basic emotions like fear or sorrow can be triggered right away by a situation, self-referential emotions require an inner comparison with a standard of feeling and behaviour. That is why they also emerge later in child development. Self-referential emotions tend to persist more like feeling guilty or jealous. If a more episodic basic emotion persists it can turn into a personality disorder like fear in the case of avoidant personality or anger in borderline. Explaining such long-lasting dispositional states is not part of the model here.

Basic emotions determine a loco-motor relation to an object. They generate action patterns to change situations. In Figure 28.2 this is referred to as approach and avoidance. On the core affective level, we can establish attraction or aversion to an object as a basic reaction on the dimension of pleasantness–unpleasantness. Core affective reactions already layout goal directed behaviour. Basic emotions, however, add a more specifically felt relation: to move towards an object like in the case of curiosity, to move away from it with fear, to keep it away from oneself with disgust, or to push it away with anger, or to pull it towards oneself with happiness. In body psychotherapy, we can explore this relation in an affect-motor dialogue with the intentional object imagined in the therapy room in scenic interaction.

Three tasks for working with emotions in body psychotherapy

On a phenomenal level the three steps cannot be distinguished in an emotional process, nor the different appraisals as following one after the other on a timeline. The model, however, shows different aspects of emotions as meaningful answers to situations. These aspects open an understanding of major tasks of working with clinically relevant emotional problems. According to the model, we can establish three different tasks in working with emotions in body psychotherapy. They correspond to three tasks Greenberg (2004) gathers from empirical research: emotion awareness, emotion regulation and emotion transformation.

The first task is to work with the awareness of a person for the perception of the inner and outer world. We do this by using body-oriented methods of enhancing self-perception and sensing or with focusing attention on breath or movements. One example is the so-called body scan in mindfulness-based stress reduction (MBSR) (Kabat-Zinn, 1990) that has been taught since the very beginnings of body therapy by Elsa Gindler in Germany under the term 'body journey' (Geuter, Heller, and Weaver, 2010). Another example is in the meditative work with mindfulness in Hakomi (Weiss, Johanson, and Monda, 2015).

A second task is working with the perception of core affective reactions and with modulating and regulating the core affect. This is one of the domains of body psychotherapy as the core affect can be modulated better by bodily means. The inner sensation of the 'felt sense' (Gendlin, 1996, p. 20) often signals if the person experiences something as pleasant or not. Exploring pleasantness and unpleasantness by putting attention to inner sensations or by letting the client make sensual experiences with breathing, moving, looking at or sensing objects often leads to a core affective change. Many methods of working with breath and movement in body psychotherapy try to raise or calm the level of activation. This has often been called working with 'charge and discharge' (Totton, 2003, p. 67) in Neo-Reichian body psychotherapy. Deeper breathing, moving or boosting muscular tension help to increase arousal and intensify emotional processes. Methods of grounding, centring or holding can decrease arousal and deactivate emotional tension. The first is more indicated in case of inhibition and over-regulated emotions, the latter in case of under-regulation. The aim is to work in the 'optimal arousal zone' of the 'window of tolerance' (Ogden, Minton, and Paine, 2006, p. 27) where arousal is high enough to make new corrective experiences possible and low enough to be able to consciously experience an emotional process. In the history of body psychotherapy, we find an emphasis on freeing over-regulated emotions. Starting with Reich (1933/1970) bodily expression was often believed to be the *via regia* of treatment. Other problems of emotional regulation were less focused, such as regulating under-regulated emotions, or re-associating dissociated perceptions.

Working on the dimensions of the core affect which Russell (2003) calls 'affect regulation' (p. 165) is in contrast to *emotional regulation* as a term for working on the attributed affect or discrete emotion. Core affect regulation can happen implicitly without consciously addressing an emotional problem (Koole and Rothermund, 2011). Thus, the core affect can be changed without connecting an emotional process to its cause, for example, calming down to a pleasant and deactivated state can make a problem fade without talking about it. This might be one factor for the effectiveness of meditative methods in emotional self-regulation as they help bringing people more into that state.

In psychotherapy in general the concept of emotional regulation has referred to discrete emotions mostly. When Greenberg (2011) argues that emotions can only be changed by other emotions, like overcoming sorrow by discovering the hidden anger, he talks about discrete emotions. Emotion-focused therapy has less of a focus on processes of emotional arousal (Carryer and Greenberg, 2010). In contrast, a central feature of body psychotherapy is working with the regulation of the core affect and working with regulating, clearing and transforming object-related discrete emotions in one therapeutic process.

Following Greenberg's three tasks, the third task of emotional transformation is working with the perception, expression, modulation or clarification of discrete emotions. On this level one needs to establish the connection between an emotion and its intentional object in order to reveal its 'subjective meaning' (Downing, 1996, p. 92f.). On a bodily level we can do this by exploring the loco-motor relation, by perceiving somatic markers (ref) or inquiring and discovering looming sensations or movements. We can also support the client to stay with the arousal of the concrete emotion, to express emotions by words, voice, gestures or movements or to express them to a person in the client's imagination or in an action dialogue. Clarification includes understanding the motivational and intentional meaning of an emotion, for example, asking questions such as: *'what is the object of my fear?'* or *'what is the reason for having that fear?'* or *'what has to happen in order to be able to let the fear go?'* This is a process of embodied self-reflection within the psychotherapeutic relationship. It can include exploring habituated affect-motor schemas acquired in childhood relational experiences and trying out more adaptive and appropriate ones (Downing, 1996).

All appraisals depend on the desires, needs and intentions of a subject. Emotions tell of desires, such as the desire for safety or easing in case of fear, for integrity or attachment in the case of anger, or for sharing in happiness. Intentions can determine whether the environment will be checked for potential danger or perceived as being basically safe. Working with emotional self-regulation, body psychotherapy therefore always tries to gain an understanding of the desire an emotion is expressing. Thus emotional regulation helps clients to regulate themselves in relating to the world in a way in which they can live better according to their desires.

The model of the affective cycle

In his concept of vitality affects Stern (1985) has introduced a further dimension of the contours of emotional processes in time and the fluctuations in their intensity, force or form. The following model described more extensively by Geuter (2015) and Geuter and Schrauth (2001, 2015) tries to see the core affective regulation of arousal and the regulation of discrete emotions as a process of change in time. The model has been developed mainly for working with basic

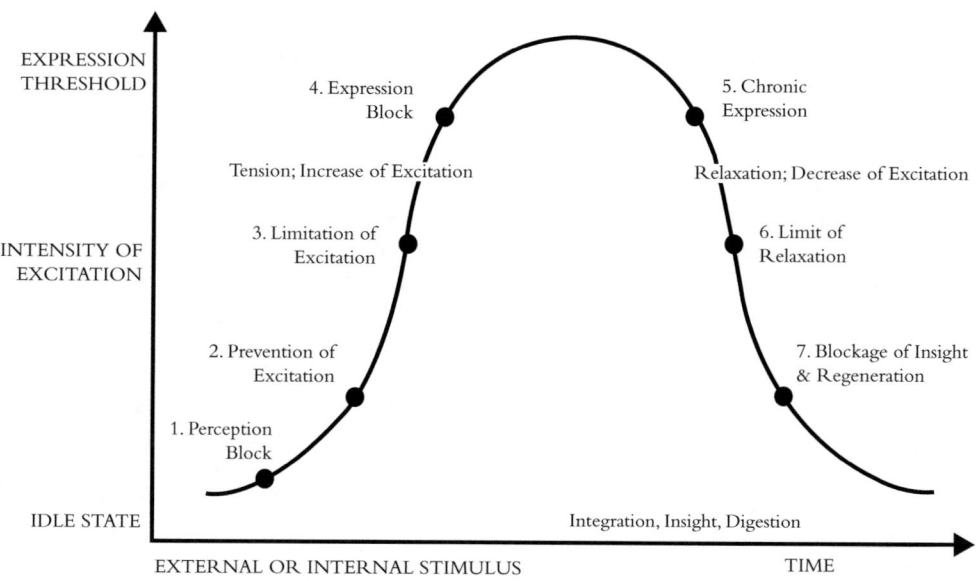

Figure 28.4 The affective cycle and the points of blockage

Source: Geuter and Schrauth, 2015, p. 549

emotions which, in contrast to self-referential emotions, mostly form a cycle of swelling up and going down. It distinguishes seven different points of blockage in an affective cycle leading to different body psychotherapeutic tasks (see Figure 28.4).

Perception block. A stimulus is not perceived. If the core affective feeling is inhibited, a person is unable to emotionally perceive a situation. This is the case in many somatoform disorders or in severe depression when situations cannot be judged as personally relevant or where no emotional reaction can be felt. In body psychotherapy, we confront this blockage by helping clients to become aware of themselves and their environment, extending their attention to noticing changes of inner sensations, movements or breath, as well as thoughts and fantasies and perceptions of the outside world.

Prevention of emotion. After perceiving an event, core affective arousal can be blocked. In this case clients need to be supported in staying with a perception, deepening their awareness and increasing activation, for example, by intensifying their breath or spontaneous gestures or by changing postures. Dancing emotions, bioenergetic stress positions or role play can be helpful in treating this blockage.

Limitation of excitation. If an emotion cannot be tolerated, clients may limit their arousal and suppress the emotional reaction, for example, by withholding tensions of anger or joy of excitement. In this case the therapist can help the patient to stay with her/his arousal and to keep the emotional process going. This can be supported by drawing attention to all signals of the emotion, by being fully present with the client, or holding her/him when he is gulping back her/his tears.

Expression block. If the arousal is felt, people may suppress the expression of an emotion due to fear or shame and thus they do not achieve their goals/desires. Here the task is to find a verbal and/or bodily expression, for example, in a role play with the intentional object of the emotion, or by intensifying the emotional experience through showing longing by stretching out the arms in front or anger by punching or hitting. The aim of this is not abreaction by acting out but deepening the emotional experience.

Chronic expression. If a client expresses his/her emotion but holds on to it or chronically repeats it without the arousal abating, the therapist has to help limiting the arousal. They can do this by offering interventions such as slowing down breathing, releasing tension or controlling movements to explore the hidden emotions and desires the client is covering up by exaggerated emotions. Techniques of grounding and centring that promote contact with reality and with oneself in the here and now as practised when treating posttraumatic over-arousal are helpful.

Limit of excitation. If a high level of arousal is maintained once an emotion and the desire behind it have been expressed, the task is to calm down the process and encourage relaxation. This can be done by soft breathing or movements; sitting still, with the therapist holding the client or speaking with a calming voice.

Blockage of insight and regeneration. When arousal has returned to a middle or deactivated state, a client can have difficulties in reflecting and integrating the emotional experience and come back to an inner equilibrium. This might be the case when s/he holds on to well-acquainted schemas of experiencing and behaving and does not manage to challenge them in the light of a new experience. Here, the therapist must work on a cognitive level to achieve integration. However, thoughts can be reconnected to the bodily felt sense to see if they feel congruent or not.

The idea of this model is that problems with emotional self-regulation start on the left side of the curve, with inhibitions in developing emotional reactions, and mainly reflect problems in clients who dissociate perceptions, inhibit arousal or repress expression. Kern (2014) has added that some clients are oversensitive in their perception or show an accelerated arousal reaction quickly leading to inner states of high emotional pressure as is the case with clients with posttraumatic disorders. In this case, the therapeutic task is to alleviate arousal from the very beginning. Similar differentiation has been proposed to this model by Eberhard-Kaechele (2017).

No emotion is solely a cognitive process. Emotion always 'involves bodily changes and serves the purpose of motivating need-specific action' (Eberhard-Kaechele, 2017, p. 47). Therefore, emotional regulation should always include working with experiencing and transforming these bodily-felt changes. Following the model of the three layers mentioned above emotions are experienced on a cognitive, a sensory-motoric and a vegetative level. Successfully regulating emotions requires forms of treatment coping with all the components and aspects of emotional experience. Body psychotherapy has many tools to offer.

References

Barlassina, L., and Newen, A. (2014). The role of bodily perception in emotion: In defence of an impure somatic theory. *Philosophy and Phenomenological Research, 89*, 637–678.

Caldwell, C. (2014). Mindfulness and bodyfulness: A new paradigm. *The Journal of Contemplative Inquiry, 1*, 77–96.

Carryer, J. R., and Greenberg, L. S. (2010). Optimal levels of emotional arousal in experiential therapy of depression. *Journal of Consulting and Clinical Psychology, 78*, 190–199.

Dalgleish, T. (2004). The emotional brain. *Nature Reviews Neuroscience, 5*, 582–589.

Damasio, A. R. (1994). *Descartes' Error*. New York: Putnam.

Damasio, A. R. (2003). *Looking for Spinoza. Joy, Sorrow and the Human Brain*. Orlando: Harcourt.

Damasio, A. R., Grabowski, T. J., Bechara, A., Damasio, H., Ponto, L., Parvizi, J., and Hichwa, R. D. (2000). Subcortical and cortical brain activity during the feeling of self-generated emotions. *Nature Neuroscience, 3*, 1049–1056.

Downing, G. (1996). *Körper und Wort in der Psychotherapie* [Body and Word in Psychotherapy]. Munich: Kösel.

Eberhard-Kaechele, M. (2017). Emotion is motion: Improving emotion regulation through movement intervention. *European Psychotherapy, 13*, 26–49.

Ekman, P. (1999). Basic emotions. In T. Dalgleish and M. Power (Eds.), *Handbook of Cognition and Emotion* (pp. 45–60). Sussex: John Wiley.

Feldman Barrett, L., and Russell, J. A. (1998). Independence and bipolarity in the structure of current affects. *Journal of Personality and Social Psychology, 74*, 967–984.

Feldman Barrett, L., and Russell, J. A. (1999). The structure of current affect: Controversies and emerging consensus. *Current Directions in Psychological Science, 8*, 10–14.

Frijda, N. H. (2007). Klaus Scherer's article on 'What are emotions?' Comments. *Social Science Information, 46*, 381–383.

Frijda, N. H. (2009). Emotion experience and its varieties. *Emotion Review, 1*, 264–271.

Garvey, A., and Fogel, A. (2008). Emotions and communication as a dynamic developmental system. *Espaciotiempo, 2*, 62–73.

Gendlin, E. (1996). *Focusing Oriented Psychotherapy. A Manual of the Experiential Method*. New York: Guilford.

Geuter, U. (2015). *Körperpsychotherapie. Grundriss einer Theorie für die klinische Praxis* [Body Psychotherapy: Outline of a Theory for Clinical Practice]. Berlin, Heidelberg: Springer.

Geuter, U. (2016). Body psychotherapy: Experiencing the body, experiencing the self. *International Body Psychotherapy Journal, 15*(1), 6–19.

Geuter, U., and Schrauth, N. (2001). Emotionen und emotionsabwehr als körperprozess [Emotions and emotional defence as body processes]. *Psychotherapie Forum, 9*, 4–19.

Geuter, U., and Schrauth, N. (2015). The role of the body in emotional defence processes. In G. Marlock, and H. Weiss (with C. Young and M. Soth) (Eds.), *The Handbook of Body Psychotherapy and Somatic Psychology* (pp. 543–552). Berkeley, CA: North Atlantic.

Geuter, U., Heller, M. C., and Weaver, J. O. (2010). Elsa Gindler and her influence on Wilhelm Reich and body psychotherapy. *International Journal of Body, Movement and Dance in Psychotherapy, 5*, 59–73.

Greenberg, L. S. (2004). Emotion-focused therapy. *Clinical Psychology and Psychotherapy, 11*, 3–16.

Greenberg, L. S. (2011). *Emotion-Focused Therapy*. Washington, DC: American Psychological Association.

Greenberg, L. S., and Bischkopf, J. (2007). Anger in psychotherapy: To express or not to express? That is the question. In T. A. Cavell and K. T. Malcom (Eds.), *Anger, Aggression, and Interventions for Interpersonal Violence* (pp. 165–183). Mahwah: Lawrence Erlbaum.

Greenberg, L. S., and Van Balen, R. (1998). The theory of experience-centered therapies. In L. S. Greenberg, J. C. Watson, and G. Lietaer (Eds.), *Handbook of Experiential Psychotherapy* (pp. 28–57). New York: Guilford.

Hertenstein, M. J., Holmes, R., McCullough, M., and Keltner, D. (2009). The communication of emotion via touch. *Emotion, 9*, 566–573.

Johnson, M. (2007). *The Meaning of the Body. Aesthetics of Human Understanding.* Chicago: The University of Chicago Press.

Kabat-Zinn, J. (1990). *Full Catastrophe Living: The Program of the Stress Reduction Clinic at the University of Massachusetts Medical Center.* New York: Delta.

Kern, E. (2014). *Personzentrierte Körperpsychotherapie* [Person Centered Body Psychotherapy]. Munich: Reinhardt.

Koole, S. L., and Rothermund, K. (2011). 'I feel better but I don't know why': The psychology of implicit emotion regulation. *Cognition and Emotion, 25*, 389–399.

Nummenmaa, L., Gelerean, E., Hari, R., and Hietanen, J. K. (2014). Bodily maps of emotions. *PNAS, 111*, 646–651.

Ogden, P., Minton, K., and Pain, C. (2006). *Trauma and the Body. A Sensorimotor Approach to Psychotherapy.* New York/London: W.W. Norton.

Panksepp, J. (1998). *Affective Neuroscience. The Foundations of Human and Animal Emotions.* Oxford: Oxford University Press.

Reich, W. (1970). *Character Analysis.* New York: Farrar, Straus and Giroux. (Original work published 1933)

Reisenzein, R. (1994). Pleasure-arousal theory and the intensity of emotions. *Journal of Personality and Social Psychology, 67*, 525–539.

Russell, J. A. (2003). Core affect and the psychological construction of emotion. *Psychological Review, 110*, 145–172.

Sachse, R., and Langens, T. A. (2014). Implikationsstrukturen von emotionen (Structures of implications of emotions). In R. Sachse and T. A. Langens (Eds.), *Emotionen und Affekte in der Psychotherapie* [Emotions and Affects in Psychotherapy] (pp. 47–55). Göttingen: Hogrefe.

Sander, D., Grandjean, D., and Scherer, K. (2005). A systems approach to appraisal mechanisms in emotion. *Neural Networks, 18*, 317–352.

Scherer, K. R. (2009a). Emotions are emergent processes: They require a dynamic computational architecture. *Philosophical Transactions of the Royal Society, 364*, 3459–3474.

Scherer, K. R. (2009b). The dynamic architecture of emotion: Evidence for the component process model. *Cognition and Emotion, 23*, 1307–1351.

Scherer, K. R. (2015). When and why are emotions disturbed? Suggestions based on theory and data from emotion research. *Emotion Review, 7*, 238–249.

Schore, A. N. (2003). *Affect Regulation and the Repair of the Self.* New York/London: W.W. Norton.

Stern, D. (1985). *The Interpersonal World of the Infant.* New York: Basic Books.

Sugamura, G., Haruki, Y., and Koshikawa, F. (2006). *Mindfulness and bodyfulness in the practices of meditation: A comparison of Western and Eastern theories of mind-body.* Poster presented at the 1st Convention of the Asian Psychological Association, Bali, Indonesia.

Tangney, J. P., and Fischer, K. W. (1995). *Self-Conscious Emotions. The Psychology of Shame, Guilt, Embarrassment and Pride.* New York: Guilford.

Totton, N. (2003). *Body Psychotherapy. An Introduction.* Maidenhead: Open University Press.

Weiss, H., Johanson, G., and Monda, L. (Eds.). (2015). *Hakomi Mindfulness-Centered Somatic Psychotherapy. A Comprehensive Guide to Theory and Practice.* New York: W.W. Norton.

Zinck, A., and Newen, A. (2008). Classifying emotion: A developmental account. *Synthese, 161*, 1–25.

29

THE EMBODIMENT OF DREAMS

Exploring mind/body connecting devices

Michel Coster Heller and Gillat Burckhardt-Bartov

Introduction

Mary[1] is a case that this author followed, using a blend of body psychotherapy technics (Heller, 2016) to treat her vaginismus. The aim of this paper is to give a practical example of how embodiment can be used and explored as a part of mental health treatment. It will also show how a concrete approach to embodiment highlights particularities that are sometimes forgotten in theoretical papers. Discussions pertaining to the treatment of vaginismus are beyond the scope of this chapter and can be explored in a more clinically oriented paper.

This case was selected because it required a particularly clear way of organising the body/mind dialogue, as if these dimensions followed parallel roads. Neurologists have provided an enormous corpus of information on the numerous *correlations* that exist between neurological, behavioural and psychological modules (Aybeck et al., 2014); yet even acclaimed Nobel prize scientists agree that our knowledge of 'the biological modulators of emotion and empathy is just beginning' (Kandel, 2012, p. 436).

Presenting the patient and the choice of treatment

Mary[1] is a woman of approximately 25 years, from the French part of Switzerland. She is the daughter of a dentist, has a twin sister and two brothers. Her mother manifested some depressive symptoms. Before Mary began her psychotherapy, she was seeing her general practitioner for recurring panic attacks that increased her cardiac activity. After examining her physical symptoms, cardiologists concluded that they were not triggered by an organic pathology. Mary has given us written permission to publish her psychotherapy sessions with me.

Mary had become involved in a love relationship which was marred by her vaginismus. The couple engaged in sexual and sensual interactions, but the patient's vagina remained tight upon penetration. Subsequent therapeutic investigation revealed that frigidity was not the issue at hand. Her general practitioner sent her to a female physiotherapist. Despite months of body therapy, the muscles of Mary's pelvis and thighs remained tight. The physiotherapist asked the author if he could be of help to this patient, using body psychotherapy. He agreed to try.

Mary was referred by her practitioner for symptom-focused psychotherapy. The rationale for this delegation was that body psychotherapists know how to loosen muscles and reframe breathing patterns, have some knowledge of sexology and could connect physical dynamics with instinctive, emotional and cognitive functions of the mind. The therapy followed a multi-dimensional approach, as was recommended by experts treating psychosexual symptoms (Crowley, Richardson, and Goldmeier, 2006; Jawdokimova, 2016; Ogden and Ward, 1995). The following is the first 18 months of a process that lasted a bit more than 2 years. The frequency of the sessions was once or twice a week.

Method used for this treatment: For Mary's case three types of treatment were combined: (1) Ordinary psycho-educational *conversation*, similar to counselling, where both parties are sitting in armchairs that are more or less facing each other. (2) A form of *dream analysis* close to Sigmund Freud's method (Freud, 1900/1978), however nonverbal items were also included in the chain of associations (Heller, 2012). In Mary's case, moving from a manifest to a latent content was a fruitful parallel to how representations and body manifestations resonate with each other and (3) body psychotherapy methods derived from the *Vegetotherapy* and the *Orgonomy* developed by Reich (1940/1967, 1951/1973), with modifications taught by Gerda Boyesen and her team during the 1970s (Boyesen, 1985; Heller, 2012).

This method aims at facilitating the emergence of emotional expressions and the orgasm reflex (Reich, 1945/1990). For the Orgonomy work, jellyfish exercises were used. These have been developed by Ola Rakness, Gerda Boyesen, her daughter, Mona-Lisa Boyesen and by this author (Heller, 1993a, 2018). These movements tend to activate an experience of deep pulsating, pleasurable sensations (Heller, 2012). A Reichian approach is designed to tackle chronic fears of pleasure, which can be relevant with patients who suffer from vaginismus (Crowley et al., 2006).

Relational issues were framed using psychodynamic models of transference (Heller, 1993b; Kohut, 1971[2]) and systemic approaches to nonverbal communication (Heller, 1997, 2004). This blend of relational models is used by psychotherapists who use psychodynamic or biodynamic psychotherapeutic approaches (Beebe and Lachmann, 2003; Westland, 2015).

Uncontrolled anger hides hidden sources of pleasure

From the very start the material presented by Mary oscillated between love and guilt, anger and compliance. These contradictory emotions could not be integrated, each one remaining in conflict with the other. These dissociated affects conflicted with the humanistic attitude of her family, which upheld the generous ideology of the Red Cross and the first ecologist movements. Mary was striving for a harmonious world and negated every suggestion that conflicts could sometimes become a form of constructive interaction. She desperately wanted the world to remain as it is. She could not accept that her needs could be incompatible with those of others. What follows are extracts of the notes taken during the psychotherapeutic process. They show how techniques, discussions and associations weaved the unplanned partition of Mary's process.

Discovering Mary's disconnected partial drives[3]: The therapeutic process began with a combination of discussions and body work, to discover and explore the geography of Mary's drives and representations. In the second exploratory session, a Gestalt exercise was proposed[4] during which she enacted a dialogue between her mother and herself. At the end, she remembered that, as a child, she had made an inner contract that she would never be angry.

In the next session, she arrived shocked, because she had been attacked by two hitchhikers, who threatened her with a gun and a knife. Her explosive reaction made them run away. Her body seemed to be stuck in a permanent startle mode (hyper-startle) (Heller, 2012). I asked her if she was willing to lay on the mattress, so that she could explore how her body reacted to this aggression. Her jaws were tight, her chest remained inflated in the inhalation position, her belly was tightly gathered to the spine as if she was exhaling, there were tension points along the spine and in the right thigh (she is right-handed). She then explored how she could move these tensions to explore the emotions that may be repressed by them. The rigidity gradually softened, leaving room for a pleasurable sensation that flowed into the whole organism. Her body began to move as if parts of her orgasm reflex had surfaced in a disordered, dispersed and ungrounded way (Heller, 2012; Reich, 1945/1990).

A week later, I used massage[5] to loosen her muscular tensions and open her restricted breathing. Again, features of what could have been parts of her orgasm reflex emerged. Spontaneous vibrations spread from the legs to the neck. However, these automatic reactions did not become associated with images, body sensations and feelings. They were for her a bizarre, uncontrollable phenomenon. At the end of this session she talked of her fear of pleasure, and her difficulty of 'being herself' with others. For many months, this oscillation between remnants of her startle reflex and remnants of her orgasm reflex recurred, resembling to what Reich calls a 'character trait' (Reich, 1945/1990, pp. 316–320). At the start of a massage session, her jaws would clench tight. When these tensions relaxed, she would suddenly experience pleasurable body sensations. These became an englobing inner warmth, which transformed itself in agreeable movements that allowed her to appreciate how nice it was to be in contact with one's flesh. A pattern seemed to unfold pointing to a strong link between the clenching of her jaws and the tightness of her vagina.

She returned with painful tensions in her belly. While I massaged her abdominal muscles, the tension in her jaws increased. She began to explore what happens if she tried to move her tense lips, and what emerged during these movements. This led to a sensation of sucking. In the next session, she described what she experienced when her boyfriend tried to penetrate her. All the muscles of her body would become particularly tense, as if she was being raped. While she was describing these sensations, her jaws clenched, once again. She moved her jaws to explore their tightness and experienced a pleasurable need to bite on something that penetrated her mouth. Once again, her gestural and verbal associations highlighted dissociated affects that shifted from mother to father, from the genital to the oral, in unpredictable ways. Gradually, a dissociated state of aggression versus pleasure became linked, as if they formed an inner polarity. The patient could begin to differentiate and then synthesise the two emotions without feeling threatened. This phase was followed by 2 weeks of holidays, during which her need to combine these disconnected experiences began to emerge.

Alternating between dream analysis and vegetotherapy: After the holidays, what had been stirred during the previous months recalibrated something in Mary's inner realm. She brought dreams to the sessions and demonstrated pleasure when she consciously explored these inner experiences. The psychotherapeutic process now combined dream analysis with body psychotherapy. During this work, I encouraged the production of verbal and body associations, sometimes proposed a synthesis of what emerged, but seldom used what psychoanalysts call an interpretation (Etchegoyen, 1991).

In a first dream, she is alone in a huge building, which belongs to her. A powerful monster is trying to force his way inside. As she fought him, she found herself flying with him close to a high ceiling. She told her dream lying on her back on the mattress. She suddenly felt an urge to move. She put herself on her hands and knees, feeling strength streaming through her. After that she lay on the mattress again. The dream analysis continued, using free associations. Her inner images introduced me to an amusing father who sometimes played at being a horse instead of telling the two sisters a bedtime story, to make them laugh. Then came the 'nasty witches' of her family (grandmothers, aunts and godmothers). The impression of falling is perceived as falling in a hole, solitude, and darkness, not feeling the presence of her mother. The flow of her associations brought back a memory of the sliding door in the room she shared with her twin sister that was often open. Sometimes she preferred that it remained closed. The end of the dream is associated with images such as Mary Poppins, whom she venerates, the impression that the monster is actually her father and horrible images of crows flying. In her childhood dreams, crows would announce that she had been condemned.

Next session she lay on the mattress and complained that her legs felt extremely tense. I asked her to explore what happened when she separated and moved her legs. She experienced this as painful. I proposed that while she explored this painful sensation, she could express what she felt with vocalisations and gestures. The tension became pleasurable once again, but she was too shy to use her voice for expressive purposes. As Mary associated on the doors in the building of her dream, she began to remember her fear of being detected by her sister when she masturbated, and of wanting the door that partitioned the room to be closed. The tightness of her jaws and vagina was now a link in a new associative chain.

She began another session by complaining about the impossibility of sharing intimate feelings in her family. She felt anger at having to manipulate her feelings to become acceptable. Her hunger must remain polite, and her feelings 'should be as delicate as lace . . .', while her experience of herself is that of a passionate being. I must say that I did not experience a woman who can make dangerous hitchhikers run away, as delicate and fragile. A childhood memory came of a moment when she took the decision that, from now on, she would 'give them nothing'. To achieve this aim, she severed herself from her feelings, to avoid being forced to lie about them.

Before the summer holidays, she told me that her boyfriend could begin to penetrate her; but that their sexual encounters had become less enjoyable. One of the issues she raised is that it was only anger and anxiety that could prevent her life from becoming boring. She also noticed that she had not experienced any tachycardia for the past few weeks.

How to be oneself with a man?

Airport and car dreams: Mary comes back from her holidays in the family's house in Greece. She was now more aware of her fear of meeting her inner space, which was gradually becoming a less chaotic entity. She brought a short airport dream. The floor and walls of this dreamed airport had cold stones. She associated them with how she experiences the centre of her being every time she sleeps in her bed, at home. In the same dream, flying led to a fear of falling into the sadness and melancholia she experienced every time her vagina remained dry, when she was in bed with her boyfriend. The corridors and the escalators of that airport conveyed impressions that were close to how she experienced her vagina at such moments: They had seemed to have no function, and to lead nowhere. She did not know for whom these corridors were designed, and where they could lead her. When I ask her to explore what she experiences in her body at the end of the session, she feels tightness in her jaws, hands and feet – and a need for vengeance. I asked her if she can explore this impression by breathing around it. She then tells me that she is also experiencing a sense akin to a reassuring feeling of strength.

At the beginning of the next session, she describes a horrible nightmare of a car accident. As we analysed it, some patterns emerge, such as the negative correlation between a sense of horror in the dream and that of pleasure in the body. We examine the disgust she experiences for men of her age, which does not prevent her from being attracted to them. She also says that it is because of her therapy with me, that she continues to face the ordeals of a sex life.

What love for a father can an adult woman dare to feel?

Mary now has the strength to tell her boyfriend she wishes to abstain from sexual relationships for a while. Having said this, she described a dream of Malaysia, which in French could be associated with bad-ease. When she associated with that airport dream, she had already told me of her idealisation of a Greek island where her family owned a house. It is paradise for her. She takes airplanes and boats to reach it. There her father is calm, while at home he is often angry and irritated. His anger became more pronounced when he fell in love. He left what Mary calls 'home', to live with his new girlfriend when Mary was 16 years old. This triggered a dramatic change in the family life. If she marries and has children, she will also be bound to leave her families' home. She is now in the process of realising how strong is her need for an ideally stable symbiosis, and how the association of having a lover and leaving her family is linked to the threat of forfeiting this deep need.

When Mary is alone with her father, he becomes playful. Sometimes they play ball games together. It is only once her father had left home that Mary actually got to know him. At home, father was bad and she said, 'I was also bad, because I wanted to go and live with him, and because I liked his girlfriend: father and I agreed that we did not like home'. She is also jealous of her father's love for her twin sister saying, 'my father loves my sister, and only loves me because I look like her'.

Learning to experience independent well-being

During the more bodily sessions, I used a combination of vegetotherapy and bioenergetics. Mary hits and stamps and screams her anger. . . but doing this becomes so pleasurable that she cannot really explore her aggression. In her boyfriend's apartment, she dares to be openly angry and sulky with him. . . sometimes excessively so. Anger is still experienced as a way of spicing up life, which could otherwise become boring. After these sessions, she feels relaxed, warm and sometimes sleepy.

During grounding exercises[6], she gradually tolerates the vibrations that invariably come, but most of the weight is on the inside of the feet, which is coherent with the tightness of her thighs. I sometimes put dance music. She then uses grounding exercises as a way to motivate dance: 'I can now make my strength circulate in all the parts of my body'. Although we are in October, she experiences a strong urge to be in a sunny landscape, like her father's Greek Island.

At the end of the term, Mary tells me of a dream where I am a nice person, and of another dream where I am mean. Her dreams mostly focus on how to separate herself from her twin sister, and on conflicts flaring up between her boyfriend and her sister. She mentions female friends she had when she was 13 years old, just before her puberty. Two of her friends were identical twins who looked alike, and another friend who had fallen madly in love with a 16-year-old boy (platonically, probably). An older woman they had known had a lesbian relationship. Slowly but surely, she was beginning to think in terms of competition between females (notably her sister) in relation to men of the same age. She is beginning to perceive herself as an adult who seeks to situate herself not only in the realm of her family, but also in the world of adults of her age.

Learning to be a pulsating being. When Mary returns from the holiday, her process continued to structure the material we had explored. She is angrily creating a space between herself and her sister, who is becoming increasingly demanding. This ostentatious possessiveness is probably activated by the tighter bonds that are being formed between Mary and her boyfriend. Sexually, she can now let him penetrate her more deeply, although not completely.

Jellyfish exercises: After Mary ends her narrative, I propose a jellyfish exercise with the hope that, as she performed it, she might discover bodily sensations that connect her vagina to the rest of her body sensations. In the exercise, one explores ways of repeatedly passing from an open to a closed position, following the rhythm of respiration (see Heller, 1993a). After a deeply relaxing exercise has been used, the organism often requires some time before it becomes fully functional for an intellectual discussion. Mary reported that she felt something like a pulsating energy.

Instead of asking for an immediate description of that impression, I suggested that the verbal feedback for this exercise could be postponed until the next session, and that, in the meantime, after the sessions, she observes how she passes from relaxation to a fully active state.

During the week, the exercise generated disagreeable reactions. She had slept badly and was sometimes afraid when walking along the street. She oscillated unpredictably from feeling adult to being a child. She also had a bad headache and a pulsating sensation in her head. She feared that her skull would explode. While she speaks, I notice that her feet keep rubbing each other in an unusual way. She tells me that repetitive gestures reassure her. They generate an impression of predictability. She then has images of her and her sister in her mother's womb, with all three hearts pulsating together. She wished it were possible to experience 'the original union' again.

The jellyfish exercise activated inner dynamics that are still reverberating 1 week later. She arrives tired and depressed: 'the world does not interest me!' She feels tensions in the legs and the belly. I follow these sensations using body techniques, like a psychoanalyst follows mental manifestations with mental techniques. In this case, I used a Chinese massage: I lift Mary's feet and shake her legs to create soft vibrations that spread up to the belly and the chest for about 10 minutes.

Memories come: She is 8 years old. There is a popular feast in Lausanne. The two sisters are dressed in a ridiculous way, but they have tremendous fun. People follow the tradition to throw coins into a particular fountain. She then remembers her birthday. Everybody loved the two sisters, and she loves her too. At the end of the session she has the impression that her legs feel so good that they are 10 years younger.

After two sessions of massage and jellyfish exercises, her wellbeing increases. Somehow, integrating her love for her sister helped her to develop a form of boundary that can be used in different situations, such as strengthening her feminine boundaries with her lover. Once she could trust her capacity to create these boundaries in an automatic way, the muscles in the area of her sex could vary their tone more easily, and sexual pleasure could become a safer form of interaction. Anger and reconciliations were no longer experienced as disconnected emotional events, but as a pulsation between affirmation and reparation. Beautiful images fill her imagination, while global pleasurable sensations fill her body.

After these sessions, she suffered from a painful dysentery, which lasts for 2 weeks. She oscillates between frightening images of sharks and oceanic visions. We notice the fluctuation between the negative and positive images maintain an inner coherent field. As with electricity, the positive and negative poles create a charge, something that could become a sensation of an intimate inner strength. She also recollects that for years, in her pre-puberty (she began menstruating when she was 14 years old) she resisted becoming increasingly a woman by wanting to be a boy, with short hair. She only played with boys, and hated her long hair imposed upon her by her parents. She ended the session with images of pyramids which were sometimes upside down and could see weeds moving in the sand of a beautiful sea.

Outcome

Although the clinical summary of the case ends here, the vaginismus disappeared 6 months later. The psychotherapeutic process continued for a little more than a year. Mary needed to integrate the affective dynamics and the flow of representations that had emerged. Having a sense of identity that can integrate her love for a loving father became a central theme.

Years later, Mary took a few months of additional psychotherapy. Her children were now at school. She could not bear to be alone at home for the whole day and did not want to abandon her maternal role. The process now involved her relationship with her mother. More than a decade later, Mary returned for treatment when her children left home to lead an adult life. We then tackled issues concerning the development of her professional career, connected with improving her independence (autonomy) from her twin sister. Mary's vaginismus had not reappeared during this period.

Conclusion: Aspects of body psychotherapy illustrated by this case

There exists a wide variety of ways of understanding a term such as embodiment. Most authors see it as the assumption that the mind is embedded in the interaction of the organism and its environment (Thomson, 2010) while some body-mind therapists define embodied awareness as a particularly mature form of self-awareness (Fogel, 2009), close to mindfulness. The term is often used in recent body psychotherapy meetings as a useful fashionable vehicle to communicate notions they developed since evolutionary psychology exists (Heller, 2016).

Three layers were distinguished for the analysis of Mary: (1) A *psychological* layer which requires a specific set of therapeutic methods such as tranquilisers, hypnosis, conversation, dream analysis (etc.), (2) A *somatic* layer which requires another set of interventions such as those proposed by Mary's general practitioner and (3) a postulated *intermediary* layer, which could explain manifest interactions between the psychological and somatic layer, and why these interactions often seem to be complex and difficult to predict.

The presentation of this case shows how combining body and psychological technics can be an efficient way of treating not only vaginismus, but of helping the patient to ingrate what emerged in her experience when this symptom cast doubts on her sexual health and identity. The body psychotherapy methods that were used activated to a creative reshuffling of psychological and physiological dynamics. Approaching intimate dynamics by becoming aware of how they connect to movements, tissue textures and words brings forth complementary information.

Experience helps a body psychotherapist to acquire predictable intuitions on how psychological and physiological dynamics tend to recalibrate each other. Recent research suggests that these mutual influences are nonconscious, complex and to require different timescales (Dum, Levinthal, and Strick, 2016). They seem to pass by a variety of connecting devices which are rarely symmetric and the impact of psychological mechanisms on physiological modes of functioning, such as muscle tone, does not seem to be of the same type as those that connect breathing patterns to moods.

The initial complaint, which was regarded as physical in nature, was treated successfully by employing body psychotherapeutic methods which perceive such complaints as pertaining to an entity in which subsystems resonate with each other. These mutual recalibrations elude quantification and paradigmatisation. The implications of my observations are that approaches that use terms such as embodiment cannot avoid being aware of how heteroclite the organism's routines can be. Not everything is connected to everything in the same way, or even in a coherent way.

Notes

1 I have changed the names and some biographical information, to ensure Mary's privacy.

2 Kohut's management of transference is used by several body psychotherapists (Marlock and Weiss, 2001).

3 These Freudian notions were integrated in what Reich (Reich, 1945, pp. 310–323) called character analysis.

4 Following the procedures of Gestalt psychotherapy (Perls and Andreas, 1969), "proposals" are exercises that can be used by patients as they wish.

5 The massage techniques are mostly those I learned with Gerda Boyesen and her team.

6 Standing on parallel feet slightly apart, with knees slightly bent. After a while vibrations automatically but gradually rise from feet to head. (Lowen and Lowen, 1977, p. 11–18)

References

Aybeck, S., Nicholson, T. R., Zelaya, F., O'Daly, O. G., Creig, T. J., David, A. S., and Kanaan, R. A. (2014). Neural correlates of recall of life events in conversion disorder. *Journal of the AMA Psychiatry, 71*(1), 52–60.

Beebe, B., and Lachmann, F. (2003). The relational turn in psychoanalysis: A dyadic systems view from infant research. *Contemporary Psychoanalysis, 39*(3), 379–409.

Boyesen, G. (1985). *Entre psyché and soma.* Paris: Payot.

Crowley, T., Richardson, D., and Goldmeier, D. (2006). Recommendations for the management of vaginismus. *International Journal for STD and Aids, 17*(1), 14–18.

Dum, R. P., Levinthala, D. J., and Strick, P. L. (2016). Motor, cognitive, and affective areas of the cerebral cortex influence the adrenal medulla. *PNAS, 113*(35), 9922–9992.

Etchegoyen, R. H. (1991). *The Fundamentals of Psychoanalytic Technique.* London: Karnac Books.

Fogel, A. (2009). *Body Sense. The Science and Practice of Embodied Self-Awareness.* New York: W.W. Norton.

Freud, S. (1978). The interpretation of dreams. In A. Richards (Ed.), *The Pelican Freud Library* (Vol. 4). Harmondsworth, UK: Penguin Books. (Original work published 1900)

Heller, M. (1993a). The jellyfish, or the Reichian world of Gerda Boyesen, I. *Energy and Character, 24*(2), 1–27.

Heller, M. (1993b). Le transfert. In J. Besson (Ed.), *Manuel d'enseignement de l'Ecole Française d'Analyse Psycho-Organique* (Vol. 3, pp. 67–122). Paris: École Française d'Analyse Psycho-Organique.

Heller, M. (1997). Posture as an interface between biology and culture. In U. Segerstrale and P. Molnár (Eds.), *Non-Verbal Communication: Where Nature Meets Culture* (pp. 245–263). Mahwah, NJ: Lawrence Erlbaum.

Heller, M. (2004). Behind the stage of interacting faces. Commentary on case study by Beatrice Beebe. *Psychoanalytic Dialogues, 14*(1), 53–63.

Heller, M. C. (2012). *Body Psychotherapy: History, Concepts, and Methods.* New York: W.W. Norton.

Heller, M. (2016). The embodied psyche of organismic psychology: A possible frame for a dialogue between psychotherapy schools and modalities. *International Body Psychotherapy Journal, 15*(1), 20–50.

Heller, M. (2018). *La méduse, ou le monde Reichien de Gerda Boyesen* [The jellyfish, or the Reichian world of Gerda Boyesen]. Montpellier: Les Éditions Biodynamiques.

Jawdokimova, V. (2016). *How Exploring Penetration in Women with Life Long Vaginismus Informs Counselling and Psychotherapy.* London: GC7404 Research Proposal, University of East London.

Kandel, E. R. (2012). *The Age of Insight. The Quest to Understand the Unconscious in Art, Mind, and Brain.* New York: Random House.

Kohut, H. (1971). *The Analysis of the Self: A Systematic Approach to the Psychoanalytic Treatment of Narcissistic Personality Disorders.* New York: International Universities Press.

Lowen, A., and Lowen, L. (1977). *The Way to Vibrant Health: A Manual of Bioenergetic Exercises.* New York: Harper Colophon.

Marlock, G., and Weiss, H. (2001). In search of the embodied self. In M. Heller (Ed.), *The Flesh of the Soul: The Body We Work With* (pp. 133–152). Bern: Peter Lang.

Ogden, J., and Ward, E. (1995). Help seeking behaviour in sufferers of vaginismus. *Journal of Sexual and Marital Therapy, 10*, 23–30.

Perls, F. S., and Andreas, S. (1969). *Gestalt Therapy Verbatim.* Lafayette, CA: Real People Press.

Reich, W. (1967). *The Function of Orgasm: Sex-Economic Problems of Biological Energy* (T. P. Wole, Trans.). New York: Bantam Books. (Original work published 1940)

Reich, W. (1973). *Cosmic Superimposition.* New York: Farrar, Straus and Giroux. (Original work published 1951)

Reich, W. (1990). *Character Analysis* (3rd ed.). New York: Farrar, Straus and Giroux. (Original work published 1945)

Thomson, E. (2010). *Mind in Life. Biology, Phenomenology and the Sciences of the Mind.* Cambridge, MA: The Belknap Press of Harvard University Press.

Westland, G. (2015). *Verbal and Non-Verbal Communication in Psychotherapy.* New York: W.W. Norton.

30

THE THERAPIST'S BODY AND THE INTERSUBJECTIVITIES OF THE UNCONSCIOUS

Tom Warnecke

Introduction

Psychotherapy is inevitably a bodied[1] process since we need a body to think and feel with, a body that also provides the basis for our subjectivities. Body psychotherapy made the body central to its focus but, with some welcome exceptions, only occasionally gives the therapist's body much attention in its literature. In the therapeutic endeavour, the therapist's body is present in multiple ways both intra-personally and inter-personally, ranging from social, cultural, gendered or racial dimensions to bodied responses, co-regulation and bodily felt experience. This chapter focuses on phenomena of established concepts such as somatic countertransference and projective identification as it considers the therapist's body-in-process as a synergistic phenomenological field that allows for intersubjectivities of the unconscious to emerge. The following is a composite vignette by way of introduction to the subject.

Evelyn: An introductory vignette

Early in my career, I received a call from Evelyn to arrange an appointment to start therapy which we scheduled for the following week. There was nothing unusual about this call except that her voice made her sound peculiarly attractive and quite powerfully so. As my sensory-affective experience *sank in after I put the phone down, I wondered if it would even be appropriate for me to work with Evelyn given the effect her voice had on me during this brief encounter. However, when I met Evelyn in person the following week there was no repeat of my previous experience. Evelyn spend the next 6 months exploring feelings of crippling low self-esteem with no discernible erotic tensions in the room or indeed indications for any sexual aspects of the traumatic disturbances in her history.*

One day, out of the blue, Evelyn disclosed an incident at the age of 12 when a psychiatrist she had been referred to exposed himself to her. Evelyn escaped and fled the scene in shock. I recall my own shocked surprise at the time, my acute awareness that I was yet another male clinician Evelyn was talking to, and my concern whether our still young therapeutic relationship would prove sufficient to contain this turbulence. Looking back, it appears that her sudden disclosure, which seemed to mirror the shocking suddenness of the violation, impacted me too profoundly, both psychically and with a sudden drop of my somatosensory anchoring I was unaware of, to register the potential precedent of her flight from the incident for our relationship. Sadly, Evelyn did not return for another session. Over the next 12 months, Evelyn contacted me twice to arrange another appointment but sadly seemed unable to follow her intention through.

With hindsight, it appears that the puzzling attraction I experienced during our initial phone conver-
sation would have been a bodied vehicle to introduce an (most likely unconscious) aspect of Evelyn that
carried both the unprocessed traumatic disturbance and any anxieties about bringing this into our rela-
tionship. With the benefit of such hindsight, Evelyn's disclosure would seem neither sudden nor surprising
but unfortunately, I had failed to recognise this as such. I have wondered what I might have done if I had
been more alert to my bodied experience as a phenomenological emergent space. I had not considered my
anxiety and concerns, following the initial phone call, as potentially some kind of co-created alert to a
hidden but acute fragment of something unsafe, or forbidden, at the birth of our working relationship. It is
difficult to think of anything I might have said to Evelyn in acknowledgement, but I believe that holding
the likelihood of something dangerous, secret and possibly something forbidden, in my awareness might
have made a good enough container. This vignette provides a good example for the kind of experiences
that inspired this chapter and I will now outline and briefly review some conceptions relevant to consider
such phenomena.

Fragmentation and dissociative dynamics

As Ferenczi already argued, 'There is neither shock nor fright without some trace of splitting of personality' (1949, p. 229). Fragmentation, cognitive-affective unlinking and dissociation are inherent in our species' psychobiology and powerfully populate our unconscious. They appear primarily driven by autonomic nervous system (ANS) fight-flight-freeze responses (Levine, 1997) to situations in which we may fear or experience threats to our subjective existence. These may be feared or perceived threats to both our physiological and our psychological integrity, including any adaptive compensatory aspects of the latter. Fight-flight-freeze dynamics narrow our consciousness (Clark, Classen, and Fourt, 2015) and affect perception or cognition, as well as our sensory-motor systems, with rapidly diminishing somatosensory experience: a numbing dynamic seeking to protect the person from overload. Such narrowing of consciousness occurs in two ways. The parasympathetic nervous system (PNS) driven 'freeze' response is associated with suppressing and inhibiting perception and mental processing that may extend to blackouts or loss of consciousness. The intrinsically polarising ('life or death') mobilisation-accelerating dynamics of the sympathetic nervous system (SNS) on the other hand, impair our capacities for multidimensional psychological-emotional perception and processing of events (also described as reflective function, or mentalisation). The SNS exerts a powerful siren on our psychobiology too compelling for reason and cognition to resist – and catapults the individual into a continuum of polarised either-or perception driven by sympathetic hyperarousal (Uvnäs-Moberg, 2006).

The concept of dissociation can be traced back to the work of Pierre Janet (1889) who also pioneered ideas that mental and physiological manifestations activate conjointly. Janet understood dissociations as adaptively altered states of consciousness arising from excessive or inappropriate physical responses to manage overwhelming or unbearable experiences (Schore, 2009). Janet also thought that such physical responses might include what we would describe today as hypo-responses, a deficiency of psychological energy that could impair a person's abilities to bind together all their mental functions into an organised unity. We have since learned that both hyper- and hypo-tension disrupt and emaciate the ability of muscle spindles, the sensorimotor system's sense organs, to 'feel themselves', and thus facilitate proprioception sufficiently (Warnecke, 2003). Muscle spindle hyper- or hypo-tension may operate as localised or context-specific as dissociative numbing or affect the person more generally as an aspect of their procedural organisation. In other words, the body's psycho-physiological organisation in space is fundamental to one's sense of self and implicit communication with others (Carroll, 2014), manifesting as general anxiety, poor confidence or low self-esteem.

The therapist's body as a clinical utility

In the therapeutic relationship, bodied dialogue occurs not only through proximity, posture, movement, tactile, eye, or voice contact but also through intersubjective bodied phenomena such as somatic resonance, co-regulation, transference and countertransference (Pallaro, 2007; Sheedy, 2013). If we accept that psychotherapy is an enquiry into the intersubjective space between client and therapist and an endeavour to bridge the dissociative gap (Bromberg, 2010), more attention is needed to the body of the therapist, an instrument which, if finely tuned, may listen to the psyche's '[. . .] subtle voice, hear its silent music and search in to its darkness for meaning' (Mathew, 1998, p. 17).

Current understanding of somatosensory significance and clinical merit builds on the work of early pioneers such as the German philosopher Theodor Lipps (1903) who argued that empathy ('Einfühlung' – to feel into) was facilitated by inner imitation and organ perception rather than some reflective state of mind. It was phenomenological philosopher Merleau-Ponty, who observed, 'It is through my body that I understand other people' (1962, p. 186) and psychoanalyst Milner (1936/1981) who developed an introspective technique for therapists which included an openness to sensory experience she called 'wide awareness' (p. 108). Furthermore, Reich proposed a concept of 'plasmatic imitation' (Sletvold, 2014). The quintessential idea that unites these early conceptions has since been confirmed by researchers. For example, Damasio (2000) proposes a primacy of somatosensory responses to psychic and external events which appear necessary for us to become conscious of these events.

Bodied intersubjectivity or intercorporeality (Gallese, 2009) is today seen as a main source of knowledge that allows one to gather information about others. Mother-infant affective neuroscience research gave rise to models of self and mutual regulation (Stern, 1985) and organising principles of interaction for body-based inter-affective systems such as the 'dyadic systems model' (Beebe and Lachmann, 2002). Such insights were acknowledged and incorporated by pioneers of the Relational paradigm (Mitchell, 1988). Field theory (Lewin, 1939) also recognised body sensation and experience as key aspects of the interactive-cooperative field (Nolan, 2014) in the therapeutic relationship.

Inter-affectivity or affect permeability, often registered as an internal bodied sense (Carroll, 2014), enables therapists to simultaneously experience both their own and their clients' affective world with a view to facilitate self-regulation, co-regulation, empathy and working with disavowed psychic fragments. Inevitably, such sensory-affective experience will be populated by, or may activate, some deeply personal meaning and thereby connect the therapist to his or her own vulnerabilities as illustrated by the clinical vignettes here. The active co-creation of resonance and consensus or dissonance and conflict by both protagonists in the consulting room as emphasised by contemporary intersubjectivity theory (Benjamin, 2005) will necessarily manifest within and through the therapist's affective, visceral, proprioceptive and sensory-affective imagery experience.

The therapist's inter-affective and somatosensory or imagery experience is informed and facilitated by psychobiological systems, particularly the sensorimotor, 'fight-flight' and 'calm and connect' (Uvnäs-Moberg, Arn, and Magnusson, 2005) systems. Researchers also established that the right brain hemisphere, which appears crucial to psychological-emotional processing through sensory-affective imagery, symbolism and interoceptive sensation (e.g. a 'gut feeling'), is dominantly linked (Schore, 2011) to the limbic system, to the two branches of the ANS and to the somatosensory network. Sensorimotor activity is reciprocal: words activate sensorimotor experience and vice versa (Sletvold, 2014). The open loop physiology of our limbic and sensorimotor systems is designed to 'penetrate' others in order to assess and predict their actions with the aid of limbic resonance (Lannon, Amini, and Lewis, 2000), as well as mirror neurons and bodied simulation (Gallese, 2009; Pineda, 2008), systems that equally serve us to facilitate empathy, resonance, co-regulation or transference.

The therapeutic *art of listening inwards to our* moment to moment somatosensory and ANS responses is particularly crucial in the work with clients fragmented by borderline dynamics or other severe early trauma, or indeed on occasions of conflict between therapist and client. Mobilising and accelerating fight-flight or numbing freeze dynamics will commonly trigger rapidly diminishing somatosensory self-experience for the therapist as Evelyn's vignette illustrates. The resulting disruptions to the therapist's somatosensory anchoring also appear to constitute a critical aspect in re-enactments of trauma dynamics and in ruptures in the therapeutic relationship (Warnecke, 2009). For example, when both therapist and client may feel like the victim of the other. On the other hand, a therapist's alertness to, and awareness of, such *'loss'* of bodied presence can help re-establish this to some degree and allow therapists to constructively engage with the enactment.

Psychobiology and psychological-emotional processing

Somatosensory anchoring and the 'calm and connect' system appear to play a crucial part in enabling psychological-emotional processing of events or stimuli. More specifically, for affective,[2] pre-verbal and pre-symbolic experience to become transformed into emotional experience and thus into intentional states of mind that are available for regulation and reflection. I regularly find implicit references to this psycho–physiological connection in psychoanalytic literature, for example when Searles (1960) associates fragmentation with a loss of distinction between the 'animate and the inanimate', (p. 147). In another example, the ANS dynamic is implicit when Benjamin, describing the therapeutic encounter, writes '. . . how we shift from this complementary structure, with its features of omnipotence and helplessness [i. e. fight-flight-freeze], into a more recognising relation [i. e. calm and connect] in which it feels possible to communicate rather than push or pull' (Benjamin, 2005, p. 450).

The therapist's body is located in the present moment. As such, the therapist's somatosensory subjectivities provide essential grounding and anchoring for the co-regulation of trauma activation or equally for some bewildering stream of psychic intersubjectivities, which may feel 'at sea', while simultaneously furnishing a theatre for the intersubjectivities of the unconscious. Somatic countertransference will often introduce what is hitherto unconscious for the client such as disavowed affective or emotional states (Lewis, 2001; Pallaro, 2007; Warnecke, 2011). In a similar fashion, bodied phenomena experienced by the therapist may connect us to a client's raw affective, pre-verbal and pre-symbolic material. Dethlefsen and Dahlke (2002) propose a model of symptomatic bodied escalation: shock or trauma that cannot be processed by the individual through cognitive or emotional higher order systems for whatever reason, may metabolise along a psychobiological spectrum. The symptomatic body, aptly portrayed as a patient's other story by Broom (2007), may present as functional affective disturbances, as illnesses and accidents, or as chronic conditions further along the escalation spectrum.

Bromberg (1998) argues that fragmented or dissociated self-states may not only occur as by-products of trauma, but also in the course of normal development. Either way, the ensuing struggle of attempting 'to feel like one, while being many' (Bromberg, 1993, p. 166), is a familiar feature in psychotherapeutic practice. Therapists are likely to encounter a confusedly intricate spectrum of disavowed, alien or unowned psychic fragments within the dynamic interplay of subjectivities, and particularly so working with unknown or pre-verbal traumatic disturbances as the following two composite vignettes illustrate.

Andreas

During most of Andreas' sessions, something not readily identifiable would trigger him into hyperarousal states. Visibly agitated, he was only able to articulate two aspects of his distress; his shame about being overcome by whatever was happening and his need for a minimum proximity between us. These hyperarousal states appeared to lead a seemingly parallel existence to the various difficult or traumatic experiences past or present we explored. Context for the hyperarousal activations remained elusive as the months went by. I noticed that Andreas' blankness seemed mirrored by my own. Quite unusually, I would not populate these recurring activations with interior experiences of my own, which, however mystifying initially, may over time gradually lead to some sense or insight into my client's inner world. I seemed unable to projectively identify[3] with any aspect of Andreas' hyper-aroused states. While Andreas' need to maintain the proximity, status quo kept me quite literally at the proverbial distance, I would not connect with any corresponding imagery, sensory or affective responses in me that might have provided us with some clue.

Eventually, it would be the blankness of my somatosensory and psychic responses that got me to wonder whether the trauma was truly his or perhaps some intergenerational transmitted trauma. When I eventually articulated this question, the visceral effect of these words was immediately salient. It was in fact the first intervention with an immediate effect on Andreas' hyperarousal. For the next few weeks, his hyper-anxiety states reoccurred with diminishing frequency and intensity and eventually disappeared altogether. This development did not seem to require further details about the nature of the trauma. Based on what Andreas had previously shared about his parents' background, there was little doubt that both would have experienced significant traumatic disturbances. But Andreas did not seem particularly curious, sensing that something of that nature was affecting him was apparently sufficient to break the cycle.

Baum (2013) uses the metaphor of a vinyl record stuck in a groove for transgenerational trauma as the groove of the wound; a repetitive bodied experience that impedes the meaning-making of the vinyl record as a whole. In hindsight, I wondered again about the prominence of proximity in this process. Did it perhaps also serve as a segregation to prevent trauma transmission and contamination in our relationship? Seen in this light, the absence of my bodied responses might have symbolised that Andreas and I could exist and relate as distinct rather than merged beings or, in other words, that transmission and contamination were not inevitable, with my body serving like a transitional object (Winnicott, 1951/1958) *for an emergent unafflicted body coming into being.*

I would like to clarify however that I am not suggesting that a therapist should not be able to tune into previous generation's intrapsychic material (Duran and Korby, 2014). In Andreas' context, the focus of attention was on his acute distress and confusion about what was so inexplicably happening within himself.

Hannah

Hannah presented a habitual disposition to look after others and neglect her own needs. She struggled with low self-esteem and lack of motivation. Hannah had been in a traumatic marriage earlier in her life but subsequently achieved qualifications and a career while raising children who had turned adult by the time we met. Her external image of a calm and competent professional woman masked anxious and depressive states. In our relationship, she regularly felt misunderstood or not seen and quickly responded defensively while

I wondered, with little success, how to engage what I suspected to be a variety of disavowed psychic fragments. I began to notice that Hannah's sessions became preceded by sensory and ANS disturbances within myself that occurred for a few minutes prior to her arrival and subsided once she had entered my consulting room. My experience varied from week to week, but always included a level of affective agitation as well as maintaining some vaguely recognisable but very subtle quality or feel I could not name. Hannah was not the first client to make herself felt just prior to arrival but others had presented themselves primarily in my affective or emotional experiences which, while not straightforward, would allow me to consider connections between what I felt and my client's presenting issues.

Hannah on the other hand presented me with what appeared to be some raw agitation of ANS arousal. Pondering these experiences, they seemed reminiscent of observing moving shadows and trying to guess the nature of the objects that cast them. Or I was reminded of high alpine landscapes seen through milky clouds with tantalising glimpses of light and shapes that briefly appear and disappear again in misty white and grey. Over many months, some reoccurring pattern seemed to condense however, and I began to register and name to myself how these disturbances seemed forcefully demanding (of my attention) as well as being conflicted about being so. But it would take me a long time to work up to the challenge of attempting to put my tentative sense-image into words.

'Hannah, I am wondering if there might be a part of you that wants to forcefully or aggressively demand?' I suggested one day. Hannah professed feeling a bit shaken by the image my words conjured for her but to my surprise, her response lacked elements of defensiveness or feeling misunderstood I had grown accustomed to. I shared with her that these were my words for an agitation I frequently experienced prior to her arrival and emphasised that these words could and should be adapted if any of this proved relevant to her. The following week, Hannah reported that she had been deeply affected and disturbed by our previous session but also acknowledged a curiosity which seemed to exist alongside an openness to let whatever was happening take its course.

During subsequent weeks, the matter transited gently into the background without any particular revelations. I noticed however that our relationship began to feel less precarious and appeared to turn into a quite robust working alliance instead. On occasions when she might have attacked me defensively earlier, she might now express her upset in a playful manner, by threatening to throw something at me for example, safe in a shared understanding that I would get the message.

Conclusion

In all three vignettes, bodied intersubjective dynamics of the unconscious unfold while yielding to their unbidden siren call. We might of course consider all three vignettes primarily as enactments and particularly so the first one, Evelyn. I suspect however that crucial subtleties might easily get missed that way. Kurtz' internal observer's passive stance (Weiss, 2009) offers an alternative perspective to psychodynamic transference phenomena paradigms which strongly resonates with me when I think of Andreas' vignette. Yet another perspective is offered by Pinkas (2016), who describes how she 'lets [her] psyche wander', (p. 206) as a therapeutic technique which appears to connect her somewhat intentionally with similar experiences to my entirely unbidden ones.

The intersubjectivities of the unconscious are, or are certainly in part, somatosensory and sensory-affective imagery experiences. This bodied characteristic is important as it provides at least some sort of anchor within the ambiguously shifting sands of inherent uncertainty about the origin and ownership of such phenomena. Jung, proposing his four orienting functions of consciousness, notes that 'sensation establishes what is actually present' (Jung, 1921/1992, par. 958). The human mind, while an excellent tool to focus on, abstracts matters or, on some singular task, needs assistance to facilitate broader awareness of the multiple and simultaneous subjectivities that characterise human existence and particularly so in a psychotherapy setting. In the clinical context, therapists are therefore reliant on the entire range of psychobiological systems to help negotiate the intricate complexities present in the consulting room. This is further exacerbated by polarisation dynamics described earlier that can profoundly narrow the therapist's consciousness within the intersubjective space and particularly at moments of rising ANS arousal. In addition, fragmentations occur in multiple ways as the following vignette by Bioenergetic Analyst Robert Lewis illustrates:

> I remember only too well how, as a Bioenergetic patient, I surrendered my body to Bioenergetic therapy and was envious of my therapist's interest in and relationship to its (my body's) vibration, and responses. I sensed this envy deep within myself (although I did not realise what it was at the time) as I bent and stretched in various positions which were intended open my body's pulsatory, spontaneous motility. I felt that my therapist was more interested in my spontaneous motility than in my inner experience of myself.
>
> *(2003, p. 35)*

Furthermore, our psychobiology will commonly metabolise simultaneous but contradictory affective or emotional states. For example, shoulders and upper arms may be intensely and expansively engaged in a state of anger or rage while, simultaneously, the chest area may be contracted in a state of fear or collapsed in some 'I don't exist' state. If I, as the therapist in such a client scenario, can at least partially avoid the inter-affective or reactive polarisations therein, my bodied experience or sensory-affective imagery might alert me to multiple subjectivities and afford me with opportunities to build containment and connections with any disavowed states. Rumble (2010) argues that the body, rather than simply overlapping with affect states, forms a distinct dimension of attunement that is accessible through imagery and sensations. The concept of 'creative indifference' which Fritz Perls (1947/1969) adopted from Friaedlander's (1918/[2009]) ideas for Gestalt therapy, is superbly suited to facilitate broad awareness that might notice unfolding aspects that are incongruent or at odds with the foreground image.

By developing the art of looking inwards and maintaining awareness for somatosensory experience, the therapist's intersubjective bodied presence may, as Rumble describes, 'offer a kind of living hypothesis on the other' (2010, p. 134). Through indwelling and meticulous observation of their own interior, therapists can develop their awareness of subtle strata and details of intersubjective dynamics at work in the therapeutic relationship as resonance, dissonance, enactments of transference dynamics, or disturbance of relational vitality. The intersubjectivities of the unconscious have the potential to bridge and interconnect a client's psychic and somatic fragments. The therapist's body may also provide a container for raw affective, or pre-verbal and pre-symbolic psychic material as Hannah's vignette illustrates or provide an anchor when acting as a character in a client's internal drama. Or, reconsidering Andreas' and Hannah's vignettes through the lens of Winnicott's (1951/1958) original transitional objects conception which highlighted their 'not me' characteristic, the therapist's body might offer a phenomenological emergent 'not me' symbolic object space to the client where transitional phenomena may creatively unfold.

Notes

1 I use the term 'bodied' in preference to 'embodied' which is typically used to acknowledge a bodily aspect or extension of another phenomena, e.g. 'embodied cognition'. This appears to imply some hierarchical dimension in contrast to conceptions such as 'conjointly activating manifestations' or 'action-thought reciprocity' I draw on in the chapter.

2 The terms affect and emotion are sometimes used inter-changeably. Here, affect refers to a basic response that is simultaneously psychological and physiological whereas emotion is reserved for complex higher order psycho-physiological processing of events and stimuli.

3 The term projective identification describes transference dynamics that enable therapists to resonate with or experience internal states (which necessarily need to have a degree of familiarity for the therapist) that are too frightening or overwhelming for a client. They characteristically appear as if originating from the therapist's personal realm.

References

Baum, R. (2013). Transgenerational trauma and repetition in the body: The groove of the wound. *Body, Movement and Dance in Psychotherapy, 8*(1), 34–42.

Beebe, B., and Lachmann, F. M. (2002). *Infant Research and Adult Treatment: Co-Constructing Interaction.* Hillsdale, NJ: Analytic Press.

Benjamin, J. (2005). Creating an intersubjective reality: Commentary on paper by Arnold Rothstein. *Psychoanalytic Dialogues, 15*, 447–457.

Bromberg, P. M. (1993). Shadow and substance: A relational perspective on clinical process. *Psychoanalytic Psychology, 10*, 147–168.

Bromberg, P. M. (1998). *Standing in the Spaces: Essays on Clinical Process, Trauma, and Dissociation.* Mahwah, NJ: Analytic Press.

Bromberg, P. M. (2010). Minding the dissociative gap. *Contemporary Psychoanalysis, 46*, 19–31.

Broom, B. (2007). *Meaningful Disease.* London: Karnac.

Carroll, R. (2014). Four relational modes of attending to the body in psychotherapy. In K. White (Ed.), *Talking Bodies* (pp. 11–39). London: Karnac.

Clark, C., Classen, C. C., and Fourt, A. (2015). *Treating the Trauma Survivor: An Essential Guide to Trauma-Care.* Hove: Routledge.

Damasio, A. (2000). *The Feeling of What Happens: Body, Emotion and the Making of Consciousness.* London: Vintage.

Dethlefsen, T., and Dahlke, R. (2002). *The Healing Power of Illness: Understanding What Your Symptoms Are Telling You.* London: Vega Books.

Duran, E., and Korby, D. (2014). *Eduardo Duran on Psychotherapy with Native Americans* (Interview). Retrieved from www.psychotherapy.net/interview/native-american-psychotherapy.

Ferenczi, S. (1949). Confusion of the tongues between the adults and the child: The language of tenderness and of passion. *International Journal of Psychoanalysis, 30,* 225–230.

Friedlaender, Salomo/Mynona. (2009). *Schöpferische Indifferenz* [Creative Indifference] (Vol. 10 of *Gesammelte Schriften*). In H. Geerken and D. Thiel (Eds.), Originally published in 1918 with a second, revised edition in 1926 (München: Ernst Reinhardt Verlag). Nordestedt, DE: Waitawhile. (Original work published 1918)

Gallese, V. (2009). Mirror neurons, embodied simulation, and the neural basis of social identification. *Psychoanalytic Dialogues, 19*, 519–536.

Janet, P. (1889). *L'automatisme Psychologique* [Automatic Psychology]. Paris: Alcan.

Jung, C. G. (1992). Psychological types (R. F. C. Hull, Trans). In H. Read, M. Fordham, and G. Adler (Eds.), *The Collected Works of C. G. Jung* (Vol. 6). London: Routledge. (Reprinted from *Psychologische Typen*, 1921, Zurich: Rascher Verlag.)

Lannon, R., Amini, F., and Lewis, T. (2000). *A General Theory of Love.* New York: Random House.

Levine, P. A. (1997). Waking the tiger – Healing trauma. Berkeley, CA: North Atlantic Books.

Lewin, K. (1939). Field theory and experiment in social psychology. *American Journal of Sociology, 109*(1), 1–49.

Lewis, R. (2001). *Projective identification revisited: Listening with the limbic system.* Conference paper presented. Retrieved from www.BodyMindcentral.com.

Lewis, R. (2003). Human trauma. *Energy and Character, 32*, 32–39.

Lipps, T. (1903). Einfühlung, innere Nachahmung und Organempfindungen [Empathy, inner imitation and Organ sensations]. *Archiv fuer die gesamte Psychologie, 1*(2 u. 3), 185–204.

Mathew, M. (1998). The body as instrument. *Journal of the British Association of Psychotherapists, 35*, 17–36.

Merleau-Ponty, M. (1962). *Phenomenology of Perception.* London: Routledge & Kegan Paul.

Milner, M. (1981). *A Life of One's Own* (2nd ed.). London: Chatto and Windus. (Reprinted New York: Puttnam, Original work published 1936.)

Mitchell, S. (1988). *Relational Concepts in Psychoanalysis.* London: Harvard University Press.

Nolan, P. (2014). The relational field of body psychotherapy. *Body, Movement and Dance in Psychotherapy, 9,* 29–40.

Pallaro, P. (2007). Somatic countertransference: The therapist in relationship. In P. Pallaro (Ed.), *Authentic Movement: Moving the Body, Moving the Self, Being Moved* (Vol. 2). London: Jessica Kingsley.

Perls, F. (1969). *Ego, Hunger and Aggression* (Reprinted 1969). New York: Vintage. (Original work published 1947)

Pineda, J. A. (2008). Sensorimotor cortex as a critical component of an 'extended' mirror neuron system: Does it solve the development, correspondence, and control problems in mirroring? *Behavioral and Brain Functions, 4,* 47.

Pinkas, S. (2016). Psychic fragments and changing bodies: Theoretical and clinical applications of bodily reverie. *Body, Movement, and Dance in Psychotherapy, 11*(4), 206–219.

Rumble, B. (2010). The body as hypothesis and as question: Towards a concept of therapist embodiment. *Body, Movement, and Dance in Psychotherapy, 5,* 129–140.

Schore, A. N. (2009). Attachment trauma and the developing right brain: Origins of pathological dissociation. In P. Dell and J. O'Neil (Eds.), *Dissociation and the Dissociative Disorders: DSM-V and Beyond* (pp. 107–141). New York: Routledge.

Schore, A. (2011). Foreword. In P. M. Bromberg (Ed.), *The Shadow of the Tsunami.* New York: Routledge.

Searles, H. F. (1960). *The Nonhuman Environment in Normal Development and in Schizophrenia.* New York: International Universities Press.

Searles, H. F. (1979). *Countertransference and Related Subjects.* New York: International Universities Press.

Sheedy, G. (2013). *Between Bodies: An Implicit Relational Model* (Doctoral thesis, Middlesex University and Metanoia Institute). Retrieved from http://eprints.mdx.ac.uk/13063/.

Sletvold, J. (2014). *The Embodied Analyst: From Freud to Reich to Relationality.* London: Routledge.

Stern, D. B. (1985). *The Interpersonal World of the Infant: A View from Psychoanalysis and Development.* New York: Basic Books.

Uvnäs-Moberg, K. (2006, September 23). *Love, Touch and Oxytocin.* Paper presented at the 10th EABP Congress for Body Psychotherapy, Askov, Denmark.

Uvnäs-Moberg, K., Arn, I., and Magnusson, D. (2005). The psychobiology of emotion: The role of the oxytocinergic system. *International Journal of Behavioral Medicine, 12*(2), 59–65.

Warnecke, T. (2003, Autumn/Winter). Some thoughts on involuntary muscle. *Association of Chiron Psychotherapists Newsletter, 25,* 20–28.

Warnecke, T. (2009). The Borderline relationship. In L. Hartley (Ed.), *Contemporary Body Psychotherapy: The Chiron Approach* (pp. 194–211). London: Routledge.

Warnecke, T. (2011). Stirring the depths – Transference, countertransference and touch. *Body, Movement and Dance in Psychotherapy, 6*(3), 233–243.

Weiss, H. (2009). The use of mindfulness in psychodynamic and body oriented psychotherapy. *Body, Movement and Dance in Psychotherapy, 4*(1), 5–16.

Winnicott, D. W. (1951). Transitional objects and transitional phenomena. In *Through Paediatrics to Psychoanalysis: Collected Papers* (pp. 229–242). London: Tavistock. (Reprinted 1958.)

31

BEING MOVED TO TEARS

Somatic and motoric aspects of self-disclosure

Asaf Rolef Ben-Shahar

Introduction: Giving myself over

The body is the source of non-verbal communication – a distracted gaze and slumped shoulders, a lively look in the eyes, or animated hand gestures. We can all see and come to understand this kind of communication through learning how to read our internal body sensations (including our intuitions) and couple them with our observation.

(Westland, 2015, p. 2)

It had been a difficult week, one when life seems too much to bear, and the glass-half-empty is all that I can see. It is the beginning of the week and I am glad to have survived the weekend. I wish to conceal my difficulty. I want nobody to see. I don't want to share it with anyone; this is such a private pain. I want it to remain my own, mine alone.

Sharon, a supervisee, who is very sensitive to her surroundings, is about to enter the room. Thinking of her sitting with me, I get angry. I know she would pick things up, she would notice my difficulty, and me. I feel neither able nor willing to share how I feel. Moreover, I resent the thought of her noticing me against my will; the possibility of her drawing attention to me. It is too raw. Before our session even begins I notice myself skinless, defensive and invaded. Please leave me alone, please leave me be. Two trained body psychotherapists in the same room, both accustomed to look for body movements, for postures, tone, resonance and energetic fluctuations. What a disaster! Will she ask how I am? Can we just focus on her and her clients?

The dreaded knock arrives. Sharon enters the room and my body hardens. There is a smile on my face, but will I be allowed to hide? She sits in front of me. I notice myself hardening and preparing. Here it comes, here it comes. Oh shit, here it is.

She asks: 'How are you, Asaf?'

I do not want to spend an hour like that. I do not want to hate her. It's hard to be seen so I finally say 'I don't know how to answer that, Sharon'. In a moment, I decide to let go of trying so hard, allowing her to see me. I soften my bodily shell, a little less control. My body speaks, heavy, just by being there. Then I take a cushion and cover myself. 'It's not easy. But let's not go there today, ok? I can be present with you but cannot go to me today'. Sharon smiles and sighs. She understands. There is tacit understanding between us, I have shown myself to her, she saw. And now we can move on. Sharon respected the dialogue and kept it in its original, bodily, language. It makes it tolerable for me.

For years, in teaching the history of body psychotherapy and particularly relational body psychotherapy, Freud's notes (1913/1958b), relaying the reasons for using the psychoanalytic couch:

> I hold to the plan of getting the patient to lie on a sofa while I sit behind him out of his sight. This arrangement has a historical basis; it is the remnant of the hypnotic method out of which psychoanalysis was evolved. But it deserves to be maintained for many reasons. The first is a personal motive, but one which others may share with me. I cannot put up with being stared at by other people for 8 hours a day (or more). Since, while I am listening to the patient, I, too, give myself over to the current of my unconscious thoughts, I do not wish my expressions of face to give the patient material for interpretations or to influence him in what he tells me.
>
> *(pp. 133–134)*

Regretfully, I mostly related to Freud's refusal to be seen from a patronising stance.

As a relational body psychotherapist, self-disclosure has become a deserving platform through which to process client's material. But increasingly, I can appreciate the desire to hide, to claim my right not only to be seen, but also not to be seen. The trained body psychotherapy client learns to perfect their attunement to themselves, and to their surroundings. We provide them with tools for scrutiny of the BodyMinds they encounter; that is – to see us. '*Please, do not see me today. Can I adopt the psychoanalytic couch and just focus on you?*'

The facilitative surrounding for surrender

Psychoanalyst Emmanuel Ghent (1990) wrote: 'Surrender is not a voluntary activity. One cannot choose to surrender, though one can choose to submit. One can provide facilitative conditions for surrender but cannot make it happen' (p. 215). This chapter will focus on the facilitative surrounding for surrender in the context of therapist's embodied self-disclosure.

Therapist's self-disclosure has been extensively discussed in psychoanalytic and relational literature (Aron, 1996; Hill and Knox, 2001; Pizer, 1997, 2006; Rachman, 2001; Rachman and Ceccoli, 1996). In fact, for many therapists self-disclosure is seen as the main characteristic of relational psychotherapy. 'No single issue illustrates more clearly the interpersonal therapist's struggle between asymmetry and mutuality than countertransference disclosure' (Burke, 1992, p. 241). Today, self-disclosure is understood as a crucial tenet in holding the tension between mutuality and asymmetry (Ziv-Beiman, 2013), which characterise relational positioning.

In body psychotherapy, the therapist's willingness to share their own body experiences, verbally and nonverbally is a skill which deserves further exploration. Orange and Stolorow (1998) differentiate the skill of self-disclosure as the therapeutic stance of self-disclosure. In this chapter, my emphasis would presuppose a relational stance: while disclosure is a psychotherapeutic act, it is also a therapeutic position (Maliach, 2016). This stance is at the heart of relational configuration, which considers mutual recognition as one of the most important elements which could be offered in psychotherapy (Benjamin, 1990/1999; Pizer, 2012).

While Hill and Knox (2001) define therapist self-disclosure as statements that reveal something personal about therapists, Aron (1992) argues that every intervention or non-intervention discloses something about the analyst. He writes, 'Inadvertent self-revelation is inevitable, and in addition, I do believe that there are many times when direct expression of the analyst's experience is useful' (p. 481). I wish to focus here on statements, both intentional and inadvertent ones, made by our bodies; on occurrences where our bodies share our stories with our clients. I would particularly like to examine the choice therein or using Ghent's words – the choice to submit.

The aftermath of love in the afternoon

Let us leave the main road of body disclosures for a moment and take a look at Jody Messler Davies' (1994) *Love in the Afternoon* which originally shook the psychoanalytic world, but is now a celebrated paper. In it she shares with her client some erotic dreams and thoughts she had about him. It was not the first paper written about the subject, but perhaps the first time a woman analyst talked about it so openly.

Twenty years later, psychoanalyst Jonathan Slavin (2013) asked us to reconsider Messler Davies' intervention. According to Slavin, the intervention should not be considered self-disclosure, since it did not introduce anything the patient did not already know. Both client and analyst knew about the erotic tension. It had waited in the room to be named. Instead, he suggested, the intervention should better be understood as a moment of truth, a naming of what both parties were aware of but yet unable to name. Integrating Slavin's argument with that of Hill and Knox (2001), when we share something with the client that they already know (even if they haven't conceptualised it), it is a moment of truth. When we share something unknown to them, it is self-disclosure.

So, what of the body? Can we decide what to share? Can we monitor what our clients know about us? Can we conceal what we want? Is there any level of informed decision in disclosing through our bodies and in our movements? It is easy to relate to nonverbal disclosure as inadvertent, particularly because many body expressions and resonance are seemingly unconscious. Yet body-awareness can increase our ability to monitor movements, expressions and even gain some command over what we show and what we don't energetically (Keleman, 2012, relates to this as forming an embodied life). I believe that the episode I shared at the beginning of the chapter with Sharon was not simply an inadvertent passive sharing. I elected to submit, to let her see something. It was, to the very least, an informed moment of truth.

There are times where we choose to not share verbally yet our bodies speak. Yet the extreme inadvertent sharing is of less interest for me here. Although much of our somatic and motoric activity is inevitably transparent to the other, we can nonetheless exercise some level of informed choice. There is a short space, I believe, where that which is shown and even known has not yet been conceptualised. During these spaces, we are able to act – to illuminate aspects of ourselves – and share our subjectivities as a therapeutic act. Missing those moments often creates a gap between what the client knows and what they hear.

Inasmuch as body psychotherapy (and DMT) bring attention to somatic and motoric aspects, respectively, they also provide another platform for language, a legitimate language for sharing (and concealing). I am curious about the therapeutic act of embodied self-disclosure and naming moments of truth. The places where we do not talk, and let our bodies speak on our behalf are highly relevant to the bodily-curious psychotherapist.

Moving back to the main embodied road, three types of bodily and motor disclosures are offered by the therapist, demonstrating these clinically as well as offering some conceptualisation: (1) passive bodily self-disclosure: allowing ourselves and our bodies to be seen, (2) active bodily self-disclosure: be it spontaneous or inadvertent, these are somatic and motoric actions of disclosure through gestures, muscular responses, facial expressions and (3) resonance: the way the other person is alive in our body, the way we are alive in the other person's body (Boadella, 1982; Pinkas-Samet, 2016). Throughout this chapter, surrender is seen as the main compass for differentiating inadvertent sharing and informing one. It is not only what we elect to show, but also an agreement to submit. Therefore, the therapist's body-awareness (or lack of) and willingness to surrender could have significant impact on the richness of therapeutic relationships, and the therapeutic outcome (Fogel, 2009; Sella, 2005).

Taking off my makeup: Passive bodily self-disclosure

In his characteristically arrogant (yet brilliant) fashion, Reich (1967) stated, 'When it becomes possible through character analysis to read emotional expressions, the patient does not have to talk. If we know the patient well enough, we know what's going on without words being spoken. You tell me what you are by the way of your expression' (p. 5). Setting aside the limitation of any typology, particularly attempts at body-reading outside of its multi-layered context (see Epstein's, 2013, excellent paper on the subject), body-oriented therapies are as educational as they are therapeutic in teaching how to notice bodies and to better understand nonverbal communication.

As a therapeutic skill, body reading carries high ethical and transferential challenges. The main one, in my opinion, is the high potential for the expert, doctor–patient transference activation. When somatic and motoric awareness are cultivated, the natural tendency of clients to attune to their therapist is strengthened by the indirect learning experience they gain as body psychotherapy clients. To that extent, Reich's statement can be just as valid when considering the clients observation of us. If our clients know us well enough, they (sometimes) know what's going on without words being spoken. We tell them what we are by the way of our facial and bodily expression. Our clients notice us much more than we would like to recognise, and often-times they exercise grace in pretending they did not notice. For example, they might comment: 'Oh, you've got a new haircut. . .'; 'Are you ok? You look strange'; 'You don't approve of my new girlfriend; I can see it in your face'. While the therapist's observation is seen as essential to the therapeutic process, the client's observations often remain in the shadows; unspoken, not allowed, impinging. Nonetheless, the gaze is there, and it is of value.

Jade returned to supervision 6 months after she gave birth to her second child. 'I cannot bear being looked at by my clients', she said, 'They can see how broken and tired and empty I feel. It's supposed to be a blissful time but look at those black circles around my eyes'. Together, we considered the possibility of not showing her clients how tired she was. Having a break from being super-relational (can self-disclosure be useful if we have to share?) by applying make-up to look fresher, not as a false-self, but, in a similar vein to the vignette at the beginning of this chapter to retain her right for not sharing. I remember a similar debate with a supervisee who went through a unilateral mastectomy. After all, to be seen in our body is so exposing.

One day Jade brought Dana to supervision. Dana came to see her with severe post-natal depression and struggled to share her difficulties with her projected 'perfect' mother (who had five children, always functioned and seemed content and happy). She considered Jade too perfect to understand. 'If only she knew how much I struggle, I am not sure she'd ever come back to therapy', said Jade.

The next time we met, Jade told me of the following intervention. Dana came into the room and was quite upset. 'You cannot possibly understand how dysfunctional I feel', she told Jade. With a sense of right-eous protest, Jade reached out for her bag, and without saying a word spent a few moments removing her makeup. 'Oh my god,' said Dana, 'but you seem so together'.

Moved to tears: Active bodily self-disclosures[1]

There is an exercise I often run with groups when teaching relational body psychotherapy. I ask trainees to pair up into therapists and clients. Each pair is asked to spend a couple of minutes in silence, just easing into the position of therapist and client. They are then asked to let go of the roles, and assume a friendship, or peer position. How does the therapeutic position manifest in the body? What kind of holding does it involve? Can you compare 'the therapist's stance' to your normal one? The holding position of the psychotherapist has embodied implications. Withholding certain bodily information is necessary when assuming the therapeutic position. Some of this withholding is defensive, the rest responsible. As therapists, we protect clients from being exposed prematurely – or too extensively – to our subjectivity, so that they might engage with their autonomy (Mitchell, 2005). This is, of course, an approximation. We cannot eradicate our subjectivity, but we can submit to withhold aspects of our subjectivity to allow the other to explore their own.

The degree to which we submit our motoric and sensory experience to the shared relationship depends on many factors, among which are our therapeutic position and our beliefs and values. In discussing self-disclosure, Pizer (1997) elucidates,

> I emphatically believe that the degree and manner of a self-disclosure by any analyst is, and must always be, inextricably linked to that analyst's conscious and unconscious dynamics. Participation through self-exposure, to whatever degree and whatever the content, is necessarily determined not only by the analyst's technical framework, but by her personal boundaries, beliefs, and sense of comfort.
>
> *(pp. 454)*

To exemplify two sensory and motoric disclosures, the first is less controlled than the second, but both represent a continuum where the therapist makes an informed decision to be seen. For example,

> "I'm having an attack" Frances says.
> "Hold my hand" I say.
> "Please don't try to make it better" she says.
> "Just be with me" I respond.

Frances suffers from fibromyalgia. Her attacks are debilitating. We spent the first year of therapy with me trying to use every technique under the sun to make her feel better and failing triumphantly. Mostly, we sit in the dark with an alarm set to indicate the end of a session. In my personal history, I had fought to transform my body of shame into an embodied celebration. By the white of my knuckles I held on to this positive approach to body. I wanted her to delight in having a body.

Sitting with Frances in the dark was getting claustrophobic for me. My hand was sweaty. A memory invaded me. I am at a military base underground. It is pitch-black and I keep falling, and injuring myself. I hurt. It feels that the temperature in the clinic has suddenly dropped. 'Is it me or did it really get cold in here?' I ask Frances. 'It's you, Asaf,' she responds.

We sit together for what must have been 20 minutes or so but feels like eternity. My body is shaking with pain, with fear, with anger and with cold. Some of it is mine, surely some resonate Frances'? Her body too is shaking. Her hand is dry and mine is sweaty. Who is holding whom? In the darkness I can hear her breathing change and she starts crying; quietly first, then louder. I am surprised to discover that my own cheeks are getting wet. I must be crying too. No words are spoken, no interpretations made. Momentarily, our hands let go of one another and my hand reaches out for her face, touching her wet cheeks. Frances does the same and she can feel my own tears. 'I really don't like being a body right now,' I say. 'I know, Asaf, that's why I came to see you. You know what it's like.'

I had no control over these tears or my terror. My body responded very strongly when I was there, with Frances. But this is not the whole story. 'One cannot choose to surrender, though one can choose to submit', writes Ghent (1990, p. 215). Over the years I sense that I can increasingly loosen the tight holding over what I allow myself to feel in the presence of another and what I do not. Submitting becomes more possible although, strangely, not less painful. It concerns a gradual exposure of the other to my subjectivity, much like I gradually expose my daughters to my subjectivity.

They can see more emotions, more complexity. There is a degree of submission to the moment. Even though the memory, the physical response and the tears caught me by surprise, I did not experience a loss of therapeutic position. And then, Frances touched my face. She knew I was crying, she knew it inside her. It was, therefore, a moment of truth rather than self-disclosure. It was exactly this kind of intervention (which I was reluctant to engage with too frequently) that brought us closer together, and that Frances found most healing. The next vignette demonstrates a slightly more informed, semi-deliberate self-disclosure.

As Adam begins to speak I immediately struggle to stay attuned. His words bore me; I find it hard to remain empathic to his defeatist attitude. Or could it be the time of the day? I swallow my yawns. Like contractions, their frequency increases. He seems either uninterested or inattentive to his impact on me.

During one session, I toy with the idea of sharing with him what is happening to me in his presence, so that we may look at it together. I am not sure how to do that, yet the opportunity presents itself quickly. Here comes the yawn and this time, instead of stifling it I let it out, without concealing it. Adam stops. 'Do I bore you?' 'I don't know', I said, 'You have this impact on me, but I am not sure what it is'. 'It's funny. I feel like I have to speak without stopping. That there is a quota I need to meet, and even though I can see that I lose you, I mustn't stop lest I will not be given another chance. I so don't want to lose you that I lose you anyways'. I reply, 'I am sorry for yawning like this, Adam. I think I also wanted to speak about it and didn't know how, and I hurt you instead'.

Searles (1979) wrote:

> For the analyst to reveal, always in a controlled way, his own feelings toward the patient would thus do away with what is often the source of our patients' strongest resistance: the need to force the analyst to admit that the patient is having an emotional effect on him.
>
> *(p. 52)*

I believe that witnessing this impact, seeing it with your own eyes, can sometimes be more persuasive than hearing it. The yawn brought us together; we were both responsible for a co-construction of a distant, careful relationship. More reminders became a part of treatment later, as we began to feel transparent to the other – we both needed to be shown that we have an impact on the other. But that was a good beginning.

Resonance[2]

'Can you hold me really tight until I fall asleep?' my eldest daughter Zohar asks, and I partly delight in the opportunity to spend some quality time with her, but another part of me wishes to have some time for myself. 'Sure,' I tell Zohar and stay. I firmly hold her small body for a few minutes. At first our contact is all that I can feel, and it is a most precious gift. But then my thoughts take over and I find myself preoccupied with the many things I need and want to do once she falls asleep. Between my arms, Zohar irritates me, she wriggles and turns – I am waiting for her to fall asleep, but she is annoyingly restless, tossing and moving and not letting go: 'I cannot fall asleep like that, daddy,' she says. 'You are not sleepy at all; your thoughts wake me up'.

And she is right, of course. I take a deep breath, allowing myself to feel more comfortable, letting my body sink ever so gently into the bed; then I close my eyes and slow down; the things I have to do can wait till tomorrow. Thoughts are still coming and going, but they too give way to quietness and slow down their pace. I can feel Zohar's little body softening, her breathing is a bit deeper, as well as my own. My mind is drifting and floating as my body surrenders, yet I am not fully asleep. Zohar has fallen asleep, smiling, and a sense of freedom envelopes me, both soothing and exciting at the same time.

The capacity to sense the other through our own bodies can sound, as it is hoped that this description does, as a most natural and innate human ability. At the same time, when skilfully honed, it can establish and contribute to highly complex communication processes. Resonance is in my opinion one of the greatest contributions of body psychotherapy to the larger psychotherapeutic milieu. Yet, like touch, resonance is bidirectional – it is not only I who sensed Zohar. She, in her highly attuned nature, easily sensed my energetic activity and was unable to sleep.

That a great deal of communication between people occurs nonverbally is both common sense and broadly agreed upon (e.g. Benjamin, 2000; Eigen, 2016; Klein, 1960; Ramberg, 2006). 'Considering that words account for as little as 7 per cent of the perceived message' Heuer (2005). He goes on to say, 'a cure exclusively relying on talking is an impossible endeavour indeed' (p. 108).

Resonance is a central therapeutic skill in body psychotherapy and constitutes a significant aspect of relational work. Resonance describes a primarily nonverbal and affective response to what is happening in the other. It is a conversation taking place in an unmediated fashion between bodies and between unconscious processes. Freud (1915/1957) was deeply curious about this phenomenon writing 'it is a very remarkable thing that the unconscious can react upon another, without passing through consciousness' (p. 194). It was also Freud (1912/1958a) who recommended that the analyst 'must turn his own unconscious like a receptive organ towards the transmitting unconscious of the patient' (p. 115). This opening of our unconscious towards the other is attained through sensory channels – it is a bodily receptivity.

Resonant self-disclosure thus happens in two ways. First, we may share (fully or in part) our resonance experiences with our clients. This is an active disclosure. Relational body psychotherapists Hadad and Rolef Ben-Shahar (2012) demonstrate:

> Daphne is sitting with me telling me with great enthusiasm that something wonderful has happened, her partner asked her to move in with him, move with him abroad for a year, all of which he would financially support. 'It's a dream come true . . .' As I sit with her, listening to her words, I deeply yearn to join her celebration and am finding myself unconsciously copying her sitting position and facial expressions, yet my primary experience is an increasing contraction in my chest and shoulders, throat pain and dried lips, as well as feeling I'm losing my balance. I choose to share this dissonant experience with Daphne, between my desire to be happy with her and my bodily sensation. Daphne remains still for a moment, and then says with a tremor: 'yes . . . it is all happening way too fast . . .' the eyes that are looking at me know express fear and apprehension. I can breathe deeper.
>
> *(p. 57)*

Elad's self-disclosure is a clear demonstration of resonance. The therapist shared his internal processes with the client, from an understanding that this belongs to the intersubjective field. But we are not only sensing, we are also sensed and just like Zohar was attuned to me, so are many of our clients attuned to us.

Rod, for example, brought a dream to a session and told me that he had dreamed of me on a plane going back to Israel. We did work with the interpretation of his abandonment anxiety but I felt like a liar, I was really leaving England to go back to Israel. A week later he came back to therapy and said: 'Asaf, I don't know what has happened to me, but I dreamed that you left to Israel with your family'. It was premature for me to share it with him, but Rod sensed it and I had to confirm his dream. Had I not named the moment of truth, it would have easily become an empathic failure.

Rod was not a mind reader. He was attentive to his body (and to me). For me, this attunement is at the heart of what it means to relate. In my eyes, the phenomenon of resonance is remarkable because we have something to do with it, we can be receptive to it. I can submit into the intersubjective field in a way that will open channels of communication between the other and myself.

Conclusion

Nothing new has been conceptualised in this chapter. Instead, this author hopes to have inspired some thoughts about surrender, self-disclosure and moments of truth as they manifest in the body. He hopes to have demonstrated that between the seeming passivity of the observed body (which makes sharing inevitable) and the active showing of ourselves, there are shade of receptivity and submission which hold great potential for therapeutic engagement and for human communication.

It is the hope that body psychotherapy can contribute skills of observation and of speaking through the body in movement, breath, resonance and touch, enriching and deepening the greatest mystery of all that very remarkable phenomenon Freud (1912/1958a) pondered about, whereupon one body (or unconscious) can react upon another, without passing through consciousness. This is the mystery that allows us to meet, against all odds, as people.

Notes

1 An earlier version of this vignette appeared in my co-edited book *Speaking of Bodies* (2016, pp. 180–181).
2 Some parts of this section are excerpts from the chapter on resonance in my book *Touching the Relational Edge* (2014).

References

Aron, L. (1992). Interpretation as expression of the analyst's subjectivity. *Psychoanalytic Dialogues, 2*, 475–507.

Aron, L. (1996). *A Meeting of Minds: Mutuality in Psychoanalysis*. Hillsdale, NJ: The Analytic Press.

Benjamin, J. (1999). Recognition and destruction: An outline of intersubjectivity. In S. A. Mitchell and L. Aron (Eds.), *Relational Psychoanalysis: The Emergence of a Tradition* (pp. 181–210). New York: The Analytic Press. (Original work published 1990)

Benjamin, J. (2000). Intersubjective distinctions: Subjects and persons, recognitions and breakdowns: Commentary on paper by Gerhardt, Sweetnam, and Borton. *Psychoanalytic Dialogues, 10*, 43–55.

Boadella, D. (1982). Transference, resonance and interference. *Journal of Biodynamic Psychology, 3*, 73–93.

Burke, W. F. (1992). Countertransference disclosure and the asymmetry/mutuality dilemma. *Psychoanalytic Dialogues, 2*, 241–271.

Eigen, M. (2016). Where is body? In A. Rolef Ben-Shahar, L. Lipkies, and N. Oster (Eds.), *Speaking of Bodies* (pp. 125–129). London: Karnac.

Epstein, S. (2013). War is a crying thing. *Somatic Psychotherapy Today, 3*, 36–42.

Fogel, A. (2009). *The Psychophysiology of Self-Awareness*. New York: Norton.

Freud, S. (1957). *The Unconscious. S. E.* (vol. 14, pp. 159–215). London: Hogarth. (Original work published 1915)

Freud, S. (1958a). *Recommendations to Physicians Practising Psycho-Analysis. S. E.* (Vol. 12, pp. 109–120). London: Hogarth. (Original work published 1912)

Freud, S. (1958b). *On Beginning the Treatment* (Further Recommendations on the Technique of Psycho-Analysis I). *S. E.* (Vol. 12, pp. 121–215). London: Hogarth. (Original work published 1913)

Ghent, E. (1990). Masochism, submission, surrender: Masochism as a perversion of surrender. In S. A. Mitchell and L. Aron (Eds.), *Relational Psychoanalysis: The Emergence of a Tradition* (pp. 211–242). New York: The Analytic Press.

Hadad, E., and Rolef Ben-Shahar, A. (2012). The things we're taking home with us: Understanding therapist's self-care in trauma work. *International Journal of Psychotherapy, 16*(1), 50–61.

Heuer, G. (2005). 'In my flesh I shall see god': Jungian body psychotherapy. In N. Totton (Ed.), *New Dimensions in Body Psychotherapy* (pp. 102–114). Maidenhead: Open University Press.

Hill, C. E., and Knox, S. (2001). Self-disclosure. *Psychotherapy: Theory, Research, Practice, Training, 38*(4), 413–417.

Keleman, S. (2012). Forming an embodied life: The difference between being bodied and forming an embodied life. *International Body Psychotherapy Journal, 11*(1), 51–56.

Klein, M. (1960). *Our Adult World and Its Roots in Infancy*. London: Tavistock.

Maliach, R. (2016). *An exploration of self-disclosure in body psychotherapy* (MA in Body Psychotherapy). Anglia Ruskin University, Cambridge.

Messler Davies, J. (1994). Love in the afternoon: A relational reconsideration of desire and dread in the countertransference. *Psychoanalytic Dialogues, 4*, 153–170.

Mitchell, S. A. (2005). *Influence and Autonomy in Psychoanalysis*. Hillsdale, NJ: The Analytic Press.

Orange, D. M., and Stolorow, R. D. (1998). Self-disclosure from the perspective of intersubjectivity theory. *Psychoanalytic Inquiry, 18*, 530–537.

Pinkas-Samet, S. (2016). Other people's movements: Ethnologic perspectives on motoric armouring in body psychotherapy. *Psychotherapy and Politics International, 14*, 144–154.

Pizer, B. (1997). When the analyst is ill: Dimensions of self-disclosure. *Psychoanalytic Quarterly, 66*, 450–469.

Pizer, B. (2006). Risk and potential in analytic disclosure: Can the analyst make 'the wrong thing' right? *Contemporary Psychoanalysis, 42*, 31–40.

Pizer, S. (2012). *The analyst's generous involvement: Recognition and the tension of tenderness*. Paper presented at the Affective relatedness and therapeutic action, The Relational training programme, Psychotherapy School at the Faculty of Medicine, Tel Aviv University.

Rachman, A. W. (2001). Beyond neutrality: The curative function of analyst self-disclosure. In J. Reppen and J. Schulman (Eds.), *Way Beyond Freud: Post-Modern Conceptions of Psychoanalysis* (pp. 127–142). London: Opengate.

Rachman, A. W., and Ceccoli, V. C. (1996). Analyst self-disclosure in adolescent groups. In P. Kymissis and D. A. Halperin (Eds.), *Group Therapy with Children and Adolescents* (pp. 155–173). Washington, DC: American Psychiatric Press.

Ramberg, L. (2006). In dialogue with Daniel Stern: A review and discussion of The Present Moment in Psychotherapy and Everyday Life. *International Forum of Psychoanalysis, 15*(1), 19–33.

Reich, W. (1967). *Reich Speaks of Freud*. Harmondsworth: Penguin.

Rolef Ben-Shahar, A., Lipkies, L., and Oster, N. (Eds.). (2016). *Speaking of Bodies: Embodied Therapeutic Dialogues*. London: Karnac.

Sella, Y. (2005). Recovering and eliciting precursors of meaning: A psychodynamic perspective of the body in psychotherapy. In N. Totton (Ed.), *New Dimensions in Body Psychotherapy* (pp. 87–101). Maidenhead: Open University Press.

Slavin, J. H. (2013). Moments of truth and perverse scenarios in psychoanalysis: Revisiting Davies' 'Love in the afternoon'. *Psychoanalytic Dialogues, 23*(2), 139–149.

Westland, G. (2015). *Verbal and Non-Verbal Communication in Psychotherapy*. New York: W. W. Norton.

Ziv-Beiman, S. (2013). Therapist self-disclosure as an integrative intervention. *Journal of Psychotherapy Integration, 23*(1), 59–74.

32

OPPRESSION AND EMBODIMENT IN PSYCHOTHERAPY

Rae Johnson

Introduction

Research has established the crucial role of the body in navigating experiences of social injustice and in mediating the complex trauma of oppression. Multicultural counseling and anthropological research show us that embodied microaggressions (everyday slights, insults, and injuries enacted nonverbally) can cause significant psychological distress to members of marginalized communities (Sue, 2010). Recent developments in traumatology (van der Kolk, 2014) have helped us understand that the body responds swiftly and strongly to relational threat, and that individuals who experience oppression[1] (the systematic mistreatment of people within a subordinated social identity group) may manifest the somatic symptoms of post-traumatic stress, exhibiting signs of somatic dissociation, body shame, and restricted movement expression (Johnson, 2009; Scott and Stradling, 1994). In short, the body is a primary locus for the reproduction of oppression, and it bears much of the burden.

Because we work directly at the site where much of the damage occurs, somatic psychotherapists are uniquely positioned to address the embodied consequences and correlates of oppression. Through movement, touch, and body awareness, we facilitate a creative exploration of how life experiences are held in the body and transformed through engaged and embodied relationship. This unique emphasis on intercorporeal[2] connection positions us to work with the client's experience of oppression in ways that other psychotherapy modalities cannot. Not incidentally, as somatic practitioners, our professional history is rooted in the work of Wilhelm Reich, Marian Chace (Chaiklin, 1975), and other pioneers – people whose ideas and practices were often considered radically counter-cultural in their time.[3]

In theory, then, somatic psychotherapists should be at the cutting edge in understanding and working with issues of social justice in psychotherapy. However, although many somatic psychotherapy practitioners have incorporated a trauma lens into their work, social justice remains a relatively unexplored territory within current somatic psychotherapy research, theory and practice. Consequently, many somatic psychotherapy training programs do not explicitly address issues of diversity in their curriculum nor provide their trainees with the knowledge and skill to address complex social issues as they arise in the consulting office. As a result, somatic therapists may very well find themselves at a loss when confronted by diversity issues in clinical work, especially when those differences come with an emotional charge or political overtones.

Drawing on current research into the embodied experience of oppression (Johnson, 2009, 2015), this chapter articulates three steps that somatic psychotherapists can take to bring themselves into an experience of fuller contact with the somatic impact of oppression. Furthermore, it may assist in becoming more aware of the complex reactions that oppression elicits in themselves and their clients and feel more confident in navigating the territory of embodied social justice, both in the therapy session and in conversations with professional colleagues.

These steps are: 1) exploration of the therapist's embodied experiences and perspectives around oppression (including how the soma has been shaped by social norms and privileges), 2) critically examining learning (or that which has yet to be learned) about the embodiment of oppression through professional training, and 3) consider how personal and current perspectives on oppression might be communicated to clients through embodied interactions with them when in the role of therapist.

Step one: Beginning with ourselves

A hallmark of excellence in somatic psychotherapy practice is the insistence that practitioners wishing to facilitate a process of exploration for a client must prepare by thoughtfully and honestly examining our own experiences with respect to the issues being addressed. In working professionally with clients who have experienced oppression, it essential to have a solid understanding of how oppression has shown up in the therapist's life, family history, and cultural background (in my own explorations this has been fundamental). This is not to suggest the therapist needs to have had identical experiences as their clients in order to be informed and helpful (for example, in my case that I have personally experienced transphobic discrimination), but should enter the facilitation with some awareness of their potential triggers, blind spots, expectations, assumptions, and projections.

Some questions that might be helpful in unpacking therapist's embodied experience and understanding of oppression include the following:

1) Taking stock of your own life history of oppression, and how the experience of being marginalized and discriminated against has shaped your relationship to your own body. How are the things you like (or do not like) about your body related to the social value these attributes hold? How is your body's appearance or function implicated in how you navigate the social world? Are there restrictions in how you move and feel in your body that are rooted in the rules about how someone in your social group(s) should behave?

2) Pay closer attention to your visceral reactions when reading the bodies of others. We are socialized to track many social differences (race, ethnicity, gender, class, age, physical ability) through their physical markers, but are not always aware of the implicit bias we attach to skin colour, weight, facial features, dress, or gait. Do you associate the jerky body movements and slurred speech of cerebral palsy with a lack of intelligence, body fat with laziness, or dark skin with violence? Does it make you uncomfortable when you are unable to identify a person's gender by their appearance? Is a person in a uniform a reassuring or intimidating sight? Researchers at Harvard University are conducting a multi-year study using the Implicit Associations Test (Smith & Nosek 2010), an online tool that measures attitudes and beliefs about social difference that we may find difficult to recognize or acknowledge. Taking one of their tests (https://implicit.harvard.edu) can be a useful place to begin exploring unconscious stereotypes about people's bodies. They also offer some excellent strategies for reducing the unwanted impact of implicit bias on behaviour.

3) Own your embodied privilege. Peggy McIntosh (1998) conceptualized privilege as a hidden, weightless package of unearned social assets. She likened it to an 'invisible knapsack'

containing an array of special provisions, maps, passports, and currency. McIntosh realized that most of us are unaware of what our own particular knapsack of privilege contains and are largely oblivious to how often we rely on its contents to help us get by. Each of us carries a unique set of privileges, depending on our assigned membership in particular social groups, and many of these privileges are body-based. For example, my white skin allows me to browse through clothing shops in the town where I live without arousing suspicion, my ability to walk means that these shops are physically accessible, and the clothing I try on will be sized to fit my body. I can go shopping for clothes without ever thinking much about it, but someone without these three body-based privileges would have a very different experience.

4) Using our own embodied experiences and responses as a foundation, our engagement with issues of diversity, equity, and inclusivity becomes grounded in what's real for us, before exploring what feels true for others. If desired, a similar set of questions to those above can be adapted to guide clients through an exploration of their own embodied experiences of oppression and privilege.

Step two: Mapping the strengths and gaps in our professional development

For many somatic psychotherapists, the professional training offered both implicit and explicit messages about oppression and social justice. For example, my own somatic psychotherapy training provided a clear conceptual framework that asked me to set aside any personal bias with respect to issues that clients brought to therapy. However, I was not shown how to identify such bias when it came to social difference and was taught by instructors whose own unexamined beliefs about power and privilege could only be described as naive. So, while the explicit message given to me as a somatic psychotherapy trainee was 'bracket your bias' and 'be authentic', the implicit message was that unconscious bias around issues of race, class, gender, sexuality, age, ability, or religion did not need to be examined. In nearly all of the training I received it was assumed that simply being present in my own body and attentive to the body of my client would somehow transcend the differences in our social identities.

Anti-oppressive educator Kumashiro (2015) refers to this phenomenon as the invisible curriculum, which means people do not always learn what they are told they are learning, and sometimes learn things that no one (including teachers) realizes are being taught. This invisible curriculum almost always conveyed implicitly and/or by omission. For example, when a somatic psychotherapy trainee asks a question, the instructor's nonverbal response (perhaps an indirect gaze and hesitant gestures) teaches the whole class something about the topic that has little to do with the words the trainer actually speaks. The same holds true for those topics that are not addressed at all – no readings, no assignments, no class discussion, and no practice sessions is implicitly understood as 'not very important' or 'not really okay'.

To be clear, the point here is not that somatic psychotherapists are not well-intentioned when examples of social injustice come up in session, or that the basic concepts and methods of somatic psychotherapy are not congruent with a compassionate and effective approach to exploring oppression. However, they are sufficient, given the complexities of modern life and rapidly changing social landscape. Here are some questions that might be useful to ask about somatic psychotherapy training, as a way to begin 'unpacking' it before considering what further training or education to undertake:

1) Are social difference, privilege, and bias explicitly addressed as part of somatic psychotherapy training and/or ongoing professional development?

2) What messages are given about differences in social and role power in the therapeutic relationship? Are trainees encouraged to recognize these differences as salient, or to minimize them?
3) Are trainees exposed to the theoretical perspectives and lived, embodied experiences of members of marginalized communities?
4) Is there instruction on how to identify the somatic impact of oppression?
5) Are supervised opportunities offered for practice in working with clinical examples of oppression (not just with marginalized or oppressed communities)?

If answering these questions has helped trainees and trainers to appreciate the gaps in professional knowledge and skill, please consider how to enhance practitioners' ability to work with clients by undertaking additional training. Although some may believe they do not work with issues of social justice in their practice, it will most likely be the case they already do. If answering these questions has helped trainees, practitioners and trainers to appreciate the degree to which professional training in BP or somatic psychotherapy has been a preparation to work with the embodied impact of oppression please consider sharing your knowledge and skill with colleagues.

Step three: Understanding the embodied dimensions of oppression

This next step represents my commitment to sharing my learning about the embodied experience of oppression since completing my initial somatic psychotherapy training. Much of my learning has come from trainings in multicultural awareness and sensitivity, and from the research colleagues and I have undertaken into the somatic impact of oppression (Johnson, 2009, 2015). Just as much has come from working directly with clients i.e. listening to their experiences of marginalization and discrimination and helping them experientially unpack the impact of their experiences on how their body feels and moves through the world. While it is important not to rely on clients to educate us about things like racism, sexism, and homophobia, being an informed and sensitive witness can often teach us more than books or presentations.

My research suggests that understanding the embodied dimensions of oppression involves the exploration of two interlocking ideas; the first is that we learn about social norms and power differences through everyday interactions with others, and the second is that these power differentials are learned, enacted and reinforced through the body (Dovidio & Ellyson, 1985). Researchers in nonverbal communication estimate that upwards of 75 per cent of all interpersonal communication is conveyed nonverbally, through posture, gesture, touch, eye contact, and use of space (Argyle, 2013). Many decades of research have also established that the embodied dimension of interpersonal communication is consistently experienced as more 'truthful' than the actual words spoken, and that when our body language contradicts our spoken words, it is the nonverbal message we believe.

Given the power of nonverbal communication to influence perception and transform meaning, it is perhaps not surprising the degree to which interpersonal power dynamics are communicated through this medium. In fact, nonverbal communication researcher Nancy Henley (1977; Henley and Harmon, 1985; Henley and Freeman 1995) has argued that the nonverbal component of everyday social interaction (rather than laws or institutional structure) is the locus for the most common means of social control.

According to Henley and her colleagues, members of socially subordinated groups are constantly reminded of their inferior social status through the nonverbal messages they receive from others. They are also required to affirm that status in their response to those messages, as well as in the messages they themselves transmit. Henley argues that the repetitive and insidious nature of these subtle exercises in dominance and submission slip below the level of awareness (if in fact they were ever conscious), effectively internalizing social conventions to the point where they may no longer even feel oppressive.

These embodied 'microaggressions' show up in our everyday interactions as nonverbal interpersonal slights, insults, invalidations, and injuries between members of different social groups. They possess a power to wound because the perpetrator most often unconsciously transmits them, and because they often remain vague and difficult to articulate. This nebulous quality makes it difficult for the victim to call them out to the perpetrator in an attempt to rectify the situation. In a way, they are like paper cuts, seemingly innocuous but painful, with a sting that often lasts well beyond the immediate moment of injury.

Multicultural counselling theory and practice has long recognized the impact of microaggressions in the everyday experience of counselling clients and in the client/counsellor dyad. These relational wounds suffered by members of socially subordinated groups have been shown to have significant and enduring impact on their mental health and wellbeing (Sue, 2010). Being able to identify and respond to the microaggressions that clients report during the counselling session is an essential clinical skill, as is the equally important ability to recognize and repair the impact of microaggressions that occur within the relational context of therapy itself.

While microaggressions take many forms, the following areas are frequent sites for the asymmetrical interactions that are a feature of the nonverbal communication between members of dominant and subordinated social groups. As such, they are a useful place to begin exploring how embodied microaggressions might be a feature of your client's everyday experience, as well as how they might occur in your interactions with them.

Intimacy and informality

A key feature of nonverbal communication patterns between individuals with differing social status or authority is an unequal access to certain behaviours related to informality and intimacy. In these cases, the individual with more power is usually acknowledged (by both parties) to have the right to exercise certain familiarities that the subordinate is not permitted to initiate or reciprocate. The prerogative to initiate or increase intimacy and informality affords the person with more status more control of the relationship.

For example, a male therapist may begin a session by leaning back in his chair in a relatively relaxed posture, while a female client might maintain a more formal, composed posture even after receiving the nonverbal signal that a more casual posture is acceptable. That same therapist may touch his female client casually on the shoulder in the course of ushering her into the consulting room, but the client probably does not feel the same license to touch the therapist back. Applying these examples to one's own professional development, some questions for reflection might include the following: Does my relaxed posture really serve to invite my client to relax with me, or does it simply underscore the privilege of my role to initiate informality? Does my office/studio policy of 'no shoes' really serve to make all of my clients feel comfortable? Even though I always ask permission before initiating touch with clients, how would I feel if a client asked to touch me?

Gestures of submission

Certain nonverbal behaviours can signal subordination and submission, depending on the sociocultural group and the relational context. For example, nodding the head may not necessarily indicate agreement, lowering the eyes may not be sign of thoughtful reflection, bowing the head or collapsing the spine may not be associated with sadness or depression, tilting the head might not signal curiosity, and smiling may not be an expression of pleasure. All of these frequent non-verbal gestures, postures, and expressions can also be indicators of submission on the part of the client. It is important for somatic psychotherapists to question whether what we assume to be a client's nonverbal indicators of assent or contemplation might really be indicators of compliance or resignation. It can also be useful to explore the flip side of this dynamic as well, especially for therapists who may unconsciously enact submissive behavioural patterns. For example, I found that my own impulse to nod and smile at clients was especially challenging. I had come to associate these movement behaviours with being empathetic and understanding, when in fact I smiled at clients at least in part because I was concerned about the relational consequences if I didn't, especially with male and masculine-identified clients.

Use of space

Social norms and preferences around interpersonal space are highly variable across cultures, but also provide another example of asymmetrical nonverbal interaction. Early studies in nonverbal communication (Sommer, 1969) showed that dominant animals and high-status human beings are usually afforded greater personal space, and those with lower status tend to yield space to those with higher status. This nonverbal indicator of dominance can complexify a common occurrence in therapy – that moment when the therapist, experiencing empathy and an impulse to make contact, leans in towards the client. Perhaps they even move their chair a little closer, in an effort to signal their presence and concern. However, a client with a history of oppression may not necessarily feel more connected and supported by this gesture.

Studies of abused children and military veterans show an increased need for personal space in response to relational trauma (Bogovic, Mihanovic, Jokic-Begic, and Svagelj, 2014; Vranic, 2003), suggesting that marginalized and socially subordinated clients may also feel an increased need for space. For example, instead of feeling comforted by an increase in physical closeness, they might feel invaded and invalidated, and they may not necessarily communicate their negative reaction directly. Accustomed to having their personal space violated by members of dominant social groups, they may become inured to its impact, or may have learned to respond to the invasion with submissive and compliant nonverbal behaviours in order to appease the invader. In these moments, it can be very helpful for somatic psychotherapists to be especially awake to the dynamics of the interaction, and to be curious (both verbally and nonverbally) about what the client is experiencing. More broadly, I have found nonverbal boundary experiments to be very useful in helping clients recover the lost bodily sensations of invasion and marginalization, and to learn how to more clearly experience, communicate, and enforce their personal space boundaries.

Embodied trauma

In addition to becoming more attuned to the body-to-body transmission of microaggressions, it is also important to consider the embodied impact of these everyday experiences. Many somatic psychotherapists are already aware that the body bears a significant burden in coping with trauma, but fewer recognize that oppression is a form of chronic trauma whose effects align with many of the criteria of post-traumatic stress disorder (Scott and Stradling, 1994). Clinicians working with members of oppressed groups should watch for the physiological indicators of trauma even in the absence of a single incident acute trauma or known child abuse or neglect. Once identified, somatic psychotherapists can use the embodied relational field to help clients feel safe and grounded as a first step toward addressing the bodily hypervigilance, dissociation, and constriction that can result from macro- and micro-aggressions.

Body image

Research into body image (Grogan, 2007) supports the common sense insight that when a person is targeted for discrimination and marginalization based (in part) on their physical characteristics, body shame is an understandable consequence. Conversely, being valued for one's physical characteristics (for example, as often occurs with women) can result in self-objectification even when body ideals have been met. As somatic psychotherapists, it is important to recognize the significance of body image issues for those who have experienced oppression, and to take them seriously. At the same time, don't assume that clients whose bodies appear normative to you will feel 'normal' to them, or that those whose bodies are marked by physical characteristics that fall outside current social norms will not have a healthy relationship to their own bodies and resilience toward social attitudes around body image. My own research (2009) and clinical work suggests that one way to help address body shame in clients who have experienced oppression based on physical traits is to help them find ways to return to a felt sense of the body as a source of pleasure, strength, and skill.

To sum up this third step, the demonstrated significance of oppression on the lived experience of the body suggests that somatic psychotherapists wishing to become more informed and skilful in working with clients from marginalized groups undertake the following:

1) Educate yourself about the embodied experiences of those whose social identifications place them in a subordinated or marginalized relationship with the dominant culture, and about the variations in nonverbal communication across cultures. Learn to recognize these differences between you and your clients, and notice asymmetries in the use of body language, eye contact, touch, and the use of space. For example, learn how eye contact is used to signal differing attitudes about authority and respect, and how much personal space is considered 'appropriate' in various cultural groups.

2) Take into account a client's social identifications and relative privilege when evaluating their stress levels and ability to cope. Recognizing the embodied impact of oppression on our clients does not mean that individual advantages and disadvantages are not at play in people's lives, or that we are utterly at the mercy of social forces that determine who we are and what kind of person we become. However, if we have not carefully examined our own privilege or learned about how members of marginalized groups are oppressed, then we will certainly run the risk of assuming our client's struggles with life are largely a consequence of their individual characteristics and personal history, rather than also the result of their membership in subordinated social groups. Every client's experience and expression of self will be unique, based on the complex intersection of their social identities, family upbringing, and multiple other factors.

Conclusion

In this chapter, a sequence of steps designed to cultivate an appreciation of how oppression shapes the embodied lives of therapist and clients alike has been outlined. Integrating key findings from psychology, traumatology, and anthropology, these steps articulated how somatic psychotherapists might become more perceptive and skilful in addressing oppression with their clients. It is my hope that issues of diversity, equity, and inclusion are foregrounded in the professional development of somatic psychotherapists, and that we become more active contributors to the evolving discourse on social justice and embodiment in psychotherapy.

Notes

1 For the purposes of this paper, oppression is defined as the unjust use of socially-assigned power. Systemically, oppression is often enacted through laws and norms that subjugate members of a subordinated social group to benefit members of the dominant group. According to anti-oppressive educator Kumashiro (2000, p. 25), 'oppression refers to a social dynamic in which certain ways of being in this world – including certain ways of identifying or being identified – are normalized or privileged while other ways are disadvantaged or marginalized'. This understanding of oppression includes both established (and socially constructed) categories of difference (such as 'race', sex, gender, ability, sexual orientation, class, ethnicity, religious belief, and age) and a range of behaviours occurring on a continuum from a lack of awareness of social privilege and a disinterest in its impact on others through to overt acts of hostility and violence. Johnson (2000, p. 20) notes that 'Oppression is a social phenomenon that happens between different groups in a society; it is a system of social inequality through which one group is positioned to dominate and benefit from the exploitation and subordination of another'. He argues that it is through our implicit values and unconscious behaviour that we most effectively collude with a system of oppression, and thereby contribute to its maintenance in a society. According to Johnson, participation in oppressive systems is not optional, but how we participate is. Accepting privilege is a path of least resistance in an oppressive system where oppression requires no malicious intent, simply a refusal to resist.

2 The term 'intercorporeality', first elaborated by phenomenologist Merleau-Ponty (1962), suggests that our subjective and embodied sense of identity depends on being with other lived bodies. Each individual exists in a multi-personal field and this field conversely inhabits the individual (Tanaka, 2013). The concept of intercorporeality implies that we remain exposed to the other and can take the other's different perspectives on ourselves (Weiss, 2013). It emphasizes the role of social interactions in the construction and behaviours of the body and simultaneously asserts that our identity in relation to others is something tangible and bodily (Csordas, 2008).

3 See, for example, Reich's *The mass psychology of fascism* (1970) and *The function of the orgasm: Discovery of the orgone* (1973), both published by Macmillan, as well as Marian Chace's 1964 article 'The power of movement with others' in *Dance Magazine* (*38*, 42–45).

References

Argyle, M. (2013). *Bodily communication.* New York, NY: Routledge.

Bogovic, A., Mihanovic, M., Jokic-Begic, N., and Svagelj, A. (2014). Personal space of male war veterans with posttraumatic stress disorder. *Environment and Behavior, 46*(8), 929–945.

Chace, M. (1964). Dance alone is not enough. *Dance Magazine*, July, 58, pp. 46–47.

Chaiklin, S. (1975). Dance therapy. In Arieti, S. (Ed.) *American handbook of psychiatry*, second edition, volume 5 (pp. 701–720). New York: Basic Books.

Csordas, T. J. (2008). Intersubjectivity and intercorporeality. *Subjectivity, 22*(1), 110–121.

Dovidio, J. & Ellyson, S. (1985). *Power, dominance and nonverbal behavior.* New York, NY: Springer-Verlag.

Grogan, S. (2007). *Body image: Understanding body dissatisfaction in men, women and children.* New York, NY: Routledge.

Henley, N. (1977). *Body politics: Power, sex, and nonverbal communication.* Englewood Cliffs, NJ: Prentice-Hall.

Henley, N., and Freeman, J. (1995). *The sexual politics of interpersonal behavior in women: A feminist perspective.* London, UK: Mayfield Publishing.

Henley, N., and Harmon, S. (1985). The nonverbal semantics of power and gender: A perceptual study. In S. L. Ellyson and J. F. Dovidio (Eds.), *Power, dominance, and nonverbal behavior* (pp. 151–164) New York, NY: Springer-Verlag.

Johnson, A. (2000). *Privilege, power, and difference.* New York, NY: McGraw Hill.

Johnson, R. (2009). Oppression embodied: Exploring the intersections of somatic psychology, trauma, and oppression. *International Journal of Body Psychotherapy 8*(1), 19–31.

Johnson, R. (2015). Grasping and transforming the embodied experience of oppression. *International Journal of Body Psychotherapy 14*(1), 80–95.

Kumashiro, K. (2000). Toward a theory of anti-oppressive education. *Review of Educational Research 70*(1), 25–53.

Kumashiro, K. (2015). *Against common sense: Teaching and learning toward social justice.* New York, NY: Routledge.

McIntosh, P. (1998). White privilege: Unpacking the invisible knapsack. *Race, Class, and Gender in the United States: An Integrated Study, 4*, 165–169.

Merleau-Ponty, M. (1962). *Phenomenology of perception*, trans. Colin Smith. London: Routledge.

Reich, W. (1970). *The mass psychology of fascism.* New York, NY: Macmillan.

Reich, W. (1973). *The function of the orgasm: Discovery of the orgone* (Vol. 1). New York, NY: Macmillan.

Scott, M. J., and Stradling, S. G. (1994). Post-traumatic stress disorder without the trauma. *British Journal of Clinical Psychology, 33*, 71–74.

Smith, C. T., and Nosek, B. A. (2010). Implicit Association Test. In I. B. Weiner and W. E. Craighead (Eds.), *Corsini's encyclopedia of psychology* (4th ed., pp. 803–804). Hoboken, NJ: John Wiley and Sons.

Sommer, R. (1969). *Personal space.* Englewood Cliffs, NJ: Prentice-Hall.

Sue, D. W. (2010). *Microaggressions in everyday life: Race, gender, and sexual orientation.* Hoboken, NJ: John Wiley and Sons.

Tanaka, S. (2013). The notion of intercorporeality and its psychology. *The Bulletin of Liberal Arts Education Center, Tokai University, 33*, 91–98.

van der Kolk, B. A. (2014). *The body keeps the score.* New York, NY: Viking.

Vranic, A. (2003). Personal space in physically abused children. *Environment and Behavior 35*(4), 550–565.

Weiss, G. (2013). *Body images: Embodiment as intercorporeality.* New York: Routledge.

33

MICROMOVEMENTS

Filling out the movement continuum in clinical practice

Christine Caldwell

Introduction

To *em-body*, the prefix *em* connoting 'to cause to be in or make', could be seen as a growing into the body, or coming into oneself. To embody implies a conscious attention to and identification with one's physical self, but it can also include the ability to non-judgmentally reflect on one's body, to coordinate functions such as thinking with feeling, sensing, and moving, and to listen to and appreciate the signals generated by the body as relevant, usable, and meaningful. From this perspective, consciously working with such processes as breathing, sensing, feeling, and most importantly moving, can be seen as the royal road to an embodied life.

Living bodies are defined partly by their ability to move under their own power, whether that movement is cellular, systemic, or locomotor (Hanna, 1987; Sheets-Johnstone, 1999). Because of this, the field of biology has long studied movement, starting with single celled organisms and ending with primates, in a phylogenetic progression. Movement is also studied ontogenetically, from zygotes and the prenatal time, to a fully-grown adult (Fentress, 1986). Biology tends to classify both phylogenetic and ontogenetic movement along a mobility gradient, from autonomic to volitional (Allen, Bekoff, and Lauder, 1998). In wildlife biology, for instance, the mobility gradient is used to map the intricacies of animal interactions, seen as non-verbal communications, and these animal 'dances' are notated and organized to an extremely sophisticated level (Golani, 1992; Fentress, 1986).

Dance/Movement Therapy (DMT), because of its locomotor roots, carefully attends to a client's body when they produce observable movement, leaving autonomic and metabolic motions to biology and medicine, much like the rest of modern Western culture. It also tends to focus more on volitional movement, likely because of its artistic roots in dance. All dance therapists, for instance, need to extensively study one or more elaborate movement observation and analysis systems, such as those associated with Laban, Kestenberg, and Bartenieff (Payne, 1992).

This tendency to attend to only part of the movement continuum may be quite sensible, as it has long been known that there is a strong correlation between volitional movement and emotion, motivation, thought, trauma, and self-regulation, all the stuff of psychotherapy (Damasio, 1999; Fosha, 2000; Ogden and Fisher, 2015). The field of body psychotherapy (BP), on the other hand, attends to gross motor movement on a less sophisticated level, but has a history of including autonomic muscle movements such as reflexes, as well as cellular, organ, and fluid movement, linking them with psychological and emotional states (Aposhyan, 1999; Heller, 2012, 2016;

Keleman, 1985; Tantia, 2015). For instance, BP tends to value the intricacies of conscious breathing, and by noting how both autonomic and volitional breathing affects cells, tissues, organs, and systems as well as emotional and psychological states, BP bridges the small to the large motions of the body into a psychosomatic whole (Caldwell and Victoria, 2011). Clinical neuroscience also weighs in on the micro level, seeing the movement of enzymes, hormones, and neurotransmitters as the flow of both conscious and unconscious processing, linking them to physical and psychological health and illness (Cozolino, 2010; Pert, 1997; Porges, 2011).

This chapter will create an argument and a plan for unifying the smaller, subtler, and more unconscious movements of the body with the intricacies of its large, locomotor actions, as a way to understand embodiment and to bridge the theory and practice of both DMT and BP. Based in biology, the architecture of this bridge will involve a reworking of biology's mobility gradient in order to apply it to embodiment. Because larger, more conscious and observable movements have been integrated into both fields, this chapter will focus more on the micromovements that can be observed all along the Mobility Gradient (MG) (Caldwell, 2017). Micromovements are defined as small, brief, barely observable movements that can occur throughout the body. They often show up during moments of transition, stress, relational contact, or emotion. They are largely untracked and below conscious awareness but can with attention be consciously felt. Micromovements can also be seen as movement signals; communication attempts that have for a variety of reasons been relegated to a barely visible form.

The Mobility Gradient

To begin, the author proposes a Mobility Gradient that can be applied to both theoretically and practically any form of psychotherapy that sees movement as significant. This can comprise the client's motions, the therapist's movements, and the largely implicit dance of movement between client and therapist. While related to biology's mobility gradient, it borrows from various neuroscience, DMT, and BP traditions in order to create clinical coherency. For instance, in the field of BP, Totton (2005) has noted that body psychotherapists are trained to track, attune to, and make use of autonomic nervous system states both in themselves and their clients. Many body-centered psychotherapists, especially those that work with trauma, are alert to client histories where their body wanted to move to act on emotions or instincts, but for reasons of safety and survival they inhibited the motion (Fogel, 2009; Levine, 1997; Ogden and Fisher, 2015). This immobilization response can become habitual, with micromovements becoming the only hint at what action responses are being suppressed. Thoughts and emotions are also involved. Aposhyan (1999) asserts 'any thought also results in at least minute muscular responses, evidencing the body's compulsion to somehow *do* the thought' (p. 22). Keleman (1985) has devoted much of his attention to the movement of fluids, cells, tissues, and organs in the body, and how these movements literally create the shape, overall motility, and identity of a person. It is because these many fields already acknowledge and include micromovements in their clinical theory that we can feel more confident that our discipline is speaking to some important therapeutic utility. The next section will briefly describe the MG, and subsequent sections will examine therapeutic applications of micromovements along the gradient (see Figure 33.1).

From left to right, this reworked Mobility Gradient begins with Immobility, which has been shown to be crucial to our understanding of trauma responses (Levine, 1997; Ogden and Fisher, 2015; Porges, 2011). While there is still controversy about the details of the Immobility Response, the author asserts that there are two types of immobility. The first is a *freeze*, involving a simultaneous contraction of agonist and antagonist muscles such that high tension is experienced but

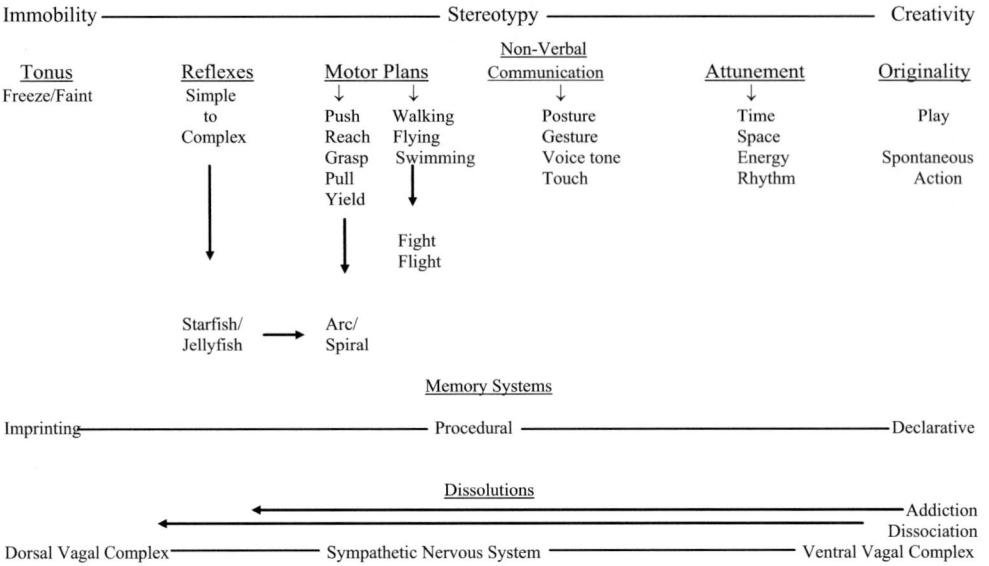

Figure 33.1 The Mobility Gradient
(Caldwell, 2017, p. 57)

no overt movement is produced; this state is typically accompanied by high sympathetic nervous system arousal. The second form of immobility is a *faint*, a powerful loss of muscle tone such that consciousness is compromised; it involves a dorsal vagal response and excessive parasympathetic nervous system dominance. While the Immobility Response is not necessarily pathological, various trauma professionals has been alert to the clinical significance of what lies underneath a client's use of very high or low tone to produce as little movement as possible. Also, important to note is that the word immobility is relative. When we include micromovements in our theoretical frame, it becomes obvious that there is no true immobility short of death. Another way to language this is that there are micromovements present even in immobility responses.

Next along the Mobility Gradient is Reflexes. Inherited and hard-wired, and from simple to complex, reflexes underlie, predate, and support all complex movement, and are associated with maintaining bodily integrity. Psychotherapies that work with reflex movement include those associated with Body-Mind Centering (Aposhyan, 1999; Hartley, 1995), with trauma (Levine, 1997; Ogden and Fisher, 2015), and with developmental movement (Frank, 2001; Marcher and Fich, 2010). In these cases, conscious movement that cooperates with and sequences the instinctual needs of reflexes can be critically important.

The next level of movement involves Motor Plans. Motor Plans are instinctual and motivationally based and comprise a set of basic movement patterns inherited by all species, such as flying in birds and walking in humans. They complement our structural body plan, yet need to be practiced in order to accomplish, perfect, and be built upon. They often involve a combining, coordinating, and alternation of complex reflexes (like flexion followed by extension) so that basic and fairly stereotypical motions such as pushing, reaching, grasping, pulling, and yielding can occur. Body-Mind Centering clinicians see these movements as crucial, associating them with organismic satisfaction, and working with clients to integrate them into more complex processes (Bainbridge Cohen, 1993; Hartley, 1995). In other body-centred psychotherapies, clinicians may not speak about motor plans, but they frequently use them. As anyone who has ever worked with a client who is reaching out or pushing away can attest, these motions have powerful symbolic and psychological meaning, and often are paired with emotional processing.

Building on Motor Plans, the next level of the gradient sequences to Non-Verbal Communication, where developmentally the infant begins to experience a connection between how they move and how their caregivers respond to them, such that they begin to use movement and sound as a communicative signal (literally their first language), and gradually become aware of and sensitive to the signals of others (Frank and LaBarre, 2011). This level of movement can be easily paired to attachment theory as well as to the implicit exchanges in the therapeutic relationship. Mary Main, one of the founders of attachment theory, was fascinated by 'the organization of the physical movements of an infant's body with respect to that of the parent' (Main, Kaplan, and Cassidy, 1985, p. 93). Trevarthen called these movement pas de deux's 'protoconversations' or action dialogues, and noted that the caregiver and secure infant were not only matching their movements, but were sharing inner states (1998). These communicative movements not only involve physical practice and trial and error, they are also contingent upon and crafted in relationship to a child's caregivers. They are powerfully interwoven with relational imprints, as well as the 'stance of the self towards experience' (Wallin, 2007, p. 1), or how we construct meaning from our experience.

When movement becomes communicative and relational as well as functional, it forms the basis of the next level of the Mobility Gradient, that of Attunement. At this level, movement is not only related to the ability to communicate, but to the capacity to feel and form a deep emotional connection to oneself, others, and the world. In non-verbal communication we form a sense that we can understand and be understood by others by shaping our sounds and movements in deliberate ways, ways that often become fairly automatic and even implicit with reinforcement. In attunement, this automaticity can be lessened, and the sophistication of movement increases, often becoming less predictable because it is much more contingent on present moment circumstances. The ability to use one's bodily movement to deliberately attune and mis-attune involves a sensitive use of time, space, energy and rhythm as the body flows into and out of contact with elements of inner and outer experience. This ability may predict such therapeutic milestones as a culturally relevant locus of control, and a sense of empowerment and embodiment.

A clinical question arising from this location on the MG might ask what happens to movements during mis-attunements. Answering this question requires further study, but developmental psychology provides us with some hints. Allan Schore (1994, 2012) and his colleagues have found that there may be a gendered quality to an infant's response to caregiver mis-attunement, such that boys use their body to protest, while girls tend to get involved with other objects, such as toys. While gender binaries are suspect, and cultural practices that solidify gender roles have been shown to be implicitly enacted and internalized starting from birth, this finding may nonetheless show that infants have multiple means of dealing somatically with mis-attunements. These researchers have also noted that infant responses to mis-attunement often occur in stages, starting with one strategy as mis-attunement begins, and switching to others when it persists. Later stage strategies often involve a kind of bodily 'giving up' on the relationship. Perhaps this involves a giving up on one's confidence that one's body signals will be seen and interpreted properly.

It has also been strongly asserted by Schore and others that mis-attunements are normal and that mis-attunements allow the caregiver to model relational repair. The ability to both verbally and non-verbally mend a relational rift may be just as important a skill to learn as the ability to attune, they note. These findings are often applied to the therapist/client relationship, noting that the non-verbal exchanges between them mimic and often directly enact relational repair and skill-building (Fosha, 2000; Schore, 2012). Clinically, this opens up a rich and complex discussion about how a therapist might use their body as a therapeutic tool, by means of movements that both attune and mis-attune to the client deliberately, for therapeutic effect.

The last level on the Mobility Gradient is called Originality. This level of movement occurs when there are minimal constraints on what must occur behaviourly, and when movement sequences are spontaneous and in the moment. This type of behaviour is often seen in artistic moments as well as play activities. The author has in other venues used the word 'bodyfulness' for this end of the mobility gradient, noting that bodyfulness can be seen as a step beyond embodiment, into a kind of embodied spirituality:

> I would define embodiment as awareness of and attentive participation with the body's states and actions. Bodyfulness begins when the embodied self is held in a conscious, contemplative environment, coupled with a nonjudgmental engagement with bodily processes, an acceptance and appreciation of one's bodily nature, and an ethical and aesthetic orientation towards taking right actions so that a lessening of suffering and an increase in human potential may emerge.
>
> *(Caldwell, 2014, p. 73)*

From the perspective of the Mobility Gradient and the micromovements imbedded within all levels of it, creativity or spirituality are not a crowning achievement, but rather are ingredients in the overall ability to oscillate along the continuum as circumstances and identities dictate. Creativity emerges from immobilities, reflexes, and motor plans just as much as non-verbal communications, attunements, and originalities.

The following characteristics exemplify the Mobility Gradient, and allow us, in the next section, to overlay micromovements onto the gradient as a way to construct clinical strategies:

- In the Mobility Gradient (MG), movement behaviour progresses along a continuum from immobility to stereotypy to increasing spatial complexity, unconstrained actions, and unpredictable sequences. This roughly parallels how movement develops from foetal stages into adulthood, as well as from one-celled organisms to social mammals (Fentress, 1986).
- The MG is a continuum, and no one place on the continuum is 'better' than another. Even though the continuum progresses from left to right both ontogenetically and phylogenetically, as humans we need automaticity just as much as we need originality.
- The MG maps movement along a continuum from actions that are the only behavioural choice an individual has, such as those related to defence and bodily integrity, to movements that can employ multiple means to achieve a single goal, an example being improvisational dance and play (Goldberg, 1992; Lorenz, 1971).
- Health is seen as an ability to adaptively shift along the continuum in a coherent, satisfying, and resilient manner.
- The MG sees movement as a product of internal motivations *and* social context. For instance, biologists assert that much of an animal's movement will only occur as a response to another animal's actions (Beck, 1992).
- Other theoretical constructs may map onto the MG. For instance, it easily creates a frame for how Porges' Polyvagal Theory operates (Porges, 2011), particularly its notion of behavioural dissolution towards increased movement stereotypy when perceived threats to bodily integrity occur. It works well with Body-Mind Centering's emphasis on the importance of reflexes that underlie voluntary movement and complex behaviour (Bainbridge Cohen, 1993), it corresponds well to findings in the trauma field regarding defensive movements (Ogden and Fisher, 2015; van der Kolk, 1994), and clarifies studies that correlate addiction

to increased movement stereotypy (Brust, 2010). On the more unconstrained end of the continuum, it may correspond to Csikszentmihalyi's (1990) concept of Flow and creative states.

- Movement along the gradient may involve different brain-based memory systems (Caldwell, 2012).
- Micromovements occur in all places along the continuum.
- This adaptation of the Mobility Gradient should not be seen as a mature theory. It is hoped that continuing discussion and research will refine it, and the author invites input about the MG's continued development.

Micromovements in clinical practice

Psychologists, from Freud and James onwards, have noted micromovements and seen them as relevant, while failing to develop a comprehensive practice that overtly includes them. For purposes of developing a clinical frame, a micromovement is here defined as a barely observable motion, accomplished with effort or the release of effort that constitutes a non-conscious or minimally conscious signal as to a person's status on the Mobility Gradient. They are individualistic, especially on the right side of the MG, and signal psychological as well as physiological status. Micromovements occur in moments of quiet in the body, as well as embed within large, whole body actions. Micromovements at the periphery of the body may hold less emotional charge than those in the core of the body, but this remains to be researched.

For example, a slight widening of the eyes, or a subtle slump of the spine may signal an immobility response. Immobility micromovements tend to initiate stillness, whether freezing or fainting. A small twitch at the base of the skull or slight curling of the fingers, may point to a reflex. These micromovements are usually flexions or extensions as well as orienting responses that are often observed when memories of sudden threats to bodily integrity arise, such as falling or being hit, etc. Of particular significance is when paired reflexes, such as flexing and extending, are out of balance, so that one dominates over the other and pulls the body into distorted shapes. A barely observable widening of the chest may be a nascent motor plan.

These micromovements look like tiny pushes, reaches, graspings, pulls, etc., that are related to motivational states such as thirst, hunger, or sex, or to organizing locomotion towards or away from something or someone desired or feared. A purse at the mouth, or a lengthening of the index finger may be the leading edge of a non-verbal communication attempt. Non-verbal communication micromovements often involve minute shifts of posture, gesture, eye gaze, head tilt, etc. that are seen around the edges of speech, or in relational contact. A minimal lean forward could signal an attunement action. Attunement micromovements use momentary shifts of timing, rhythm, space, and effort to match or synchronize self to self and/or other. And a tiny whole-body wiggle or a twitch at the corner of the mouth could be a play signal that presages originality. Originality micromovements contain small signals of readiness to play, invitations to play, and/or spontaneous motions that are done solely for the pleasure of doing them.

It is important to stress how small these movements can be. It is very easy to miss them completely in the traffic noise of larger gestural and locomotor movements. In fact, our non-conscious or barely conscious tracking of these micromovements may be how we experience our intuition as therapists. Rather than intuition being seen as some ill-defined sixth sense, we may be able to support what researchers such as Ekman and Rosenberg (1997), Hall (1981), and Montague and Matson (1979) have posited; that our intuition is driven by an attuned, subtle reading of another's micromovements, especially those in the face, and those related to emotion and arousal. Because many micromovements are strongly related to affect and intention, the conscious inclusion of micromovements may be the royal road to experiential processing in psychotherapy, processing that is based in what the client really feels rather than what they think they should feel or do.

An interesting question is why micromovements are not more visible. One way to think about this question is through the lens of post-modern identity theory, which holds that we are multiple selves and hold multiple identities, all of which express their own narratives (Atkins and Mackensie, 2008). These narratives are embodied and moved as well as being verbally expressed, yet we privilege some of these narratives while we suppress or oppress others (Caldwell, 2016). It is the privileged narratives that live in gross motor actions, where they can be seen by others and reinforced. The marginalized aspects of our identity remain in the shadows, where the movement expressions of these narratives can only peek out in small ways, much like a verbal 'Freudian slip'. In any system of oppression, it is not safe to express oneself honestly, so these incipient movements stay hidden and un-integrated; when evoked they result in barely discernable actions that can tell a vastly different narrative than the more visible aspects of identity. Micromovements in this sense represent defended against, suppressed, and affect-laden material that can be easily ignored, yet continually reasserts itself, and that any psychotherapy longs to access.

Clinically, micromovements can be seen as movement impulses that need attention and support to develop into movement sequences. They are body whispers that could, with assistance, become full, rich body narratives. In the authors work, called the Moving Cycle, they are focused on and gently centralized, then supported to develop at their own pace, and in their own way. This ability to tell the body's stories, its remembrances, its sorrows and its pleasures in its own original language system – movement – without having to be translated into verbal language systems that have their own, often distorting interpretations, may be one of the finest ways that body-centred psychotherapies can operate.

Support for this movement sequencing comes from therapist attention and bodily attunement, along with the client's high quality, focused attention. The author suggests that the therapist avoid getting into the business of interpreting and diagnosing micromovements. For one thing, it can be an abuse of power on our part (Caldwell, 2013). For another, interpretation by the therapist is clinically unnecessary, as the therapeutic power of micromovements lies in their ability to become conscious, held in non-judgmental attention, and supported to tell their story on their own terms. Meaning-making comes afterwards, at the client's direction, and as a by-product of the lived experience of the session.

Micromovements also develop into body narratives by aligning with their tendency to oscillate. They often organize in waves of effort and the release of effort (work and rest). They also respond well to being held in a balance between moving, breathing, and sensing, what the author calls The Therapeutic Triangle. In this framework, the therapist helps the client to self-regulate by making sure that breathing supports moving. If we move more than we breathe we dis-regulate due to low oxygen levels. If we breathe more than we move, we dis-regulate due to too much oxygen. If we are not tracking our sensations we do not know our current status, and therefore cannot regulate it. It is not an issue of how much we breathe and move and sense/feel, but how these three critical systems work together for self-regulation.

Within a session, the first task is to *identify* micromovements, gently and without interpretation. The therapist or the client will likely see multiple micromovements and must use clinical judgment as to which ones are more relevant at the moment. Because micromovements often signal marginalized aspects of a client's identity, they are often defended against, so it is extremely important that the therapist note them to the client in a friendly, open, and curious way. With practice, the client can identify many of his or her own micromovements. If the client assents, both individuals then focus on the small movement, giving it high quality attention, similar to the Focusing practice developed by Eugene Gendlin (Weiser Cornell, 2013) or Kurtz's Hakomi mindfulness (Weiss, Johanson, and Monda, 2015). This alters consciousness in ways that access the right hemisphere, relax left hemisphere storylines, and focus attention in the present moment.

Next, the therapist helps the client to *find associations* (rather than explanations) to the movement. Is there an image, a sound, a sensation, an emotion, a memory that comes up when the movement is done deliberately? The association is braided into the embodied experience of moving, so that the client can hold right hemisphere-based memories in their attention while moving. Often this combining of micromovements with their associations will begin to organize a more coherent movement impulse, such as a push, an upper body extension, or a playful grin. The impulse is then *nurtured* and allowed to carefully sequence and develop on its own, with support rather than direction from the therapist. This allows macromovement to be integrated with the micro in a safe and accepting environment, in the crucible of right hemisphere processing.

It may be useful to consciously repeat the micromovement, to play with its shape and size, transfer it to a less threatening part of the body, let the whole body do the motion, or to intensify the action. In any of these cases, the movement is experimented with so that it can be supported to more fully tell its story. It may be that classic forms of BP called this sequencing a *discharge*, or it could also be seen in DMT as an *enactment* (Koch and Fischman, 2011), but from a pragmatic standpoint the movement is encouraged to develop into a full, accurate, and visible expression. It does not involve 'getting an emotion out', as that makes the emotion more important than the body story. Emotion is felt, certainly, but the feeling is used to direct and inspire the movement rather than rule over it, a hallmark of emotional intelligence (Goleman, 1995).

It is important to once again emphasize that the therapist is not making assumptions about the micromovements. On a micro level, movement is NOT predictable, coherent, or obedient to therapeutic interpretation. It is highly symbolic, affect-laden, and right-hemisphere dominant, and needs its own authority to emerge, be supported, and to begin to speak through the moving body. In terms of the movement itself, again, more is not necessarily better. The movement is supported to have its own shape, size, rhythm, and effort patterns, ones that accurately tell the body story rather than develop into a demonstration of what the therapist thinks is healthier. Golani (1992) notes, for instance, that there is a difference in movement repertoire between two individuals when there is a difference of status between them. A high status person has a greater range of movement than a lower status person, and an individual's mobility decreases in the presence of a higher status individual as well as becoming earlier developmentally. This important assertion may have implications for how therapists understand their role in the relationship, and how they understand how dominance, hierarchy, and privilege can constrain client movement due to the inherent power differential in the therapeutic relationship as well as oppressive social forces. It will be important to research and write about the micromovement exchanges between the therapist and client; to see them as vital to an attuned and secure relationship, as well as a potential source of enacting bias and privilege.

As a movement sequence emerges and organizes and the session comes to a close, the therapist assists the client to appreciate and care for the nascent identity statements embedded in the motions. The end of the session involves a co-creation of ways to integrate the movement sequence, the new identity statements, and the derived client-centered meanings, into daily life. Thus, the client can *embody* the session.

Micromovements form the tip of an intrapsychic as well as an interpersonal iceberg, and as such can be leveraged for embodiment purposes in any body-centred psychotherapy. Micromovement work is currently specialized towards working with individuals and needs development in order to be applied to group formats. By integrating micromovements into clinical practice, and by appreciating their relationship to the client's status on the mobility gradient, body-centred healing can be enriched.

References

Allen, C., Bekoff, M., and Lauder, G. (1998). *Nature's purposes: Analyses of function and design in biology*. Cambridge, MA: MIT Press.

Aposhyan, S. (1999). *Natural intelligence: Body-mind integration and human development*. Baltimore, MD: Williams and Wilkins.

Atkins, K., and Mackensie, C. (Eds.). (2008). *Practical identity and narrative agency*. New York: Routledge.

Bainbridge Cohen, B. (1993). *Sensing, feeling, and action: The experiential anatomy of Body-Mind Centering*. Northampton, MA: Contact Editions.

Beck, C. (1992). The environment modulates the mobility gradient, temporarily if not sequentially. *Behavior and Brain Sciences, 15*(2), 268–269.

Brust, J. (2010). Substance abuse and movement disorders. *Movement Disorders, 25*(13), 2010–2020.

Caldwell, C. (2012). Sensation, movement, and emotion: Explicit procedures for implicit memories. In S. Koch, T. Fuchs, M. Summa, and C. Mueller (Eds.), *Body memory, metaphor and movement* (pp. 255–266). Amsterdam: John Benjamins.

Caldwell, C. (2013). Diversity issues in movement observation and assessment. *American Journal of Dance Therapy, 35*, 183–200.

Caldwell, C. (2014). Mindfulness and bodyfulness: A new paradigm. *Journal of Contemplative Inquiry, 1*, 69–88.

Caldwell, C. (2016). Body identity development: Definitions and discussions. *Body, Movement and Dance in Psychotherapy*. Advance online publication.

Caldwell, C. (2017). Conscious movement sequencing: The core of dance movement psychotherapy experience. In H Payne (Ed.), *Essentials in dance movement psychotherapy: International perspectives on theory, research and practice* (pp. 53–66). London: Routledge.

Caldwell, C., and Victoria, H. (2011). Breathwork in body psychotherapy: Towards a more unified theory and practice. *Body, Movement and Dance in Psychotherapy*. Advance online publication.

Cozolino, L. (2010). *The neuroscience of psychotherapy: Healing the social brain*. New York: W.W. Norton.

Csikszentmihalyi, M. (1990). *Flow: The psychology of optimal experience*. New York: HarperCollins.

Damasio, A. (1999). *The feeling of what happens: Body and emotion in the making of consciousness*. New York: Harcourt Brace and Co.

Ekman, P., and Rosenberg, E. (Eds.). (1997). *What the face reveals: Basic and applied studies of spontaneous expression using the Facial Action Coding System (FACS)*. New York: Oxford University Press.

Fentress, J. (1986). Development of coordinated movement: Dynamic, relational, and multileveled perspectives. In M. Wade and H. Whiting (Eds.), *Motor development in children: Aspects of coordination and control* (pp. 77–105). Dordrecht: Martinus Nijhoff Publishers.

Fogel, A. (2009). *The psychophysiology of self-awareness: Rediscovering the lost art of body sense*. New York: W.W. Norton.

Fosha, D. (2000). *The transforming power of affect: A model for accelerated change*. New York: Basic Books.

Frank, R. (2001). *Body of awareness: A somatic and developmental approach to psychotherapy*. Cambridge, MA: Gestalt Press.

Frank, R., and LaBarre, F. (2011). *The first year and the rest of your life: Movement, development, and psychotherapeutic change*. New York: Routledge.

Golani, I. (1992). A mobility gradient in the organization of vertebral movement: The perception of movement through symbolic language. *Behavioral and Brain Sciences, 15*(2), 249–308.

Goldberg, G. (1992). Dynamical systems theory and the mobility gradient: Information, homology, and self-similar structure. *Behavioral and Brain Sciences, 15*(2), 278–279.

Goleman, D. (1995). *Emotional intelligence: Why it can matter more than IQ*. New York: Bantam Books.

Hall, E. (1981). *The silent language*. New York: Anchor Books.

Hanna, T. (1987). *The body of life*. New York: A.P. Knopf.

Hartley, L. (1995). *Wisdom of the body moving: An introduction to Body-Mind Centering*. Berkeley, CA: North Atlantic Books.

Heller, M. (2012). *Body psychotherapy: History, concepts, methods*. New York: W.W. Norton.

Heller, M. (2016). The embodied psyche of organismic psychology: A possible frame for a dialogue between psychotherapy schools and modalities. *International Body Psychotherapy Journal, 15*(1), 20–50.

Keleman, S. (1985). *Emotional anatomy*. Berkeley, CA: Center Press.

Koch, S., and Fischman, D. (2011). Embodied enactive dance/movement therapy. *American Journal of Dance Therapy, 33*, 57. doi:10.1007/s10465-011-9108-4

Levine, P. (1997). *Waking the tiger: Healing trauma*. Berkeley, CA: North Atlantic Books.

Lorenz, K. (1971). *Studies in animal and human behavior* (Vol. 2). Boston, MA: Harvard University Press.

Main, M., Kaplan, N., and Cassidy, J. (1985). Security in infancy, childhood, and adulthood: A move to the level of representation. *Monographs of the Society for Research in Child Development, 50*(1–2), 66–104.

Marcher, L., and Fich, S. (2010). *Body encyclopaedia: A guide to the psychological function of the muscular system*. Berkeley, CA: North Atlantic Books.

Montague, A., and Matson, F. (1979). *The human connection*. New York: McGraw-Hill.

Ogden, P., and Fisher, J. (2015). *Sensorimotor psychotherapy: Interventions for trauma and attachment*. New York: W.W. Norton.

Payne, H. (Ed). (1992). *Dance movement therapy: Theory and practice*. London: Routledge.

Pert, C. (1997). *The molecules of emotion: The science behind mind-body medicine*. New York: Touchstone.

Porges, S. (2011). *The polyvagal theory: Neurophysiological foundations of emotions, attachment, communication, self-regulation*. New York: W.W. Norton.

Schore, A. (1994). *Affect regulation and the origin of the self: The neurobiology of emotional development*. Hillsdale, NJ: Lawrence Erlbaum Associates.

Schore, A. (2012). *The science of the art of psychotherapy*. New York: W.W. Norton.

Sheets-Johnstone, M. (1999). *The primacy of movement*. Philadelphia: John Benjamins.

Tantia, J. (2015). The interface between somatic psychotherapy and dance/movement therapy: A critical analysis. *Body, Movement and Dance in Psychotherapy*. Advance online publication.

Totton, N. (Ed.). (2005). *New dimensions in body psychotherapy*. Berkshire, UK: Open University Press.

Trevarthen, C. (1998). The concept and foundation of infant instersubjectivity. In S. Bråten (Ed.), *Intersubjective communication and emotion in early ontogeny* (pp. 15–46). Cambridge, UK: Cambridge University Press.

van der Kolk, B. (1994). The body keeps the score: Memory and the evolving psychobiology of posttraumatic stress. *Harvard Review of Psychiatry, 1*, 253–265.

Wallin, D. (2007). *Attachment in psychotherapy*. New York: Guilford Press.

Weiser Cornell, A. (2013). *Focusing in clinical practice: The essence of change*. New York: W.W. Norton.

Weiss, H, Johanson, G., and Monda, L. (2015). *Hakomi mindfulness-centered somatic psychotherapy: A comprehensive guide to theory and practice*. New York: W.W. Norton.

34

SAFETY IN PSYCHOTHERAPY

The body matters

Helma Mair

Introduction

Regardless of their theoretical orientation, the issue of safety in psychotherapy is generally considered important by clinicians, yet rarely explicitly discussed between therapist and client. As a practicing somatic psychotherapist and through my own experience as a psychotherapy client, I observed time and again how essential it is for the client to feel safe in order to benefit from therapy. This led me to explore the question of the client's experience of safety in psychotherapy as part of my PhD dissertation. Through this study, a complex and multi-faceted picture emerged, elucidating the components contributing to safety and the meaning participants attributed to their experience of safety in psychotherapy.

Considering the focus of the current handbook, this chapter will present two themes that were identified in the larger study (Mair, 2015): (a) the language of safety, and (b) connection and disconnection processes. From the perspective of embodiment, which can be understood as the ability to be present in the body, being aware of the sensations and energy flow through the body and using this to connect with the environment (Aposhyan, 2004), these themes are particularly relevant. They show that safety is primarily experienced in the body and that clients' responses to signals of safety and danger increase or diminish the degree of connection clients experience to themselves and/or to their therapist. A deeper understanding of these processes will help therapists become more attuned to their clients feeling safe or unsafe in the session and will benefit clients if their therapists are proficient in the use of interventions that foster client safety.

Background

Psychotherapists across modalities and theoretical orientation generally agree on the importance of client safety for the process of therapeutic self-inquiry (Dallos, 2006; Gendlin, 1996; Kurtz, 1990; Levine, 2010; Ogden and Fisher, 2015; Rogers, 2003; Sampson, 1990; Yalom, 2005). This view is supported by several qualitative studies, which have revealed the significance of safety for positive participant experiences and successful therapy outcomes (Davis and Piercy, 2007; Giorgi, 2011; Payne, 2001).

The issue of safety is particularly relevant in trauma therapy and requires therapists to stay closely attuned to their clients' experience of safety and danger during the session (Courtois and

Ford, 2013; Herman, 1992). Over the last two decades, somatically oriented trauma therapists have drawn on Porges' (1995, 2003, 2004, 2007) polyvagal theory to better understand how the autonomic nervous system is involved in responding to signals of danger and threat in the environment (Heller and LaPierre, 2012; Levine, 2010; Ogden and Fisher, 2015; van der Kolk, 2014). Incorporating polyvagal theory, they have devised useful tools that facilitate the return to homeostasis of an autonomic nervous system that has become dysregulated by the impact of trauma. The polyvagal theory will be briefly described in the following section as an explanation of the neurophysiological mechanisms underlying individuals' responses to signals of safety and danger.

Conceptual framework

From a clinical perspective, an understanding of the neurophysiological processes involved in how individuals perceive safety and danger is essential for the development and use of appropriate interventions that increase client safety. The most significant contributions in this area stem from Porges' (1995, 2003, 2004, 2007) polyvagal theory. In this theory, Porges explains how phylogenetically three different neural circuits have evolved with which humans respond to safety and threat in their environment. When individuals feel safe, the ventral branch of the vagus nerve activates the social engagement system that allows humans to connect with each other via eye contact, facial expressions, and vocalizations. When individuals feel threatened, they first turn to this system in order to try and avoid the threat by looking for support and help from others. If unsuccessful, the sympathetic nervous system initiates fight and flight responses to ward off an attack or get away from it. If escape is not available, the dorsal vagal branch of the vagus nerve mediates shutdown and freeze responses. Porges (2004) uses the term *neuroception* to refer to a neurobiological process operating outside conscious awareness that detects safety and threat and enables individuals to respond quickly and adaptively to their environment.

An understanding of the neuroception of safety can help clinicians provide a safe environment and interventions that activate their clients' social engagement system. This system's regulatory capacity can then be used to reduce maladaptive fight, flight, or freeze responses, which are particularly pronounced in clients with a history of trauma (Porges, 2004, 2007).

Qualitative inquiry

Interpretative Phenomenological Analysis (IPA; Smith, Flowers, and Larkin, 2009) was chosen as the qualitative approach epistemologically best suited to answer the research question of how clients experience safety in psychotherapy and what meaning they make of this experience. Influenced by the work of the phenomenological philosophers Husserl, Heidegger, Merleau-Ponty, and Sartre, IPA rests on the three pillars of phenomenology, hermeneutics, and idiography. In keeping with its phenomenological roots, it acknowledges the subjective nature of individuals' lived experience. The hermeneutic influence in IPA can be seen as the acknowledgment that observation involves interpretation. In IPA, this gets expressed as a double hermeneutic, whereby the researcher attempts to make sense of the participant attempting to make sense of his or her experience. Finally, IPA's commitment to idiography values a detailed and nuanced analysis of a small number of participants' accounts.

Participants and sampling

Consistent with IPA's requirement for a purposive and homogeneous sample (Smith et al., 2009), ten participants (nine female and one male) were selected from a pool of psychotherapy trainees enrolled in a psychotherapy training course at an Irish university or psychotherapy training institute. Nine participants responded to an advertisement for participation in the study circulated by training coordinators via email and/or posted on bulletin boards, and one participant was identified via snowball sampling. Participants were required to be actively engaged in their own personal psychotherapy with a minimum of 20 sessions completed.

Data collection and data analysis

A semi-structured interview schedule was used to interview participants a single time about their experiences of safety as a psychotherapy client. The interviews of approximately 1 hour duration were recorded and transcribed verbatim by the researcher. Names and identifying characteristics were altered for reasons of confidentiality and privacy.

The transcribed textual data were then analysed in accordance with IPA recommendations (Smith et al., 2009), following Smith's (2011) guidelines for ensuring quality. Each participant's transcript was read repeatedly to get a feeling for the flow of the interview, followed by exploratory coding and the identification of emergent themes. These were subsequently organized for each participant, and finally patterns in the form of super- and sub-ordinate themes were identified across accounts. N-Vivo software was used to help with the organization of themes.

Findings

The interpretative phenomenological analysis of the ten participant interviews yielded four superordinate themes with four subordinate themes each. The superordinate themes of (a) the language of safety, (b) safety as a process, (c) the transformative power of safety, and (d) the therapist's role in creating and maintaining safety point to a multitude of factors that affect clients' experience of safety. The findings show that safety can be understood as a language that consists of specific signals and develops over time in a process that is subject to disruptions. They also indicate that the presence of safety in the therapeutic encounter facilitates change and is mediated by the therapist's personhood and behaviour. Two subordinate themes relevant to the somatic aspects of experiencing safety will be presented here: the somatic language of safety as a subtheme of the language of safety, and connection and disconnection processes as a subtheme of safety as a process.

The somatic language of safety

The somatic language of safety refers to signals that are exchanged between client and therapist and are processed in the client's body as an indication of safety or danger. Participants who felt safe reported the presence of specific sensations that signalled safety to them:

> I can feel it in my body, I can feel my breath is quite even, kind of thing, slow and deep, you know, my heart rate is steady, you know, yeah. It feels kind of unhurried, yeah, still, hm, yeah. Like it's not effortful, if that makes sense, it just is, do you know what I mean, yeah, peaceful and there's a kind of a warmth in it, too, yeah, hm.
>
> *(Rita)*

Rita observes a slowing down of certain body functions, such as her breath and her heart rate. Coupled with sensations of peacefulness and warmth, this points to a physiologically calm and restful state. At the same time, Rita recognizes that these changes happen without her volitional input. Her comment that 'it just is' indicates that this state is not achieved through conscious effort but arises naturally and organically. When participants described their physical experience of feeling safe, a slow breath, a steady heart rate, a feeling of warmth, and a relaxed state were the markers that were most easily identifiable.

Conversely, a feeling of unsafety during the session manifested as hypervigilance, alertness, pressure building up in the body, muscular tension, tingling sensations, a rapid heartbeat, or a feeling of numbness or paralysis. Overall, the embodied experience indicated diminished integration and increased disorganization, as Fiona's experience shows: 'If you're not safe internally or don't experience that safeness, you're just too fragmented, you never feel whole'.

Although a history of childhood trauma has left Julia confused about the issue of safety, there are early warning signs when she shifts from a safe to an unsafe state:

> And I suppose that's why, you know my body tells me lots of things that I don't know, you know. Like I get redder, I get pressure up my neck, or different symptoms, you know, I could get tingling in my leg, or you know. So I know I'm alerted to something but I don't know what, I mightn't know what it is then, you know. I know I'm uneasy and I'm uncomfortable.
>
> *(Julia)*

Julia reports a range of symptoms that are indicative of heightened physiological arousal. She has a vague bodily sense that she needs to be alert to a change in her environment, but in the moment when it happens she does not have the capacity to reflect on it and make sense of it. A similar state of increased alertness in response to feeling unsafe is reported by Kay, who notes that her 'embodied experience was watchful, kind of analysing'. In order for her to make sense of why she is feeling unsafe in the session she allows her body to take the lead:

> And I think once I came more in touch with my embodied experience of bracing and pushing, it was almost, it's quite hard to put words on it really, it was through realizing what I was doing on a nonverbal level, I came into touch, and I was able to drop, just drop into why did I have that boundary, why did I not feel safe or why did I feel threatened.
>
> *(Kay)*

Both Julia's and Kay's experiences attest to the fact that somatic awareness may occur long before cognitive awareness. The body understands the whole of a situation before the rational brain can dissect, analyse, and conceptualize the individual parts. Like other participants, Julia and Kay respond to feelings of threat without having a clear sense of where the threat might originate from or what it might mean.

This efficiency of the body to pick up signals of safety and danger was considered by many participants as a reliable signpost to what they were experiencing in the session. They generally trusted their visceral and sensory experiences, or felt sense, as a dependable source of information. Rita explains how she knows that she feels safe:

> I think I could be, you know, a hundred thousand years looking for sort of cerebral evidence of safety, you know. And I don't think anyone could ever actually meet the criteria, whatever they are, you know. I don't think I can or anybody could, you know. So when I experience it, it's kind of somatic, you know, it's in my body. It's in that kind of 'Ahhh,' (sigh of relief) stillness and ease that I feel. And so then I know that it's there, some part of me then knows that it's there.
>
> *(Rita)*

Rita's view that safety is first and foremost located in the body was shared by many participants. Her comment that 'a hundred thousand years' are required to find evidence of safety via cognitive understanding attests to her disbelief that safety could ever be found via that route. When she explains how she becomes aware of the presence of safety and later qualifies this by stating that it is 'some part' of her that has this awareness, she yet again emphasizes the distinction between somatic and cognitive knowledge.

The benefit of including the body in the therapy session is highlighted by Jacinta, when she expresses her view that 'with a somatic awareness of what's going on, it's much more possible to create safety'. Like many other participants, she knows what helps her achieve a sense of safety more easily:

> That, coming back to this place of centredness, was just using the breath, and like one or two breaths with a certain kind of awareness were enough to come back to a place of being centred in the body, and once I'm centred in my body, I feel—and I'm very centred now—, I feel safe with anything, you know.

> *(Jacinta)*

Focusing on the breath was mentioned by several participants as a useful tool to help them return to safety. For Jacinta, breathing helps her feel more centred, which in her experience equates with feelings of safety. Similarly, Julia tries to find ways to cope with feelings of threat and unsafety when she explains that 'maybe what would help me to stay with it differently, would be to feel the support of my feet or, you know, my bottom in the chair or just something like that'.

These extracts show that participants are aware of how they can influence their sense of safety by attending to their physiological state. Breathing and grounding are two simple ways to achieve this.

Connection and disconnection processes

This theme shows that safety is not static but gets dynamically created between therapist and client. In the presence of safety, participants felt a deeper sense of connection to themselves and their therapist, whereas an absence of safety resulted in greater disconnection and intensified the various defence strategies participants used in the face of threat.

The link between feeling safe and feeling connected was observed by several participants. For some, feeling connected was a prerequisite to feeling safe, as for Jacinta, who comments that 'I feel more safe in the relationship now because my connection to myself is much better'. For others, the reverse was true, and greater connection arose from feeling safe. In Avril's experience, 'if you're safe, you're more, I think, connected to different parts of you, like your senses and your thinking and what's happening in your body'.

Jacinta's and Avril's reflections indicate that there is a close relationship between feeling safe and feeling connected to oneself and that these two experiences mutually influence and strengthen each other. A sense of internal connection leads to increased feelings of safety, and feeling safe deepens a sense of internal connection. As can be seen in the accounts of other participants, greater internal connection manifests as a linking of thinking and feeling, an integration of the mind and the body.

In addition to improved internal connection, participants also experienced changes in the connection between themselves and their therapist in an atmosphere of safety. Niamh describes the ease of connection she has with her therapist, which allows them to 'seamlessly move from the personal to the professional without there being any jarring in our contact'. This reflects the experience of other participants who felt that safety narrowed the divide between client and therapist. The safer they felt with their therapist, the easier they found it to relate to their therapist not from the perspective of the client, but from one person to another. A sense of light-heartedness and the ability to laugh about one's own or the therapist's foibles were common features.

All this was liable to change, however, when participants started to feel unsafe. A common coping strategy mentioned by many participants to deal with feelings of unsafety was to dissociate or shut down. In response to a therapeutic intervention that Niamh did not feel comfortable with, she remarks that she was 'shutting down internally, I suppose'. She explains what happened to her:

> I didn't feel I could express that, and I think perhaps it's only in retrospect that I realize it made me feel unsafe. I think at the time I think I probably disassociated from, you know, maybe feeling unsafe or whatever. But I did, retrospectively looking at it, I did feel unsafe, I suppose, in that situation.
>
> *(Niamh)*

Like other participants, when Niamh feels unsafe, she experiences an internal change that occurs rapidly at a bodily level. At the moment it is happening, she has no control over it and lacks a cognitive understanding of the cause and meaning of her sensations. It is only upon later reflection that these become clear to her. She expresses her newly discovered understanding twice, first tentatively by using the qualifier 'probably', and later more emphatically when she asserts that she 'did feel unsafe' in that moment. Her immediate response, however, is one of disconnection.

For many participants, disconnection served a specific purpose. Talking about her therapist's understanding of her reactions, Susan, for example, states: 'She knows how I break the connection and how I self-preserve and that's all because I don't feel safe in that moment'. Similarly, Liam observes: 'If I didn't feel safe, I would disconnect'. The degree of his disconnection is 'not to the point necessarily of dissociation, but I'm disconnecting sufficiently to protect myself'. As these extracts show, disconnection was seen as a useful defence strategy to ensure emotional safety.

For participants with a history of childhood trauma, the degree of disconnection was often quite pronounced. Julia, for example, notes that when she feels 'in some way threatened' she dissociates to the point of leaving her body. She describes her experience as 'I used n't to be present at all, you know. I'd go and I'd observe from outside. So I could be up there looking down, you know, that sensation'. The level of dissociation that Julia and some other participants with a history of trauma report diminishes over time as they start to feel safer in their sessions. For these participants, dissociation is a fast and efficient response to situations of perceived threat. Although Julia's double use of 'I'd' (go and observe) seems to make her an active agent of her actions, the work she does with her therapist around her tendency to disconnect shows that her dissociation is an involuntary and immediate reaction that does not require conscious thought or an action plan.

Other defence strategies that participants used to establish some distance between themselves and their therapist in response to feeling unsafe were fight or flight responses. Tara describes how difficult she finds it to stay with her process once feelings of unsafety have been triggered. She describes how she wants 'to get out the door, run away from it, run away from what I'm experiencing or what I'm feeling or what I think might be about to come'. The unsafety Tara experiences resides inside herself, yet she responds as if the threat was coming from her environment. Her urge to escape is reflected three times in her statement, attesting to the intensity of her experience. Not only does she want to run away from her present-moment sensations, feelings, and thoughts, but she also imagines them to take an even worse trajectory, adding to her anticipatory fear and flight response.

The impulse to fight as expressed through anger is also commonly seen as a useful strategy to keep potential threats at a distance. Tara comments on the advantages of this line of defence: 'It's kept me quite safe in the past, because obviously when you get angry, people will want to move away, you know'. Similarly, Susan observes: 'Like I didn't realize how much anger I had until I started therapy and how it would get expressed with her in the sessions, but that was all a way of trying to keep myself safe'.

Participants described various ways in which their therapists helped them work through episodes of disconnection. Focusing on breathing, grounding, and the therapist's supportive presence were all considered helpful. Jacinta, who due to her history of childhood trauma has a tendency to dissociate quickly, mentions the power of touch to reconnect her with herself and her therapist. She and her therapist have agreed that she can hold his hands if her sense of safety gets compromised during the session:

> That's been actually vital and when I can do it, you know, in those situations where I had gone so far away, it started to bring me back into my body again a little bit. But he offers his hands and then I can hold them if I want, so I have complete choice within it and it allowed me to start developing some sense of physical safety in the context of an intimate relationship.
>
> *(Jacinta)*

Whereas for some participants the emotional connection with their therapist was enough to navigate episodes of disconnection, Jacinta required safe physical touch to reconnect with her body. Through this, she was able to experience a level of safety with another person that was largely absent from her childhood.

Discussion

The findings show that the physical sensations associated with feeling safe are consistent with descriptions in the literature of decreased sympathetic arousal and heightened parasympathetic tone and ventral vagal engagement (Levine, 2010; Ogden and Fisher, 2015; van der Kolk, 2014). Safety allowed participants to stay within their *window of tolerance* (Ogden and Fisher, 2015; Siegel, 1999), which denotes the optimal zone between states of excessive or insufficient nervous system arousal. This zone correlates with Porges' (2003) social engagement system, which supports calm and relaxed states and connection with others. Participants' accounts showed that these states were conducive to linking the brain and the body, thereby fostering neural integration. According to Siegel (1999), such an integrated state contributes to health and well-being.

Participants' accounts showed that sense- and meaning-making often starts at the level of the felt sense, providing strong support for psychotherapeutic modalities that include the body as an equally important source of information as cognition (Aposhyan, 2004; Gendlin, 1996; Heller and LaPierre, 2012; Kurtz, 1990; Levine, 2010; Ogden and Fisher, 2015). The fast and involuntary nature of evaluating safety and danger described by participants is entirely consistent with the concept of neuroception as described by Porges (2004). The neuroceptively influenced move toward social engagement or defensive manoeuvres as outlined in Porges' (1995, 2003, 2004, 2007) polyvagal theory manifested as connection with oneself and the therapist in states of safety or as a break in the connection through fight, flight, and shutdown responses. There was, however, a substantial amount of variation in the degree of disconnection that participants experienced, ranging from emotional distancing to out-of-body experiences.

Implications for clinical practice

Clients' experience of safety on the level of the felt sense can serve as a guidepost for clinicians to track where on the continuum between safety and danger a client is (open to social engagement, ready for fight/flight, or going into a freeze). This is particularly important when working with traumatized clients, who may experience rapid and radical shifts in the direction of unsafety, coupled with high physiological arousal.

Somatically oriented modalities and trauma therapies in particular offer a variety of techniques and tools to deal with physiological arousal caused by clients' neuroceptive perception of danger (Heller and LaPierre, 2012; Hoskinson, 2015; Levine, 2010; Ogden and Fisher, 2015; van der Kolk, 2014). van der Kolk (2014) explains that breath, touch, and movement are three ways in which a dysregulated autonomic nervous system can be regulated. Participants experienced all three of these as helpful tools to reestablish safety. In their accounts, they mentioned focusing on their breath, feeling their feet on the ground or their back against the seat, or holding their therapist's hands as simple, yet helpful interventions that reduced the high sympathetic or parasympathetic arousal associated with unsafety.

Conclusion

The two themes of safety as a language and connection and disconnection processes are significant in that they show that the body does indeed matter when it comes to clients' subjectively experienced sense of safety in psychotherapy. Because safety and unsafety are first and foremost experienced as a felt sense in the body, it is essential that therapists develop an awareness and understanding of the signs and meaning of these state shifts in order to move the therapeutic process in the direction of increased safety. Porges' (1995, 2003, 2004, 2007) polyvagal theory serves as an excellent framework for understanding how the unconscious evaluative process of neuroception induces the fluid movement between states of connection and disconnection that clients experience during psychotherapy sessions. This is particularly helpful when working with traumatized clients, for whom these state shifts occur rapidly and frequently. It is therefore recommended that psychotherapy training programmes place greater emphasis on clients' bodily experience and raise therapists' awareness of the emotional and behavioural concomitants of clients' neuroception of safety and danger.

References

Aposhyan, S. (2004). *Body-mind psychotherapy: Principles, techniques, and practical applications*. New York, NY: W.W. Norton.

Courtois, C. A., and Ford, J. D. (2013). *Treatment of complex trauma: A sequenced, relationship-based approach*. New York, NY: The Guilford Press.

Dallos, R. (2006). *Attachment narrative therapy: Integrating narrative, systemic and attachment therapies*. Maidenhead, UK: Open University Press.

Davis, S. D., and Piercy, F. P. (2007). What clients of couple therapy model developers and their former students say about change, part II: Model-independent common factors and an integrative framework. *Journal of Marital and Family Therapy, 33*(3), 344–363.

Gendlin, E. T. (1996). *Focusing-oriented psychotherapy: A manual of the experiential method*. New York, NY: The Guilford Press.

Giorgi, B. (2011). A phenomenological analysis of the experience of pivotal moments in therapy as defined by clients. *Journal of Phenomenological Psychology, 42*(1), 61–106. doi:10.1163/156916211X567497

Heller, L., and LaPierre, A. (2012). *Healing developmental trauma: How early trauma affects self-regulation, self-image, and the capacity for relationship*. Berkeley, CA: North Atlantic Books.

Herman, J. (1992). *Trauma and recovery: The aftermath of violence—from domestic abuse to political terror*. New York, NY: Basic Books.

Hoskinson, S. (2015, October). *Working the physiology using trauma, not working the trauma using physiology, part 2* [Blog post]. Retrieved from www.organicintelligence.org/oi-blog/working-the-physiology-using-trauma-part2/

Kurtz, R. (1990). *Body-centered psychotherapy: The Hakomi method.* Mendocino, CA: LifeRhythm.

Levine, P. A. (2010). *In an unspoken voice: How the body releases trauma and restores goodness.* Berkeley, CA: North Atlantic Books.

Mair, H. (2015). *Making the implicit explicit: An interpretative phenomenological analysis of the client's experience of safety in psychotherapy* (Doctoral dissertation). Available from ProQuest Dissertations and Theses database. (UMI No. 3684563)

Ogden, P., and Fisher, J. (2015). *Sensorimotor psychotherapy: Interventions for trauma and attachment.* New York, NY: W.W. Norton.

Payne, H. (2001). Student experiences in a personal development group: The question of safety. *European Journal of Psychotherapy, Counselling and Health, 4*(2), 267–292.

Porges, S. W. (1995). Orienting in a defensive world: Mammalian modifications of our evolutionary heritage. A polyvagal theory. *Psychophysiology, 32*(4), 301–318.

Porges, S. W. (2003). Social engagement and attachment: A phylogenetic perspective. In J. A. King, C. F. Ferris, and I. I. Lederhendler (Eds.), *Roots of mental illness in children* (Annals of the New York Academy of Sciences, 1008) (pp. 31–47). New York: New York Academy of Sciences.

Porges, S. W. (2004). Neuroception: A subconscious system for detecting threat and safety. *Zero to Three: Bulletin of the National Center for Clinical Infant Programs, 24*(5), 19–24.

Porges, S. W. (2007). The polyvagal perspective. *Biological Psychology, 74*(2), 116–143.

Rogers, C. R. (2003). *Client-centered therapy: Its current practice, implications, and theory.* London, UK: Constable.

Sampson, H. (1990). How the patient's sense of danger and safety influence the analytic process. *Psychoanalytic Psychology, 7*(1), 115–124.

Siegel, D. J. (1999). *The developing mind: How relationships and the brain interact to shape who we are.* New York, NY: The Guilford Press.

Smith, J. A. (2011). Evaluating the contribution of interpretative phenomenological analysis. *Health Psychology Review, 5*(1), 9–27.

Smith, J. A., Flowers, P., and Larkin, M. (2009). *Interpretative phenomenological analysis: Theory, method and research.* London, UK: Sage.

van der Kolk, B. (2014). *The body keeps the score: Mind, brain and body in the transformation of trauma.* New York, NY: Viking.

Yalom, I. D. (with Leszcz, M.). (2005). *The theory and practice of group psychotherapy* (5th ed.). New York, NY: Basic Books.

35

TOUCH AND EMBODIMENT

Body-oriented psychotherapeutic applications of clinical touch

Michael Changaris

Introduction

Touch is one of the core nutrients in human development, yet it is ignored and often poorly understood by therapists. The first sensory experience to develop in the womb is touch. The first warmth of human connection is expressed in the wordless language of shared physical contact between a parent and a child. We develop our experience of emotions, self-efficacy, wishes, and cognitions, and even our sense of meaning and purpose emerges through contact with the world. The lack of physical touch in infancy can lead to death. In childhood, absence of caring touch has been found to impact development and increase risk for suboptimal academic performance, depression, disruptive behaviors, and anorexia, to list a few (Feldman, Rosenthal and Eidelman, 2014; Jakubiak and Feeney, 2016). Touch remains a vital human nutrient throughout the lifespan.

Touch and developing body awareness

In the womb, prenates learn the boundaries of their own hand through the rush of amniotic fluid on the skin and the feeling of tension and release of muscles in a cartography of motion and feedback from the world. Early motor activity drives the development of the somatosensory cortex. When a hand moves, it also activates the body's sensory neurons, feeding information back to the brain. This in turn gives the brain a better awareness of the hand, enhancing its ability to modulate movements. This learning process lays the foundation for the more complex self-in-world experience, known as embodiment.

Areas of the body, such as the back, often have fewer neurons in the brain devoted to them. This restriction is largely due to the lesser need for input from the back in how one navigates life. However, more insidiously, it may also be caused by simply not attending to, or 'inhabiting', the back with conscious attention. Sensation can remap the brain even in adulthood. Fibromyalgia (a centralized pain condition) can lead to fundamental alterations in the somatosensory cortex (Kim et al., 2015). Developing a sense of one's body in space and the different ways to engage with the world creates the relationship with one's self, others, and the world.

Touch and affect regulation

Affect regulation is the ability to engage flexibly with the demands of a wide range of emotional states. Affect or emotions have a cognitive component (thoughts, memories, etc.), emotion-related bodily states (muscle tone, heart rate, endocrine system, etc.), emotion-related physical state indicators (sensation, tension, gut motility, etc.) and emotion-related behavioral action patterns (e.g., clenching fists when angry, jaw tightening, etc.) (Schore, 2015). In his work at Yale University, Bracket focused on five core components of emotion regulation, using the acronym RULER: *recognizing* emotions, *understanding* the consequences of emotions, *labeling* emotions, *expressing* emotions, and *regulating* emotions (Rivers, Brackett, Reyes, Elbertson, and Salovey, 2013).

Touch plays a central role in affect regulation (Hertenstein and Weiss, 2011). First, touch can increase the brain growth in areas related to emotion regulation, leading to the development of affect regulation skills (Jakubiak and Feeney, 2016). Second, touch can help increase emotional regulation capacity through scaffolding an individual's current ability to regulate emotions. Safe compassionate touch increases the functioning of emotional regulation centers of the brain (orbital medial pre-frontal cortex, cingulate cortex, insular cortex, etc.) helping the brain to regulate emotions more effectively (Bjornsdotter, Gordon, Pelphrey, Olausson, and Kaiser, 2014; McGlone, Wessberg, and Olausson, 2014). Third, emotional regulation can be improved by touch through self-soothing activities, such as rubbing the outside of one's legs, stroking one's own shoulders, and touching one's hair (Gentsch, Crucianelli, Jenkinson, and Fotopoulou, 2016).

Affect regulation: Core components

Affect regulation can be further classified in terms of the regulation of emotional states as: (1) cognitive regulation skills, (2) co-regulation ability, and (3) implicit regulation capacity. Cognitive regulation of affect includes any skill that is chosen and applied through conscious or effortful action, whereby an individual, for example, takes a deep breath in response to the sensations of stress in the body. Co-regulation pertains to the interactional regulatory processes that occur between individuals or people and animals. Implicit emotional regulation is exerted through the automatic processes stored in procedural memory that modulate emotional intensity. Some aspects of implicit regulation are thought-based (e.g., automatic thoughts), some are body-based such as self-touch (rubbing shoulders or wringing hands), while some are based on conditioned reactions, such as certain smells triggering the fight/flight response.

Table 35.1 Types of affect regulation and affect regulatory touch

Affect regulation type	Common affect regulatory touch
Cognitive regulation skill	1. Petting an animal when stressed 2. Warm bath, shower, soft clothing or putting on lotion 3. Taking a deep breath to regulate
Co-regulation processes	1. Putting hand on friend's back 2. Seeking a hug 3. Massage or bodywork 4. Regular physical contact between members of a couple
Implicit emotion regulation capacity	1. Rubbing outside of legs when stressed 2. Twirling hair in hand 3. Rubbing arms, face or eyes

Embodiment in physical and mental health

The challenge in understanding embodiment is that it represents a fundamental shift in the ways of knowing. A good working definition of embodiment is provided by the computer scientists who work with embodied cognitions. Embodied cognition holds that intelligent behavior is an emergent property of the interaction between the brain, the body, and the world.

Thus far, the main challenge with understanding the embodiment has been that it always has a context, while scientific research is typically conducted in a decontextualized and highly limited frame. This approach has resulted in neglecting entire aspects of the interiority that drives behavior. In one such study, Skinnerians attempted to get a mouse to sit on a chair through operant conditioning, failing to appreciate that sitting is an adaptive behavior for the human (and a not very mouse-like) body. Embodiment is rooted in the qualia of our self as it is premised on the moment-to-moment dialog with inner and outer changes. In other words, embodiment is both a personal and contextual process. Exploring some of its core aspects can help in elucidating its role in how touch interacts with health and self.

Awareness: Embodiment is rooted in interoceptive and exteroceptive awareness. Interoceptive awareness tracks the changing inner states of self, whereas exteroceptive awareness engages with the fluid movements of external events. The integrated dance as attention saccades (see mental saccade) through inner sensations and perceptions stiches together the felt experience and an embodied state. Safe clinical touch can draw awareness into a neglected area of the body while simultaneously activating affect regulation centers of the brain, leading to a new experience of embodied self. In a family therapy session, a therapist can support a parent to put a hand on the bowed back of a child who weeps after saying how overwhelmed he/she is. The touch begins to soothe and smooth the tearful convulsions of the child's body, thereby increasing coherent regulated motions.

Skillfulness/mastery: Increased awareness of self-states and their relationship with context leads to opportunity for growth in coping skills and mastery experiences. For instance, young children may not have any understanding of what to do with the intensity of sadness that grips their chest when they have to say goodbye to a friend as they move. A parent can help scaffold awareness of the bodily state by holding the child as she cries. Through the experience with the parent the child gradually learns how to cope with this difficult feeling and gains skills and mastery in coping with the inner states.

Coherent integration: Extending one's hand to grab a glass of water requires a symphony of coherent rhythms of cells that fire, cells that don't fire, and feedback from the world. There is a tight choreography in each motion in the body, from the coherent contraction and relaxation of peristalsis in the gut, to the rhythm of facial expressions, vocal tones and bodily states present in any human communication. When this coherence is disrupted, it places stress on the body, relationships, and the self-state. Payne, Levine and Crane-Godreau (2015) described stress reactions as the inability for a body to shift in a coherent manner between what they called preparatory sets. They identify preparatory sets that prime action through a coherent interaction between posture, breathing, autonomic functions, motivational/emotional states, attention and expectation of outcomes. Stress is induced when the body has a preparatory set that is rigid, fixed or not appropriate to context.

Clinical touch deprivation

There are limits to what can be said in words. The provocative title 'Cognitive affect regulation fails the stress test' of the study conducted by Raio, Orederu, Palazzolo, Shurick, and Phelps (2013) speaks to this clearly. Upon exploring the limits of verbal impact on regulation, these authors concluded that cognitions have limited impact on cortisol levels. A therapist's attempt to verbally support their client to regulate their emotions may be lacking a key nutrient in the interpersonal dynamic that enhances its bodily aspects (Jakubiak and Feeney, 2016). Although a client may not be able to articulate it, the lack of a particular nutrient can be felt as a profound absence in relatedness.

Touch as a key nutrient in human psychobiological change

As touch is one of the core 'atomic' components of self-regulation, it is a key element in the development of self-regulatory capacities (Gentsch et al., 2016). We can easily communicate and understand emotions through physical contact. Early life interactions educate the body (including the brain), the endocrine system, and other regulatory processes about what is required to function in and respond to the world (Fleming, O'Day, and Kraemer, 1999; Schore, 1996).

The science of psychology has traditionally been based on a cognitive-centric view of the self, and a brain-centric view of the mind, neither of which is supported by the currently available data. A non-verbal dialog between the body of a parent and that of child teaches the child's endocrine system and tunes the autonomic nervous system, just as the child learns from parents how to say 'ma ma'. For instance, skin-to-skin contact between pre-term infants and their parents supports the establishment of the development and maturation of the infant's heart rate (Feldman and Eidelman, 2003).

Table 35.2 Key impacts of touch in development of embodied affect regulation

Biological impacts of touch	*Social impacts of touch*	*Psychological impacts of touch*
Setting sleep cycles and circadian rhythm.	Development of Theory of Mind (ToM) permits understanding of one's own inner state and making predictions about others.	Stability in bodily felt states, e.g., pleasure, discomfort, stress, frustration, cold, tiredness.
Metabolic regulation: • Diurnal cortisol. • Metabolism. • Heart rate. • Cortisol reactance.	Co-regulation established: Self-other dyads are felt as safe and responsive to needs.	Neurocognitive development: • Increased ability to habituate to stimuli. • Maturation of attentional capacity.
Development affect regulation brain structures: • Insular Cortex (bodily sensations of affect). • Cingulate Cortex (mediates between bodily and cognitive aspects of affect). • Dorsal Lateral Pre-Frontal Cortex (pleasure).	Communication and openness to others in stress states: • Turning towards others for comfort vs. independent self-soothing. • Serve-and-return interactions.	Experience of efficacy in the developmental moment and coping strategies: • Turning towards others in stress. • Self-soothing actions, e.g. self-touch. • Communication of need state.
Changes in neuromodulators: • Oxytocin levels. • Dopamine levels. • Serotonin levels. • Norepinephrine levels. • Leptin/Ghrelin levels.	Self-awareness of bodily states when in a difficult state while in social contact.	Expectancies related to negative affect states e.g. difficult emotions are paired with soothing.

The neuroendocrine programing that occurs in early years can change the direction of health for a lifetime (Cicchetti, Rogosch, Toth, and Sturge-Apple, 2011). Profound lifetime changes in cortisol levels have been noted in primates that were removed from their parents for even a short time when they were infants. Children who experience more than four adverse childhood events on the ACEs scales have increased risk of developing heart disease and diabetes in their lifetime, respectively (Felitti et al., 1998). Some of the biopsychosocial impacts of touch are in Table 35.2.

Body-oriented touch treatment for development of the embodied self

Multiple systems of touch are examined in research and are adopted in body psychotherapy and other forms of touch therapies. Some researchers have focused on types of touch, differentiating, for example, affectionate touch, coercive touch, and mechanical touch. For instance, in intensive care units (ICUs), there is a tendency to use mechanical or instrumental touch, which is always goal-oriented, i.e. its objective is to restore patient's health (Henricson, Ersson, Määttä, Segesten, and Berglund, 2008).

Touch communicates emotions, offers regulation, teaches about muscle tension, and provides a scaffolding as the individual enters into contact with his/her emotional state – a clinician who can reflect in direct physiology-to-physiology communication. Safe clinical touch confers new emotional regulation capacity in its primary language, the language of sensation and experience.

Embodied touch: Five core types of touch

In this section, three core components of touch and the pertinent five core applications of touch in treatment are explored. The three core components of touch are: (1) attention and intention, (2) attunement/serve-and-return style, and (3) emotional dialog and resonance:

1   *Attention and intention:* Attention and intention are key aspects of effective clinical touch. Attention has multiple components, one of which pertains to the focus of attention in the contact. In some forms of clinical touch, attention is placed at the boundary of contact. This creates a sensation that increases orientation and safety through the felt experience of one's boundary being respected.

In touch work, there is a need to make micro adjustments in contact. The attention to small braces or changes in tone can indicate the patient's inner state, allowing the clinician to adjust the contact to mirror a clearer respect for the level of pressure that supports the boundary of contact. However, in many cases, while the physical pressure is appropriate, the quality of the attention needs to be adjusted. To the client, it can feel like the attention itself is pushing past a boundary. In order to address this issue, the clinician can, while leaving his/her hand at the same level of pressure, move his/her inner attention back and away. Attention allows the clinician the ability to highlight changes that support growth in the same way that a well-formulated question highlights aspects of client experience.

While attention supports processes that are already in motion, intention guides the interaction in a desired direction. Intention during safe compassionate clinical touch is conveyed through the quality of the touch. The intention behind the touch is like vocal tone to verbal communication. It sets the emotional quality. The intention behind touch in effect communicates at the limbic level of the brain what the quality of the relationship is at this time. For instance, if a clinician evokes an inner state of open and receptive listening, this communicates to the client's tissues some qualia of relatedness that is respectful.

2   *Attunement/serve-and-return:* Attunement is the experience of being reflected in one's current state. It is in essence mirroring of the current state, thus promoting safety and maintaining connection. The serve-and-return style allows for differences in states between two or more individuals to be experienced as safe, and for one's boundaried experience to be respected. In this interactional pattern, the experience (the serve) is met by the other, who reciprocates while adding his/her own spin (return). At times, in a therapeutic interaction, an individual requires high amounts of attunement in order to tolerate and experience the self-state in a relationship. A good clinical measure of relational resilience is how much attunement an individual requires.

3   *Emotional dialog and resonance:* Physical touch is the basic building block of the experiences of emotional dialog and resonance. These experiences start in infancy and continue through a lifetime. As such, touch affects the growth of innate self-regulation and allows new states of organismic functioning to develop. For example, in a study of twins receiving skin-to-skin contact, the mother's body would match the temperature of each of her infants on resting on different sides of her body.

Clinical example: Emotional dialog and resonance

A patient lies down on the table gazing up softly. The clinician asks where contact would feel good, and the patient indicates the shoulder. Through a series of micro-adjustments of attention and intention, the tissues begin to respond by relaxing and the patient verbally communicates that the contact 'feels right'. This allows the clinician to enter more deeply into a resonant emotional dialog.

As the client describes his/her challenges, muscles in the shoulder brace and tremble. The clinician, without changing the physical pressure, adjusts his/her attention to an emotional state that is soothing and containing. As this process continues, the client begins to include more resourced and empowered information into their story. The clinician verbally supports this process to deepen their awareness by asking the client to describe a sensation in detail. The clinician then allows their bodily state to mirror the emotional shift occurring in the client supporting deepening of state.

The clinician then begins to track an ongoing movement to reduction in tension in the client's shoulder. Gradually, the tissues become more robust to the touch (there is greater qualia of contact in the physical contact). The next pattern in the sequence begins to emerge. The clinician notices a bracing pattern under his/her hand. The client begins to lightly tear up and states, 'I always had to fight so hard. I just wanted to feel safe'. The clinician mirrors the statement saying, 'you always had to fight so hard and there is part of you starting to feel safe'. The client begins to shake slightly, tears well up and the shoulder movement begins to organize into a motion. The clinician supports the integration of that movement by guiding the patient's attention. Stating, 'Did you notice that tension? Let it move where it wants to move'. Moving his/her inner intention (using a guiding intention for the motion to complete). Next there is an increase in the coherent smooth organization of motion (balance between the pyramidal and extra-pyramidal modulation of motion). This is a change in the way the somatosensory map of this movement pattern had been paired with fight-or-flight reactions.

Embodied touch: Five core types of clinical touch

Five core types of clinical touch are used in multiple body-oriented approaches to psychotherapy. These core types of touch are an attempt to develop a trans-theoretical approach to touch-based interventions. Each of these types of touch can be modulated by the processes discussed above (intention/attention, attunement, emotional resonance/dialog):

1   *Listening touch:* In listening touch, the attention is maintained right at the edge of contact, the place where one's skin meets that of another. As it is not focused on the skin, it can result in the felt experience of being safe and respected. The clinician does not intrude into the boundary of the individual, but rather respects that boundary. The quality of intention is one of receptivity and trust. The listening touch is not aimed at an outcome or following a movement. Rather, listening touch is receptive and mirroring of current states. In employing this type of touch, the clinician does not demand the client to become 'healthy'. The quality of listening touch is analogous to the holding environment described by Carl Rogers as, unconditional positive regard (Rogers, 1957).

2   *Guiding touch:* The hallmark of guiding touch is the ability to shape the direction and connection with intention, attention, and contact itself. Whereas in listening touch, one takes a following stance and channels the attention to aspects of the experience shaping the change. In essence, guiding touch works like a guide through a nature preserve. Guiding touch allows the unfolding of individual experience to take its course while supporting the movement towards a path, giving direction.

3   *Containing/soothing touch:* This type of touch works with soothing and containment – two main properties of the body in emotional life. Soothing occurs when a person shifts into a lower activation state or a parasympathetic rest state. A mother holding a crying baby soothes the emotional experience through contact. The quality of touch provides a boost to the parasympathetic system. Soothing works with two main aspects of emotional regulation: increased parasympathetic tone and distraction of attention from the negative emotion. The physical contact shifts the mental attention away from the internal negative self-state/sensations of the difficult emotions, focusing it onto the contact, thereby allowing the state to settle.

The body itself is a container for emotions. For example, an angry person would often grit his/her teeth, signifying that the emotional intensity is both expressed and contained in physical tension. Containing touch allows for an external support to take over the bodily tension (e.g., holding the arm in such a way that the person does not need to hold it up themselves). Containing touch works with three main factors: namely, (1) increased parasympathetic tone (relaxation response); (2) distraction/shifting attention away from negative self-states and channeling it towards periphery (faster myelinated neurons); and (3) externally supporting/increasing tension pattern, which allows for the body to reduce its tension and develop new ways to contain its own affective states.

4   *Unwinding/following touch:* Many times the body is looped in a sequenced pattern of tension and movement that leads to ineffective responses to the environment. Unwinding touch works with an existing pattern of movement and tension by following through the pattern and finding more effective, coherent, and resourced movements. Trauma is a looped pattern of feelings, behaviors, and experiences that are acted out in each new situation (van der Kolk, 2015). Unwinding touch works by prompting the development of more adaptive movement sequences, allowing for the completion of affective states, paired with a movement pattern, and unfolding into new possibilities in the inner space.

5   *Sequencing touch:* The body is a sequenced pattern of movement, a choreography of neurons firing and resting, our breath moving in an out and endocrine system, going through patterns of activation and deactivation. Memories are not about our relationship with the past. Rather, they teach us how to respond to the present moment. The body needs to be sequenced and responsive to the environment. In order to grab a glass of water, a fine-tuned series of muscle movements need to occur to allow the glass to reach the lips. When the sequence of neurons and muscles do not fire in a coherent manner the water might spill or the hand could simply overshoot the mouth. When the sequence of movements is not coherent all movements require more effort.

Table 35.3 Touch-based treatment plan and intervention

Safe compassionate clinical touch treatment plan

LN is a 35-year-old Latina woman. Her family has lived in California for five generations. She was admitted to the hospital for an elective cosmetic surgery. During the application of the anesthesia, she had an intense allergic reaction that resulted in her nearly dying. Since that time, LN has struggled with sleeping and has not been able to work due to her exhaustion. She is presently on leave of absence from her work as an accountant.

Her therapist referred her for a brief course of touch-focused somatic therapy to help her treatment process. She reports waking up multiple times in the night and, as she falls asleep, she jolts awake into a state of what she refers to as panic. She says that she cannot fall asleep unless she is "extremely tired." She attended six sessions to address increased comfort with the self-states related to sleep and somnolence. The clinician provided an explanation of the role and aims of touch in treatment in their informed consent form and developed a treatment plan in collaboration with LN to address her sleep disturbance and feelings of panic.

Presenting problem: LN came to therapy to address difficulty with sleeping. Her sleep latency is two hours at sleep onset and she has multiple arousals at night. At intake, she reported that she had a near death experience during a surgery. As she is falling asleep, she jolts awake and feels that she cannot breathe.

Theory of change: Reducing triggers to the self-state of somnolence will improve sleep latency and sleep quality. Experiencing the self-state of sleepiness through imaginal exposure paired with the strong resource of physical contact could reduce the conditioned trigger of somnolence, leading to intense fight-or-flight reaction. Clinician can use listening touch to recognize changes in affective state and to help client begin to attend to shifts towards increased regulation of intense affect.

Objectives:
1. Increase ability to evoke resourced or ventral vagal parasympathetic state when approaching sleep.
2. Empowerment to complete defensive strategy that the body mobilized during near death experience.
3. Increased safety during self-state of somnolence.

Interventions:
1. Develop ability to evoke resourced or empowered parasympathetic state (self-touch, somatic mindfulness, mindfulness of resourced states).
2. Graded Imaginal Exploration Identifying Resource: Starting with seated mental imagery and moving to laying on a table, patient verbally explores attempts at sleeping. Clinician offers supportive soothing touch as an anchor for the patient.
3. Self-Soothing Touch: Patient is given skills to self-soothe through self-touch. When affective spikes are noted, patient is encouraged to use soothing self-touch to regulate.
4. Listening Touch: Clinician listens and mirrors changes in affective states. Clinician uses attention focus to begin to highlight with touch and verbal reinforcement the shifts from trigger states to relaxation states.

Sequencing is the skill of allowing the body to tell its story. A person that has witnessed something horrific upon turning his/her head may create a bracing pattern of rigidity against performing this bodily motion. Sequencing allows for: (1) completion of defensive strategies (fight, flight, tend and befriend, freeze); (2) emergence of new more efficient learning movements and patterns of protection and self-regulation; as well as, (3) reduction in the background tension from bracing patterns underlying movement. Table 35.3 is a clinical case formulation that applies these skills to an embodied biopsychosocial treatment plan integrating touch interventions.

Conclusion

Touch is one of the fundamental nutrients in the human ecological milieu. The lack of healthy touch increases the risk of disease and can contribute to challenges with emotion regulation and mental health. Touch is a key factor that supports the development of the embodied self through supporting somatic awareness, mastery experiences in engaging with self-states and coherent integration of somatic and cognitive systems. There are multiple types of touch, and touch can be adapted to a diverse set of clinical presentations.

References

Bjornsdotter, M., Gordon, I., Pelphrey, K. A., Olausson, H., and Kaiser, M. (2014). Development of brain mechanisms for processing affective touch. *Frontiers in Behavioral Neuroscience, 8*, 24.

Cicchetti, D., Rogosch, F. A., Toth, S. L., and Sturge-Apple, M. L. (2011). Normalizing the development of cortisol regulation in maltreated infants through preventive interventions. *Development and Psychopathology, 23*(3), 789–800.

Feldman, R., and Eidelman, A. I. (2003). Skin-to-skin contact (Kangaroo Care) accelerates autonomic and neurobehavioural maturation in preterm infants. *Developmental Medicine and Child Neurology, 45*(4), 274–281.

Feldman, R., Rosenthal, Z., and Eidelman, A. I. (2014). Maternal-preterm skin-to-skin contact enhances child physiologic organization and cognitive control across the first 10 years of life. *Biological Psychiatry, 75*(1), 56–64.

Felitti, V. J., Anda, R. F., Nordenberg, D., Williamson, D. F., Spitz, A. M., Edwards, V., and Marks, J. S. (1998). Relationship of childhood abuse and household dysfunction to many of the leading causes of death in adults: The Adverse Childhood Experiences (ACE) Study. *American Journal of Preventive Medicine, 14*(4), 245–258.

Fleming, A. S., O'Day, D. H., and Kraemer, G. W. (1999). Neurobiology of mother–infant interactions: Experience and central nervous system plasticity across development and generations. *Neuroscience and Biobehavioral Reviews, 23*(5), 673–685.

Gentsch, A., Crucianelli, L., Jenkinson, P., and Fotopoulou, A. (2016). The touched self: Affective touch and body awareness in health and disease. In *Affective Touch and the Neurophysiology of CT Afferents* (pp. 355–384). New York: Springer.

Henricson, M., Ersson, A., Määttä, S., Segesten, K., and Berglund, A. L. (2008). The outcome of tactile touch on stress parameters in intensive care: A randomized controlled trial. *Complementary Therapies in Clinical Practice, 14*(4), 244–254.

Hertenstein, M. J., and Weiss, S. J. (Eds.). (2011). *The handbook of touch: Neuroscience, behavioral, and health perspectives.* New York: Springer Publishing Company.

Jakubiak, B. K., and Feeney, B. C. (2016). Affectionate touch to promote relational, psychological, and physical well-being in adulthood: A theoretical model and review of the research. *Personality and Social Psychology Review.*

Kim, J., Loggia, M. L., Cahalan, C. M., Harris, R. E., Beissner, F., Garcia, R. G., and Napadow, V. (2015). The somatosensory link in fibromyalgia: Functional connectivity of the primary somatosensory cortex is altered by sustained pain and is associated with clinical/autonomic dysfunction. *Arthritis and Rheumatology, 67*(5), 1395–1405.

McGlone, F., Wessberg, J., and Olausson, H. (2014). Discriminative and affective touch: Sensing and feeling. *Neuron, 82*(4), 737–755.

Payne, P., Levine, P. A., and Crane-Godreau, M. A. (2015). Somatic experiencing: Using interoception and proprioception as core elements of trauma therapy. *Frontiers in Psychology, 6,* 93.

Raio, C. M., Orederu, T. A., Palazzolo, L., Shurick, A. A., and Phelps, E. A. (2013). Cognitive emotion regulation fails the stress test. *Proceedings of the National Academy of Sciences, 110*(37), 15139–15144.

Rivers, S. E., Brackett, M. A., Reyes, M. R., Elbertson, N. A., and Salovey, P. (2013). Improving the social and emotional climate of classrooms: A clustered randomized controlled trial testing the RULER approach. *Prevention Science, 14*(1), 77–87.

Rogers, C. R. (1957) The necessary and sufficient conditions of therapeutic personality change. *Journal of Consulting Psychology, 21,* 95–103.

Schore, A. N. (1996). The experience-dependent maturation of a regulatory system in the orbital prefrontal cortex and the origin of developmental psychopathology. *Development and Psychopathology, 8*(1), 59–87.

Schore, A. N. (2015). *Affect regulation and the origin of the self: The neurobiology of emotional development.* London: Routledge.

van der Kolk, B. A. (2015). *The body keeps the score: Brain, mind, and body in the healing of trauma.* New York: Penguin Books.

36

TRAUMATIC DIS-EMBODIMENT

Effects of trauma on body perception and body image

Maurizio Stupiggia

Introduction: Phenomenology

When an abusive event occurs, the ability for self-identification as our inner mirror in which we can usually recognize ourselves and allow us to feel our body and our thoughts as our own, crashes down. In short, everything about 'feeling at home' is taken away. Freud (1919) used to define this kind of unease with the word *unheimlich*, literally meaning 'not-at-home', usually translated to 'non-familiar'. This is a central feature about living with abuse: the feeling of being taken away from oneself, ripped out, as if by magic by an unknown, tremendous power that can transform a person into an outsider. In addition, the person can be robbed of the ability to control and manage their comportment under unforeseen situations. In essence, the abused person lives in a constant sense of exposure, as if his inner drama were public knowledge. What a paradox!

To confirm this paradoxical situation, we can think about the etymology of *umheimlich* in *heim*: the ancient root of the word 'home', and we can find it in a different word, *geheim. Es ist geheim* means 'it is a secret' and in this sentence, we can understand the close connection between feeling at home and the possibility of keeping a secret. The experience of abuse immediately breaks down one's inner protection, and the person is bound to be feel great risk. "I feel like I cannot find a way to hide my 'disability'", one of my patients used to say during the first few therapy sessions. 'It's like everybody knows there's something wrong with me. I'm always tense, never relaxed, careful of how I move, watching what others do, trying to constantly understand if I'm acting well or doing something wrong'.

When a secure and safe inner place is missing for a person, they live in a constant state of unrest and concern, and the body shows symptoms that make it look like a little scared fawn, or an animal who doesn't want to be approached. In addition, there is another result of this exile: abuse influences the patient's self-knowledge, relegating the patient himself into a kind of cognitive vagueness, fearing their own emotional awareness, and body sensations.

'I am terrorized, but don't know about what' said one of my patients during our first session, 'I'm often scared, but not quite sure of what I fear'. These words are emblematic of some patients' state of uncertainty and reveal the separation between corporeal sensations and cognitive functions. For instance, a person can sense a deep muscular tension re-enacting the fear, but without connected congruent mental representations. Such a separation is very common in these cases:

memory has split in two, one side physical and the other side mental and the reunification of these components is the only hope of healing, otherwise our patient's already fragile and disorganized mindset is at great risk. 'When I speak about that, I start feeling bad, not feeling relieved at all', say patients after they share their story, 'even worse than before, I feel heavier'. Reporting to a therapist usually comforts a patient, but not in the case of abuse. Even talking about it increases a sense of anguish, and the patient often asks to suspend and turn to another topic. However, in such a situation, a body-and-breathing-based therapy only would not be enough: during therapy sessions with abused patients, they report that they experience a lack of corporeal identity, a gradual loss of self-consciousness and an empty feeling inside. 'If I keep on shaking my arms – some patients say – I feel kind of weird . . . as if they don't belong to me . . . like I'm losing them . . . I feel dizzy, almost like fainting'.

These kinds of sentences are common during therapeutic sessions: a therapist who is treating a sexually abused patient has to work with symptoms that are difficult to categorize: in some cases, a patient might report that doing rapid and strong arms movements, might have the uneasy feeling that his arms belong to someone else, or at least from his wrist down. In other cases, a patient might report that it's impossible to raise their tone of voice when the situation demands, even if the situation is not important, or thereafter notice that using a higher tone of voice, or even a low scream, they would be terrorized by their own voice as though it came from somebody else, within or outside themselves. In other words, when the patient moves differently or if arousal increases, they experience that their body is no longer their own.

From a phenomenological point of view, the threatening feeling that is experienced when a patient is listening to the internalized traumatized voice, the 'Selves' begin to split within the patient. It becomes obvious that this split is connected to the abuse experience, although it's not so obvious how to relieve this sense of alienation and reunify even a minimum sense of identity.

Chiara: The devil in my belly

Chiara came to psychotherapy at a time of despair. After so many years of difficulty in having sexual intercourse and intimate moments with her previous partners, she was recently experiencing a totally new relationship with her new mate, Antonio, who's sweet, caring and in love; he doesn't mind too much about the troubles Chiara faced in the past and he's very respectful during their awkward moments in bed. Everything seems to be going smoothly, until Chiara found out that she was pregnant. Antonio was on top of the world, as he had been hoping for it to happen for a long time and they had already talked about it.

But the day after finding out she was pregnant, Chiara woke up in a different mood: she felt kind of weird; she couldn't stand Antonio's physical proximity and felt disappointed in seeing his joy. She tried to conceal her negative emotions, and tried to think of a medical explanation, blaming her hormonal changes. Indeed, hormonal changes are part of pregnancy, but not exactly the way Chiara thought; what has dramatically changed is how she perceives Antonio. Only a few days previously, he was like an angel that had fallen from the sky, but now he's a demon, who introduced his gift into her womb, like an invader burning his mark upon conquered territories. Antonio's joy sounded like a disgusting victory-cry in front of a humiliated enemy. 'I can't sleep anymore, because I'm afraid of my belly demon, I'm worried that he can get out and catch me at night', Chiara reported.

During one of our therapy sessions, Chiara said that she still has her wits and realizes that she is probably delirious, but she can't help it. I realized that Chiara was experiencing a typical distortion of reality, which is very different from a psychotic delirium, but no less pervasive.

Chiara's experience was very common amongst abused women: they conflate their invasive traumatic experience with a possible pregnancy and cannot bring it to term because it's viewed as an illness, like a violent experience. Chiara's hatred for Antonio was tempered only by a voluntary termination of pregnancy, twenty days later, after going through emotional hell that affected both of their lives. It took another four years of hard emotional work for Chiara to fulfill her dream of having a baby; an example of how abuse can influence the ability for the couple to accomplish their own biological desire of having a child. These difficulties can therefore disrupt different life stages important to an individual and for a couple, and the possibility to live in harmony with nature. It is also a clear example of detachment between body and emotional processes, generating scary and delusional thoughts.

Neurobiology of somatoform disorder

The dissociative symptoms of detachment refer directly to an individual's experience of feeling alienated from their emotions, from their body, from the usual sense of their own identity, and from the sense of familiarity (van der Hart, Nijenhuis, and Steele, 2006). Dissociative symptoms and some types of somatoform symptoms have common roots in dissociative processes, a concept that Nijenhuis (2004) has proposed to introduce the diction *somatoform dissociation*. Patients with some types of somatoform disorders have demonstrated high levels on scales that measure dissociation and present dissociative symptoms coexisting with the somatoforms symptoms. (Farina, Mazzotti, Pasquini, and Mantione, 2011). In addition, there is evidence that physically and sexually abused people have a higher risk of developing somatoform disorder (Paras et al., 2009).

Furthermore, Barsky (1992) describes a cognitive style called 'somatosensory amplification' (p. 28), which can be applied to many patients with somatoform disorder (SD). Patients with somatoform disorder often exhibit a heightened focus on their own bodies, perceiving their bodily complaints as illness quicker than healthy people do. The term *central sensitization* (Bourke, Langford, and White, 2015) has recently been used to describe a neurobiological process which assumes that symptom onset is associated with a hyper-responsive neural network in high-risk individuals. Patients with SD rate normally innocuous stimuli as painful stimulation due to an alteration of the brain's neural network and perceive their complaints as illness and thus display augmented bodily attention (Barsky, 1992).

The insula is known to be important for pain processing (Fitzek et al., 2004) and in tests where painful stimulation was administered (Sawamoto et al., 2000); activation of the insula has been reported primarily for cutaneous pain rather than visceral pain. However, it seems that central mechanisms like central sensitization might have a higher impact than a peripheral one. This unspecific network of higher brain functions was also called a *neuromatrix* (Melzack, 2001). This network, previously called *painmatrix* (Iannetti and Mouraux, 2010) is not specific for pain as it is active in various conscious processes (Melzack, 2001). The results seem aligned with the hypothesis of central sensitization (Bourke et al., 2015) as mentioned above (Perez, Barsky, Vago, Baslet, and Silbersweig, 2015).

Body image: Insula at work

We just discussed the relevance of the insula in somatoform disorders as it is connected to dysfunctional perception of pain and to somatosensory amplification. Another crucial aspect of those disorders is the distortion of body image. The insula is just one of the places where body maps are generated. We have also seen that in people with dissociative PTSD, the insula is involved in de-regulation, since the insula is necessary to perceive the internal sensations of the body, map them in terms of the body, and is an essential bridge between the motor areas of the mirror neurons and the amygdala.

Forms of body depersonalization also modify body image, sometimes clamorously, and can be observed in eating disorders and in body dysmorphic disorder (Nijenhuis, 2004). One distinctive aspect of the brain is in the prodigious skill to create maps. When the brain creates maps, it informs itself. Action and maps, movement and mind are part of an endless cycle. The human brain is a born cartographer and the cartography begins with the mapping of the internal body. These are probably the mind's primordial constituents based on afferent nerves coming directly from the body.

It is interesting to observe that body maps are also essential and primordial components which constitute for the mind the very first revelation that its organism is alive. Briefly, while the brainstem nuclei would ensure basic level sensations, the insular cortices would provide a more differentiated version of them and most importantly, they would be able to put sensations into relation with other cognition aspects based on the brain activity taking place somewhere else. For all these reasons, we can say that clinical work deals with body sensations, body image and the integration between the two.

Synthesis

In short, while the dissociative phenomenon of detachment corresponds to a lack of integration between higher structures of the brain, and the deficit in the regulation of emotions is due to the lack of top down modulation of the neocortical structures of the limbic system, some types of dissociative somatoform symptoms seem to show an integrative deficit of bottom up modulation between the centers of the visceral brain and neocortical areas. In other words, the disconnection of the experience in the somatoform dissociation would be due to the lack of integration of the information from the lower nerve centers, branches of the afferent and of the somatovisceral memories, with the information processed with the maps in higher brain related to the representational capacities of consciousness and reflexiveness. In particular, somatoform dissociation leads to a lack of integration between consciousness and explicit somatovisceral memories that form the basis for the perception of the body, and the representation of what may appear to the others.

The clinic

Usually in the field of psychotherapy, clinical pictures are traditionally traced to a single defensive reaction of the mind that would protect it from overwhelm and intolerable pain caused by trauma. The brain will also dissociate from consciousness the memory of the event, its meaning, its value of reality to avoid the experience of the pain. This explanation of the linear relationship between trauma and dissociation, despite its undeniable plausibility, is not so evident: many cases show an inadequate vision of the relation between trauma and dissociation, the latter as a purely intrapsychic defense from the mental pain caused by the former.

Some studies (Cantor, 2005; Liotti, 2011) suggest for example, that the type of exchange of affection between a disorganized attachment figure and a child is the primary cause of this dissociative dynamic. The healing will not depend so much on the clinical work of the reworking of individual traumatic memories, but from the fact that such work is carried out in specific interpersonal contexts capable of allowing the recovery of a sufficiently safe and organized experience (Liotti, 2011). In a secure attachment the dissociative processes resulting from trauma are not the source of particular relevant dissociative symptoms, but only transient changes of the integrative functions of memory and consciousness (arising from the defense system operations designed to reduce the physical pain and inhibit the higher brain activity) (Andrews, Brewin, Rose, and

Kirk, 2000; Cantor, 2005) In order to understand more fully this complexity, we must explore a dynamic that is both intrapsychic and intersubjective; where intersubjectivity is viewed first and foremost as *intercorporeality* (Gallese, 2005).

Maria

Maria, who was 37 years old when she consulted me, was aware of a traumatic child abuse incident which occurred when she was between 7 to 10 years old. At the age of 11 Maria started complaining about abdominal pain, diagnosed as chronic irritable bowel syndrome. Since she was 14, she had been suffering from a thyroid dysfunction that made her gain weight rapidly and in an uncontrolled way. When she was 22, she started having sudden fevers that weakened her for long periods of time. Doctors thought the symptoms were similar to rheumatoid arthritis with unknown origin.

Maria rarely had romantic relationships, excluding a very long relationship with a priest that never turned into a sexual relationship, but there had always been an ambivalence between them regarding friendship and something deeper. Maria reported that she often felt as if her body didn't belong to her; sometimes she vomited unexpectedly or would become paralyzed by muscular heaviness while in difficult situations. In the moments of paralysis, she feels 'weird' and 'not in control of her arms and legs'. This is a significant symptomatology that does not appear to correspond to any reasonable medical diagnosis, but that can be included under the somatoform disorders category.

During one of the first sessions, Maria started talking about her history of abuse, but as soon as she got to the core of her story, she stopped and reported that she was in a high agitated state. I asked her to stop and put her right hand on her chest, where she was feeling agitated, and breathe gently; I did the same and we gradually catch the same breathing rate, which becomes like a sort of gentle wave. Maria began to calm down: her face gets more relaxed, her shoulders relaxed and she can take a couple of deep breaths. She seemed to be better, but suddenly, I see the contorted look on her face when she says, 'It's absurd! I can see you, but I see your penis, in front of me'. Her whole body got extremely stiff and rigid with tension, and the atmosphere became tougher and suspended, like a harbinger of imminent danger.

I stayed still, only moved by my breathing, until I caught a subtle hand gesture that looked like a distancing movement, trying to push away something or somebody in front of her. I started nodding and mirroring her gesture, encouraging her to widen it and continue that sensorimotor pattern of constructing boundaries (Stupiggia, 2013). Meanwhile, I bent my head to the side and leaned on the backrest of my armchair to show a distancing motion. After 1 minute of a significant silent dance, I noticed Maria's gentle breathing start again, her shoulders relax and a peaceful expression on her face. 'Now everything returned to normal, you look like your usual self, I feel better'.

A week later

A week later, Maria reported that since the last session, she felt 'more energetic, more alive', especially in her arms and hands. She talked about her moments of generic fear that she suffered in the past (not necessarily related to the abuses), and began to show the same kind of agitation she experienced during our previous session, this time including a choking knot in her throat. We start the same work over again (self-contact and breath mirroring with me), and got into a relaxed state exactly the same way as before, but this time, almost in the same moment, she said that she could not feel her feet and legs up to her knees. She became afraid and her body tensed up again, showing the anaesthesia/analgesia and movement disorder states, which are typical of somatoform dissociation symptoms (Nijenhuis, 2004).

I started to slow down my movements, my rate of speech, and lowered my tone of voice, asking her to look at her legs and feet and make physical contact with those parts of her body. Maria, wide eyed, looked at her legs and feet as if they are foreign objects; it seemed like a never-ending moment until she finally stretched her shaking hand out on her leg, in an extremely slow motion. It felt like a very long time, and, while I observe the scene, I think about how she must have felt when she was a child, when her uncle used to touch her little body!

Similar to our last session, I also made contact with my legs, trying to imitate her movements in a sort of partial mirroring. After several minutes in this state, Maria seemed to be slowly feeling confident in her legs; her breathing rate gradually connected with the movements of her hands and her whole body became involved in a tender self-massage. 'I have never touched myself in this way ... I have always hated my body ... or feared it. And I have never allowed anyone to touch it! I had almost forgotten to tell you that I've had a numb sensation in my feet for so many years, that I was almost unable to feel my shoes or the ground beneath me'. Maria looked very surprised by her new sensations and continued touching her legs and feet.

We spent a little more time feeling such a new experience until I noticed that the excitement level reduced. I then suggested to her to take a step further: 'Close your eyes half way, and try to visualize the image of the external shape of your entire body and put it in front of you. Then take your time ... in your own way ... keeping in touch with your sensations ... continue touching your body with your hands, ... try to let your newly perceived body into that pictured silhouette'. Maria focused on her task, her face seeming to follow the imagination process for a full minute until she took a deep breath that shakes her gently. 'I feel better ... I feel safe ... protected'.

Conclusion

Two years have passed since these two sessions when Maria addressed her past traumatic events, and after these 2 years of continued therapy with me, her life has significantly changed: she feels calm, has new friends, she feels more productive at work and has begun a loving relationship with a man. Above all, she has changed her relationship with her body and no longer has anesthetic, numb feelings in her feet and legs. In addition, she has started to try the pleasure of touching and caressing herself and feels surprisingly complete: no longer has that terrible feeling of living in a 'foreign body'.

Body psychotherapy treatment with Maria was obviously complex and full of obstacles, moving backwards and forwards. This chapter highlighted the core aspects of these sessions, illuminating the first part of the work to describe the type of care provided for symptoms of SD.

In the two sessions described above some guiding principles of body psychotherapy treatment were applied. First, Polyvagal Theory (Porges, 2009) guided the treatment by decreasing arousal whenever Maria came into contact with emotional content that was too intense and disturbing. Second, the principles and methodology of Sensorimotor Psychotherapy (Ogden, Minton, and Paine, 2006) helped to focus attention on Maria's sensations and movements and to wake up the bottom-up process that forms the basis of treatment. In addition, the methodology of key-gesture (Stupiggia, 2013) helped to detect, amplify, intensify and then turn microgestures, that represent internal resources, into new sensorimotor patterns that were not yet known by Maria.

A third aspect, the importance of body image (which in these cases were compromised), became a key part of the treatment. A small example is represented in the latter part of the second session, when I asked Maria to imagine her body and to connect it with the body sensations in that moment. The body image is a crucial aspect of the construction in personal identity.

Fourth, the importance of doing all of this inside a relational frame which, as Liotti (2011) says, is a big factor in the production of dissociative disorders and is also the main therapeutic factor.

Fifth, and closely linked to the relational dimension, is the way of working with *mirroring*, which becomes the clinical application of mirror neurons (Gallese, 2005) in their interpersonal paradigm of neurobiological foundations. Dance/movement therapist Marian Chace first used the term mirroring when describing her clinical work during the 1940's and 1950's (Chaiklin and Schmais, 1993). Chace distinguished mirroring from simple imitation which is a duplication of the external shape of movement without the emotional content. She had the clear intuition that answering movement in similar forms can build a strong and deep relationship and can dissipate the feeling of loneliness or apartness.

In relation to the sessions illustrated, mirroring was applied in a specific way in body psychotherapy; not only the partial or almost total mirroring of the movement of the patient, but also the complementary participation of the therapist's involvement in the process. In the first session there is an example of this that we can define as 'following mirroring', a concept which I am defining for this type of technical work. When Maria freezes because of her hallucinatory vision of the therapist's penis, the therapist tries to tune in to the immobility of Maria and her respiratory rate while she, at the same time, produces a series of small movements that are representative of gestures trying to distance themselves from a hazard or a hostile person. Seen from the outside, this looks like an interactive dance, where one person (the therapist) follows and adapts to the movement of the patient, thus producing an obvious effect and conduction process of the dance and of the management of the process, on the part of the patient (Gallese, 2014).

It is important that the patient leads this interactive dance and above all it is essential that she is aware of having a clear effect on the therapist. In the cases of traumatized patients, we work by concentrating on the inversion of the past traumatic situation of the patient, who had to obey the oppressive power of someone else (or event) that was overwhelming for the individual. In this form of mirroring the therapist comes in and acts as a subordinate by mirroring partly the movements of the patient, and partly adapting the movements into a complementary or subordinate way.

This technical variation allows the patient to recover the power lost during the traumatic event, and to lead and take control of the process: for these reasons I decided to define this technical process 'following mirroring'.

In summary, trauma can rip a person from their body, and cause disembodiment which can alter the capacity to tolerate intense experiences; alter the ability to regulate emotional states through the use of the body, distort body image and tear apart the capacity for relationships. The result is an individual who is distanced from themselves, from their body, and from healthy relationships with others. The body psychotherapist's job is to help the patient 'return home' and reconnect the story and their body into a new dimension of intimacy with others, but above all, with themselves.

References

Andrews, B, Brewin, C. R., Rose, S., and Kirk, M. (2000). Predicting PTSD symptoms in victims of violent crime. *Journal of Abnormal Psychology, 109*, 69–73.

Barsky, A. J. (1992). Amplification, somatization, and the somatoform disorder. *Psychosomatics, 33*, 28–34.

Bourke, J. H., Langford, R. M., and White, P.D. (2015). The common link between functional somatic syndromes may be central sensitization. *Journal of Psychosomatic Research, 78*, 228–236.

Cantor, C. (2005). *Evolution and post traumatic stress: Disorder of vigilance and defence.* London: Routledge.

Chaiklin, S., and Schmais, D. (1993). The Chace approach to dance therapy. In S. Sandel, S. Chaiklin, and A. Lohn (Eds.), *Foundations of dance/movement therapy: The life and work of Marian Chace* (pp. 75–97). Columbia, MD: Marian Chace Memorial Fund of the American Dance Therapy Association.

Farina, B., Mazzotti, E., Pasquini, P., and Mantione, G. (2011). Somatoform and psychoform dissociation among women with orgasmic and sexual pain disorders. *Journal of Trauma Dissociation, 12*(5), 526–534.

Fitzek, S., Huonker, R., Reichenbach, J. R., Mentzel, H. J., Witte, O. H., and Kaiser, W. A. (2004). Event-related fMRI with painful electrical stimulation of the trigeminal nerve. *Magnetic Resonance Imaging, 22*, 205–209.

Freud, S. (1919). *Das Unheimliche* [The Scary]. Vienna: Imago.

Gallese, V. (2005). Embodied simulation: From neurons to phenomenal experience. *Phenomenology and the Cognitive Sciences, 4*, 23–48.

Gallese, V. (2014). Bodily self, affect, consciousness and the cortex. *Neuropsychoanalysis, 15*(1), 42–45.

Iannetti, G., and Mouraux, A. (2010). From the neuromatrix to the pain matrix (and back). *Experimental Brain Research, 205*, 1–12.

Liotti, G. (2011). Attachment disorganization and the clinical dialogue: Theme and variations. In J. Salomon and C. George (Eds.), *Disorganization of attachment and caregiving* (pp. 383–413). New York: The Guilford Press.

Melzack, R. (2001). Pain and the neuromatrix in the brain. *Journal Dental Education, 65*, 1378–1382.

Nijenhuis, E. (2004). *Somatoform dissociation: Phenomena, measures and theoretical issues.* New York: W.W. Norton.

Ogden, P., Minton, K., and Pain, C. (2006). *Trauma and the body.* New York: W.W. Norton.

Paras, M. L., Murad, M. H., Chen, L. P., Goranson, E. N., Sattler, A. L., Colbenson, K. M., . . . Zirakzadeh, A. (2009). Sexual abuse and lifetime diagnosis of somatic disorders: A systematic review and meta-analysis. *Journal of American Medical Association, 302*, 550–561.

Perez, D. L., Barsky, A. J., Vago, D. R., Baslet, G., and Silbersweig, D. A. (2015). A neural circuit framework for somatosensory amplification in somatoform disorders. *Journal of Neuropsychiatry Clinical Neuroscience, 27*, e40–e50.

Porges, S. (2009). The polyvagal theory: New insights into adaptive reactions of the autonomic nervous system. *Cleveland Clinic Journal of Medicine, 76*(2), 86–90.

Sawamoto, N., Honda, M., Okada, T., Hanakawa, T., Kanda, M., Fukuyama, H., . . . Shibasaki, H., (2000). Expectation of pain enhances responses to non-painful somatosensory stimulation in the anterior cingulate cortex and parietal operculum/posterior insula: An event-related functional magnetic resonance imaging study. *The Journal of Neuroscience, 20*, 7438–7445.

Stupiggia, M. (2013). From hopeless solitude to the sense of being-with. *International Body Psychotherapy Journal, 11*(1), 25–40.

van der Hart, O., Nijenhuis, E. R. S., and Steele, K. (2006). *The haunted self: Structural dissociation and the treatment of chronic traumatization.* New York: W.W. Norton.

37

RESEARCH INFORMING BODY PSYCHOTHERAPY CLINICAL WORK

A spotlight on emotions

Margit Koemeda-Lutz

Introduction

Human beings depend on their senses to perceive the environment and on their whole bodies to interact with it (Fuchs, 2011, 2013; Scheurle, 2016). They encounter reality through their bodies and build memories of what they encounter (Damasio, 1994, 1999). Experience forges personality (Freud, 1917/1969, Johnson, 1994). Precipitations of experience as explicit memories or implicit cognitive, emotional and behavioural dispositions influence future decisions and how individuals cope with new situations (Ciompi, 1997; Fuchs, 2011; Markowitsch, 2009). They shape all consecutive interactions with the environment (as preferences, by emotional attitudes and cognitive styles) while being modified themselves by each new experience and situation. Physiological patterns in our bodies and the neuronal architecture of our brains keep building and declining throughout our lives (Hebb, 1949; Jäncke, 2013).

As clinicians, our main focus is on how we perceive our clients, what resonates in us when they tell us what happened to them, when we watch them move or see how they hold themselves, what we feel when we interact with them or what they tell us about how they perceive us. For two to three decades around the millennial turn we have been witnessing a proliferation of neuroscientific findings, fierce theoretical debates on their philosophical premises (Bauer, 2015; Roth, 1994, 2001) and impressive advances in research techniques (Damasio, 2005; Filler, 2009). As clinicians we have been facing an increasing challenge of how to relate details of microbiological, neurochemical, neuroanatomic and functional knowledge to more general questions of our therapeutic work (Koemeda-Lutz, 2012).

From (epi-) genetics we know that while DNS sequences, i.e. the genetic "texts" are fixed for all organisms (Chial, 2008; Venter et al., 2001), the expression (activity) of most genes is subject to regulation in interaction with environmental as well as with intero- and proprioceptive stimuli (Bauer, 2002, p. 29). Can we volitionally, purposefully and selectively influence the activation or absorption of promotors, i.e. the regulatory sequences on specific genes? There are researchers, for example, in the field of oncology, who try to do so, (Brahmer et al., 2010) but as for psychotherapists, this must be doubted.

Neurobiological research has demonstrated, however, that the quality of our social relationships does influence the activity of our genes (Bauer, 2002) and that early experiences shape our somatic functioning, our postural habits, reaction-patterns of our inner organs, our behaviour and the neuronal architecture of our brains. Attuned positive bonding in early childhood can, for example, protect stress genes from over-reactivity later in life.

As clinicians we perceive our clients and interact with them on several levels, many of them beyond consciousness. By mirror neurons (Bauer, 2005), muscular tensions, posture and gestures one person can influence the muscular patterns and feelings of others. When two or more organisms interact, there are always biochemical, psychological and behavioural processes involved, and processes on each of these levels influence each other, bottom-up as well as top-down. They evolve parallel in time and resonate with each other – intra-, as well as inter-individually.

Below are a few clinical moments from a session based on bioenergetic analysis (Heinrich-Clauer, 2009; Koemeda-Lutz, 2002; Lowen, 1958), an approach for which two prospective effectiveness studies (Crameri et al., 2014; Crameri et al., 2016; Koemeda-Lutz et al., 2006; von Wyl, Tschuschke, Crameri, Koemeda-Lutz, and Schulthess, 2016) resulted in effect sizes comparable to treatments based on Cognitive Behaviour Therapy.

Case vignette 1

When Sarah entered therapy, she was 50 years old. After almost one year of treatment she opened her 24th session by complaining about her aching body. 'Pain all-over', she says. Originally, this patient had sought treatment to get help with her partner, whom she described as intolerable. She shared an apartment with him and their 5-year-old son. The couple was unmarried.

Sarah described her partner as withdrawn from the relationship, his behaviour as infantile, spiteful and defiant. There were moments when he softened somewhat and expressed his own desperateness. But most of the time he was emotionally cold, he hardly communicated with Sarah, cooperation between him and her was practically non-existent. Although Sarah had repeatedly tried to initiate couples' therapy, which in two cases had worked for a few sessions, the relationship obviously was beyond hope. Eventually Sarah took her son and moved into an apartment of her own.

Unfortunate disagreements about finances and residency battles concerning their son kept the patient busy for months. After the situation had calmed down, feelings of abandonment and loneliness arose in Sarah. She thought of asking friends to buy a house with her, so their daily lives could be shared. Some of them seemed interested and were actually enthusiastic about the project. But in the end, they all withdrew. Nothing tangible developed, as none of them was really ready to make a commitment.

In the session I invite Sarah to concentrate on her pain and ask her if it were connected to certain other sensations, thoughts or images, or if there were any impulses to move. Sarah closes her eyes. Her breathing deepens.

After a while she says that she would need to lash about. I ask her if she needs to get up for this, or would she rather lie down, or sit. She decides to stand. After we made sure that she had enough space around her, she starts to push back with her right elbow, saying, 'With this I should scream, but you know me, I'm not capable of shouting or screaming'.

I invite her to at least imagine the scream, which she feels would go with her movement; and try to just give a hint of how it might sound. I myself give her a few tones, just as a suggestion. Sarah starts uttering some sounds, then words: 'Go away! Piss off!' Sarah is struggling with her balance. I ask her if she needs to enhance her grounding. But she answers that she is alright using her legs. A little later she realizes that her left side is completely immobile (paralyzed).

Indeed, her left arm limps. 'It would be great if this arm could move', she says '. . . but I can only move my fingers a tiny little bit'. She then adds, 'No! I need to go on lashing'. And she goes on. She then stops to say, 'I think, like with genuine paralysis I need to grasp and operate my left arm with my right hand'. For the next moment it looks as if she were holding a baby in her right arm.

'Almost like a preterm baby', I utter, an idea that had just popped up in my mind. 'This little creature, I am holding here ... must be very tiny', she continues. I ask her how she feels in this moment. 'Lonely and sad', she says. And after a while: 'But now I feel some defiance arising: I can hold myself alone. I don't need anyone'.

The session ends here. We make a promise to her right hand and left arm; 'mother' and 'child' (treating them as if they were real, distinct persons), that we will be back in the next session and that we will want to know how they have been doing in the meantime.

Commentary

Focussed attention on a current complaint (her aching body) leads Sarah by deepening her breathing and intensifying her body awareness to follow some interesting behavioural (lashing) and expressive impulses (wanting to shout). She thereby re-enacts an early mother-infant inter-action which informs her about her own limpness or even paralysis as a baby (we do not know yet why), her need to be held and helped with her movements and her self-protective, defensive reaction of defiance ('I don't need anyone').

On the body level we observe a dissociation of aggressive impulses on one hand and an inclination to give up on the other or perhaps this a re-enactment of an interaction between perpetrator and victim. Associations from the patient's and the therapist's side, as well as verbal accounts of what she remembers from her early childhood help to model hypotheses about what may have contributed to her current re-enactment.

She reports that neither her mother nor her former partner had ever had much empathy for her. Both were mainly self-centred and pretty much wound up with their own problems. Very early in her development longing feelings and movements of reaching out were left unanswered and, by consequence, died down (limpness). Any further development of connection-seeking movements and affiliated emotional programs was obviously hampered. Accordingly, she did not manage to convince her friends into her project of a shared house.

Babies who are deprived of adequate nurturance, love, warmth and holding first express their frustration and rage by screaming. Maybe these were the impulses in her right arm wanting to lash about. But with time these babies get exhausted and desperate. And after a while they give up. They turn silent, and their bodies collapse in weakness, or, in Sarah's case, get trapped in the conflict between rage and defeat. Bauer (2002) reports that more than anything, interpersonal relationships influence somatic processes. This influence reaches as deep as to the regulation of gene activity. It is effective in adult human beings, but even more so during infancy and prenatal development (Schindler, 2011).

As psychotherapists we know that early experiences shape our feeling, thinking and behav-ioural patterns. But neurobiological research has demonstrated that early experiences also shape our somatic functioning, such as physiological patterns and the neuronal architecture in our brains (Bauer, 2002; Hüther, 2006; Spitzer, 2002). Attuned positive bonding in early childhood protects stress genes from over-reactivity in later life. Positive human relationships constitute, as Bauer (2002, p. 13) writes, the best 'medication without side effects' for coping with psychic and somatic stress.

Early in life neuronal networks develop that later determine how a person appraises his or her environment and how he/she copes with challenging events (Ramsay and Lewis, 1995). The architecture of neuronal networks and their functional patterns depend on early (relational) expe-riences (Liu et al., 1997). If they are positive, they foster resilience, if they are detrimental (such as neglect, abuse, violence), they may lead to dissociative patterns and contribute as etiological factors to the evolution of psychiatric disorders (Bauer, 2002; Kirschbaum, Wolf, May, Wippich, and Hellhammer, 1996).

In the described session, Sarah was able to mobilize what was left from her protest and rage elicited by chronically experiencing her needs unmet. Her right arm expressed this by lashing about, and her voice by shouting and swearing. And at first she relapsed into her defensive mode (saying "Piss off," "I don't need anyone"). But with time she created a new and constructive interactional pattern, where part of herself took over the role of a good-enough mother, fairly grounded on her own feet, holding the baby in her arm, caressing and helping her with her needs to move and to grasp and to make a meaningful connection. She committed herself to attend to this lonely and unnourished part in herself, to attune herself and give her love to it.

From epigenetics we learn that human beings share the same genetic blueprints to the incredible amount of 99.9 per cent! (Chial, 2008; Venter et al., 2001) The obvious variation between individuals therefore must be due to the interaction between environmental, including cellular and proprioceptive signals and genes. According to Bauer (2002, p. 31f), only 1–2 per cent of all human diseases are caused by gene mutations. The overwhelming remainder is due to dysfunctional communication processes on biological, social and/or psychological systemic levels. Certain environmental factors, such as nutrition, different sorts of radiation, perceived relational situations, transcription factors, etc. absorb or activate promoters, i.e. the regulatory sequences on specific genes (Schubert, 2011). Our genetic text, i.e. the totality of all human genes comprising over 3 billion nucleotides was decoded in 2000 (International Human Genome Sequencing Consortium, 2004). The expression and activity of most of our genes, however, are subject to regulation in interaction with contextual stimuli (Bauer, 2002) and still need to be explored. Individual experiences provoke and form reaction-patterns which influence this regulation (Hüther, 2006; Spitzer, 2002).

One level of observation, where epigenetics is relevant, is neuronal information processing. Our brain translates sensory into biological input. Nerve cells get stimulated and genes in these cells become activated. They elicit the production and release of neurotransmitters, growth factors or hormones and cause nerve cells to grow or decline. Active synapses enhance their structure, while inactive synapses dissolve. Frequent and intense experiences strengthen the interconnection of cell assemblies. Simultaneous, synchronic, rhythmical bioelectric activities (ca. 40 Hz) in cells create networks. Neuroscientific findings have taught us that perceptions and notions are based on synaptic connections between nerve cells and that mental operations are facilitated by the interconnections of nerve cell assemblies. In addition, we learned that the neuronal architecture of our brains is subject to change throughout our lives (plasticity: Bauer, 2002; Spitzer, 2002; Damasio, 1994; Hebb, 1949; Hüther, 2006; Jäncke, 2013).

The good news to psychotherapists is that it is therefore never too late for psychotherapeutic work, i.e. practising and learning new things. Bauer (2002) reviews and reflects on an immense body of microbiological, psychiatric and psychosomatic research literature to demonstrate how life experiences, especially early in life, interact with the genetically designed human potential, in order to shape individual personalities on different levels. He further demonstrates that, more than anything, interpersonal relationships influence somatic processes. This influence reaches as deep as to the regulation of gene activity. It is effective in adult human beings, but even more so during infancy and prenatal development.

In the following section emotions will be highlighted as one specific aspect of human experiencing, communication and functioning, which crucially depends on us being embodied (Koemeda-Lutz, 2009). Imagine feeling sad <u>without</u> feeling your body, without being embodied.

Emotions

Human beings are body and mind (Damasio, 1994, 1999; Roth, 2001). Emotions seem to particularly lend themselves for illustrating this dual nature. Most psychopathological disorders include emotional dysfunction (Saß, Wittchen, and Zaudig, 2000; Thoits, 1985). Emotion-oriented work therefore is key to (body) psychotherapeutic treatment. Any decision we take, involves emotional processing. Movement, besides other components, is emotionally motivated as in the approach or withdrawal from objects or persons.

Sometimes we notice an unusual tension in our neck, or that our palms get sweaty, we feel our face blush, a slight tingling in the belly. We spot heart rate changes, vasoconstriction, an acceleration or deceleration of gut motility etc. And at the same time, we feel sad, scared or angry.

We constantly appraise external and internal stimuli, situations and events as relevant or irrelevant to ourselves, as pleasant or aversive. Our states of arousal adapt accordingly. And this helps us to prepare actions like fight, flight, freeze or desire.

Emotional processes can be observed from the outside and at the same time are subjectively experienced. They negotiate between us and the outside reality. They highlight sensations, perceptions and events, which are meaningful to us and adapt our current physiological states. By this means they help structure our perceptions, cognitions and our mnestic functions. Recurring experiences, appraised as relevant to us, elicit similar reactions and get wired into our predominantly unconscious implicit procedural memory. They are imprinted as cognitive, emotional and behavioural dispositions and can repeatedly be elicited by similar stimuli. Personality structure builds from such dispositions.

If a person basically feels and behaves aggressively and stressed, he will most likely encounter critical, irritable and unfriendly fellow human beings. If he tries to remember his past, his memories will confirm, that it has always been like this. Our basic prevailing moods coin our perceptions and memories in a way, that we encounter and remember things that match it and blend out events and situations which do not.

Emotions occur in the present. They involve our bodies and connect us to our vitality (Lowen, 1958, 1995). Emotions are processes, which observably originate in certain (limbic) structures of our brain (Roth, 2001). They impact other areas of the central nervous system, elicit changes in organs, vessels and muscles, and go with specific facial expressions, gestures, and behaviour (Koemeda-Lutz, 2009).

Our language provides for a great number of words for different feeling states. Some languages offer finer gradations for some sections of the spectrum of feelings and fewer words in other sections as compared to other languages (Russell, 1994). There is anxiety, defiance, gratitude, envy, stress, rage, love, pride, shame, grief and many others. Some authors claim that there are only a few basic emotions, from which all others develop: fear, anger/rage, nausea, sadness, surprise, acceptance/trust, curiosity/interest and joy (Ekman and Friesen, 1969; Plutchik, 1991).

In order to characterize and distinguish emotions from each other two basic dimensions seem to be most useful, they are arousal and valence. Boredom in this two-dimensional matrix is characterized by low arousal and unpleasantness, rage is highly activated and unpleasant, love highly activated and pleasant, serenity is pleasant with low arousal. However, not even these simple examples are unequivocal. Someone can love another person calmly or passionately (different levels of arousal), love can be connected to pain and suffering (unpleasant), especially if it is not reciprocated. Mild states of aggression can be experienced as pleasant, if the person feels self-confident and trusts her self-effectiveness. Peak values on both dimensions have been shown to have detrimental effects on other functions such as cognitive, perceptual, mnestic functions, or the capacity to empathize with others. Intermediate states of activation define a window of tolerance for each individual in which they can communicate and successfully interact with their environment.

Emotions usually are object-related (Frijda, 1986; Lazarus, 1991). In order to describe them we therefore need an additional spatial component, the tendency to approach an object or a person, to withdraw or to freeze in panic. Fight, flight, freeze and faint behaviour can also be observed in mammals and reptiles. In lower species stimulus-response patterns seem to be hard-wired (Ledoux, 1996). In human beings, emotions offer choices of behaviour and modulate reactions to allow for better situational adaptations.

Emotional processes develop over time (Andrade, 2011; Geuter and Schrauth, 2001). They arise from the background of a prevalent feeling, they interrupt ongoing activities, make the focus of attention change (Damasio, 1994). Changes in the level of arousal, the relevance for the self must be appraised (concerning needs, motivations and intentions) and the valence of the situation (pleasant or unpleasant) (Geuter, 2015). At the same time, and mainly subconsciously, a number of physiological and muscular reactions occur (a preparation for an attack, for fight or flight). The organism approaches the other person/the object, withdraws or freezes in panic and shock. A certain act may follow (hitting, screaming, touching, clinging, invading, kissing, devouring, vomiting, etc.). Then follows a withdrawal from the interaction, concentration on the own self, processing and integration of what happened; and still later relaxation and regeneration (Andrade, 2011; Geuter, 2015).

Problems and deficits can manifest in any of these phases (Geuter, 2015; Traue, 1998). Some people cannot accurately perceive their own or other people's emotions. Others try to avoid any emotional turmoil, they suppress their anger and joy, try to keep cool in all situations. Still others do feel sadness and joy, but try to hide their feelings. They would never admit they love someone and would do anything to not have to tell their neighbour that they are angry at him. Some people get stuck in their feelings; for example, they cannot stop being sad. They cry even in situations when they should actually feel furious. Some of these people have lost the link to the event or person, to whom their feelings had been connected. And they do not understand why they feel how they feel (Koemeda-Lutz, 2009). Finally, there are people who are chronically over-aroused, who never relax or recover. Usually these are trauma survivors, who have not had an opportunity to process their experience and got stuck in a state of overwhelming threat to their lives (van der Kolk and McFarlane, p. 37 in: van der Kolk, McFarlane, and Weisaeth, 1996).

Below is a second case vignette, which is meant to demonstrate, how listening to one's body, i.e. following its impulses, can lead out of a depressive state and help hypothesize how this state may have resulted from a long story of emotional deprivation, starting in the patient's childhood, and perpetuated by her compensating defences.

Case vignette 2

Due to the holiday season Barbara's treatment had been suspended for a longer period of time. After having entered the present session (32nd), she takes her seat and gazes at me in silence.

"How have you been?" I ask her after a while.

"Well, the old story," she says, "I am not capable of anything, I am nothing, always off-target. I see no progress whatsoever. I feel like a raw egg without its shell."

Barbara is a lawyer, 59 years old, shortly before ending her quite successful professional career. She is married and financially well-off. She feels depressed and unhappy.

"And in my last dream," she adds, "I was outdoors and naked and felt very scared to meet anyone. I was surprised that I didn't run away." I ask the patient, what exactly scared her when thinking of someone coming across.

"My profound vulnerability," she says. Saint Martin comes to my mind and I ask:

"What if Saint Martin came across to share his coat with you? Would a person like him also make you run away?"

She remains silent, but seems to ponder. After a while of silence I add that there are periods in our lives during which we all are naked, incapable of almost everything, where we literally are nobodies, particularly in the prenatal stage of development, but also during early infancy, and then again, when we get old and need assistance and care in our everyday lives.

"Yes" she agrees, more to herself than to me, "I was too much for my mother." She was quite swamped at the time when my brothers and sisters and I were children.

I ask her if she could think of a body position that would match her current state. I spread a blanket on the floor. And offer her another one to cover. She straightforwardly curls herself up in a foetal position. And pulls the second blanket over her whole body. I ask her where she wants me to sit. No answer. I sit next to her front side, but feel uncomfortable. I ask if it were okay to move to her backside.

I hear a very timid "mhm," and see something from below the blanket that could be interpreted as nodding. I change my position. This feels much more appropriate. I ask Barbara to observe any impulses to move or change things and to follow these, or if anything came to her mind, to speak up and tell me, if she needed me doing anything, but that, of course, it would also be fine, if nothing happened. I hear a little murmur. It sounds like consent. Then, for quite a while, nothing happens.

A little later she uncovers her head and I see minimal movements in her shoulders and her back. I ask if she would allow me to touch her back. She agrees.

My hands begin to dialogue with her back. Quite pronounced and firmly at times. I feel reminded of conversations between a foetus and the abdominal wall of her mother.

"This is amazing," she says, "It feels good"!

I watch her digging for something, and offer her the Kleenex box.

"Thank you, I don't need this. Brought my own."

Then she smiles, indicating that she had caught herself in an old pattern and accepts one from my box. She uncovers herself some more and turns on her back. Her head comes to lie on the plain floor. I offer her a cushion.

"I don't need one. It's perfect."

Silence.

"Maybe a cushion would be comfortable," she then says.

I take and hold her head and put a cushion underneath it. Tears come to her eyes.

"I never thought of the possibility," she starts to ponder, "that someone could share his coat with me. When I was a child, I defied them all and tried to accomplish everything by myself."

She abruptly sits up and grabs her feet. I ask her if they were cold. She nods. I propose to cover up one foot and to massage the other one.

Her immediate reaction is defensive with a tiny withdrawal. But she keeps herself from expressing it. I wait. Then she nods and seems to agree. She does not say so.

I touch her feet. I can see and feel that her whole body is alert. Her legs and feet are stiff, but while I am carefully beginning to massage them, her muscles gradually soften.

"How warm your hands are," she says after a while and again begins to sob.

Before we end the session, Barbara mentions, what an effort it took on her side to receive this massage, to really let it in. I ask her what she may have been afraid of.

"It could have become abysmal."

So far she had prevented her breath to really get deep, while experiencing this new kind of contact and dialogue. It seems like she needs to watch and stay in control. She is afraid of becoming overwhelmed by her own feelings of deprivation and desperation. Choking one's breath is a technique to restrict and control emotions which infants apply at quite an early age. She also admits that she had wished to have me at her back side instead of her front, but that she had not dared to say so. Barbara's oral conflict (when she says "I need," but at the same time "I must avoid the pain of frustration, abandonment and mother's potential rejection") had been compensated by her pronounced rigidity and pretended autonomy. The defence around her true neediness has begun to gradually melt in this session.

Conclusion

This chapter has demonstrated that, as body psychotherapists we focus on listening to what our patients say, on perceiving their bodies, and on feeling what resonates in ourselves. From time to time we invite them to leave the cognitive level of reflection, analysis and narration and, instead, explore, observe and follow their muscular impulses, postural changes and nonverbal vocalizations and dialogue with them on that level.

Symptoms and processes of change may be observed on many different levels of structure and function in an organism: If we help a patient to increase her assertiveness, we may at the same time strengthen her immune system (Schubert, 2011). If we are deeply empathic with another person who is grieving a severe loss and teach her to limit grieving when needed, this will most likely correlate with observable changes in the dynamics of her cerebral blood flow. Relaxation training has been shown to correlate with increased cellular immunity (McGrady et al., 1992, cited in Hall and Olnes, 2011).

But the connections are far more intricate and complex than simple causal relationships, as for example, when a person is taught to express anger and her lymphocyte titre may go up. However, the change in lymphocyte titre could have been caused by an infection instead.

If practising body psychotherapists learn to understand as much as possible about how human beings function on different levels, we will integrate this with our subconsciously stored body of implicit clinical expertise and will intuitively organize our therapeutic behaviour from one moment to the next by staying present with our patients and remaining available for our relationship with them in the best way possible.

References

Andrade, P. (2011). *Emotional Medicine*. Lexington: Tenacity Press.

Bauer, J. (2002). *Das Gedächtnis des Körpers – Wie Beziehungen und Lebensstile unsere Gene steuern* [Body memory – the regulation of our genes by relationships and life styles]. Frankfurt a.M: Eichborn.

Bauer, J. (2005). *Warum ich fühle, was du fühlst – Intuitive Kommunikation und das Geheimnis der Spiegelneurone* [Why I feel what you feel – Intuitive communication and the mystery of our mirror neurons]. Hamburg: Hoffmann und Campe.

Bauer, J. (2015). *Selbststeuerung. Die Wiederentdeckung des freien Willens* [Self-regulation – The rediscovery of free will]. München: Blessing.

Brahmer, J. R., Drake, C. G., Wollner, I., Powderly, J. D., Picus, J., Sharfman, W. H., . . . Topalian, S. L. (2010). Phase I study of single-agent anti-programmed death-1 (MDX-1106) in refractory solid tumors:

Safety, clinical activity, pharmacodynamics, and immunologic correlates. *Journal of Clinical Oncology, 28*, 3167–3175.

Chial, H. (2008). DNA sequencing technologies key to the Human Genome Project. *Nature Education, 1*(1), 219.

Ciompi, L. (1997). *Die emotionalen Grundlagen des Denkens* [The emotional foundations of reasoning]. Göttingen: Vandenhoeck and Ruprecht.

Crameri, A., Koemeda-Lutz, M., Tschuschke, V., Schulthess, P., and von Wyl, A. (2014). Ergebnisqualität ambulanter Psychotherapie: Ergebnisse aus der Grundversorgung in der Schweiz [Evaluation of the outcome of out-patient psychotherapy. Results from primary health care in Switzerland]. *Psychotherapie-Wissenschaft, 2*, 96–107.

Crameri, A., Schuetz, C., Andreae, A., Koemeda-Lutz, M., Schulthess, P., Tschuschke, V., and von Wyl, A. (2016). The Brief Symptom Inventory and the Outcome Questionnaire-45 in the assessment of the Outcome Quality of Mental Health Interventions. *Psychiatry Journal*, 1–14.

Damasio, A. R. (1994). *Descartes' Error. Emotion, Reason and the Human Brain.* New York: Putnam.

Damasio, A. R. (1999). *The Feeling of What Happens. Body and Emotion in the Making of Consciousness.* New York: Harcourt Brace and Co.

Damasio, H. (2005). *Human Brain Anatomy in Computerized Images.* Oxford: Oxford University Press.

Ekman, P., and Friesen, W. V. (1969). The repertoire of nonverbal behaviors: Categories, origins, usage, and coding. *Semiotica, 1*, 49–98.

Filler, A. (2009). The history, development and impact of computed imaging in neurological diagnosis and neurosurgery: CT, MRI, and DTI. *Nature Precedings, 7*(1), 1–85.

Freud, S. (1969). Allgemeine Neurosenlehre [A general model of neurosis]. In S. Freud (Ed.), *Studienausgabe, Bd. 1, Vorlesungen zur Einführung in die Psychoanalyse und Neue Folge* [Student edition, vol. 1, Introductory sections to psychoanalysis and new section] (pp. 245–445). Frankfurt a.M.: S. Fischer. (Original work published 1917)

Frijda, N. H. (1986). *The emotions.* Cambridge: Cambridge University Press.

Fuchs, T. (2011). Body memory and the unconscious. In D. Lohmar and J. Brudzinska (Eds.), *Founding Psychoanalysis. Phenomenological Theory of Subjectivity and the Psychoanalytical Experience.* Dordrecht: Kluwer.

Fuchs, T. (2013). Zwischen Leib und Körper [Between body and soma. Body and life]. In M. Hähnel and M. Knaup (Hrsg.), *Leib und Leben* [Body and life]. *Perspektiven für eine neue Kultur der Körperlichkeit* (S. 82–93) [Perspectives for a new culture of physicalness] (pp. 82–93). Darmstadt: Wissenschaftliche Buchgesellschaft.

Geuter, U. (2015). *Körperpsychotherapie: Grundriss einer Theorie für die klinische Praxis* [Body-psychotherapy. Foundations of a theory for clinical practice]. Berlin: Springer.

Geuter, U., and Schrauth, N. (2001). Emotionen und Emotionsabwehr als Körperprozess. *Psychotherapie Forum, 9*, 4–19.

Hall, H. R., and Olness, K. (2011). Hypnose, Imagination, Selbstregulierung und Immunaktiviät [Hypnosis, imagination, self-regulation and immune activity]. In C. Schubert (Ed.), *Psychoneuroimmunologie und Psychotherapie* (pp. 228–257). Stuttgart: Schattauer.

Hebb, D. O. (1949). *The organization of behavior: A neuropsychological approach.* New York: Wiley.

Heinrich-Clauer, V. (Ed.). (2009). *Handbook Bioenergetic Analysis.* Gießen: Psychosozial Verlag.

Hüther, G. (2006). *Bedienungsanleitung für ein menschliches Gehirn* [Instruction manual for a human brain]. Göttingen: Vandenhoeck and Ruprecht.

International Human Genome Sequencing Consortium. (2004). Finishing the euchromatic sequence of the human genome. *Nature, 431*, 931–945.

Jäncke, L. (2013). *Lehrbuch Kognitive Neurowissenschaften* [Textbook cognitive neurosciences]. Bern: Huber.

Johnson, S. (1994). *Character Styles.* New York: W.W. Norton.

Kirschbaum, C., Wolf, O. T., May, M., Wippich, W., and Hellhammer, D. H. (1996). Stress- and treatment-induced elevations of cortisol levels associated with impaired declarative memory in healthy adults. *Life Sciences, 58*(17), 1475–1483.

Koemeda-Lutz, M. (Ed.). (2002). *Körperpsychotherapie – Bioenergetische Konzepte im Wandel* [Body-psychotherapy. Further developments of bioenergetic concepts]. Körper und Seele (Body and Soul), Sonderband [Special issue]. Basel: Schwabe.

Koemeda-Lutz, M. (2009). *Intelligente Emotionalität. Vom Umgang mit unseren Gefühlen* [Intelligent emotionality. How to deal with emotions]. Stuttgart: Kohlhammer.

Koemeda-Lutz, M. (2012). Integrating brain, mind, and body: Clinical and therapeutic implications of neuroscience. *Bioenergetic Analysis, 22*, 57–77.

Koemeda-Lutz, M., Kaschke, M., Revenstorf, D., Scherrmann, T., Weiss, H., and Soeder, U. (2006). Evaluation der Wirksamkeit von ambulanten Körperpsychotherapien – EWAK. Eine Multizenter-Studie in Deutschland und der Schweiz [Evaluation of the effectiveness of out-patient body-psychotherapies – EEBP. A multi-center study in Germany and Switzerland]. *Psychotherapie, Psychosomatik, Medizinische Psychologie PPmP, 56*, 480–487.

Lazarus, R. S. (1991). *Emotion and adaptation.* New York: Oxford University Press.

Ledoux, J. (1996). *The emotional brain. The mysterious underpinnings of emotional life.* New York: Simon and Schuster.

Liu, D., Diorio, J., Tannenbaum, B., Caldji, C., Francis, D., Freedman, A., . . . Meaney, M. J. (1997). Maternal care, hippocampal glucocorticoid receptors, and hypothalamic-pituitary-adrenal responses to stress. *Science, 277*(5332), 1659–1662.

Lowen, A. (1958). *The Language of the Body.* New York: Grune and Stratton.

McGrady, A., Conran, P., Dickey, D., Garman, D., Farris, E., and Schumann-Brzezinski, C. (1992). The effects of biofeedback-assisted relaxation on cell-mediated immunity, cortisol, and white blood cell count in healthy adult subjects. *Journal of Behavioral Medicine, 15*, 343–354.

Markowitsch, H. J. (2009). *Das Gedächtnis. Entwicklung, Funktionen, Störungen* [Memory. Development, functions, disorders]. München: Beck.

Plutchik, R. (1991). *The emotions.* Lanham, MD: University Press of America.

Ramsay, D. S., and Lewis, M. (1995). The effects of birth condition on infants' cortisol response to stress. *Pediatrics, 95(4)*, 546–549.

Roth, G. (1994). *Das Gehirn und seine Wirklichkeit: kognitive Neurobiologie und ihre philosophischen Konsequenzen* [The brain and its reality: Cognitive neurobiology and its philosophical implications]. Frankfurt a.M: Suhrkamp.

Roth, G. (2001). *Fühlen, Denken, Handeln: Wie das Gehirn unser Verhalten steuert* [To feel, to think, to act: How our brain regulates behaviour]. Frankfurt a.M: Suhrkamp.

Russell, J. A. (1994). Is there universal recognition of emotion from facial expression? A review of cross-cultural studies. *Psychological Bulletin, 115*, 102–141.

Saß, H., Wittchen, H. U., and Zaudig, M. (2000). *Diagnostisches und Statistisches Manual Psychischer Störungen DSM-IV* (deutsche Bearbeitung). Göttingen: Hogrefe. (APA American Psychiatric Association: Diagnostic and statistical manual of mental disorders).

Scheurle, H. J. (2016). *Das Gehirn ist nicht einsam. Resonanzen zwischen Gehirn, Leib und Umwelt* [The brain is not lonely. Resonances between brain, body and environment]. Stuttgart: Kohlhammer.

Schindler, P. (2011). Am Anfang des Lebens. Neue körperpsychotherapeutische Erkenntnisse über unsere frühesten Prägungen durch Schwangerschaft und Geburt [At the beginning of life. New body-psychotherapeutic findings concerning earliest imprints during pregnancy and birth]. SGBAT *Körper and Seele Bd.7* (Body and Soul, vol. 7), Basel: Schwabe.

Schubert, C. (2011). *Psychoneuroimmunologie und Psychotherapie* [Psychoneuroimmunology and psychotherapy]. Stuttgart: Schattauer.

Spitzer, M. (2002). *Lernen. Gehirnforschung und die Schule des Lebens* [Learning. Brain research and the school of life]. Heidelberg: Spektrum Akademischer Verlag.

Thoits, P. A. (1985). Self-labelling processes in mental illness: The role of emotional deviance. *American Journal of Sociology, 91*(2), 221–249.

Traue, H. C. (1998). *Emotion und Gesundheit* [Health and Emotion]. Heidelberg: Spektrum Akademischer Verlag.

van der Kolk, B. A., McFarlane, A. C., and Weisaeth, L. (Eds.). (1996). *Traumatic stress: The effects of overwhelming experience on mind, body and society.* New York: Guilford Press.

Venter, J. C., Adams, M. D., Myers, E. W., Li, P. W., Mural, R. J., et al. (2001). The sequence of the human genome. *Science, 291*, 1304–1351.

von Wyl, A., Tschuschke, V., Crameri, A., Koemeda-Lutz, M., and Schulthess, P. (Eds.). (2016). *Was wirkt in der Psychotherapie?* [What works in psychotherapy?]. Gießen: Psychosozial-Verlag.

APPENDIX

Post graduate education and non-validated training

Dance movement therapy

Bachelors programmes

The Netherlands

ZUYD
Bachelor of Art Therapies Program
www.creatievetherapie.hsz.nl/
0031 (0)464006330

NIJMEGEN: HAN UNIVERSITY OF APPLIED SCIENCES (HAN)
Bachelor of Arts (art, drama, music, or psychomotor therapy)
Hogeschool van Arnhem en Nijmegen
Institute of Art Therapies, Psychomotor Therapy and Applied Psychology
Postbus 6960
6503 GL, Nijmegen, NL
Tel +31 648382329
www.han.nl
robert.vandenbroek@han.nl.

Masters programmes

Argentina

CAECE UNIVERSITY
Buenos Aires
Tel: 54/1 52522812 or 43/1 48070828
eroisen@caece.edu.ar
Maralia Reca, PhD, reca.maralia@gmail.com
Postgraduate training program in DMT

South Korea

KOREAN DANCE THERAPY ASSOCIATION OF ARTS THERAPY ACADEMY OF
   KOREA, SOUTH KOREA
269 Changgyeonggung-ro, Jongno-gu, Seoul
Tel: 82-2-744-5157 Fax: 82-2-744-5159
Boon Soon Ryu, PhD,
kdmta@naver.com
www.kdmta.com/eng/
Two years training program to prepare a dance therapist

SEOUL WOMEN'S UNIVERSITY GRADUATE SCHOOL OF PROFESSIONAL THER-
   APEUTIC TECHNOLOGY
Seoul, South Korea
Tel: 82-2-970-5887
Na Yung Kim, PhD,—nayungkim@swu.ac.kr
www.swu.ac.kr/special/eng/new/en_about_01.html
Master and PhD degree in DMT major of Expressive Arts Therapy Department.

SOON CHUN HYANG UNIVERSITY GRADUATE SCHOOL OF PSYCHOTHERAPY
   DEPARTMENT
Major in Dance Therapy, South Korea
22, Soonchunhyang-ro, Sinchang-myeon, Asan-si, Chungcheongnam-do
Tel: 82-10-3007-9682
Boon Soon Ryu, PhD,
kdmta@naver.com
https://homepage.sch.ac.kr/egradu/02/03.jsp
Three years training program, MA and PhD degrees major in Dance Therapy, Department
   of Psychotherapy.

Europe

BELGIUM

ARTEVELDE UNIVERSITY COLLEGE
Advanced Bachelor Degree in Arts Therapies (incorporating art therapy, dance movement
   therapy, dramatherapy or music therapy.
Part-time program consisting of 6 modules

AGAPE
Located in Koolskamp
4-year dance movement therapy training which leads to a certificate.
Programme is approved by BVCT-ABAT
www.agapebelgium.be

Estonia

TALLINN UNIVERSITY
Räägu 49, Tallinn 11311, Estonia
Eha Rüütel, PhD
+372 56475876
www.tlu.ee/et/kunstide-instituut/kunstiteraapiate-osakond
eha@tlu.ee
Creative Arts Therapies Program
Two-year Master's Program
Dance Movement Therapy, School of Natural Sciences and Health

France

UNIVERSITY SORBONNE, PARIS
MA Professional and Research in Artistic Creation
Specialization in Dance Therapy
Contact: Prof. Todd Lubart
Université Paris Descartes/ Sorbonne Paris Cité
Institut de Psychologie
Scolarité Master
71 avenue Edouard Vaillant
921090 Boulogne-Billancourt
scol-master-creation-artistique@psychologie.parisdescartes.fr
University website: www.parisdescartes.fr

Germany

SRH UNIVERSITY HEIDELBERG
Maria-Probst-Str. 3, 69123 Heidelberg, Germany
Faculty of Therapy Sciences, Creative Arts Therapies
www.hochschule-heidelberg.de/en/academics/masterstudium/dance-movement-therapy/
+49 (6221) 8223-013 Email: therapiewissenschaften@hochschule-heidelberg.de www.hoch
    schule-heidelberg.de
MA in Dance Movement Therapy (German and English study track)

Israel

ACADEMIC COLLEGE OF SOCIETY AND THE ARTS, ISRAEL
10b Ha'Orzim Street, P.O. Box 13335, Netanya, Israel 42379
Tel: 011-972-9-8656501
Samuel Schwartz, PhD sschwar@asa.ac.il
www.asa.ac.il/

KIBBUTZIM COLLEGE OF EDUCATION
149 Namir, Tel Aviv 62507, Israel. College: 03 6902345
Tel: 036412766
einya@mofet.macam98.ac.it
Coordinator: Yael Barkai
The Creative-Expressive Therapies Training Center

UNIVERSITY OF HAIFA
Dita Federman, PhD ditafederman@gmail.com
Website: http://artherapy.haifa.ac.il/index_eng.html
MA Graduate School of Creative Art Therapies.
Training program in DMT.
University of Haifa, Israel is launching a new international MA program in creative art therapies (including dance/movement therapy) taught in English. Haifa International.

Latvia

STRADINS UNIVERSITY RIGA
Medical School
MA in healthcare, art therapy specialization dance movement therapy
www.dkt.lv/en/

Slovenia

THE UNIVERSITY OF LJUBLJANA
Faculty of Education
University of Ljubljana
Kardeljeva ploščad 16
1000 Ljubljana
T: +386 1589 22 00
F: +386 1589 22 33
E: referat@pef.uni-lj.si (study affairs)
E: tajnistvo@pef.uni-lj.si (general)
MA Arts Therapies with a Dance movement therapy route.

Spain

AUTONOMOUS UNIVERSITY OF BARCELONA
Coordination: Heidrun Panhofer,
Assumpta RatAcs Edifici d'Estudiants (R) PlaAa CAvica Campus de Bellaterra
Telephone: 93 581 2990
Fax: 93 581 3099
Contact: master.dmt@uab.es
Master and Postgraduate Diploma in DMT

The Netherlands

ROTTERDAM DANCE ACADEMY
Postal Address: Kruisplein 26. 3012 CC Rotterdam, The Netherlands
Telephone: +31 (0)10 2171100
Contact (Coordinator): N. Wentholt
Department of Codarts, University of Professional Arts Education. Master's in Dance Therapy—2 year part-time programme taught in English.
www.codarts.nl/pragrammes/dance/dancetherapy/

UK

UNIVERSITY OF DERBY
MA Dance Movement Psychotherapy
Dr. Jill Bunce
j.bunce@derby.ac.uk
www.derby.ac.uk/courses/postgraduate/dance-movement-psychotherapy-ma/

GOLDSMITHS COLLEGE, UNIVERSITY OF LONDON
MA Dance Movement Psychotherapy
Caroline Frizell
c.frizell@gold.ac.uk
www.gold.ac.uk/pg/ma-dance-movement-psychotherapy/

UNIVERSITY OF ROEHAMPTON
MA Dance Movement Psychotherapy
Dr. Beatrice Allegranti
b.allegranti@goehampton.ac.uk
www.roehampton.ac.uk/postgraduate-courses/dance-movement-psychotherapy/index.html

United States

ANTIOCH UNIVERSITY, NEW HAMPSHIRE
40 Avon Street
Keene, NH 03431-3516
Telephone: 603-283-2137
Website: www.antiochne.edu/applied-psychology/dance-movement-therapy/
Contact: admission@antiochcollege.edu
Master's Program in Dance/Movement Therapy and Counseling, Department of Applied Psychology.

DREXEL UNIVERSITY, PHILADELPHIA, PA
Mail Stop 7905, Three Parkway, 7th Floor, Suite 7103, 1601 Cherry Street
Philadelphia, PA 19102
Telephone: 267-359-5511
Website: http://drexel.edu/cnhp/academics/graduate/MA-Dance-Movement-Therapy-Counseling/
Contact: Kristen Scatton, Dept. Recruitment—kristen.scatton@drexel.edu
MA Dance/Movement Therapy and Counseling, Creative Arts Therapies Department.

LESLEY UNIVERSITY, CAMBRIDGE, MA
29 Everett Street
Cambridge, MA 02138
Telephone: 617-349-8413
www.lesley.edu/master-of-arts/expressive-therapies/dance-therapy/mental-health-counseling/
Nancy Beardall—beardall@lesley.edu
MA In Clinical Mental Health Counseling: Specialization Dance/Movement Therapy

NAROPA UNIVERSITY, BOULDER, CO
2130 Arapahoe Avenue

Boulder, CO 80302-6697

Telephone: 303-546-3572 and 800-772-6951

www.naropa.edu/academics/masters/clinical-mental-health-counseling/somatic-coun
  seling/dance-movement-therapy/index.php

Stephanie San German, Admissions—ssangerman@naropa.edu or Wendy Allen—wallen@
  naropa.edu

Master of Arts in Clinical Mental Health Counseling Concentration in Somatic Counseling:
  Dance/Movement Therapy

PRATT INSTITUTE, BROOKLYN, NY

200 Willoughby Avenue

Brooklyn, NY 11205

Telephone: 718-399-4274

www.pratt.edu/academics/school-of-art/graduate-school-of-art/creative-arts-therapy/
  creative-arts-therapy-degrees/dance-movement-therapy-ms/

Joan Wittig, Assistant Professor—jwittig@pratt.edu

MSc in Dance/Movement Therapy, Creative Arts Therapy Department.

SARAH LAWRENCE COLLEGE, BRONXVILLE, NY

1 Mead Way

Bronxville, NY 10708

Telephone: 914-395-2371

Website: www.sarahlawrence.edu/dance-movement-therapy/#.TxnU6bNnV6c.email

Contact: Jennifer Lemiech-Iervolino, Coordinator: jlemiechiervolino@sarahlawrence.edu

Emanuel Lomax, Graduate Admissions: elomax@sarahlawrence.edu

MSc Degree Program in Dance/Movement Therapy.

Doctoral programmes

Australia

THE UNIVERSITY OF MELBOURNE

Creative Arts Therapies Research Unit,

Building 862,

234 St Kilda Road,

Southbank,

Victoria 3006,

Australia

Kim Dunphy, PhD k.dunphy@unimelb.edu.au

https://finearts-music.unimelb.edu.au/research/our-research/creative-arts-therapies-
  research-unit

PhD Program, Creative Arts and Music Therapy Research Group

Master's Creative Arts Therapies in development stage—Dance Movement/Drama Therapies.

UK

UNIVERSITY OF HERTFORDSHIRE

de Havilland Campus,

Hatfield Business Park,
Hatfield,
Hertfordshire
AL10 9EU
Tel: 0044 (0) 1707 285861
Contact- Professor Helen Payne, PhD
H.L.Payne@herts.ac.uk
Doctorate by research in dance movement psychotherapy/body psychotherapy/arts therapies
www.herts.ac.uk

UNIVERSITY OF ROEHAMPTON
PhD in All Arts Therapies
Beatrice Allegranti, PhD
b.allegranti@goehampton.ac.uk
www.roehampton.ac.uk/postgraduate-courses/dance-movement-psychotherapy/index. html

United States

DREXEL UNIVERSITY
1601 Cherry Street, Mail Stop 7905
Philadelphia, PA 19102
http://drexel.edu/cnhp/academics/doctoral/PHD-Creative-Arts-Therapies/
Nancy Gerber, Director, PhD Program in Creative Arts Therapies
ng27@drexel.edu or 267-359-5502
Admissions Coordinator, Department of Creative Arts Therapies kristen.scatton@drexel.edu or 267-359-5511
Creative Arts Therapies PhD Program, College of Nursing and Health Professions, Drexel University.

LESLEY UNIVERSITY
29 Everett Street
Cambridge, MA 02138
Telephone: 617-349-8166
https://lesley.edu/academics/graduate/expressive-therapies-phd
Michele Forinash, DA, MT-BC, Director, Expressive Therapies PhD Program—forinasm@ lesley.edu
Low residency PhD Program, Expressive Therapies Division, Graduate School of Arts and Social Sciences
Alternative Route Programmes
Information for the alternative route can be found at:https://adta.org/alternate-route-training/

Non-academic programmes

Argentina

Quesada 3470. (1430) Buenos Aires, Argentina
Tel: 541/542-4623

Diana Fischman, PhD—dfischman@brecha.com.ar
DMT Argentina Training Program includes BC-DMT trainers

Asia

CHINA

CHINA-GERMANY PROFESSIONAL DANCE THERAPY TRAINING, Beijing
Susanne Bender, MA; Weixiao Li, PhD.
EZETTHERA—Europaeisches Zentrum fuer Tanztherapie, GERMANY
Tel: +49/89/54662431
www.tanztherapie-zentrum.eu

INSPIREES DANCE MOVEMENT THERAPY TRAINING
Certificate and American Dance Therapy alternative route to registration
Ocean Express Building F, Xiaguangli 66, 100027, Beijing
+86 (0)10 8446 7947
+86 (0)10 8446 7847
Katee Shen, 15911509565
dmt@inspirees.com
www.dancetherapy.cn
Blog: www.weibo.com/dancetherapy

HONG KONG

Flat C1, 20/F, Mai On Industrial Bldg, 17–21 Kung Yip St., Kwai Chung,
+852 9087 7043
lifeoriginhk@yahoo.com.hk
www.lifeoriginhk.com

INDIA

KOLKATA SANVED AND THE CENTER FOR LIFELONG LEARNING, TATA INSTITUTE OF SOCIAL SCIENCES, MUBAIPOSTAL
60 Dasnagar, P.D.-Lake Gardens, Kolkata-700045m West Bengal, India
Tel: (033) 24993126; Mobile: 09836469932
Kolkata Sanved—kolkatasanved@gmail.com; Namrata Kanuga
www.kolkatasanved.org
Director: Sohini Chakraborty
Diploma course in DMT of 660 hours

CREATIVE MOVEMENT THERAPY ASSOCIATION OF INDIA
25-C Prithviraj Road, behind 25-A & near Tata House, New Delhi—110011, India
Tel: +91 9819886649
info@cmtai.org; reetu@cmtai.org
www.cmtai.org
Reetu Jain
Certificate course in DMT in New Delhi and Bangalore

Australia

INTERNATIONAL DANCE THERAPY INSTITUTE
P.O. Box 5168, Mordialloc,
Victoria 3195,
Australia
Tel: 61-439 330 008
admin@idtia.org.au
www.idtia.org.au

Europe

Finland

EINO ROIHA INSTITUTE, JYVÄSKYLÄ,
Seminaarinkatu 15
PL 35 (M)
40014 University of Jyväskylä
tel. +358 50 441 9787
www.ers.fi/content/eino-roiha-säätiö
jouni.kettunen@ers.fi
Basic studies (30 ECTS); Professional/Clinical studies (90 ECTS)

SUMMER UNIVERSITY OF NORTHERN OSTROBOTHNIA,
Torikatu 22 A, 2nd floor
PL 2437, 90014 Oulun yliopisto
kesayo@pohjois-pohjanmaa.fi
+358 44 465 2205 and +358 44 465 2206
www.pohjois-pohjanmaankesayliopisto.fi
Basic studies (30 ECTS)

KOKOS THEATRE ACADEMY, HELSINKI
P.O. Box 1
FI-00097 UNIARTS
+358 294 47 2000
www.uniarts.fi/en/contact
Basic studies (30 ECTS)

Germany

GERMAN ACADEMY FOR PSYCHODYNAMIC DANCE THERAPY AND EXPRESSIVE THERAPY
Bonn, Germany
Dance Therapist and Expressive Therapist Certified DITAT
Sabine Trautmann-Voigt, PhD
www.tanztherapie.de

EUROPEAN CENTER FOR DANCE THERAPY (EZETTHERA)
Munich, Germany

Certified Dance Therapist BTD (equals European MA)
Susanne Bender
www.tanztherapie-zentrum.eu
info@tanztherapie-zentrum.eu

FRANKFURT INSTITUTE FOR DANCE THERAPY
Frankfurt am Main, Germany
Certified Dance/Movement Therapist
www.tanztherapie-fitt.de
info@tanztherapie-fitt.de

HAMBURG INSTITUTE FOR GESTALT ORIENTED EDUCATION
Hamburg, Germany
Certified Dance/Movement Therapist
Inge Matties
www.higw.de
info@higw.de

INTERNATIONAL INSTITUTE FOR DANCE THERAPY (IIDT)
Tenerife/Canary Islands (Spain) & Germany
Certified Dance Therapist BTD & Teacher for the "Dance of Life"
Petra Klein, Psychologist and Dance Therapist BTD
www.dancetherapy.com, www.tanztherapie.com, www.danzaterapia.com, www.Jardin-Mariposa.com
info@Jardin-Mariposa.com , info@dancetherapy.com

LANGEN INSTITUTE
Düsseldorf, Germany
Dance/Movement Therapist
Martina Piff
www.langen-institut.de
angen-institut@praeha.de

PANTARHEI-INSTITUTE FOR THERAPY, INTERACTION AND DANCE
Friedland/Göttingen, Germany
Certified Dance/Movement Therapist
Thomas Wetzorke
www.pantarhei-institut.de
info@pantarhei-institut.de

PSYCHOLOGICAL DANCE THERAPY
Hamburg
Psychotherapeutische Tanztherapeutin
www.pitth.de
pohlmann@pitth.de

DANCE THERAPY CENTRE BERLIN
Berlin, Germany

Certified Dance/Movement Therapist
Imke Fiedler
www.tanztherapie-zentrum-berlin.de
tanztherapie.zb@t-online.de

HUNGARY

TRAINING INSTITUTE OF HUNGARIAN ASSOCIATION FOR MOVEMENT AND DANCE THERAPY PSYCHODYNAMIC MOVEMENT AND DANCE THERAPY (PMDT)

6 years (12 semesters) of training
www.tancterapia.net/kepzes_pdmt.htm

INSPIREES DANCE MOVEMENT THERAPY TRAINING

Certificate and American Dance Therapy Association alternate route to registration
Europe
A v Scheltemaplein
2624PJ, Delft
The Netherlands
+31 (0)15 8795501
Nuo Yang +31 (0)64744 5687

ITALY

FORMAZIONE TRIENNALE IN DANZATERAPIA CLINICA VITT3

Lyceum Formazione e Aggiornamento
Dott.ssa Laura Pezzenati
Milano, Via Carlo Vittadini, 3
02 36553846–338 2236684
formazione@arteterapia.info
www.arteterapia.info

SCUOLA DI FORMAZIONE IN DANZAMOVIMENTOTERAPIA DEI PROCESSI EVOLUTIVI PSICOCORPOREI ARDEIDAE

Associazione per la ricerca e lo studio della danzamovimentoterapia e delle tecniche a mediazione corporea
Dott.ssa Daniela Di Mauro
Palermo, Piazza Europa, 13
327 1684824
info@associazioneardeidae.org
www.associazioneardeidae.org

SCUOLA DI PEDAGOGIA DELLA MEDIAZIONE CORPOREA ED ESPRESSIVA AD INDIRIZZO SIMBOLICO-ANTROPOLOGICO

Ass.ne Culturale Eurinome A.S.D.—Perugia
Prof.ssa Alba G. A. Naccari
Sede di Perugia: Via dei Narcisi 41/A 06126—Perugia
Sede di Palmi (RC): Via Virgilio n°78 cap. 89015
338 3442140

alnacc@tin.it
ambrarospo@yahoo.it
www.danzasimbolica.altervista.org

SCUOLA DI FORMAZIONE PROFESSIONALE IN DMT ESPRESSIVA E PSICOD-INAMICA

Genova Associazione MetamorfoSidanza
Dr.ssa Cinzia Saccorotti
Sede principale di Genova Associazione MetamorfoSidanza
333694860
cinzia.saccorotti@libero.it
info@metamorfosidanza.com
www.metamorfosidanza.com

SCUOLA DMT "MARIA FUX" CENTRO RISVEGLI

Scuola DMT "Maria Fux" Centro Risvegli
Dr. Pietro Farneti
Milano, Italia, via Ventura, 4
0283241125
0232066746
risvegli@fastwebnet.it

SCUOLA DI DANZAMOVIMENTOTERAPIA DEL CENTRO DI FORMAZIONE NELLE ARTITERAPIE DI LECCO

Centro Artiterapie
Dott.a Annapaola Lovisolo
Via Lorenzo Balicco, 11, Lecco, LC, Italia
0341 350496
0341 285012
info@artiterapie.it
www.artiterapie.it/index.php/sections/la-scuola-di-danzamovimentoterapia/

SCUOLA FORMAZIONE PROFESSIONALE DMT GESTALT

Centro Metafora Gestalt Genova
Dott.ssa Mafalda Traveni Massella
Genova—Via Trento, 20/10-16145
010 364955
010 3107147
danzaterapia@metaforagestalt.it

SCUOLA DI SPECIALIZZAZIONE AFGP-SARABANDA IN DMT, DMT TRA ORIENTE ED OCCIDENTE E METODO FUX. TECNICHE E METODICHE ESPRESSIVE PER INTERVENTI NEL SOCIALE

Centro Formazione Professionale AFGP-Sarabanda, accreditato dalla Regione Lombardia
Elena Cerruto
Milano—Via Pusiano 52 20123 (MM2 CIMIANO)
02 89404056, 339 2910117
info@associazionesarabanda.it

elenacerruto@gmail.com
www.associazionesarabanda.it

SCUOLA DI FORMAZIONE PROFESSIONALE IN DANZAMOVIMENTO TERAPIA INTEGRATA

Coop. Soc. Centro Studi Danza Animazione Arte Terapia
Dott. Vincenzo Puxeddu
Cagliari—via Principe Amedeo, 13
070 650349/665967
070 650349
Cagliari, Milano, Palermo, Roma
csdanza@tin.it
www.danzamovimentoterapia.it

SCUOLA DI FORMAZIONE PER OPERATORI IN DANZATERAPIA "M. FUX" E SPECIALIZZAZIONE IN DMT CHIAVE SIMBOLICA®

Centro Toscano di Arte e Danza Terapia
Dott.ssa Paola De Vera D'Aragona
Firenze—Borgo degli Albizi, 16-50122
055 243008
055 243008
Firenze
info@centrotoscanodanzaterapia.it
www.centrotoscanodanzaterapia.it

ART THERAPY ITALIANA

Associazione Art Therapy Italiana
Dott.ssa Piera Pieraccini
Bologna—Via Barberia, 13-40123
Roma—c/o Art Therapy Studio—Via Flaminio Ponzio, 18-00145,
Firenze—Via San Gallo 79-50129
Torino—Viale Curreno, 41
Milano—Piazzale Baiamonti, 2-20154
051 6440451
051 6440451
Bologna, Roma, Firenze, Torino, Milano
associazione@arttherapyit.org
www.arttherapyit.org

SCUOLA DI ARTI TERAPIE

Associazione "Scuola di Arti Terapie"
Dott. Vincenzo Bellia
Roma
Via Costantino, 41-00145
Catania
Via San Michele, 4-95131
339 1784620-06 40802272
329 6639960

Poland

POLISH INSTITUTE FOR DANCE MOVEMENT PSYCHOTHERAPY
4-year postgraduate training in Dance Movement Psychotherapy
Diploma of completion
www.instytutdmt.pl

Russia

INSTITUTE OF PRACTICAL PSYCHOLOGY AND PSYCHOANALYSIS
Dance Movement Psychotherapy Postgraduate Professional Training (3 years)
tdt-edu.ru/programs/tancevalno-dvigatelnaya-psixoterapiya/
atda.ru/professionalnoe-obuchenie/tancevalno-dvigatelnaya-psihoterapiya
Director: Irina Biryukova, BC-DMT iradmt@gmail.com
Advisor: Patrizia Pallaro, BC-DMT

Switzerland

INSTITUTE FOR DANCE THERAPY AT THE LAKE
CH 8593 Kesswil, Switzerland
Ana Bella Nosa-Quaas
www.tanztherapie-am-see.ch
infor@tanztherapie-am-see.ch

Dance movement therapy professional associations

CZECH DANCE AND MOVEMENT THERAPY ASSOCIATION (TANTER)
www.arttherapies.cz/eng/the-czech-dance-and-movement-therapy-association.html
beatealbrich@seznam.cz

EUROPEAN CONSORTIUM OF ARTS THERAPIES TRAINING AND EDUCATION
    (ECARTE)
www.ecarte.info

EUROPEAN ASSOCIATION FOR DANCE MOVEMENT THERAPY
www.eadmt.com/
info@eadmt.com

FINNISH ASSOCIATION FOR DANCE MOVEMENT THERAPY
c/o Riita Parvia, Chairperson, Alveveien 45 N 9016, Tromso
tngstad@online.no
www.dancetherapy.no

GERMAN PROFESSIONAL ORGANISATION FOR DANCE THERAPISTS
www.btd-tanztherapie.de/BTDengl/_E_index.htm
info@BTD-taztherapie.de

GREEK ASSOCIATION OF DANCE THERAPISTS
http://gadt.gr/english.htm
dancetherapy@gadt.gr

HUNGARIAN ASSOCIATION FOR DANCE MOVEMENT THERAPY
http://mozgasterapia.net/
konferencia@tancterapia.net

PROFESSIONAL ASSOCIATION OF DANCE MOVEMENT THERAPY, ITALY
www.apid.it/info.htm
segreteria@apid.it

LATVIAN DANCE MOVEMENT THERAPY ASSOCIATION
http://dkt.lv/en/
dkt.valde@gmail.com

DANCE MOVEMENT THERAPY ASSOCIATION, RUSSIA
www.atdt.ru/desc_text.php?menu=english
tdtatdt@mail.ru

THE ASSOCIATION FOR DANCE MOVEMENT THERAPY, SPAIN
www.danzamovimientoterapia.com/
admte@danzamovimientoterapia.com

SWEDISH ASSOCIATION OF DANCE THERAPY
www.dansterapi.info/?fref=gc&dti=1800806250176943
styrelsen@dansterapi.info

THE NETHERLANDS ASSOCIATION FOR DANCE MOVEMENT THERAPY
www.nvdat.nl/
nvdat.info@vaktherapie.nl

ASSOCIATION FOR DANCE MOVEMENT THERAPY, UK
https://admp.org.uk/
chair@admp.org.uk

Body psychotherapy

European programmes

Academic programmes

UK

CAMBRIDGE BODY PSYCHOTHERAPY CENTRE
28 Ditton Walk
Cambridge
CB5 8QE

UK
00 44 (0) 1223 214658
www.cbpc.org.uk
gillwestland@cbpc.org.uk
Diploma in Body Psychotherapy; Humanistic and Integrative Psychotherapy College (HIPC) of the United Kingdom Council of Psychotherapy
Post qualifying MA Body Psychotherapy Anglia Ruskin University, Cambridge (2 years part time)

Non-academic programmes

Bulgaria

BULGARIAN INSTITUTE OF NEOREICHIAN ANALITYCAL PSYCHOTHERAPY (BINAP)
5, Chernomen str., Sofia, Bulgaria
office@ibpt.eu
www.binap.eu

Denmark

BODYNAMIC INTERNATIONAL
Ådalsparkvej 3, 3rd. floor.c/o bahlawan, Horsholm, Denmark
ditte@dittemarcher.com
www.bodynamic.dk

INSTITUTE FOR EMOTIONAL INTEGRATION
Kastanie allé 18, Venlose, Denmark
mail@emotionelintegration.dk
www.emotionelintegration.dk

France

ECOLE BIODYNAMIQUE
1400 ch. de Moulares, Montpellier, France
cl@psychologie-biodynamique.com
www.psychologie-biodynamique.com/

INSTITUT DE FORMATION EN THÉRAPIE PSYCHOCORPORELLE
102 route du Polygone, Strasbourg, France
secretariat@ifcc-psychotherapie.fr
www.ifcc-psychotherapie.fr

Germany

AUS- UND FORTBILDUNGSZENTRUM TRANSFORMATIVE KÖRPERPSYCHO-THERAPIE
Nassauische Str. 26, Berlin, Germany
bettinaschroeter@freenet.de
www.transformative-koerperpsychotherapie.de

EUROPAISCHE SCHULE FÜR BIODYNAMISCHE PSYCHOLOGIE (ESBPE)
Dragerkoppel 7, Gronenberg, Germany
esbpe@web.de
www.biodynamik.de

HAKOMI INSTITUTE OF EUROPE
Weissgerbergasse 2/A, Nürnberg, Germany
info@hakomi.de;
www.hakomi.de

INSTITUTE FOR CORE EVOLUTION
Postfach 143206, Essen, Germany
siegmar.gerken@gmail.com
www.CoreEvolution.com

ZENTRUM FÜR INTEGRATIVE KÖRPERPSYCHOTHERAPIE UND HUMANIS-
TISCHE PSYCHOLOGIE
Bachmannstrasse 2–4, Frankfurt, Germany
Ilse.Schmidt@mac.com
www.zikp.de

UNIVERSITY OF MARBURG
Motologie, Schwerpunkt Körperpsychotherapie
Barfüßerstraße 1, 35032 Marburg
Tel. +49 6421/28-23970, Fax +49 6421/28-28946
Director: Prof. Dr. Martin Vetter
wolfb@staff.uni-marburg.de

GREECE

GREEK INSTITUTE OF VEGETOTHERAPY & CHARACTER ANALYSIS
12 Athinas St, Monastiraki, Athens, Greece
info@kentroraix.gr
www.kentroraix.gr

ISRAEL

KARKUR COLLEGE OF HOLISTIC THERAPY
Hamoshav St 40, Karkur, Israel
info@spirit.co.il
www.spirit.co.il

REIDMAN INTERNATIONAL COLLEGE—SCHOOL FOR BODY-CENTERED
PSYCHOTHERAPY
26 Haim Levanon st., Tel-Aviv, Israel
sally@reidman.co.il
www.reidman.co.il/

ITALY

EUROPEAN SCHOOL OF FUNCTIONAL PSYCHOTHERAPY (SEF)
P.Co Comola Ricci 41, Napoli, Italy
info@psicologiafunzionale
www.psicologiafunzionale.it

SOCIETÀ ITALIANA DI ANALISI REICHIANA
Via Valadier 44, Roma, Italy
siar@analisi-reichiana.it
www.analisi-reichiana.it

SOCIETÀ ITALIANA DI BIOSISTEMICA
Pzza S.M. Liberatrice 18, Rome, Italy
info@biosistemica.it
www.biosistemica.org

SPAIN

ESCUELA ESPANOLA REICHIANA
c/ Rep. de Guinea Ecuatorial 4 1c, Valencia, Spain
xserrano@mac.com
www.esternet.org

SWITZERLAND

INSTITUT FÜR KÖRPERZENTRIERTE PSYCHOTHERAPIE
Kanzleistrasse 17, Zurich, Switzerland
helene.helwing@ikp-therapien.com
www.ikp-therapien.com

THE NETHERLANDS

BODYMIND OPLEIDINGEN
1/e Pijnakkerstraat 135/a, Rotterdam, The Netherlands
info@bodymindopleidingen.nl
www.bodymindopleidingen.nl/

NEDERLANDS INSTITUUT VOOR BIODYNAMISCHE PSYCHOLOGIE
Paramaribostr. 11, NL-1058 AN Amsterdam, The Netherlands
jlbvisser@gmail.com
www.biodynamischepsychologie.nl

United States programmes

Masters programmes

CALIFORNIA INSTITUTE OF INTEGRAL STUDIES
MA in Counseling Psychology, Somatic Psychology Concentration
Lindsay Roth, admissions counselor

lroth@ciis.edu (415) 575-6291
www.ciis.edu/academics/graduate-programs/somatic-psychology/apply

NAROPA UNIVERSITY
MA in Somatic Counseling: Body Psychotherapy
Wendy Allen, Chair- wallen@naropa.edu: 303-245-4844
www.naropa.edu/academics/masters/clinical-mental-health-counseling/somatic-coun
    seling/body-psychotherapy/index.php
Doctoral programmes

PACIFICA GRADUATE INSTITUTE, SANTA BARBARA, CA
Doctorate in Somatic Studies
Rae Johnson, Chair- RJohnson@pacifi ca.edu
www.pacifi ca.edu/degree-program/somatic-studies/

Body psychotherapy professional associations

Austria

AUSTRIAN ASSOCIATION FOR BODY PSYCHOTHERAPY
www.aabp.at/
President: Elfriede Kastenberger, PhD
e.kastenberger@aon.at
Marchetstrasse 10, A-2500 Baden, Austria
Tel: +43-676 911 71 70
Secretary: Dr Eva Wagner-Margetich
margetich@aon.at
Treasurer: Anna Gruber-Laumer
praxis@koerper-therapie.at
Secretariat: Lisa Holzweber
office@aabp.at

Bulgaria

BULGARIAN NEOREICHIAN PSYCHOTHERAPY SOCIETY
Str. Klokotnica, Sofia, Bulgaria
info@neoraihianstvo.org
www.neoraihianstvo.org

France

ASSOCIATION PROFESSIONNELLE DE PSYCHOLOGIE BIODYNAMIQUE
c/o Ecole Biodynamique 1400 Chemin de Moulares, Montpellier, France
president@appb.org
www.appb.org/

ASSOCIATION EUROPÉENNE DE THÉRAPIE PSYCHOCORPORELLE ET
    RELATIONNELLE
102, Route du Polygone, Strasbourg (Neudorf), France

secretariat@aetpr-psychotherapie.org
www.aetpr-psychotherapie.org/

Germany

DEUTSCHE GESELLSCHAFT FÜR KÖRPERPSYCHOTHERAPIE
www.koerperpsychotherapie-dgk.de/
President: Manfred Thielen, PhD
ma.thielen@gmx.de
Crellestr. 14, D-10827 Berlin,
Germany Secretary: Axel Schulz
sekretariat@koerperpsychotherapie-dgk.de
Hellmut-v.-Gerlach-Str. 8, D-34121 Kassel, Germany
Treasurer: Thomas Harms
info@zepp-bremen.de
Bremen, Germany Secretariat: DGK/ c/o Axel Schulz
sekretariat@koerperpsychotherapie-dgk.de
Vice President: Dagmar Rellensmann
dagmar.rellens@t-online.deDGK-Sekretariat
Tel: 0049(0)561-286 13 67

Greece

GREEK ASSOCIATION FOR BODY PSYCHOTHERAPY
www.pesops.gr
President: Eri Basiouka
ebasiouka@yahoo.gr
16 Lakonias Str, 11523 Athens
Secretary: Constantine Panayotopoulos
cpan54@yahoo.gr
Treasurer: Eleni Mavromati
mavromatielen@gmail.com
Vice President: Ioannis Korkotselos
korkotselos@hotmail.com
Members: Antigone Oreopoulou—antigone@althaia.gr
Mariella Sakellariou—mosakellariou@gmail.com
Despina Mavropoulou—info@somapsychotherapy.org

Israel

ISRAEL ASSOCIATION FOR BODY PSYCHOTHERAPY
www.ilabp.org/
President: Amir Leibman
bodyenergetics@gmail.com
Secretary: Irena Markus
luna.scorp@gmail.com
Treasurer: Asaf Avraham
assafav1172@walla.co.il

Membership Secretary: Roi Maliach
roimaliach@gmail.com

Italy

ASSOCIAZIONE ITALIA PSICOTERAPIA CORPOREA
www.psicoterapiecorporee.it
President: Genovino Ferri
genovino.ferri@gmail.com
via Altino 16 sc.C/2 (c/o Filoni Rosaria) Secretary: Paola Mancini
Treasurer: Francesco Mallardi
International contact: Fabio Carbonari
fabio.carbonari@istitutoreich.it
Board Members: Francesco Mallardi, Paola Mancini, Simona De Stasio, Rosaria Filoni (Vice-
President), Christoph Helferich and Fabio Carbonari.

Serbia

SERBIAN ASSOCIATION FOR BODY PSYCHOTHERAPY
http://telesnapsihoterapija.org/sr/
President: Ana Ristovic
anarista@sbb.rs
Dimitrija Tucovica br.42, stan br.4
Secretary: Biljana Jokic
jokic.bi@gmail.com
Vojvode Savatija 14/17, Belgrade, Serbia
Treasurer: Ljiljana Jovanovic
ljlipra@gmail.com
Smederevska 5, Belgrade, Serbia

Spain

ASOCIACIÓN DE PSICOTERAPIAS CORPORALES Y CARACTEROANALÍTICAS
DEL ESTADO ESPAÑOL
http://apcce.es
President: Tair Paredes
taireparedes@yahoo.es
Secretary: Juan Antonio Colmenares
colgja@yahoo.es
Treasurer: Xavier Serrano Hortelano
xserrano@mac.com

Switzerland

DER SCHWEIZERISCHE VEBAND FÜR KÖRPERPSYCHOTHERAPIE
www.ch-eabp.ch
President: Christina Bader-Johansson

bader.johansson@bluewin.ch
Secretary: Evi Monti
info@ch–eabp.ch

The Netherlands

EUROPEAN ASSOCIATION FOR BODY PSYCHOTHERAPY
Rob van Schaik
Tintorettostraat 29/1
1077 RP Amsterdam
The Netherlands
+31(0)6 30439755
secretariat@eabp.org

NEDERLANDSE VERENIGING VOOR LICHAAMSGEORIËNTEERDE PSYCHO-
THERAPIE
www.nvlp.nl/
President: Angela Terpstra
angelacmyterpstra@live.nl
Treasurer: Eline de Man
info@stresstelijf.nl
Postal address:
Galjoenstraat 53a
5017 CL Tilburg

UK

WWW.BODY-PSYCHOTHERAPY.ORG.UK
President: Steve Elliott
chair@body-psychotherapy.org.uk
Phone: +44 20 7731 7730
Treasurer: Russell Rose
admin@body-psychotherapy.org.uk
Secretariat: Kerensa Martin
admin@body-psychotherapy.org.uk
International contact: Steve Elliott
chair@body-psychotherapy.org.uk
Ethics Committee Chair: Michaela Boening
ethics@body-psychotherapy.org.uk
For membership enquiries, please contact the CABP Administrator:
admin@body-psychotherapy.org.uk
If you are living in the UK, please email CABP for application forms

Journals

International Journal of Body, Movement and Dance in Psychotherapy
An academic journal, four issues per anum, peer reviewed and published by Taylor and Francis
www.tandfonline.com/toc/tbmd20/current

American Dance Therapy Journal
An academic journal, four issues per anum, peer reviewed and published by Elsevier
https://adta.org/american-dance-therapy-journal/

International Body Psychotherapy Journal
Published by the EABP
www.ibpj.org

The Arts in Psychotherapy
An academic journal, four issues per anum, peer reviewed and published by Springer
www.sciencedirect.com/journal/the-arts-in-psychotherapy

Creative Arts Therapies
Published by the German Scientific Association of Creative Arts Therapies (http://wfkt.de/)
www.egms.de/static/en/journals/index.htm

INDEX

Page numbers in italics refer to figures and those in bold refer to tables.

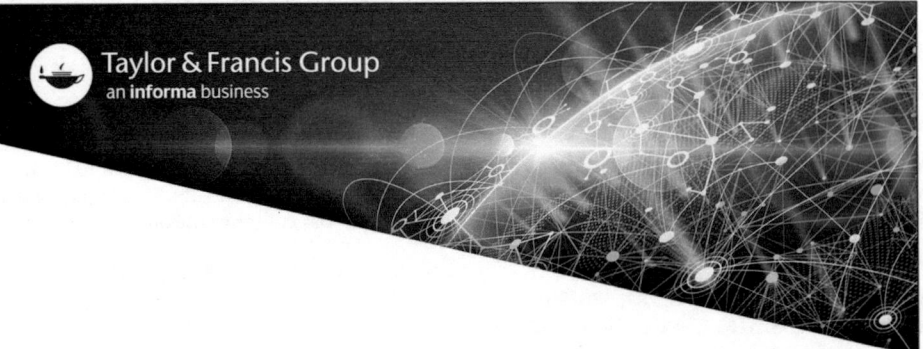
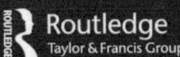
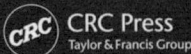